Living with
renal failure

Travenol Laboratories are pleased to have been associated both with this symposium and the publication of these proceedings.

The treatment of chronic renal failure is a field of ever-increasing complexity to the manufacturer of the essential equipment and to the medical and paramedical groups involved in the treatment and welfare of the patient.

This was the first truly national multi-disciplinary symposium on chronic renal failure to take place in the U.K. and the publication of these proceedings emphasises this company's continuing belief in the importance of co-operation between the medical profession and industry in the interest of increasing knowledge.

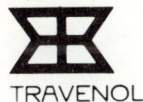

TRAVENOL

Living with renal failure

Proceedings of a Multidisciplinary Symposium
held at the University of Stirling, 7–8 July, 1977

Edited by
J. L. Anderton
Consultant Renal Physician, Western General
Hospital, Edinburgh
F. M. Parsons
Consultant Nephrologist, General Infirmary,
Leeds
D. E. Jones
Nursing Officer, Renal Unit, St. Bartholomew's
and St. Leonard's Hospitals, London

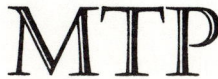

Published by
MTP Press Limited
St. Leonard's House
Lancaster, England

ISBN : 0 85200 197-5

Printed in Great Britain by R. & R. Clark Limited, Edinburgh

Contents

v

SECTION FOUR

Psychological and Personal Aspects
Chairman: M. Carmody

SECTION FIVE

Practical Management
Chairman: A. C. Kennedy

List of Contributors

Dr J. L. ANDERTON
Consultant Physician in Renal Diseases, Nuffield Transplant Unit, Western General Hospital, Edinburgh

Mr J. BAILLIE
Director, Tullis Neill Limited, Mayfield, Dalkeith, Edinburgh

Dr J. D. BRIGGS
Consultant Physician in Renal Diseases, Western Infirmary, Glasgow

Mrs MARY BROWN
Home Dialysis Sister, Renal Transplant and Dialysis Unit, Manchester Royal Infirmary, Manchester

Professor J. S. CAMERON
Professor in Renal Medicine, Guy's Hospital, London

Dr M. CARMODY
Consultant Nephrologist, St. Mary's Hospital, Dublin

Dr W. R. CATTELL
Consultant Nephrologist, St. Bartholomew's Hospital, London

Dr T. G. FEEST
Senior Registrar, Royal Victoria Infirmary, Newcastle-upon-Tyne

Mrs JEAN K. GIBBINS
Renal Unit, Royal Infirmary, Sunderland

Mr D. N. H. HAMILTON
Lecturer in Surgery, Western Infirmary, Glasgow

Dr J. A. HENRY
Senior Registrar, Department of Medicine, University College Hospital, London

Dr D. S. JAMES
Department of Child and Family Psychiatry, Royal Hospital for Sick Children, Glasgow

Mrs DEIRDRE E. JONES
Nursing Officer, Renal Unit, St. Bartholomew's and St. Leonard's Hospitals, London

Mr A. McL. JENKINS
Senior Lecturer in Surgery, Royal Infirmary, Edinburgh

Dr J. A. KANIS
Wellcome Senior Clinical Research Fellow, Renal Unit, The Churchill Hospital, Oxford

Professor A. C. KENNEDY
University Department of Medicine, Royal Infirmary, Glasgow

Miss KIRSTY M. MARSHALL
Senior Fieldwork Teacher, Training and Development, Social Work Headquarters, Lothian Region, Edinburgh

Dr A. M. MARTIN
Consultant Physician, Renal Unit, Royal Infirmary, Sunderland

Miss KATHLEEN NICHOLSON
Nursing Officer, Renal Unit, Western Infirmary, Glasgow

Dr D. M. PARKIN
Community Physician, Leeds Area Health Authority, Leeds

Dr F. M. PARSONS
Consultant in Clinical Renal Physiology, The General Infirmary, Leeds

Dr B. H. B. ROBINSON
Consultant Physician, Department of Renal Medicine, East Birmingham Hospital, Birmingham

Professor J. S. ROBSON
Professor of Medicine, The University of Edinburgh and Director of the Medical Renal Unit at the Royal Infirmary, Edinburgh

Miss HELEN ROSENTHAL
Home Dialysis Administrator, St. Leonard's/St. Bartholomew's Regional Renal Unit, London

Dr A. W. SIEMSEN
Director, Institute of Renal Diseases, Saint Francis Hospital, Honolulu, Hawaii

Miss SALLY TABER
Nursing Officer, Professorial Unit, Addenbrookes Hospital, Cambridge

Dr T. WALMSLEY
Dept. of Psychiatry, Royal Infirmary, Edinburgh

Dr M. K. WARD
Lecturer in Medicine, University of Newcastle-upon-Tyne

Dr R. J. WINNEY
Senior Registrar, Medical Renal Unit, (University of Edinburgh), The Royal Infirmary, Edinburgh

Preface

The management of chronic renal failure by dialysis and transplantation has now become an established form of treatment in many parts of the world. However, these forms of treatment have brought with them problems in relation to the selection of patients, economics, clinical problems such as hypertension, encephalopathy, anaemia and renal bone disease, and psychological and social problems. The management of haemodialysis has changed over the years with developments in dialysers, vascular access and the duration of dialysis. Although the overall survival from renal transplantation has changed little in the past four or five years, there are hopes of improvements in relation to tissue typing and enhancement.

Perhaps the most important aspect in the management of chronic renal failure is the multi-disciplinary approach. Nursing and medical staff work closely with dialysis technicians, engineers, dietitians, local authority personnel, social workers and with the relatives of the patients.

The symposium was planned to draw together representatives from all disciplines involved in the care of patients with chronic renal failure. One of the most relevant sessions was that in which two patients with chronic renal failure described their experience.

Travenol Laboratories Limited sponsored the symposium and provided the administrative services. The contributors and editors are deeply grateful for the opportunity that this has given them to reach a wider public with a message whose importance grows daily. The editors acknowledge the helpful collaboration of our publisher and the skill of Mrs Judy Fagleston who transcribed the discussions. Finally, they wish to thank Peter Irving of Travenol Laboratories who organized the symposium and who enabled us all to respond to the challenge of "Living with Renal Failure".

JLA
FMP
DEJ

Introduction
F. M. Parsons

Two hundred years ago Cotunnius[1] associated oedema with coagulable substances in the urine. These observations were brilliantly extended by Richard Bright 50 years later[2] who, in collaboration with his chemist Dr Bostock, demonstrated a disturbance in excretion of urea associated with a full pulse, oedema, albuminous urine and contracted kidneys. One year later, in 1828, Wohler was the first to synthesize urea from inorganic radicles and wrote to Berzelius: 'I must tell you that I can prepare urea without requiring a kidney or an animal, either man or dog'[3].

In 1832 another landmark occurred. Thomas Thompson, Professor of Chemistry, University of Glasgow, who was also medically qualified, investigated the biochemical imbalance produced by malignant cholera[4], which was then endemic in the United Kingdom. Dr O'Shaughnessy[5] both extended and reported Professor Thompson's work in the *Lancet* and concluded that salts and water left the blood to enter the rice stools. Dr Latta, a clinician from Leith who probably worked in the Drummond Street Cholera Hospital, Edinburgh (situated close to the Old Royal Infirmary), logically interpreted the data of Thompson and O'Shaughnessy with amazing insight for that era and 'resolved to throw the fluid immediately into the circulation'[6] in extreme cases when the deficit could not be corrected via the gastrointestinal tract. Dr Latta recorded several examples of the beneficial use of intravenous therapy in his report to the Central Board of Health, London[6]. It would appear that he suffered the fate that many pioneers of newer forms of successful therapy encounter. In the management of one patient found *in extremis* and given intravenous fluid in her home he recorded[7]: 'A female, aged 50, very destitute, but previously in good health, was on the 13th instant, at four a.m., seized with cholera in its most violent form, and by half-past nine was reduced to a most hopeless state. The pulse was quite gone, even in the axilla, and strength so much exhausted, that I had resolved not to try the effects of the injection, conceiving the poor woman's case to be hopeless, and that the failure of the experiment might afford the prejudiced and the illiberal an opportunity to stigmatize the practice; however, I at length thought I would give her a chance, and in the presence of Drs Lewins and Craigie, and Messrs. Sibson and Paterson, I injected one hundred and twenty ounces, when like the effects of magic, instead of the pallid aspect of one whom death had sealed as his own, the vital tide was restored, and life and vivacity returned'.

Presumably Messrs Sibson and Paterson were solicitors and had been asked to attend as independent witnesses to this very new and controversial therapy. The patient made an excellent recovery and was then 'for better accommodation, carried to the hospital'. In 1832 this must have been considered a highly scientific exercise based, as it was, on an accurate assessment of the biochemical abnormality induced by cholera and exhibited all the criteria of correct fluid and electrolyte therapy as used today.

Dr Craigie, a colleague of Dr Latta, recorded the treatment of another patient[7]. 'Martha Smith, aged 38, a noted drunkard, thin and debilitated in sixth month of pregnancy, admitted into the hospital at 8 p.m., May 16th, 1832'. She was treated conventionally with 'saline' enemas but at 11.30 a.m. the findings were: 'Breathing becoming much affected; extreme restlessness; cramps severe in legs, and every symptom of sinking. Let the following saline solution be injected into one of the veins of the arm.

> ℞   *Muriat. sodæ* ʒi ;
> *Carbon. sodæ* gr. **x** ;
> *Aq. calid.* ℔iij, *solve temp.* **105°**
> *Fahr.*

Noon. When about ℔i [i.e. about 450 ml] had been thrown in, the pulse was perceived to flutter at the wrist, and gradually strengthened as the injection was proceeded with. By the time ℔iiiss [i.e. about 1,5 l] had been injected, the countenance, which was before quite death-like, now beamed with the appearance of health, and she began to converse freely. Pulse 96, moderate. To have ʒi gin in warm water with sugar.

Half-past one. The gin was immediately rejected'.

She required two further intravenous injections, making a total of about 4 litres in all, and then Dr Craigie reported: 'Has passed about ℔j [i.e. about 450 ml] of urine, of natural appearance; this is the first she has made since she was brought in'.

The composition of the fluid given intravenously was NaCl 45.0 mEq/l and NaHCO$_3$ 5.3 mEq/l. Thus, these accounts of the world's first intravenous fluid therapy also include the first known correction of a pre-renal failure.

In 1830 Thomas Graham (Figure 1), a Scot, was appointed to the first independent chair of chemistry at Anderson's University, Glasgow. He moved to University College, London, in 1837 and became Warden and Master Worker of the Mint in 1855[8]. Graham was one of the great scientists of the nineteenth century (see Graham's Law on the Diffusion of Gases) but to nephrologists he will be remembered for his experiments with

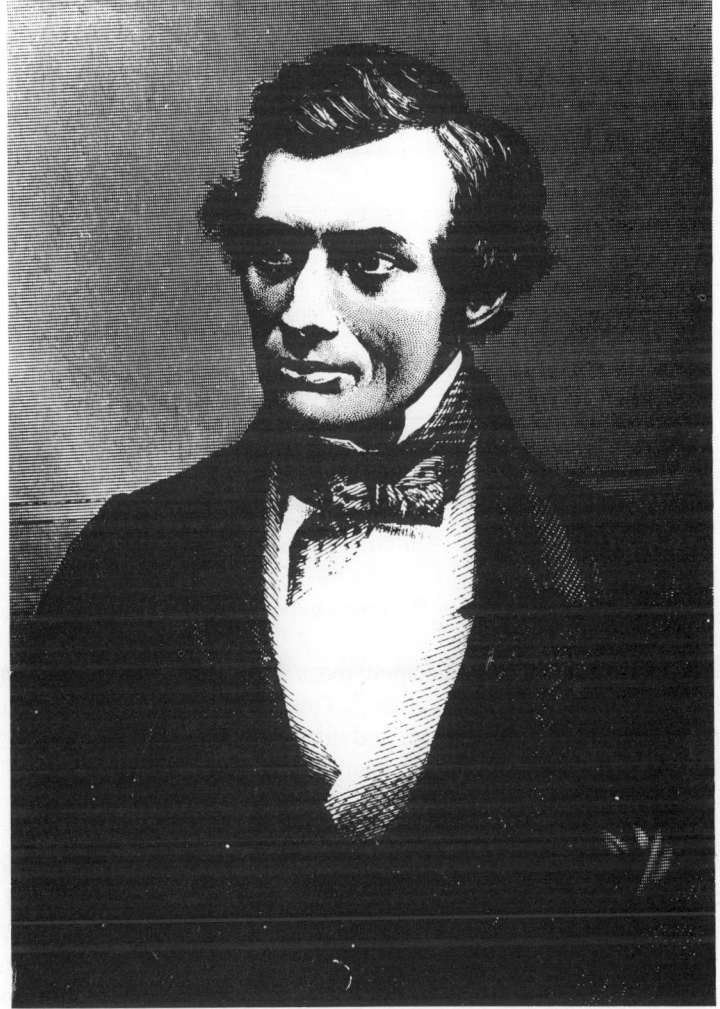

Figure 1   Thomas Graham (1805–69)

the membrane parchment (manufactured by the firm of Messrs De la Rue) which he attached to a wooden or (preferably) a guttapercha hoop (Figure 2) which was then floated on water – the 'Graham hoop dialyser'[9]. He demonstrated that when colloids and crystalloids were placed in the hoop only crystalloids passed through to enter the water. He coined the phrase 'dialysis' (from the Greek *dia*, through and *luein*, to loosen) to describe the

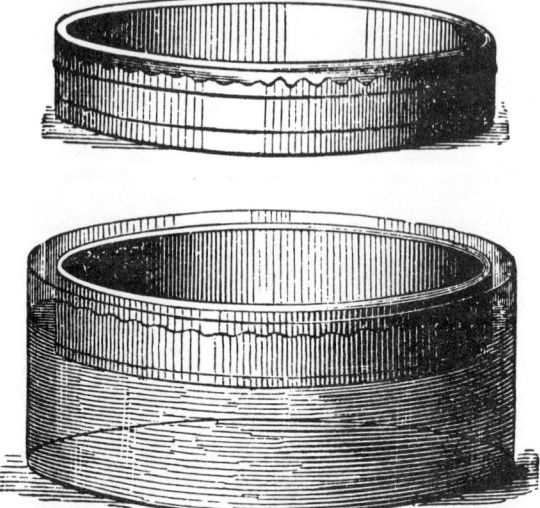

Figure 2   The Graham hoop dialyser

process. He used his 'dialyser' for much experimental work on crystalloids and colloids.

It was not until 1912 that haemodialysis was used experimentally on the dog by Abel, Rowntree and Turner[10]. This dialyser, which used celloidin as a semipermeable membrane and hirudin as an anticoagulant, was further developed by Haas in Germany[11] who was the first person to perform haemodialysis on the human. Technical problems, though, were plentiful.

In the 1940s four groups took up the challenge, each working independently. Kolff[12] must take the initial honours with the design and development of the rotating drum artificial kidney but the valuable contributions made by Alwall[13], Murray et al.[14] and Skeggs and Leonards[15] cannot be ignored. By the early 1950s haemodialysis was well established for the management of patients with reversible types of renal failure and in 1956 the first artificial kidney unit in the United Kingdom was opened in the General Infirmary at Leeds. Treatment then settled down to a relatively quiet peaceful routine until the development of the Scribner Shunt in 1960[16]. Overnight the scene changed, for in this single, but simple, breakthrough the long-term management of patients with irreversible types of renal failure became possible. It must be remembered, though, that it had taken over 200 years of progressive endeavour by scientists and physicians to achieve this desirable goal.

As the life of patients with terminal renal failure has now been usefully extended by intermittent dialysis new problems have inevitably emerged and many of these will be discussed during this symposium. Pre-existing disease processes have become exacerbated. New syndromes have developed whilst technical problems have been lessened or even solved. What are the inner thoughts of patients who spend many hours strapped to a machine? Is it a bearable life? Is transplantation desired by patients? What are the social and economic implications? For we are all too conscious that none could afford therapy without financial help from the community.

Speakers have been chosen to introduce these and other topics but it is hoped that everyone will join in the subsequent discussions.

ACKNOWLEDGEMENTS

Figure 1 was kindly supplied by Edith Frame, Sub-Librarian, University of Strathclyde.

Figure 2 is reproduced by permission of the Librarian of the Royal Society and the quotations are reprinted by permission of the Editor of the *Lancet*.

References

1. Robson, J. S. (1967). The nephrotic syndrome. In D. A. K. Black (ed.). *Renal Disease*, pp. 275–308. (Oxford: Blackwell Scientific Publications)
2. Bright, R. (1827). *Reports of Medical Cases*, Vol 1 (London: Longmans Green)
3. Feiser, L. F. and Feiser, M. (1961). *Advanced Organic Chemistry*, p. 3. (New York: Rheinhold Publishing Corporation)
4. Thompson, T. (1832). Chemical Analysis of the Blood of Cholera Patients. *Philosophical Magazine and Annals*, 11, 345
5. O'Shaughnessy, W. B. (1832). Chemical pathology of cholera. *Lancet*, ii, 225
6. Latta, T. (1832). Documents communicated by the Central Board of Health, London, relative to the treatment of cholera by the copious injection of aqueous and saline fluids into the veins. *Lancet*, ii, 274
7. Craigie, T. (1832). Details of two cases of malignant cholera treated by venous injection. *Lancet*, ii, 277
8. Frame, E. (1970). Thomas Graham: A Centenary Account. *Trans. R. Soc. Glasgow*, 7, 116
9. Graham, T. (1861). Liquid diffusion applied to analysis. *Phil. Trans. R. Soc.*, 151, 183
10. Abel, J. J., Rowntree, L. G. and Turner, B. B. (1913). Some constituents of the blood. *J. pharmacol. exp. ther.*, 5, 611
11. Drukker, W. (1978). Haemodialysis—A Historical Review. In W. Drukker,

      F. M. Parsons and J. Maher (eds.). *Replacement of Renal Function by Dialysis*. (The Hague: Martinus Nijhoff, B. V.) (in press)

12.   Kolff, W. J. (1947). *New Ways of Treating Uraemia*. (London: J. & A. Churchill)

13.   Alwall, N. (1947). On the artificial kidney. I. Apparatus for dialysis of the blood *in vivo. Acta Med. Scand.*, **128**, 317

14.   Murray, G., Delorme, E. and Thomas, N. (1947). Development of an artificial kidney. *Arch. Surg.*, **55**, 505

15.   Skeggs, L. T. and Leonards, J. R. (1948). Studies on an artificial kidney. I. Preliminary results with a new type of continuous dialyzer. *Science*, **108**, 212

16.   Scribner, B. H., Hegstrom, R. M. and Buri, R. (1961). Treatment of chronic uremia by means of hemodialysis: a progress report. In G. Richet (ed.) *First International Congress of Nephrology*, p. 616. (Basle: S. Karger AG)

SECTION ONE

Meeting the Needs
Chairman:
J. S. Robson

1

Selection of patients for dialysis and transplantation
B. H. B. Robinson

1.1 EARLY DEVELOPMENTS AND SELECTION

The success of Scribner's group in Seattle, in overcoming the problem of repeated vascular access for haemodialysis and making possible regular dialysis for chronic renal failure[1], came not only as an exciting new venture for nephrologists but as a challenge for those who have to decide financing and priorities in health care. The inevitable and unpleasant death in uraemia for those in chronic renal failure was averted and the patients returned to active life. It soon became clear that regular dialysis therapy would pose many problems. These were economic and political on the one hand – for here was a dramatic and effective treatment for an inevitably fatal disease, but a very expensive treatment – and medical on the other. Which patients would prove most suitable for therapy and rehabilitation? What complications were to be expected? The latter question was answered in part after only a few years, as renal bone disease, ectopic calcification, neuropathy and dialysis-associated hepatitis began to appear.

At the same time as regular dialysis treatment (RDT) was being developed, new progress was made in renal transplantation by the application of relatively safer and more effective immunosuppressive regimens. At first, dialysers and transplanters seemed to be apparently in competition, but during the past decade have worked in very close cooperation in offering an improved outlook for patients with chronic renal disease. The relative indications for treatment have changed as facilities have become more generally available. The economic aspects of treatment are to be dealt with in a later session, but with our present dearth of facilities medical criteria will be important in determining priorities.

In many western countries facilities have been developed to treat all subjects with end-stage renal failure, and selection is a thing of the past. Some of us are less fortunate[2]. After a promising start in the UK the lack of any politically or administratively directed policy from the centre, as much as economic stringency, has resulted in a considerable shortfall of treatment facilities, despite the urgings of nephrologists.

I propose to examine the various factors which we have to consider when a patient presents in advanced renal failure, and discuss the way in which these factors affect suitability for treatment and the method of treatment chosen.

1.2   TYPE OF PRIMARY RENAL DISEASE AND SELECTION

Dialysis treatment was initially confined to patients with uncomplicated renal disease. Those with systemic disease such as amyloidosis and diabetes were excluded. Patients in the former group still constitute the vast majority undergoing treatment. The largest single diagnostic group of patients is included in the miscellaneous classification of glomerulonephritis, with pyelonephritis and the various forms of interstitial nephritis second. Polycystic disease and primary hypertension account for large minority groups. The influence of hypertension upon selection will be discussed below. Several reports have emphasized the exceptionally good results obtained with RDT in the treatment of patients with polycystic disease. Their prognosis and rehabilitation are better than average, and most patients have normal or near normal haematocrits in happy contrast with most of their fellows. European experience[3] suggests that results in polycystic disease are less impressive for renal transplantation, results being similar or even a little worse in age-matched controls with other renal disorders.

One might suppose that some forms of glomerulonephritis, particularly those in which an active immunopathogenic mechanism is strongly suspect, would recur in transplanted kidneys, yet no consistent pattern has been reported even for rapidly progressive glomerulonephritis[4]. In 300 transplants we have seen recurrences of crescentic glomerulonephritis in only two, leading to graft failure after 6 and 8 months respectively. In several other patients it has not been possible to distinguish between recurrent glomerulonephritis and chronic rejection. Early and severe recurrence of focal glomerulosclerosis (FGS) has been reported in allografts[5]. In our limited experience with transplantation in this condition we have seen one patient in whom heavy proteinuria led to a nephrotic syndrome within a month of grafting but in another similar patient there has been no recurrence after 18 months. Recurrence has not been universal[4,6] and this diagnosis need not debar at least one attempt at transplantation. Although the histological changes of membrano-proliferative with dense deposits may recur in allografts[4], the clinical significance of this is not yet apparent.

Thus it seems that with the possible exception of FGS, which may sometimes recur in the transplant, the initiating renal disorder *per se* has little influence on selection, and little or no influence on selection as between dialysis or transplantation, although massive polycystic kidneys, recurrent infection or an abnormal lower urinary tract may require preliminary surgery. A bladder severely affected by tuberculosis or other pathology may bias one in favour of dialysis, although the ureter may be implanted into an ileal-loop conduit.

Analgesic nephropathy has been considered a relative contraindication in some centres because it suggests a personality disorder in the individual. In practice we have found that these patients do well on dialysis. One patient, having given up his analgesics, recovered sufficient renal function after five months RDT to be taken off the programme and to survive in comparatively good health on mild protein restriction alone, until he died 20 months later following a myocardial infarction. A few patients unfortunately continue to take analgesics after transplantation, and may endanger their graft. There is also an increased risk of carcinoma of the renal pelvis in this condition[7], and we have lost one dialysis patient from this cause.

1.3 HYPERTENSION AND CARDIOVASCULAR PROBLEMS IN SELECTION

Hypertension has been present in more than half the patients we have accepted for the dialysis programme and in 15% has been in the accelerated (malignant) phase. Hypertension has been easily controlled by dialysis in nearly all patients. We have found bilateral nephrectomy necessary only for dialysis-resistant hypertension with grossly elevated plasma renin levels in three patients out of nearly 500 entering our combined programme. Several other patients have had a bilateral nephrectomy with only moderate effect on the hypertension. These proved to be individuals who abused fluid restriction. These patients can be a serious problem in a dialysis unit but they are not easy to identify before starting therapy.

Diazoxide is a valuable drug for reducing the very high blood pressure of malignant hypertension, and minoxidil is of value in the resistant blood pressure associated with chronic renal failure. More recent experience with diafiltration suggests that we may have another valuable tool[8].

Hypertension is often a complication of chronic renal disease and, unless prolonged, has not significantly altered prognosis in our group, although most, but not all, deaths from cerebral infarction or haemorrhage have been in patients previously hypertensive. Prognostically, a large heart and angina have been unfavourable selection criteria. None of our patients starting dialysis with angina have survived 5 years. But care must be taken to distinguish angina from the pain and apparent cardiomegaly of uraemic pericarditis, for this condition is responsive to dialysis – although initially we prefer peritoneal dialysis to diminish the risk of haemorrhagic effusion and tamponade. If we have selected a patient for dialysis we endeavour to commence therapy before pericarditis develops.

Few would plan dialysis or transplantation for those who have had severe strokes but limited experience of patients who have had transient ischaemic attacks or even a minor, largely recovered, hemiparesis has been encouraging. Nevertheless myocardial infarction and cerebral vascular accidents are major causes of late mortality in dialysis and transplantation[3]. Perhaps we should pay more attention to the hyperlipidaemia which is so common in uraemic subjects.

Peripheral vascular disease may be so severe as to make vascular access for dialysis almost impossible, even with newer techniques for grafting vascular prosthesis (bovine carotid, umbilical vein or expanded polytetrafluoroethylene (PTFE). Vascular calcification associated with hyperparathyroidism is an important factor in many patients, and another indication for early management of uraemia and avoidance of overenthusiastic vitamin D therapy.

There is no more tragic situation than the progressive loss of all available access sites in a patient on dialysis. We have seen gross occlusive vascular disease leading to gangrene of finger tips in a 19-year-old with advanced primary glomerulonephritis. We consider careful assessment of peripheral vessels a vital part of patient selection, and since the iliac vessels may be patent in the presence of severe distal arteriopathy, a factor in balancing choice between dialysis and transplantation. We include in our preliminary care a stern warning to other clinicians to 'keep off the veins'.

1.4 THE INFLUENCE OF SYSTEMIC DISEASE IN SELECTION

For a long period renal replacement was confined to patients without generalized systemic disorders because of shortage of facilities, and later because of a natural reluctance to be involved with further problems in a treatment already complicated enough. The commoner disorders in this group are amyloidosis, systemic lupus and diabetes. Results in the treatment of amyloidosis are encouraging in our personal experience and in that of others, even though amyloid changes may occur in a grafted kidney[9]. Results have been even more encouraging in systemic lupus.

The treatment of renal failure in diabetics has been more controversial. So often, as with a patient we are considering now, diabetic nephropathy reaches end-stage only when a patient is blind from retinopathy, with muscle weakness and with distal gangrene from peripheral neuropathy and when the access sites are virtually unavailable because of vascular occlusion. Rapid progression of retinopathy in the first year has been a major problem[10] and survival on haemodialysis relatively short[3], although results may be better with peritoneal dialysis. Transplantation seems to offer more favourable chances for rehabilitation. Overall survival figures in Europe for these diseases, taken from the EDTA Registry[3], are summarized in Table 1.1. There is no doubt that physician-effort and rehabilitation-failure are greater in diabetics than others and they are likely to rate a lower priority when dialysis places are limited.

TABLE 1.1   Survival rates of patients with diabetes, amyloidosis and lupus erythematosus in hospital dialysis

	Number	6 months	1 yr	2 yrs
Diabetes	491	83.2 ± 1	68.2 ± 3	50.0 ± 4
Amyloidosis	212	78.2 ± 3	64.4 ± 4	52.6 ± 5
Lupus erythematosus	139	84.1 ± 3	73.7 ± 5	65.4 ± 6

From the Combined Report of the European Dialysis and Transplant Association Registry 1975[3].

A word should be included about hepatitis B. In some countries this is taken relatively lightly, but in the UK strict isolation and screening of patients has virtually eliminated this problem from renal units, apart from special 'yellow' units and a few home patients. Unfortunately a new patient found to be hepatitis B positive will have great difficulty finding a place in a UK dialysis/transplant programme. Hopefully the new hepatitis vaccines may help to solve the problem.

1.5   AGE IN SELECTION

Perhaps the most controversial factor in selection is the age of the patient. During the early years of renal replacement most centres concentrated upon treating the 15–45 age group and regrettably in parts of Britain we are still nearly as restrictive. Whilst this younger group has the best survival and rehabilitation rate, several studies have now confirmed the success of dialysis in the older age groups[11] – even into the seventies. For older patients expectations should necessarily be more restricted and sensible judgement is demanded. Transplantation too is promising in the over-fifties, but survival rates to date are poorer than for younger patients or for dialysis and there is a tendency to consider dialysis as offering a better survival prospect for most older patients.

Dialysis and transplantation in children has also been an emotive issue.

There is little doubt about the success of these techniques in children although the problems of ensuring normal growth and puberty have yet to be solved. Most feel that transplantation offers better chances for full rehabilitation. Parental, if not sibling, donations are most frequently available for this group. Nephrologists once felt reservations about putting children through demanding regimens with uncertain long-term prospects, but the successes recorded for the 10-plus age group have been reassuring. These doubts still linger for very small children, with their lack of understanding, prospects of dwarfing and uncertain long-term prognosis. The techniques need to be improved.

In terms of psychological and social rehabilitation our worst prospects have been in the 13–17 age group, surprisingly. Alternation between over-dependance, distorting the whole family, and bitterness – with an often aggressive expression of the desire not to compete in a life for which they can see little long-term hope – has blighted technically successful treatment. Perhaps we have paid insufficient attention to the psychological and social needs of this group.

1.6 PSYCHOLOGICAL AND SOCIAL FACTORS

Attempts to select patients on psychological grounds have proved particularly difficult. While one tends to exclude those who are frankly psychotic, we have had considerable success in patients with a background of intermittent depressive illness. Psychiatrists often express the view, even in prospective studies, that their assessment of suitability differs little from that of the experienced clinician, although perhaps couched in more elegant terms. To some extent this reflects the natural disinclination of the psychiatrists to be cast in the role of executioner – for 'unsuitability' may equal death in uraemia. Certain personality characteristics, difficult in the management of most illnesses, are particularly troublesome in renal replacement therapy. The most worrying are over-dependance, denial – with the inevitable difficulty in collaborating with dialysis or the immunosuppressive regime of transplantation – and aggression. The patient who voices his resentment against his illness by aggression towards family and nursing staff or towards himself, is particularly difficult to manage in the close and regular contact of a renal unit. Self-aggression may take the form of fluid over-indulgence or the more dramatic form of separating shunts, cutting fistulae or discontinuing immunosuppression. Neurotic pre-morbid personalities often settle well. The remarkable stability of most individuals despite the chronic stress of a life threatening illness is one of the most interesting and heartening aspects of dialysis and transplantation.

We have not found it easy to predict reactions to dialysis and transplantation from early response to dietary restriction – a factor some centres have stressed. Whilst one may be able to observe the aggressive, the obviously 'psychopathic' or the frankly stupid, we have had patients, most uncooperative on modified Giovanetti diets, who have flourished on dialysis and vice versa. One might anticipate better rehabilitation with a good transplant, but one lonely country lass, who coped with home dialysis well, down on the farm, and hardly ever bothered the unit, has become almost totally dependant now she has a graft with a creatinine clearance of 90 ml/min. A most valuable factor in success is a stable family background and suport from either spouse, relatives or friends. Intelligence helps (more than education) but even those of low IQ can cope.

1.7   CHOICE OF TREATMENT

Selection involves not only admission to the treatment programme, but the type of treatment to be considered. Most UK centres run an integrated home/hospital dialysis/transplant programme. The unstable, with poor support or inadequate housing, are clearly best treated at hospital or transplanted. For those who live far away home treatment has proved highly successful. We have touched on the medical indications for treatment selection between dialysis and transplantation. The interesting difference

TABLE 1.2   Home patients as a percentage of total on haemodialysis (if more than 10.0%)

	Country	1975	(1974)	(1973)	(1972)
1	United Kingdom	65.8	(64.8)	(61.6)	(58.8)
2	Ireland	36.6	(41.2)	(31.7)	(31.9)
3	Fed. Rep. of Germany	29.5	(29.0)	(27.2)	(24.2)
4	Sweden	23.1	(24.2)	(24.7)	(18.7)
5	Switzerland	21.8	(18.7)	(18.2)	(11.7)
	EUROPE	19.2	(18.8)	(18.5)	(17.6)
6	Denmark	15.4	(10.0)	(4.3)	(2.1)
7	Norway	14.1	(10.0)	(21.7)	(23.8)
8	France	12.5	(9.4)	(11.2)	(10.0)
9	Netherlands	11.4	(11.2)	(9.1)	(8.2)

in philosophy or social customs between nations is shown in Table 1.2 which reflects the percentage of dialysis patients treated at home. It is interesting to speculate whether in the UK enthusiasm for and emphasis on home dialysis has actually slowed up the development of new hospital centres, thereby contributing to our present shortfall in facilities.

The choice between home dialysis and transplantation may be difficult. Considerations of age, family support or availability of dialysis access sites may influence this choice but, despite the relative survival figures[2], most patients opt to have a transplant should one become available.

1.8 TIMING OF TREATMENT

Finally, selection should include a proper assessment of the correct timing for each phase of treatment. Where dialysis places are limited there is a risk that patients may develop severe cachexia, pericarditis, fluid overload or die before treatment is started. No hard and fast rules can be given, but the stage at which the patient is likely to lose time from work, or is becoming disabled by uraemic symptoms unresponsive to diet or is moving into negative nitrogen balance with steady loss of muscle (excluding any nephrotic phase with preservation of adequate GFR) is the time to start regular dialysis. This often corresponds to a serum creatinine greater than 1000 μmol/l, or a glomerular filtration rate below 10 to 15 ml/min. Many centres would start sooner. There is a very definite place for considering transplantation without preliminary dialysis if a suitable donor kidney becomes available. As transplantation results improve, this approach may become more commonplace.

1.9 CONCLUSIONS

For most or all of us, the unhappy early period of restricted availability of dialysis and transplantation, requiring careful selection of patients on grounds of medical and social suitability, cooperation, personality, etc., is a thing of the past. Yet in many centres, certainly in the UK, facilities remain inadequate and selection criteria still operate with regard to age and complicating medical conditions, despite the success of these treatments for a wide spectrum of age and primary illness. This shortage has the added disadvantage that treatment may be started late and patients with failing transplants may not be returned to dialysis in time. Since renal replacement therapy has a better success rate than treatment provided without question for many other fatal disorders, it is incumbent upon nephrologists to plead their cause to those responsible for selecting health care priorities. The very accurate costing of our therapies when compared with the ignorance about costing in so many other fields of medicine is an undoubted disadvantage.

ACKNOWLEDGEMENTS

I am grateful to the Editors of the Proceedings of the European Dialysis and Transplant Association for permission to reproduce Figures 1.1 and 1.2.

References

1. Quinton, W. E., Dillard, D. H., Cole, J. J. and Scribner, B. H. (1962). Eight months' experience with Silastic-Teflon bypass cannulas. *Trans. Am. Soc. Artif. Int. Organs,* **8,** 236
2. Jacobs, C., Brunner, F. P., Chantler, C., Donckerwolcke, R. A., Gurland. H. J., Hathway, R. A., Selwood, N. H. and Wing, A. J. (1977). Combined report on regular dialysis and transplantation in Europe, VII, 1976. *Proc. Eur. Dial. Transpl. Assoc.,* **14,** 4
3. Gurland, H. J., Brunner, F. P., Chantler, C., Jacobs, C., Schärer, K., Selwood, N. H., Spies, G. and Wing, A. J. (1976). Combined report on regular dialysis and transplantation in Europe, VI, 1975. *Proc. Eur. Dial. Transpl. Assoc.,* **13,** 3
4. Cameron, J. S. and Turner, D. R. (1977). Recurrent glomerulonephritis in allografted kidneys. *Clin. Nephrol.,* **7,** 47
5. Huyer, J. R., Raij, L., Vernier, R. L., Simmons, R. L., Najarian, J. S. and Michael, A. F. (1972). Recurrence of idiopathic nephrotic syndrome after renal transplantation. *Lancet,* **ii,** 343
6. Couser, W. G., Idelson, B. A., Stilmant, M. M., Migdal, S. D. and Davis, R. C. (1975). Successful renal transplantation in focal glomerular sclerosis: report of two cases. *Clin. Nephrol.,* **4,** 62
7. Bengtsson, U. (1974). Phenacetin and renal pelvic carcinoma. *Clin. Nephrol.,* **2,** 123
8. Quellhorst, E., Schuenemann, B. and Doht, B. (1977). Treatment of severe hypertension in chronic renal failure by haemofiltration. *Proc. Eur. Dial. Transpl. Assoc.,* **14,** 729
9. Wilson, R. E. (1976). Transplantation in patients with unusual causes of renal failure. *Clin. Nephrol.,* **5,** 51
10. Silfkin, R. F., Neff, M. S., Baez, A., Gupta, S., Mattoo, N. and Haimov, M. (1976). Maintenance dialysis in diabetic patients. *Proc. Eur. Dial. Transpl. Assoc.,* **13,** 377
11. Brunner, F. P., Giesecke, B., Gurland, H. J., Jacobs, C., Parsons, F. M., Schärer, K., Seyffart, G., Spies, G. and Wing, A. J. (1975). Combined report on regular dialysis and transplantation in Europe, V, 1974. *Proc. Eur. Dial. Transpl. Assoc.,* **12,** 3

DISCUSSION

R. Gabriel (London): Dr Robinson said a clearance of 5–10 ml/min. for taking people on dialysis. Did he really mean that?

Robinson: Yes, I did. I purposefully did not mention figures because I think that it is very difficult. One could certainly take higher rates, 15–20 ml/min.

Robson: What was the concentration of creatinine in the blood of your dialysis patients prior to going on to the programme?

Robinson: About 1000 μmol/l.

J. M. Bone (Liverpool): Until recently we had no hospital facilities for sustaining patients awaiting a transplant, and we had to take patients on the waiting list for transplantation without prior dialysis. This was not very successful. The transplant operation carried a 25% mortality and the waiting list itself carried a 60% mortality because patients used to die before kidneys became available. At present this is not a very good substitute for adequate supporting dialysis facilities for the transplant programme.

Robinson: I entirely agree. To get good results from transplants one must be prepared to take the patients back. We have noticed this very much within the last year or two. We have been comparing the results of patients treated by home dialysis alone with those transplanted from home dialysis. There is no doubt that the mortality rate of the transplanted group is higher and yet, nevertheless, the vast majority of patients still wanted to be considered for transplantation. Since we have been more inclined to take patients back on to a dialysis programme when the transplant has failed, and not to push immunosuppression too far, results in terms of patient survival – if not graft survival – have been much better.

One may transplant a patient before he comes on to a dialysis programme, but if good survival rates are to be achieved one must be prepared to start dialysis should the graft fail.

H. Elliott (Glasgow): Has peritoneal dialysis any value as a maintenance form of treatment, particularly in the diabetic group?

Robinson: It probably has. We have very little experience of this. We have had few patients on peritoneal dialysis. Those who have gone into it enthusiastically have claimed some very good results and there are claims that for diabetics it may be the treatment of choice. They may fare better on peritoneal dialysis than on haemodialysis, but I have no experience myself.

Has Dr Elliott any experience?

Elliott: It is very limited. Perhaps two patients.

2

The status of haemodialysis
W. R. Cattell

2.1 INTRODUCTION

Twelve years ago the potential for saving life by artificial means was the subject of great controversy[1]. In respect of kidney machines the profession was suspicious and divided; the lay public emotional and vociferous. Regular haemodialysis was being pioneered on soft money and often in the teeth of opposition from the establishment. Newspapers carried banner headlines and committees were set up to assess its acceptability. In 1965 the then Minister of Health, Kenneth Robinson, agreed that regular dialysis had passed from being a research undertaking to a proven and acceptable form of treatment which should be provided within the National Health Service. Twelve years later where have we got to? How readily available is regular dialysis treatment and how successful has it proved to be?

2.2 SUPPLY AND DEMAND

The first and perhaps crudest approach is to examine the number of patients receiving treatment at the present time. Statistics are provided by the excellent work of the EDTA Registration Committee, to whom I am indebted for the figures for the year ending 1975[2] and the provisional data for the year ending December 1976[3]. From this information we see (Table 2.1) that in December 1976 there was a total of 2409 patients receiving

TABLE 2.1   Patients receiving haemodialysis in the UK in December 1976[3]

Hospital	802
Home	1607
Total	2409
Total/mill. pop	43.0

haemodialysis treatment in Great Britain of whom 1607 or 67% were being treated in the home. Relating this to our population, a figure of 43.0 per million is obtained. I had hoped to give updated comparisons between the British performance and that in other European countries in December 1976. Unfortunately the cross-checking of this information by the EDTA Registration Committee is not yet complete and we must, therefore, be content with the 1975 data. Table 2.2 shows the rating as of December of that year. The United Kingdom comes 12th in the list, providing treatment for fewer patients than the European average. This table tells its own tale. Looking at the preliminary data for 1976 the league table is much the same.

TABLE 2.2   Comparison of haemodialysis statistics in Europe in 1975[2]

	Pop. in mill.	Hospital	Home	Total	Total/ mill.
Israel	3.4	341	14	355	104.4
Luxemburg	0.3	28	—	28	93.3
France	52.8	4067	583	4650	88.1
Switzerland	6.4	437	122	559	87.3
Fed. Rep. Germany	61.8	3565	1491	5056	81.8
Italy	55.8	3889	300	4189	75.1
Belgium	9.8	701	30	731	74.6
Netherlands	13.6	799	103	902	66.3
Denmark	5.0	247	45	292	58.4
Sweden	8.2	269	81	350	42.7
Greece	9.0	365	—	365	40.6
United Kingdom	56.0	741	1427	2168	38.7
Europe	491.4	18116	4305	22421	45.6

The position is, however, even worse than this! The data we are looking at relates to patients established on haemodialysis – some possibly for years. In assessing the adequacy of our programmes we should, however, relate supply to demand. Several studies in the United Kingdom have calculated that there are some 33 patients per million per year up to the age

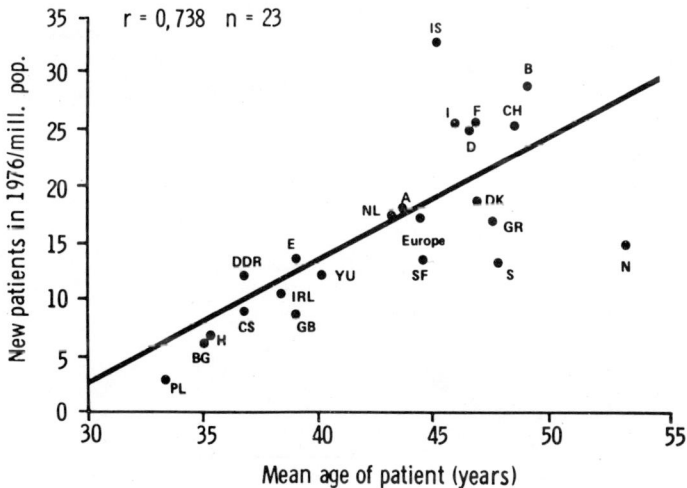

Figure 2.1   Number of new patients commencing haemodialysis in 1976[3]

of 55 requiring and suitable for regular dialysis treatment. If supply is to meet demand a comparable number of patients should start regular dialysis treatment each year. Looking at the recent EDTA data, however, (Figure 2.1) we see that in Great Britain less than 10 patients per million commenced dialysis in 1976, i.e. a third of the calculated number requiring treatment. This compares with almost three times that number starting treatment in 1976 in France, Germany, Italy, Switzerland and Belgium. Interestingly, only Israel among the EDTA countries approaches the stated required level.

Another interesting point deduced from these statistics is that, with some exceptions, the fewer the patients accepted for treatment, the younger their age. This is open to several interpretations. It could be that some

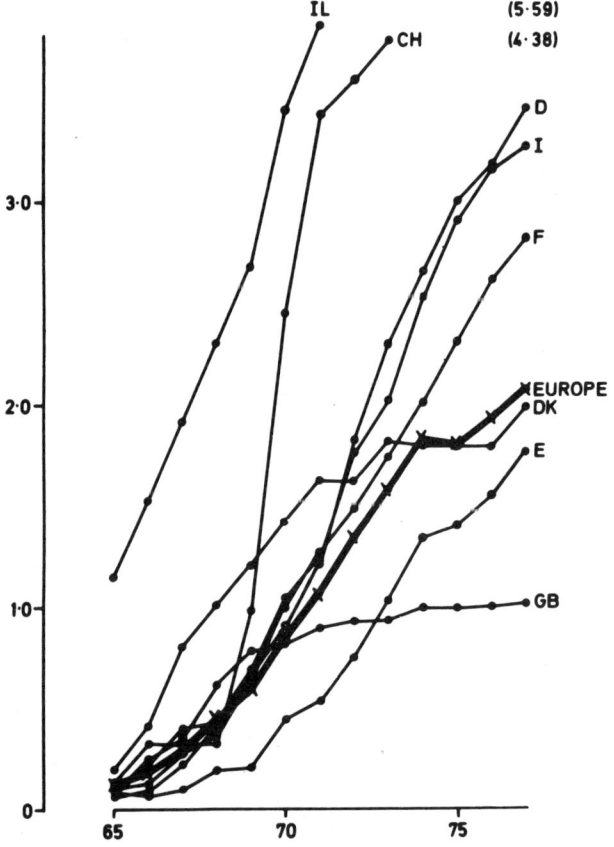

Figure 2.2   Number of centres in European countries 1965–76[3]

countries, at an early stage of development of regular dialysis facilities, elected to take older patients. Examining the countries in question this cannot apply to Holland, Ireland and United Kingdom, all of whom have been undertaking dialysis for many years. There are many other possible interpretations but the most probable is that where resources are limited, clinicians practice selection and in this age is an important factor. The more generous the facilities the greater the number of older patients that can be reasonably accepted for treatment.

This, of course, implies that we are trying to match the need. The statistics suggest we are indeed working quite hard. Thus (Figure 2.2) the United Kingdom has fewer centres per million population than most other countries, yet (Figure 2.3) we treat more patients per centre than any other European country.

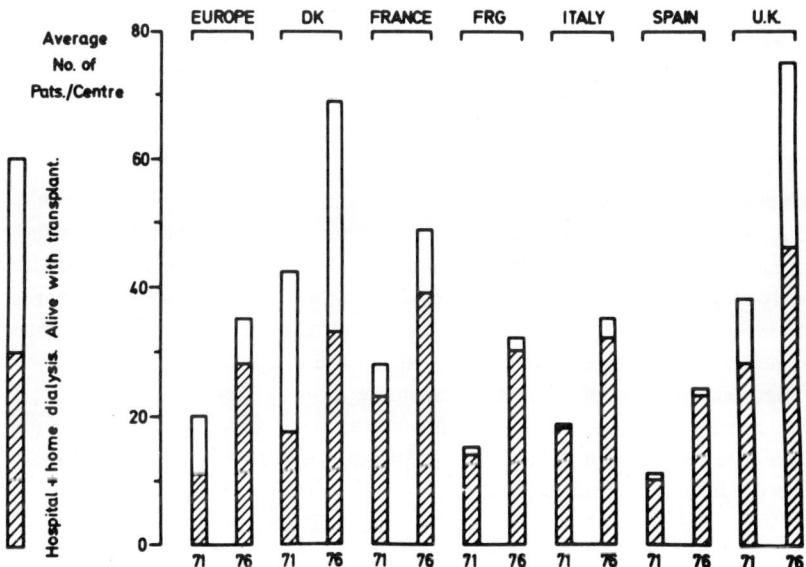

Figure 2.3   Number of patients per centre, 1971–76: all Europe and some countries[3]

The message would, therefore, seem to be that in the UK we are not in any way matching the demand for treatment despite a high workload per individual centre. As a so-called industrialized nation we should be doing better. Looking at the European data it is difficult to escape the conclusion that what we need is more centres. Thus we already have a high workload per centre and from personal experience we are all too well aware of immense demands made on staff – medical, nursing and ancilliary – to sustain this workload. To expand it further could well break the back of the system and is unlikely, rapidly, to match supply to demand.

2.3   THE QUALITY OF TREATMENT

Crude statistics on the *quantity* of dialysis provided does not, of course, necessarily reflect the *quality* of treatment. In discussing the position of haemodialysis it is thus also appropriate to ask how good is it? It is difficult to assess the quality of treatment in an otherwise life and death situation. At the risk of oversimplification I have chosen to examine it in terms of effectiveness and acceptability.

2.3.1   Effectiveness

In terms of effectiveness I have used the parameters of survival, rehabilitation, patient well-being and freedom from complications.

2.3.1.1   *Survival*

Over the past seven years the EDTA Registration Committee has carefully documented the survival statistics of patients on regular dialysis treatment in Europe. These have stayed remarkably constant over recent years with an overall 5-year survival of between 70 and 80%. Patently, when compared with other killing disease such as malignant disease or chronic bronchitis which require long-term treatment, these are excellent results. On superficial examination of the statistics, home dialysis would seem to have a better survival record than hospital dialysis but this is almost certainly qualified by selection policies and local expertise. In centres providing both there is little difference in results.

2.3.1.2   *Rehabilitation*

What, however, is the quality of this survival? One measure of this is the degree of rehabilitation as judged by the return to full-time work by those *capable and wishing* to undertake full employment. This year's analysis by the EDTA Registration Committee gives the results set out in Figure 2.4.

It can be seen that some 65% of home dialysis patients wishing to do so returned to full-time employment – essentially the same as those with successful cadaver transplants. It should, however, be pointed out that further analysis shows that, with time, patients with successful transplants over-

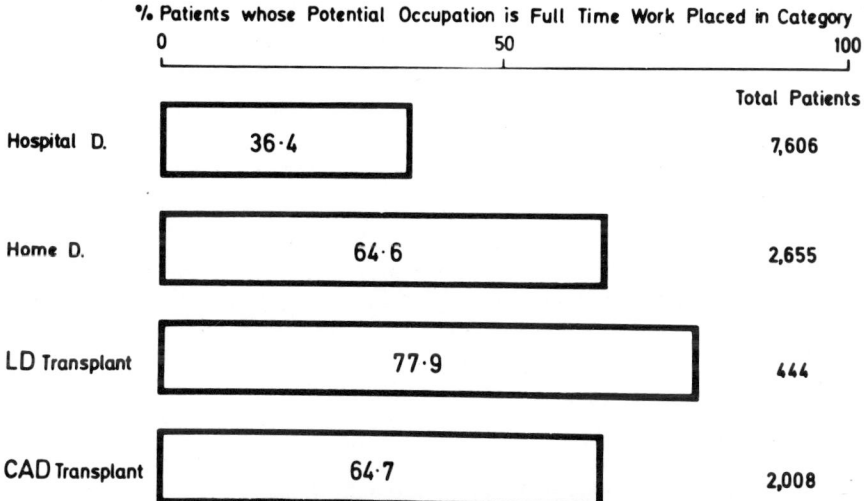

Figure 2.4 Rehabilitation of patients able and wishing to return to work[3]

take patients on home dialysis in terms of rehabilitation, reaching a 71% return to full-time work after 2 years. Hospital dialysis has a much poorer showing in terms of rehabilitation, but this almost certainly relates to selection, complications and possibly age. It is also true that many patients not rehabilitated on regular dialysis treatment, including hospital dialysis, can be returned to full-time work after successful transplantation.

2.3.1.3 *Patient well-being*

Well-being also means 'how do you feel'? We must admit that a significant proportion of patients feel less than fit. Many factors, both physical and psychological, are involved. High among these is the chronic anaemia of renal failure. Despite claims for androgen therapy or the use of cobalt, I believe that across the country as a whole we still fail to achieve really satisfactory correction of the chronic anaemia of dialysis patients and that this is one of the most important limiting factors in returning our patients to a sense of complete well-being.

2.3.1.4 *Freedom from complications*

This brings me to complications and the great success story in the UK with respect to viral hepatitis. Alone in Europe, or indeed in the world, we seem to have conquered the yellow peril. This has only been possible, however, by strict attention to preventive measures. There is a feeling abroad that we may be becoming complacent and lax. This must be guarded against. Thus it may well be less dangerous and possibly, with respect to transplantation, even advantageous to ease up on our policy of minimal transfusion, but this should only be allowed with the strictest control of screening of transfused blood for hepatitis B antigen.

What is the present situation in respect to other complications? Bone disease, dialysis dementia and hypertension will all be dealt with later. Aside from 'Newcastle bone disease' I believe that we have the increased understanding and potential to both prevent and treat bone disease and hypertension. With respect to the control of hypertension and fluid overload the selective use of ultrafiltration has been a major recent advance. Its tremendous value is already accepted in acute renal failure and in patients starting regular dialysis. Its role in the management of long-term haemodialysis is yet to be assessed, as is that of diafiltration.

What few of us have yet faced up to, however, is the prospect of ageing dialysis populations. Experience in long-established centres indicates that with advancing age of our patients and the increased incidence of vascular disease we are almost certainly going to have problems and a significant return of home patients to centre or limited care dialysis. This will be inevitable and will demand increased hospital resources.

2.3.2 Acceptability

Turning to the acceptability of regular dialysis, this may be considered under a variety of headings.

2.3.2.1 *Ease of treatment*

First and foremost, how easy is it? We have more than 10 years' experience in dialysis for chronic renal failure in the UK and should by now have refined our practice both in terms of safety and ease of operation. Have we? Critical to the performance of regular haemodialysis is satisfactory access to the circulation. This was the first important breakthrough made by Scribner and his colleagues[4] in 1960 when they introduced the Teflon shunt. Shunts have their problems and were replaced in the 1960s by the Cimino–Brescia arterio-venous fistula[5]. This in turn was an important advance but we cannot pretend that we don't have fistula problems. Indeed the ease of needling fistulae, the adequacy of blood flows obtained and fistula failure are still considerable problems. Single-needle dialysis was introduced as long ago as 1970[6] but has not received universal acceptance. Why? Partly cost and partly doubt as to its efficacy. I suspect many of us have not pursued this practice with sufficient vigour or enthusiasm. A national reappraisal of both the fistula problems and single needle dialysis would be immensely valuable in highlighting possible areas for improvement. For the present I fear that access to the circulation is still an important factor limiting the ease and efficiency of dialysis.

Regarding the hardware available, there is no doubt this has improved considerably in the past 12 years. More reliable electronic circuitry, effective deaeration, compact high performance dialysers and automated re-use equipment have all made the practice of haemodialysis *potentially* much simpler and safer. Sadly new capital equipment is expensive and many of us are still struggling with equipment bought 10 years ago with no money to replace it. More than that, modern equipment and especially disposable dialysers are associated with high running costs. With multiple reuse of dialysers costs can be reduced. With automated closed systems reusing both dialysers and lines the needs for expensive major home conversions may also be reduced. The cost effectiveness and ease of dialysis must therefore take account not only of individual units of equipment but of the whole system. However, with the possible exception of work done by Mansell and Wing[7] on the Redy system there has, as yet, been no systematic study of interrelated capital and revenue costs with modern systems. We suspect that in the United Kingdom a whole variety of different systems are in use and that dialysis costs vary considerably from centre to centre. While in no way suggesting restriction in choice of system I believe that there is an urgent need for a nationwide assessment of running costs with different systems to assess how we can best provide the easiest effective dialysis with the smallest acceptable expenditure. Individual units cannot themselves test out each different system but a multicentre analysis might well give us the answer.

This is the second time I have mentioned national multicentre studies. I think this also reflects the status of haemodialysis in the United Kingdom. Ten years ago we were all obsessed with getting our departments running and proving that we could successfully undertake regular dialysis. In those days we had the 'Dialysis Group' in this country. This met occasionally and was a forum for exchanging experience. As we got confident, the dialysis group wound up. Now, however, we could, with great benefit, pool our national experience on the various outstanding problems with great profit to our patients.

2.3.2.2   *Duration of treatment*

Aside from the ease with which treatment can be carried out, an important feature of acceptability is the duration of dialysis. This is a very confused area. In the very early days of regular dialysis disastrous results with poor rehabilitation and the so-called 'under-dialysis syndrome' led to the belief that it was essential to dialyse for at least 28–30 h per week. It became accepted that dialysis time was required to remove toxic compounds. There followed passionate interest in the 'middle molecule' as the offending toxin. In the past 5 years however we have seen such concepts stood on their heads. Thus we have seen a steady reduction in dialysis time with none of the dire complications predicted. Part of this may relate to more efficient dialysers with high blood flows but this is not the whole story. The importance of middle molecule in the uraemic syndrome is being seriously questioned and indeed we are really no further forward in precisely identifying what we are or should be removing by dialysis. Possibly the most important factor is control of fluid and electrolyte balance and adequate nutrition.

Whatever the theoretical implications of short-hour dialysis, in practice it seems to work and reduction in the time required for treatment has improved the acceptability of dialysis immensely. Conservative Britain is still, however, very cautious. Partly this may be because we make more extensive use of Kiil type dialysers than hollow-fibre or multiple-layer high performance dialysers. The impression gained is that we are certainly not doing less than 5 h thrice weekly or anything near the 3 h thrice weekly practised in some European centres. I suspect we are too cautious and must move with the times.

Related to short hours is of course the need to individualize dialysis. It is naive to believe that all patients, whatever their size, require or desire the same duration of treatment. It is also naive to believe that patients require the same amount of dialysis at all times. This is especially important as we reduce the hours. We must all be alert to the fact that short hours is basic treatment. If there is intercurrent infection or illness, hours must be temporarily increased. The normal kidney has reserve capacity. The artificial kidney does not.

2.3.2.3   *Social convenience*

Also related to the acceptability of dialysis practice is its social convenience. Assessing this is again difficult and must be related to individual circumstances. If you live in a large mansion, the butler runs your dialysis, and your social secretary plans your week. It can be organized very nicely. If you live in a two room council house with four children it is not so easy. Overall advances in the ease of treatment and reduction in hours have led to improved social acceptance. The British policy of home dialysis, dictated primarily by cost, has been successful. It is, however, too rigid. Just as duration of dialysis should be individualized so too should the site of treatment. Some patients are best suited by home dialysis while others would be happier with limited care centre dialysis. This must be equated with the financial resources available but I believe we should now be moving to more flexibility into how and where we treat our patients both for social as well as for economic reasons.

2.3.2.4 *Dietary freedom*

Finally, we cannot consider the acceptability of regular dialysis without consideration of dietary freedom. A principal function of the normal kidney is to get rid of waste material from our diet. Kidney failure demands restriction in our diet. How well does dialysis restore the freedom to eat? I think there can be no doubt that over the past 12 years we have all moved to more sensible and liberal diets for our patients. Aside from restrictions in water, sodium and potassium most patients should now be free to eat a pretty normal diet. Certainly the expensive high calorie diets formerly recommended are unnecessary in the well treated subject. In part this relates to better management of chronic renal failure prior to dialysis but mainly it relates to confidence in our dialysis capability.

2.4 CONCLUSION

In conclusion how would I summarize the status of haemodialysis in the UK? I think it reflects our national character and economic climate. It may be summarized as being responsible, reasonably industrious, decidedly conservative, definitely under-financed but successful against the odds.

ACKNOWLEDGEMENTS

I am grateful to the Editors of the *Proceedings of the European Dialysis and Transplant Association* for permission to reproduce Tables 2.1 and 2.2, and Figures 2.1, 2.2, 2.3 and 3.4.

References

1. Fox, R. C. and Swazey, J. P. (1974). *The Courage to Fail. A Social View of Organ Transplants and Dialysis.* (London: University of Chicago Press Ltd.)
2. Gurland, H. J., Brunner, F. P., Chantler, C., Jacobs, C., Schärer, K., Selwood, N. H., Spiers, G. and Wing, A. J. (1976). Combined Report on Regular Dialysis and Transplantation in Europe, VI, 1975. *Proc. Eur. Dial. Transpl. Assoc.*, **13**, 3
3. Jacobs, C., Brunner, F. P., Chantler, C., Donckerwolcke, R. A., Gurland, H. J., Hathway, R. A., Selwood, N. H. and Wing, A. J. (1977). Combined Report on Regular Dialysis and Transplantation in Europe, VII, 1976. *Proc. Eur. Dial. Transpl. Assoc.*, **14**, 3
4. Quinton, W., Dillard, D. and Scribner, B. H. (1960). Cannulation of blood vessels for prolonged hemodialysis. *Trans. Am. Soc. Artific. Inter. Org.*, **6**, 104
5. Brescia, M. J., Cimino, J. E., Appel, K. and Hurwich, B. J. (1966). Chronic hemodialysis using venipuncture and a surgically created arteriovenous fistula. *N. Engl. J. Med.*, **275**, 1089
6. Panter, H. R., Kopp, K. F., Gutch, C. F. and van Dura, D. (1972). Single needle dialysis. *J. Extracorp. Technol.*, **4**, 41
7. Mansell, M. A. and Wing, A. J. (1976). Long term experience of home dialysis with sorbent regeneration of dialysate. *Proc. Eur. Dial. Transp. Assoc.*, **13**, 275

DISCUSSION

A. C. Kennedy (Glasgow): I would agree with both the previous speakers in their analysis of why we have fallen down the league table in respect of the number of patients treated. Over-dependence on home dialysis may well be a factor and we do not have enough centres. It is not that we do not work hard enough.

There is, I believe, a further factor. To a certain extent we operate under career restraints. Those who are in charge of dialysis units were themselves trained as physicians and nephrologists, and we lack the facility to have dialysis centres run by career dialysers who would only do dialysis. It is that kind of a possibility that has allowed, say, Italy to take off in an upward direction and to increase markedly the number of patients on dialysis. I am not advocating that we should do this. I doubt if we could under our career structure and training system, but it is a factor.

Robson: I was delighted to hear Dr Cattell identify a role for the community physician. They certainly need a role and it would be nice to be able to offer them some suggestions.

B. H. B. Robinson (Birmingham): The figure showing the development of new centres is really quite striking – the change in the slope for the UK, which occurred when the Ministry of Health stopped financing directly and left everything to the regions. There was a slowdown then, and there has been total stasis since the reorganization of the Health Service.

It is not just the money. There is a blanket of bureaucracy at the moment.

Cattell: I accept Professor Kennedy's first point. If he means a career dialysis doctor, then there are one or two in Britain who are first class. I am a great believer in the barefoot doctor and we have reached the level of sophistication in dialysis where we could probably run several dialysis centres without the doctor involvement that we have at the moment, and I should like to see this happen.

There has been a restriction on the number of new centres since reorganization. It is difficult to interpret. The original committees set up by the DHSS to plan home dialysis set certain targets. There were to be so many centres per unit of population and home dialysis would serve a hundred-plus patients. Possibly the nephrologists have been slightly 'hoist with their own petard' in that they thought that each centre could handle far more patients than it does.

Robson: But I am sure it was the way to begin. There was no other way. The issue is whether it is the way to go on.

3

Current status of
renal transplantation
D. N. H. Hamilton and J. D. Briggs

3.1 INTRODUCTION

In an ideal transplanter's world any patient on regular dialysis would prefer an offer of a living donor transplant or a well-matched healthy cadaver kidney. In the real world organizational and immunological problems prevent this ideal, and clinical compromise is essential. Even renal physicians, who are unhappy about renal transplantation, are forced by economic and organizational problems to accept transplantation in order to increase the number of patients treated because of limited dialysis capacity. There is also unanimous pressure from the patients themselves to obtain a transplant.

Thus the current status of transplantation is not the result of an overall plan, but is a shifting balance produced by two shortages – of dialysis facilities on the one hand and of donor kidneys on the other.

In discussing the status of transplantation one is thus aware of being controlled by events rather than being in control. The supply of donor kidneys, the results of transplantation and two major areas for improvement of the results will be described.

3.2 LIVING DONORS

A kidney transplanted from a relative is still the best therapy for chronic renal failure, not because of immediate function, nor entirely because of good HLA matching, but because of the success in (co-incidentally) matching non-HLA factors. Taking the figures from the European experience[1], kidney survival at one year is best with a 'full house' sibling transplant (72.5%) but less successful with only one haplotype match or with a parent to child graft (66.2%) or vice versa. Each type of living donor gives concern to the transplant surgeon for the consequences to the donor. Parents may be frail or have vascular disease; siblings may be wage earners or mothers of young children, and the willingness of informed consent from younger donors may be in doubt. It is perhaps for these reasons that in the UK the percentage of living donors is only 12% and transplant units have avoided an aggressive hunt for living donors in a family.

3.3 CADAVERIC DONORS

3.3.1 Supply

The National Organ Matching Scheme works well for distribution and matching of donor kidneys. The supply of kidneys is less than the demand,

and in 1976 the numbers of donors in the UK dropped for the first time and the number of transplants done annually seems stuck at about 300. The rate-limiting step in this supply is not the general public's attitude (all surveys show a general willingness to donate), but a disinclination of the doctors looking after the prospective donor to consider kidney donation. Transplant surgeons themselves cannot be absolved from responsibility for some of these sensitivities and perhaps private discussion and re-assurance may succeed where public remonstration has failed.

Not only are there concerns about the number of kidneys available but also about the quality.

3.3.2 Quality

While the shortage of supply of cadaveric kidneys certainly occasionally forces surgeons to use unsuitable kidneys (e.g. those with vascular or parenchymal damage or anomalies), the idea that 'dead' kidneys are being used (i.e. kidneys with severe irreversible ischaemic damage) is less soundly based. Seventeen per cent or so of cadaveric kidneys in the UK never work[2], and this figure is rising. However these kidneys may not have been killed by ischaemia. They may instead have rejected during the period of acute tubular necrosis and the available evidence, such as the good function of the partner of these 'dead' kidneys, supports this view[3]. Further investigation of this problem is important since, if 'dead' kidneys do exist, it is necessary to improve methods of collection and to use more 'heart-beating' brain-dead donors. It would also be necessary to use tests of kidney viability and to decide among the conflicting claims for these tests[4,5] (such as ATP levels, K/Na ratios, [^{125}I]iodohippuran). On the other hand, if kidneys are being rejected more frequently in the period of acute tubular necrosis, then the investigation must shift to possible changes in the immunological status of the recipient.

3.4 TRANSPLANTATION ROUTINE

The usual procedure for obtaining cadaveric kidneys, tissue typing and transplantation have been standard for some years and have been reviewed elsewhere[6]. Indeed the practice of transplantation has changed little since 1970 and many of the improvements suggested have failed to win a routine place in practice. Dr T. E. Starzl, a pioneer in kidney transplantation, recently observed in a reflective moment that the 'failure of radically new methods to be developed in the last 10 years has relegated progress to the shuffling of details'[7].

3.4.1   Selection and preparation of patients

Dialysis patients going forward for transplantation should be under 50 and reasonably fit. Excluded are those with systemic disease likely to shorten life (malignancy or severe vascular disease) or recur in the transplanted kidney (polyarteritis or oxalosis). Patients with peptic ulcers require prophylactic surgery (though some dispute this) but all agree that chronically infected or polycystic kidneys should be removed prior to transplantation and that the same procedure should be carried out in hypertensive patients. Doubts have been raised whether home dialysis patients, who have excellent survival, should be transplanted but as the majority live in hope of a transplant, it is hard to actively exclude them from this possibility. Priority for transplantation can be given to patients who have problems on dialysis (such as repeated thrombosis of access devices) though successful transplantation fails to reverse dialysis dementia. Though it is tempting to transplant patients in renal failure before any dialysis is required, the results are poor.

As for tissue typing, most units in the UK accept that tissue typing is of value to transplantation and a two-match kidney is the minimum accepted or offered.

3.4.2   Kidney preservation

In spite of considerable research efforts expended on kidney preservation, both in variants in the type of fluid used to flush the kidney and machines to maintain viability of the kidney, the majority of renal units find a simple flush with an intracellular type solution (e.g. Perfudex) is sufficient, though recently the European Cooperative Scheme have recommended Collins solution. Few units use perfusion machines as the original claims of improved kidney function and ability to be able to discriminate damaged kidneys as a result of using such machines have met a sceptical response. While it is true that the use of the preservation machine can allow transplant surgery to be carried out at leisure during office hours, most units still find it suitable to transplant within 12 hours of donation. Perfusion machines also require trained supervision, though the latest Gambro machine has many simplifications.

There are many variables involved in transplantation, making the effects of various perfusion fluids or machine preservation difficult to assess.

3.5 IMMUNOSUPPRESSION

The original, empirically derived, combination of steroids and azathioprine has been the routine therapy for 20 years. Experience with cyclo-
phosphamide as an alternative has been disappointing and it is not now
recommended[7]. There have been enthusiastic reports on the immunosuppressive properties of unsaturated fatty acids and carragenan, but full
reports are awaited. Though anti-lymphocyte globulin (ALG) is a potent
immunosuppressive agent in experimental animals its value in human
renal transplantation has been controversial with only some centres report-
ing success. The method of preparation, the dosage and timing may
be crucial. The problem of establishing that any ALG batch is indeed
immunosuppressive in human patients is formidable, though if it gives
depression of lymphocyte function or prolongation of monkey allografts,
then the ALG may be judged to be effective.

3.6 TREATMENT OF REJECTION

Increased steroid dosage is always employed but local radiation to the
kidney has been shown to be valueless in the management of rejection[8].
Much effort has been expended to devise tests which anticipate rejection,
but though the value of some in the early detection of rejection has been
established the work load required in any centre to test the whole group of
recently transplanted patients each day is formidable. There also remains a
suspicion that early detection of rejection may not change the outcome of
a rejection episode. Direct evidence on this point would be useful.

3.7 ROLE OF TISSUE TYPING

Cooperative kidney sharing schemes like the National Organ Matching
Service (NOMS) and Eurotransplant have, as their *raison d'être*, the
assumption that successful matching improves the results of transplantation. The results, though, are still controversial, and large series in America
and the collected data for Europe (Figure 3.1) show little or no benefit of
tissue typing. Paradoxically the results from smaller cooperative groups or
from individual centres (who often form part of the bigger series) show a
marked benefit of tissue typing (Figure 3.2). Thus the literature on the role
of tissue typing in first cadaveric transplants is confusing, but the explanation may lie in the obfuscation produced by pooling data from many
centres and the variation introduced in other factors influencing the outcome. It may therefore be that the results from individual centres represent
the truth of the matter.

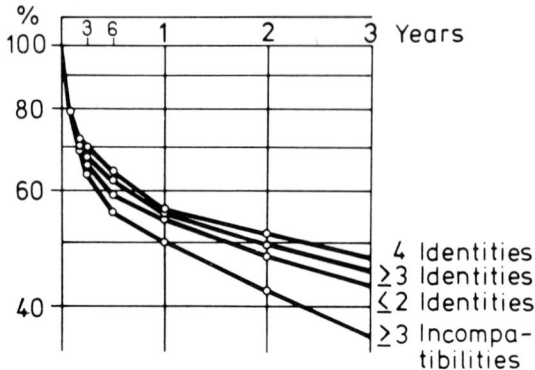

Figure 3.1   Effect of tissue typing on first cadaver kidney transplant results in collected figures from European Dialysis and Transplant Association 1975[1]

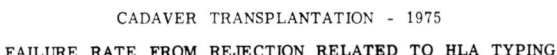

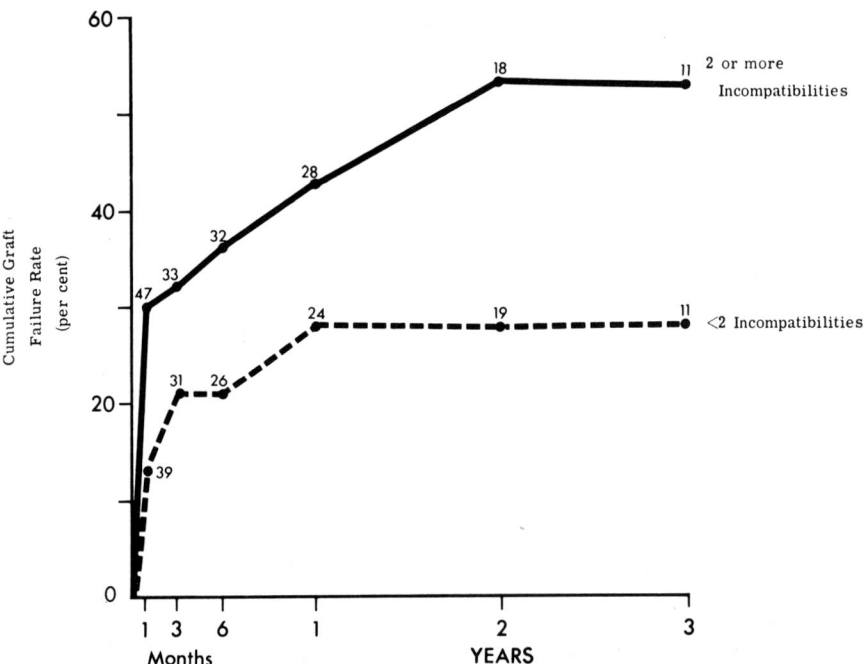

Figure 3.2   Effect of tissue typing on first cadaver transplant results in Glasgow (unpublished). In both this and the EDTA series two or more incompatibilities are compared with less than two

One well established finding from all studies is that in second cadaveric transplants tissue typing is a major determining factor, and as good a match as possible is desirable for these second transplants.

3.8 RESULTS BY YEAR OF TRANSPLANTATION

Though continuous improvement in many of the factors influencing transplantation has been made, this has not been reflected in the results. Indeed there has been a suspicion that some additional factor has been changing to hold back progress. In our unit we are concerned that kidney transplants are being rejected more vigorously than before. Though the results of large cooperative groups tend to obscure such changes, nevertheless the figures from the Kidney Transplant Registry in the USA also show a slight decline in survival rate. Both these figures are shown in Table 3.1. The trend in Glasgow is rather depressing but analysis shows that factors such as technical failure, poorer tissue typing or alterations in policy for recipient selection cannot be blamed. An increased immunological attack on the allografted kidney seems likely, and we have looked at two possible explanations, namely the effects of blood transfusion and the role of endogenous cell-mediated immunity.

TABLE 3.1   Percentage kidney survival at one year, by year of operation, of first kidney allografts in Glasgow and from the USA Kidney Transplant Register[9]

	USA	Glasgow
1969	53.7 ± 1.7	75
1971	53.0 ± 1.2	60
1973	49.5 ± 1.1	46
1975	NA	44

These two new factors give hope for progress and the hints came not from laboratory, but from clinical observations. The first was the effect of prior blood transfusion on the transplant results and the second from investigations of the endogenous cell-mediated immunity (CMI) on patients receiving regular dialysis treatment.

3.8.1   Effect of blood transfusion

It was an early finding that blood transfusion could prolong allograft survival in dogs[10] and rabbits[11]. Dosseter[12] had made a similar claim for human allografts. However, it was not until Terasaki[13] called attention to

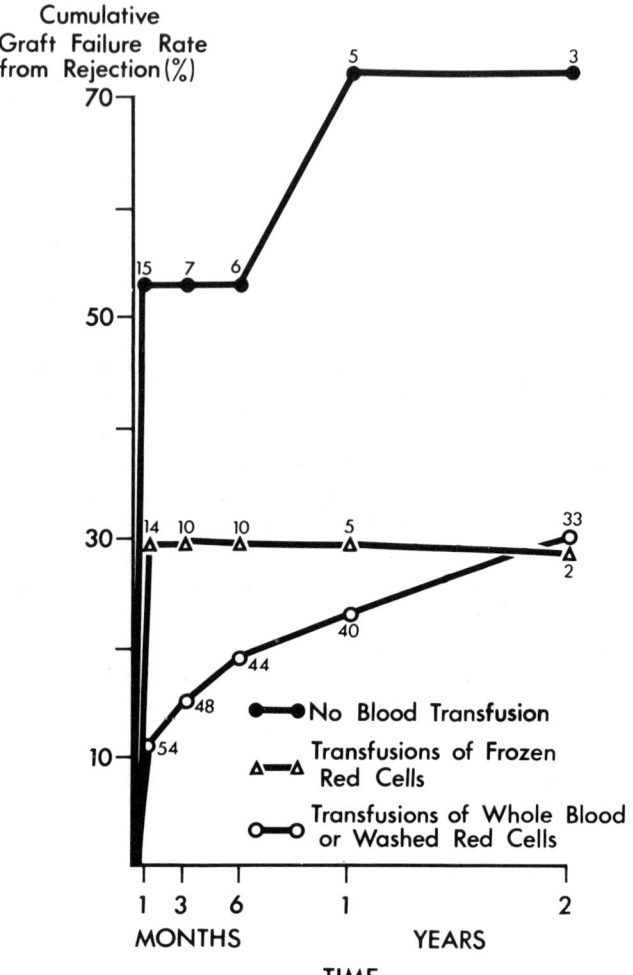

Figure 3.3   Effect of previous blood transfusion (whole or leukocyte poor) on the results of cadaveric transplantation in Glasgow (unpublished)

better kidney transplant results in transfused RDT patients that the matter was taken seriously. This finding has been confirmed in a number of studies from individual centres (Figure 3.3), though the pooled European data showed no benefit of prior blood tranfusion.

These findings do make some immunological sense since a unit of whole blood contains leukocytes bearing HLA antigens which can and do raise cytotoxic antibodies in normal and to a lesser extent in RDT patients. To explain *prolongation* of an allograft it is postulated that in some patients transfusion produces enhancing antibodies or tolerance (possibly 'low zone' in type). The suggestion however that blood transfusion *causes* prolongation of graft survival is subject to the following criticisms:

(1) Blood transfusions are not given randomly to RDT patients but for good reasons (e.g. elective surgery, gastro-intestinal bleeding or because of anaemia due to previous bilateral nephrectomy). Hence the transfused and non-transfused groups are not similar and may thus have different results after kidney transplantation.

(2) The data shows that even one small transfusion[14] is related to a better result, which would be difficult, though not impossible, to explain immunologically.

3.8.2   Immune depression and transplant results

The marked depression of CMI in RDT patients was an early finding[15] and possibly explains the unexpectedly good results in the early days of transplantation. However the outcome of kidney transplantation in indi-

TABLE 3.2   Table showing 6 month survival of first cadaver allografts according to DNCB skin reactivity prior to transplantation. Results from Johns Hopkins[16] and Glasgow (unpublished). Initial sensitization was with 2000 μg of DNCB and testing was with 200 μg

	Hopkins	Glasgow
DNCB negative	85% ($\hat{N}=45$)	84%
DNCB positive	56% ($\hat{N}=10$)	33%

vidual patients in relation to their CMI levels has not been analysed until recently (Table 3.2). Using skin testing with dinitrochlorobenzene (DNCB) as a test of cell-mediated immunity, these two studies show that RDT patients with no reaction to DNCB had a 6 months kidney allograft survival of about 80% while those with any degree of response had only a 30% kidney survival. These studies therefore shift attention away from the donated kidney and tissue typing to the host factors in allograft survival. It also shows that the CMI of RDT patients may vary and emphasizes that little is known of the biochemical or other changes in RDT patients which depress CMI though some experimental studies suggest the suppressor cells are responsible[17].

These studies also suggest that some patients may paradoxically be too fit and hence unsuitable for transplantation.

These findings on CMI levels in RDT patients and the effects of blood transfusion may offer an explanation of any recent worsening of the results of transplantation, since it may be that CMI levels in RDT patients have been rising in recent years, or that the policy of reducing whole blood transfusion during RDT has prejudiced the chance of kidney survival. Both factors do not exclude the other as an explanation and blood transfusion into anergic RDT patients may produce markedly different immunological changes compared with normal human patients.

3.9 REHABILITATION

The assessment of the results of transplantation by mortality and morbidity gives only part of the answer to the value of transplantation.

The results of transplantation are variable. Some patients have an excellent clinical result with a near normal quality of life, but some despite an excellent functioning kidney have a serious chronic disability such as repeated affliction with bone disease. Some patients, who have rejected a kidney, return to dialysis as if nothing had happened but there are those whose health and spirits are broken by the loss of the kidney and the therapies necessary to try to save it. Any attempt to assess the contribution made by transplantation in the management of patients with chronic renal failure must weigh up all clinical factors and also attempt to measure the 'quality' of life. So far assessment of results has been primitive and mainly confined to simple assessment of working capacity. As expected, of the patients covered by the EDTA Survey[1], 85% of the living-donor transplant patients were at full-time work and 76% of the cadaver donor patients were also working full-time; the corresponding figures for home and hospital dialysis were 73% and 37%. A more systematic evaluation of the 'quality' of life would be of help in attempting to assess objectively the contribution of transplantation. A successful kidney transplant is a therapeutic triumph, restoring physical and mental vigour, restoring sexual potency and function and liberating patients from the constraints of their dialysis life. Tables of graft and patient survival do not tell the whole story.

ACKNOWLEDGEMENTS

We are indebted to the Editors of the *Proceedings of the European Dialysis and Transplant Association* for permission to reproduce Figure 3.1.

References

1. Parsons, F. M., Brunner, F. P., Burk, H. C., Graser, W., Gurland, H. J., Harlen, H., Schärer, K. and Spies, G. W. (1975). Statistical Report. *Proc. Eur. Dial. Transpl. Assoc.*, **11**, 3
2. British Transplantation Society Report (1975). *Br. Med. J.*, **1**, 251
3. Hamilton, D. N. H. and Briggs, J. D. (1975). Kidneys for transplantation. *Lancet*, **ii**, 461
4. Williams, G., Peet, T. N. D. and Hamshere, R. J. (1976). Assessment of a test of renal viability. *Br. Med. J.*, **ii**, 75
5. Sells, R. A., Mcloughlin, R. A. and Tyrrell, I. (1974). Renal cortical cation composition as an index of human kidney graft viability. *Br. J. Surg.*, **61**, 326
6. Briggs, J. D. and Hamilton, D. N. H. (1976). Transplantation in Scotland. *Hlth. Bull.*, **34**, 190
7. Starzl, T. E., Weil, R. and Putnam, C. W. (1977). Modern trends in kidney transplantation. *Transpl. Proc.*, **9**, 1
8. Godfrey, A. M. and Salaman, J. R. (1976). Radiotherapy in treatment of acute rejection of human renal allografts. *Lancet*, **i**, 938
9. 13th Report of Human Renal Transplant Registry (1977). *Transpl. Proc.*, **9**, 9
10. Halasz, N. A. (1963). Enhancement of skin homografts in dogs. *J. Surg. Res.*, **3**, 503
11. Billingham, R. E. and Sparrow, E. M. (1955). The effects of the prior intra-venous injections of dissociated epidermal cells and blood on the survival of skin homografts in rabbits. *J. Embryol. Exp. Morph.*, **3**, 265
12. Dosseter, J. B., Mackinnon, K. R., Gault, M. H. and Maclean, L.D. (1967). Cadaver kidney transplants. *Transplantation*, **5**, 844
13. Opelz, G. and Terasaki, P. I. (1974). Poor kidney-transplant survival in recipients with frozen-blood transfusions or no transfusions. *Lancet*, **ii**, 696
14. Van Es, A. A., Marquet, R. L., Van Rood, J. J., Kalff, M. W. and Balner, H. Blood transfusions induce prolonged kidney allograft survival in Rhesus monkeys. *Lancet*, **i**, 506
15. Dammin, J. (1956). Prolongation of skin graft survival in uremia. *Ann. N.Y. Acad. Sci.*, **64**, 967
16. Rolley, R. T., Sterioff, S., Parks, L. C. and Williams, G. M. (1977). Delayed cutaneous hypersensitivity and human renal allotransplantation. *Transpl. Proc.*, **9**, 81
17. Johnston, M. F. M. and Slavin, R. G. (1976). Mechanism of inhibition of adoptive transfer of tuberulin sensitivity in acute uremia. *J. Lab. Clin. Med.*, **87**, 457

DISCUSSION

F. M. Parsons (Leeds): Are the effects of blood transfusion an artefact? May I expand on that?

A patient who has not been transfused has not been challenged with foreign protein. If a patient is transfused there is an immunological challenge. Are we perhaps picking up that challenge in the form of circulating antibodies and discarding such patients from transplantation? In other words, are we selecting in such a way that the so-called 'weak responders' are transplanted? Has this anything to do with it?

Hamilton: I do not know whether originally we distinguished between responders and non-responders. But now, looking at the whole group of transfused patients, including those who may have had some cytotoxic antibodies, if they are transplanted after careful cross-matching they do better as well.

The responder/non-responder idea seems to have faded a little. What might be interesting is to try to relate the response to blood transfusion with the skin testing results. The anergic patients are unlikely to respond with cytotoxic antibody, but they may make another kind of antibody. The whole problem keeps coming back to the immunological state of the dialysis patients and their response to blood transfusion.

Robson: Mr Hamilton's results are quite remarkable, and very like six or seven others in the literature. I have heard it asked whether it is ethical to conduct controlled trials of the effect of blood transfusion. There have now been six reports, all pointing in the same direction.

Hamilton: I do think that it is ethical. This is the last chance to do a controlled trial − just at this point. There are so many artefacts possible, especially the selection of patients, that we must do it.

Wallace (Glasgow): We should remember that the main reason for introducing frozen red cells into the dialysis and transplant units was to reduce the risk of hepatitis. We have had a warning (today) that the hepatitis may be lurking just around the corner. We sometimes place too much emphasis on hepatitis B and we forget that there are other infective agents, such as cytomegalovirus, and that there are good reasons for continuing to use frozen blood cells to reduce the dangers of infection. I doubt whether we have enough evidence to discontinue their use. I am in favour of multi-centre trials.

Hamilton: I take the point. CMV virus is not thought to be the major cause of morbidity considering the number of transplant patients that are infected with it, although I am not minimizing it.

Robson: A controlled trial cannot be carried out with frozen red blood cells because they do not have the immunological effect.

Hamilton: It is the white cells, of course, that may give the effect.

R. Gabriel (London): On the frozen blood story, could I ask whether it is the patient's own blood that is being taken and put under nitrogen, or anybody's blood, and with or without white cell separation.

Hamilton: It is certainly not the patient's own blood. It is donated blood and the white cells are separated physically.

Wallace: The best method of producing so-called leukocyte-poor and platelet-poor blood is to use red cells recovered from frozen banks. One must never use the term 'leukocyte-free' or 'platelet-free'. It is leukocyte-poor and platelet-poor so that there is still the possibility of immunization to HLA antigens or other antigens which may be more important than HLA within the nature of the histopathological complex.

Robson: It is surely true that where frozen red cells are used for transfusion there is apparently no immunological advantage over those patients given no blood. There have been several reports pointing in that direction. If a controlled trial is to take place it has to be with blood, not frozen.

It is rather ironic that as time has passed and we have reduced the reasons for not putting people on dialysis, e.g. systemic disease, or multiple myeloma, we are forcing ourselves into a much more difficult moral position. Ten years ago it was a great relief to find a patient with chronic renal failure who could not be transplanted because of a myeloma, or a little bit of lupus, or some other reason for not doing it. Now that this is being removed, the ethical dilemma becomes much worse in relation to the shortage.

Parsons: I have a further comment to Dr Cattell.

Having been in the European Registry, I have some inside information. One of the reasons why the UK is falling behind its neighbours is — regrettably — the gross national product. If the number of patients per million of population is plotted against the gross national product of any country, then the UK is slap on the line. In other words, we are living up to our income, as it were. If we want to get across the need for more money for patient care — may I be political? we must get it across to the miners that it is no good their asking for £135 per week. We need more money in the Health Service. How are we to do that?

Robson: I am sure that is so, but it seems extraordinary. The UK is among the industrial nations on superficial social assessments, and yet dialysis-wise it ranks with Greece, Portugal, and the unindustrialized nations.

Parsons: Which is correct on a comparison with the gross national product. I do not believe that we in the UK appreciate that we are so poor!

W. R. Cattell (London): This is from an analysis which correlates GNP per head of population. What Parsons says is correct. A slope showing many of the so-called industrialized nations on it has the UK way along the line. However, it is not fair to say that any of the so-called industrialized nations are allocating out of their GNP an appropriate amount for replacement therapy. I have only seen the slide once, but I believe that Israel is way off the line, spending far more per million population than it ought to do along the line made up by the other poorer nations. Is that correct?

Parsons: No, it is not. Israel is a special case. It so happens that during the past 2 years expansion of the number of dialysis centres has been phenomenal, hence the new intake has been phenomenal as well. A fall-off can be expected in future years.

Robson: And that is a sad state of affairs.

SECTION TWO

Economics and Limited Care
Chairman:
Sally Taber

4

The economics of treating chronic renal failure
D. M. Parkin

4.1   INTRODUCTION

Effective treatment for chronic renal failure became a reality in the early sixties with the development of intermittent haemodialysis and renal transplantation. By 1975, it was apparent that there were considerable international differences in the proportion of potential patients who received treatment. It seems likely then that there are constraints which limit the development of treatment programmes, one of which is certainly the level of finance available. This paper will consider some of the economic aspects of treating chronic renal failure.

4.2   SIZE OF THE PROBLEM

The potential number of patients requiring treatment must be estimated from epidemiological surveys of renal failure. There have been several in the UK[1-3], the most recent of which in Scotland suggested that about 96 patients per million total population under the age of 65 die annually from chronic renal failure. Of this number 52 per million have no intercurrent disease which would tend to contraindicate treatment. Under the age of 55 corresponding numbers are 63 per million total, and 38 per million 'suitable' for treatment.

In the UK in 1975 the number of new patients commencing treatment was about 14.5 per million population, which is a much lower proportion than in any other EEC country (except Ireland)[4]. Figure 4.1 shows the number of patients actually receiving treatment (prevalence) in the years 1972 to 1975, and, with the current annual mortality rate of 11%, the numbers who will be receiving treatment in each of the next 5 years with differing assumptions of 'intake'. The lower line represents 14.5 new patients per million population, the central line the numbers expected if the population of patients commencing treatment continues to increase at the rate experienced since 1972, and the upper line the number on treatment if intake is increased to 38 per million per year (a level already exceeded in North America, Japan and Israel).

Kerr in 1967[5] was the first to examine the economic implications of offering treatment to this number of new patients. He assumed 2300 new patients under 55 per year, and a 10% annual mortality on dialysis. With fairly modest estimates of the costs of running a hospital dialysis unit he came to the conclusion that annual expenditure would rise to £17$\frac{1}{2}$ million after only five years. Changes in survival on therapy, and the development of home dialysis and transplantation as alternatives to hospital care, render the conclusions of the analysis less valid today. Nevertheless it elegantly

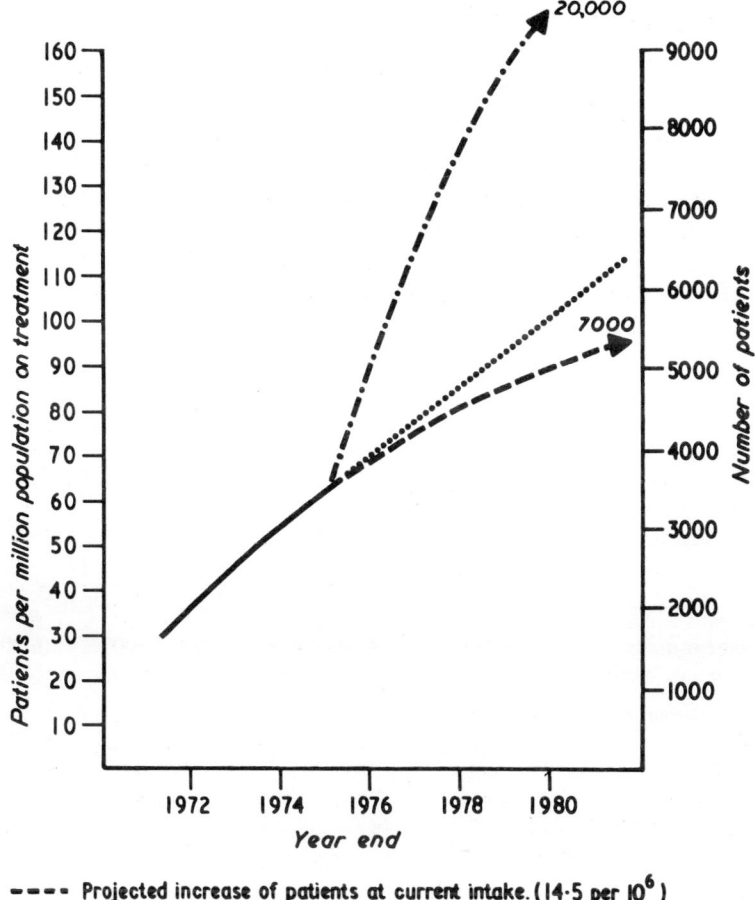

Figure 4.1   Actual and projected numbers treated (dialysis and transplant) UK, final equilibrium at 7000 and 20 000 respectively

demonstrated the principle that the development of effective therapy for a chronic disorder leads to a rapid increase in prevalent cases requiring treatment, until new cases (represented by the incidence rate) are balanced by deaths, or transfers to other forms of treatment (transplants). A complex model illustrating the full development of this principle has been developed by Farrow et al.[6].

4.3 COST OF TREATMENT

A study of the economics of managing renal failure requires that some costs are put upon different modalities of treatment. Chronic intermittent haemodialysis was developed as a hospital technique and there have been attempts to estimate the costs of treating patients in hospital. There are great difficulties in doing so, not least because of problems of apportioning capital costs (machines, buildings) on a 'per patient per year' basis. For what they are worth figures from different centres are shown in Table 4.1, together with estimates of running costs (excluding capital equipment) for the UK.

TABLE 4.1 Costs of hospital dialysis

Author	Year of estimate	Place	Annual cost (1975 £ equivalent)	
A: Annual total cost per patient				
Klarman et al.[7]	1968	USA	$14 000	(11 000)
Pearson et al.[8]	1972	USA	$14–25 000	(9–16 500)
Douglas[9]	1972	USA	$20–30 000	(13–20 000)
Schippers and Kalff[10]	1973	Netherlands	$26 000	(16 000)
Stewart et al.[11]	1973	Australia	$A 7 400	(6 000)
Buxton and West[12]	1972	UK	£5 600	(8 800)
B: UK Annual revenue costs only				
Kerr[5]	1967		£1 470	($3 175)
DHSS[13]	1970		£2 000	($3 710)
Farrow et al.[6]	1971		£2 500	($4 200)
Buxton and West[12]	1972		£3 900	($6 100)

Treatment at home is undoubtedly less expensive than treatment in hospital, in addition to having other advantages. Costs are easier to estimate than those of hospital care, since a price for equipment and home adaptation is relatively easy to obtain. The only problem is in apportioning part of the cost of the 'back up' hospital unit to each home dialysis patient, since all patients require initial training in a hospital unit, and some will require subsequent readmission for complications. Some estimates of capital costs and maintenance are shown in Table 4.2. Approximate present costs in Leeds are £4000 for equipment (machine, monitor, dialyser) £1500 for home adaptations and an annual running cost of £2250 per patient per year.

Obtaining the cost of a renal transplant is even more of a problem, and since there are no units which are devoted entirely to this activity, separat-

TABLE 4.2 Costs of home dialysis

Author	Year of estimate	Place	Capital cost*†	Maintenance*
Klarman et al.[7]	1968	USA	—	$5 000 (4 000)
Pearson et al.[8]	1972	USA	—	$5 600 (3 700)
Rae et al.[14]	1972	Canada	$8 750 (5 700)	$5 854 (3 800)
Douglas[9]	1973	USA	—	$4–6 000 (2 500–4 000)
Stewart et al.[11]	1973	Australia	$A6 000 (4 800)	$A2 600 (2 100)
Hull[15]	1975	USA	—	$15 600 (7 600)
Kerr[5]	1967	UK	£3 500 (7 600)	£1 150 (2 500)
DHSS[13]	1970	UK	—	£1 500 (2 800)
Farrow et al.[6]	1971	UK	—	£1 000 (1 700)
Robinson[16]	1971	UK	£2 450 (3 600)	£1 300 (1 900)
Buxton and West[12]	1972	UK	£3 800 (5 900)	£2 700 (4 200)
Ogg[17]	1973	UK	£3 000 (4 400)	£2 000 (2 900)

* 1975 sterling equivalent in brackets.
† Includes equipment, home adaptation and 'training'.

TABLE 4.3 Costs of a renal transplant

Author	Year of estimate	Place	Cost of operation	Cost of follow-up
Klarman et al.[7]	1968	USA	$13 000 (10 000)	—
Kountz[18]	1969	USA	$10 000 (7 500)	—
Douglas[9]	1972	USA	$13–16 000 (8 500–10 500)	—
Schippers and Kalff[10]	1973	Netherlands	$18 000 (11 300)	$3 200 (2 000)
Stewart et al.[11]	1973	Australia	$A8 900 (7 100)	$A800 (700)

Figures in brackets = approx. 1975 sterling equivalent.

ing the cost of a transplant patient from hospital running costs is almost impossible. No one in the UK has ever published a guess. Some figures from other countries are produced in Table 4.3. The actual values by themselves mean little, but comparing them with dialysis costs it can be seen that a transplant operation probably costs less than dialysis for one year in hospital.

4.4   IS IT WORTH IT?

The foregoing discussion has indicated the enormous potential expenditure on treatment for chronic renal failure. The implicit question therefore arises about the proportion of our health service finance that should be spent on such treatment. In a wholly logical world a health service planner would be faced with a series of independent programmes and could choose between them, one element guiding his choice being the return on the money he invests. This is the basis of the cost-benefit approach to medical care. Some weighing of benefit against cost goes on in many fields of medical decision making, and although many doctors reject such a notion as somehow unethical, I believe it is better to be as explicit as possible about the basis of our decisions, rather than relying upon subjective value-judgements.

There have been two attempts at relating costs to benefits in regard to treatment of chronic renal failure. The first of these by Longmore and Rehahn (1975)[19] involved some curious assumptions and calculations. These authors markedly underestimated costs of treatment, assumed that all patients treated return to full-time employment, made no allowance for mortality of treated patients, and did not 'discount' the value of a patient's future earning to their present value[20,21]. A more satisfactory analysis was performed by Buxton and West (1975)[12]. I will not discuss their methods in detail, but merely present here some of their assumptions and conclusions. They examined a theoretical cohort of 1000 patients commencing therapy by dialysis, either in hospital, or at home, and utilized mortality rates and rehabilitation rates provided by EDTA for 1972. The costs of treatment at 1972 prices were estimated for hospital as £5600 per year per patient, and for a home dialysis patient £3390 per annum with an initial cost of £1300. Benefit to society was assessed in terms of average earnings for males and females respectively, in the proportion of patients able to work. The use of those earnings which would have been lost as a result of premature death as a means of assessing benefit to society has been challenged[22], but although unsatisfactory in many ways, this is a perfectly reasonable way of estimating what are termed 'indirect benefits' of a programme[23]. Buxton and West do however fail to consider the 'direct benefits' of treating patients – that is the immediate, tangible savings to the health service. In this case these savings would be the excess cost of caring for 1000 patients dying of renal failure at present as compared with their terminal care as they die, on treatment, over the ensuing 20 years under consideration.

At the time of their analysis the conclusions reached were that the 1972 value of benefit of treating 1000 patients was about £3.6 million for hospital dialysis, and £6.3 million for home dialysis (the latter figure is higher because of better survival/rehabilitation on home dialysis, this of course reflecting selection criteria for home dialysis training). The 1972 cost of maintaining the same cohort on treatment for 20 years was £23 million for hospital dialysis, and £20 million for home dialysis. This yields cost-benefit ratios of 6.4 : 1 for hospital care, and 3.2 : 1 for home care.

As already discussed Buxton and West exclude consideration of 'direct' benefits. Percentage survival and rehabilitation have also increased since 1972 (see EDTA 1975 data[4]), and improvements in hardware and techniques have probably resulted in a relative lowering of costs. These factors will all lower the cost-benefit ratio. In addition, as the authors admit, no mention is made of renal transplantation as a possible 'cheap' option in treatment. Nevertheless, I believe that the conclusion that there is no positive economic return from the treatment of renal failure is valid.

Society is in fact tacitly agreeing to pay for 'intangible benefits'[23], that is the avoidance of pain, discomfort, grief and the premature loss of human life. These are exceedingly hard to measure in financial terms, and though economists may attempt it, the medical profession is on the whole averse to doing so. I believe it is this that makes cost-benefit so difficult to apply in the health field.

4.5 VALUE FOR MONEY

Assuming that treating patients with renal failure is not a financially rewarding exercise, but that society is prepared to do so for the sake of the intangible benefits, the next question is how to get 'the best value for money'. Here we are concerned with cost-effectiveness of treatments and procedures: what is the most economical way of achieving a given outcome? This type of analysis is much easier than cost-benefit, since benefits do not need to be costed in financial terms. In its simplest form we can examine the cost of one life-year saved by different forms of treatment. Pioneering work by Klarman et al. (1968)[7] took this approach, in comparing haemodialysis with transplantation. The authors in addition allowed for the putatively superior quality of life after transplantation, valuing such

TABLE 4.4   Present value of expenditure and life-years gained per member of cohort embarking on transplantation and in-centre and home dialysis

Modality	Present value of expenditure	Life-years gained	Cost per life-year
Dialysis			
Hospital	$104 000	9	$11 600
Home	$38 000	9	$4 200
50–50 programme	$71 000	9	$7 900
Transplantation			
Unadjusted	$44 500	17	$2 600
Adjusted for quality	$44 500	20.5	$2 200

Note: Cost of transplantation incorporates $24 500 for dialysis based on a 50–50 distribution of patients between hospital and home.

(After Klarman *et al.* 1968[7])

a life-year 25% more highly than one on haemodialysis. The results are demonstrated in Table 4.4. This work is now almost 10 years old, and it is perhaps not surprising that many of the assumptions it contains require revision, in particular the projected results for transplantation appear optimistic both in terms of graft and patient survival, and the 'life-years gained' figure is certainly too high. Nevertheless, others have reached the same conclusions about the relative expense of dialysis and transplantation, for example DHEW in the USA estimates a life-year costs $6300 on dialysis, and $3500 after transplantation (cited in Douglas 1973[9]).

4.6   CONCLUSIONS FROM COST DATA

The most economical method of treating renal failure appears then to be by transplantation. This has a high (and difficult to estimate) initial cost of operation and post-operative care, as well as an initial outlay on dialysis whilst awaiting a suitable organ. After operation, costs are relatively small (drugs and out-patient attendances), but mortality is quite high, 40% at 3 years; in addition the majority of grafts will fail in the same period (Figure 4.2)[4], so that many of the surviving patients will require a return to dialysis care. Even allowing for this, however, cost per life-year is lowest for this form of treatment, as well as offering the most satisfactory quality of life.

All workers agree that home dialysis is cheaper per patient-year than hospital dialysis. There are however considerable differences in the relative costs depending upon what is counted under each heading, and the proportion of a hospital unit costs which are allotted to 'necessary support' for a home dialysis programme. Survival in hospital (65% at 3 years) is poorer than that at home (81% at 3 years), although this of course largely reflects selection of patients; survival rates on home dialysis can only be calculated

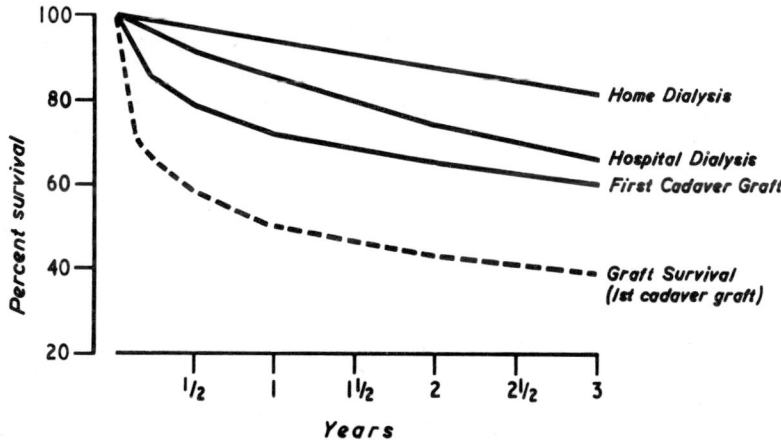

Figure 4.2   Cumulative patient survival. Europe 1975
(After Gurland *et al.*[4])

after the patients have already been treated in hospital, cases who are 'poor risks' will either die in this period, or continue in hospital care (Figure 4.2). Likewise the degree of rehabilitation achieved by patients is better for home dialysis than hospital care, and is almost as good as that of trans-

TABLE 4.5   Rehabilitation and mode of treatment
Europe 1975[4]

Mode of treatment	Total patients	Working full-time (%)	Working part-time (%)	Able to work, not doing so (%)	Unable to work (%)
Hospital dialysis	15 489	33.8	24.8	20.9	20.4
Home dialysis	3 827	64.1	15.7	14.0	6.2
Transplant	4 083	67.7	12.0	13.2	7.1

plant patients (Table 4.5). One of the many reasons for the better rehabilitation of patients treated by home dialysis is probably because the timing of treatment can be individually adjusted to be outside normal working hours.

4.7   THE BALANCE OF TREATMENT METHODS

The discussion so far has looked at the economic implications of different forms of treatment as if these were independent. Of course this is not so, and in practice it is necessary to adopt a mixture of different methods. Hospital dialysis is an expensive procedure, and by itself could not support a treatment programme of any size without an enormous increase in facilities. In practice patients are removed from the hospital dialysis pool by transplantation, by transfer to home dialysis, or to some form of limited care. Farrow et al.[6] constructed a model of a treatment programme for renal failure involving dialysis (hospital and home) and transplantation, and were able to study the theoretical effects of varying the proportions receiving different treatments.

Although their costing data is rather inadequate, they used their model to look at the economic implications of different treatment programmes[24]. Reliance on dialysis (home and hospital) alone produces an expensive programme, with good survival figures. The addition of transplantation leads to poorer overall survival, but there are advantages in terms of lower costs, and increased numbers of patients who can be treated with fixed facilities.

4.8   INTERNATIONAL COMPARISONS

It is instructive to look at the treatment of renal failure in different countries, and how the different methods of financing treatment has led to differing balances in the use of resources. The UK is now (1975) 17th in an international league table comparing patients on treatment per million population, behind all the EEC countries, Scandinavia, the USA and Japan[4]. It is impossible to say exactly what this means in terms of total national resources devoted to treating renal failure without knowledge of incidence rates, but there is a suggestion of a rough correlation between a nation's wealth and the amount spent on renal disease (Figure 4.3).

The UK had 53 centres offering dialysis in 1975, a ratio of 0.9 per million population, much lower than any other Western nation. This policy of restricting the number of dialysis places in hospital has undoubtedly been responsible for the UK having the largest proportion of dialysis patients on home treatment (65.8% of all dialysis patients in 1975). The more abundant hospital facilities elsewhere mean that a smaller proportion of patients have been trained for home dialysis, despite the undoubted economic benefits of doing so. An additional effect of restricting hospital facilities has been to increase the proportion of renal failure patients treated

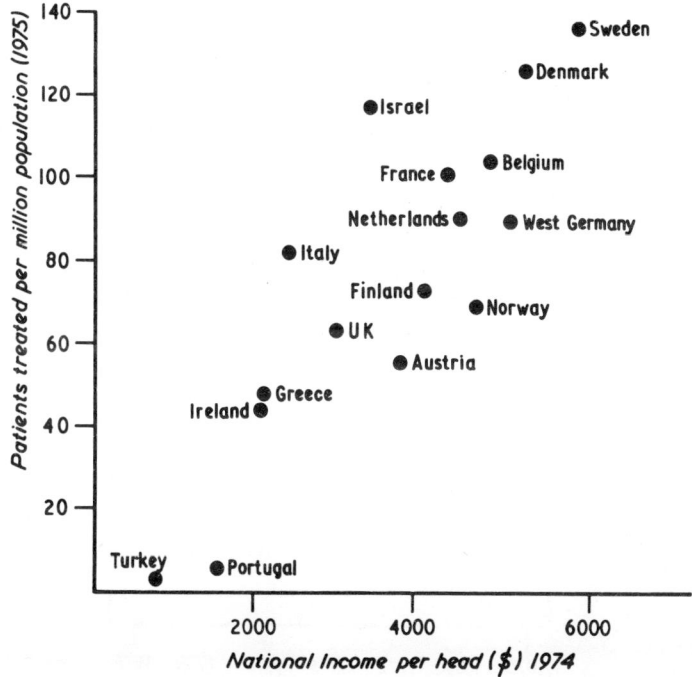

Figure 4.3   Treatment for renal failure in relation to national income

by transplantation. The UK is the only European country to demonstrate this cost-effective trend between 1971 and 1976[25].

The influence of finance on treatment patterns can be seen from recent US experience (Figure 4.4). In 1973 the Federal Government began to finance dialysis and transplantation via Medicare. Prior to this the financial advantages of home dialysis had been evident in the increasing proportion of patients using this modality. Since 1973 a patient attempting home dialysis is faced with expenses which are not covered under Medicare, but which would be covered if he was an out-patient at a facility[26]. The result has been a fall in the proportion of home dialysers and an increasing proportion using 'limited care' facilities. The economics of 'limited care' are considered later, but according to Jenkins et al. [27], the result of this change is an increased cost of treatment, the burden of which falls upon federal tax-payers.

The economic advantages of transplantation as a form of therapy have already been described; the limitations upon this form of treatment seem to be the supply of suitable donors' organs. In Australia early formulations of

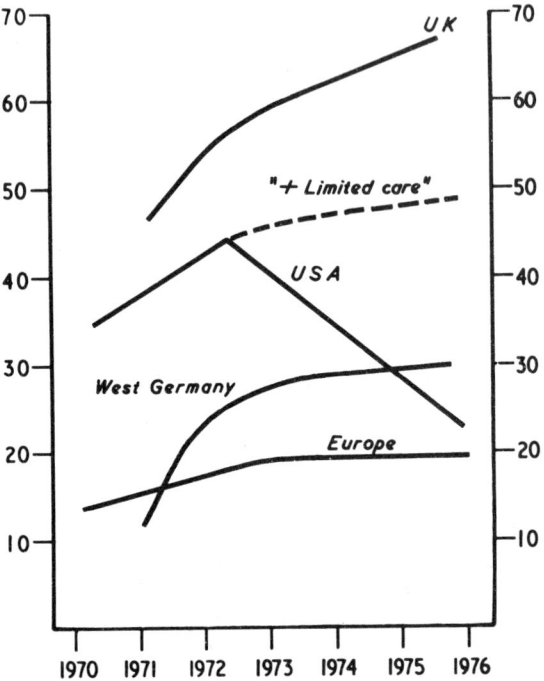

Figure 4.4   Proportion of patients on dialysis treated at home (1975)
(After Gurland et al.[4])

policy for treating renal failure sought to use a combination of hospital
dialysis with early transplantation[28], both of which were government
financed, in contrast to home dialysis, which was not. Stewart et al.[11] have
shown the medical and economic implications of this 'early transplant'
policy as opposed to home dialysis with elective transplantation. Interestingly this produces similar conclusions to those reached by Farrow et al.[24]
with their theoretical model, i.e. hospital plus early transplant leads to
poorer survival, but the cost per surviving patient is considerably less than
the home dialysis/elective transplant model.

4.9   THE ECONOMICS OF LIMITED CARE

Limited-care dialysis involves the patient attending a 'facility' as an out-
patient, and in the USA these facilities have developed as 'Satellite Centers'
outwith hospitals[29,30]. Reduced expenses on buildings and staffing means
that such centres are considerably cheaper to operate than hospital units.

They have an advantage over self-dialysis at home in that capital costs, including equipment, are shared by more than one patient and that death or successful transplantation do not mean relocation. However, staffing and travel costs generally make it more expensive than home treatment in the long term. Bilinsky et al.[31] estimate costs per dialysis as $128 hospital, $65–69 in satellites and $46 at home. The proportion of patients dialysing in limited care facilities has shown a remarkable increase in the USA in recent years. As already discussed this has probably developed as a relatively cheap alternative to hospital care in the face of the financial disincentive to home dialysis.

4.10 CONCLUSIONS

From an economic viewpoint, renal transplantation is the most effective method of treating chronic renal failure. However, the number of transplants per year in the UK, just over 6000, accounts for only $\frac{1}{3}$ to $\frac{1}{4}$ of the renal failure patients who require treatment. The number of transplants performed is not increasing[32]. The results of transplantation will probably improve with more effective tissue matching and better immunosuppressive therapy, but currently it is scarcity of donor organs that limits the number of operations. Six years ago Crosby et al.[33], in a retrospective survey of hospital deaths, found a potentially adequate supply of donor kidneys. Efforts to eliminate this constraint on treatment would undoubtedly be worthwhile.

Other than transplantation the only practical long-term solution to treatment lies in dialysis, either at home or in limited care satellites. There is little experience of limited care in the UK, but there is no reason to suppose that they would be more cost-effective than home dialysis for long-term treatment, since lower capital costs per patient would be rapidly overtaken by greater running costs. Limited care units may well be a useful alternative to hospitals for certain patients who are unable to manage themselves at home and also possibly an economical proposition in the short-term management of patients awaiting a transplant.

Cost-benefit study tends to suggest that there is no overall financial gain to society from treating patients with renal failure. This in no way implies that we should not seek to do so, it merely adds a piece of information which assists in the attempt to achieve some rationality in the use of health care resources. It is for health professionals to persuade society to allot as many resources as possible for health care, so that maximum help can be given to sufferers from renal failure, amongst other groups.

ACKNOWLEDGEMENTS

My thanks are due to Dr A. M. Davison, Renal Unit, St. James's Hospital, Leeds, and Dr J. L. Anderton, Medical Renal Clinic, Western General Hospital, Edinburgh, for their helpful comments and criticisms of the draft of this paper. I am indebted to the Editors of the *Proceedings of the European Dialysis and Transplant Association* for permission to reproduce Figures 4.2 and 4.4.

References

1. Branch, R. A., Clark, G. W., Cochrane, A. L., Jones, J. H. and Scarborough, H. (1971). Incidence of uraemia and requirements for maintenance haemodialysis. *Br. Med. J.*, 1, 249
2. McGeown, M. G. (1972). Chronic renal failure in Northern Ireland, 1968–1970. A prospective survey. *Lancet*, ii, 307
3. Pendreigh, D. M., Heasman, M. A., Howitt, L. F., Kennedy, A. C., Macdougall, A. I., Macleod, M., Robson, J. S. and Stewart, W. K. (1972). Survey of chronic renal failure in Scotland. *Lancet*, i, 304
4. Gurland, H. J., Brunner, F. P., Chantler, C., Jacobs, C., Schärer, K., Selwood, N. H., Spies, G. and Wing, A. J. (1976). Combined Report on Regular Dialysis and Transplantation in Europe, VI, 1975. *Transpl. Assoc.*, 13, 3
5. Kerr, D. N. S. (1967). Regular haemodialysis. *Proc. R. Soc. med.*, 60, 1195
6. Farrow, S. C., Fisher, D. J. H. and Johnson, D. B. (1971). Statistical approach to planning an integrated haemodialysis/transplantation programme. *Br. Med. J.*, 2, 671
7. Klarman, H. E., Francis, J. O. and Rosenthal, G. D. (1968). Cost effectiveness analysis applied to the treatment of chronic renal disease. *Med. Care*, 6, 48
8. Pearson, D. A., Stranova, T. J. and Thompson, J. D. (1976). Patient and program costs associated with chronic hemodialysis care. *Inquiry*, 13, 23
9. Douglas, R. A. (1973). The costs of kidney transplantation and hemodialysis. *Transpl. Proc.*, 5, 1043
10. Schippers, H. M. A. and Kalff, M. W. (1976). Cost comparison hemodialysis and renal transplantation. *Tissue Antigens*, 7, 86
11. Stewart, J. H., Topp, N. D., Martin, S., Schawrowas, E., Flaus, Y., Sheil, A. G. R. and Mahony, J. F. (1973). The costs of domiciliary maintenance haemodialysis: a comparison with alternative renal replacemet regimens. *Med. J. Aust.*, 1, 156
12. Buxton, M. J. and West, R. R. (1975). Cost-benefit analysis of long term haemodialysis for chronic renal failure. *Br. Med. J.*, 2, 376
13. Editorial (1970). Demand for machines and organs. *Nature (London)*, 225, 1183
14. Rae, A., Craig, P. and Miles, G. (1972). Home dialysis; its costs and problems. *Can. Med. Assoc. J.*, 106, 1305
15. Hull, A. R. (1976). 1976 concepts of hemodialysis. *Arch. Intern. Med.*, 136, 365

16. Robinson, B. H. B. (1971). Intermittent haemodialysis in the home. *Br. Med. Bull.*, **27**, 173
17. Ogg, C. (1973). Priorities in medicine: society should be better informed. *Br. Med. J.*, **4**, 648
18. Kountz, S. L. (1969). Cited by Pearson *et al.* (reference 8)
19. Longmore, D. B. and Rehahn, M. (1975). The cumulative cost of death. *Lancet*, i, 1023
20. Buxton, M. J. and West, R. R. (1975). The cost of death (letter). *Lancet*, ii, 38
21. Glass, N. (1975). The cumulative cost of death (letter). *Lancet*, i, 1341
22. Roberts, J. A. (1975). Cost-benefit analysis of long-term haemodialysis for chronic renal failure (letter). *Br. Med. J.*, **3**, 230
23. Klarman, H. E. (1974). Application of cost-benefit analysis to health systems technology. *J. Occup. Med.*, **16**, 172
24. Farrow, S. C., Fisher, D. J. and Johnson, D. B. (1972). Dialysis and transplantation: the national picture over the next five years. *Br. Med. J.*, **3**, 686
25. Jacobs, C., Brunner, F. P., Chantler, C., Donckerwolche, R. A., Gurland, H. J., Hathway, R. A., Selwood, N. H. and Wing, A. J. (1977). Combined Report on regular dialysis and transplantation in Europe, VII, 1976. *Proc. Eur. Dial. Transp. Assoc.*, **14**, 3
26. Levine, C. (1976). Home dialysis and the Medicare gap. *Hastings Centre Report*, **6**, 5
27. Jenkins, P. G., Gutmann, F. D. and Rieselbach, R. E. (1976). Self-hemodialysis: the optimal mode of dialytic therapy. *Arch. Intern. Med.*, **136**, 357
28. National Health and Medical Research Council (1968). Report of the ad hoc committee on rationalisation of facilities for organ transplantation and renal dialysis. *Med. J. Aust.*, **2**, 1200
29. Johnson, W. J., Hathaway, D. S., Anderson, C. F. and Carlson, R. A. (1970). Hemodialysis: comparison of treatment in the medical center, community hospital and home. *Arch. Intern. Med.*, **125**, 462
30. Neff, M. S., Baez, A., Slifkin, R. and Schupak, E. (1973). Out-patient dialysis. *Arch. Intern. Med.*, **131**, 717
31. Bilinsky, R. T., Morris, A. J. and Klein, H. R. (1971). Satellite dialysis: an economic approach to the delivery of hemodialysis care. *J. Am. Med. Assoc.*, **218**, 1809
32. Tovey, G. H. (1976). Annual Report 1975–76 of the National Organ Matching Service of the UK.
33. Crosby, D. L., West R. R. and Davies, H. (1971). Availability of cadaveric kidneys for transplantation. *Br. Med. J.*, **4**, 401

DISCUSSION

W. R. Cattell (London): I find it very interesting that Dr Parkin has tried to tackle the question of costs. May I have clarification? When he says it costs so much to provide a transplant, is that the cost of a successful transplant, and what about the costs of the patient with a failed transplant who has to go back on dialysis? Are those costs added to the cost of the successful transplant?

Parkin: The figures I gave included the failures. If there was a transplant unit doing nothing else we could work out the number of life-years we succeed in getting by doing the operation and divide that into the money-costs. Patients whose transplants fail and who need to continue on dialysis have to be taken into account.

Cattell: So that if they fail and go back on dialysis, the money that is spent on that is added to the cost-benefit for the successes.

Parkin: Yes.

J. S. Robson (Edinburgh): The cost-benefit approach is fascinating. Sir Douglas Black has done some work on trying to assess the shape of the National Health Service in terms of life-years saved or lost by various diseases.

However, take mental deficiency, which is an enormous burden on the Health Service. I would not like to say how much it costs, but it can be expressed as 5% of the cost of the Health Service. There are no, or virtually no, life-years lost. On Dr Parkin's analysis, these patients are alive, they have to be equated with the average national income, yet they do not work. The cost-benefit to the nation of the enormous expense of keeping mental defectives alive is a higher ratio, a worse ratio, than dialysis where the patients die and cost nothing after they are dead.

I am rather challenging the validity of relating the benefit in terms of the average working input, or we must begin to compare it with different disabled groups in society.

Parkin: I have no wish to try to defend cost-benefit analysis in general. It is by no means the answer to everything. To try to assess the benefit to society in financial terms of a programme to treat chronic renal failure is an incredibly difficult thing to do. I happened to pick on one paper – the only one that has ever attempted to do it – and I then used the method to assess the indirect benefits by calculating the income, proportion of gross national product, or whatever that would be lost if patients were not treated. It is not a very satisfactory way of doing things, but it is incredibly difficult to think of any other way of doing it.

The point about mental deficiency is that there is no particular saving. It might be argued that in a totally cost-benefit orientated medical field, the *only* benefits are the direct financial benefits, and that therefore patients with mental deficiency should not be treated.

I did stress that there are other benefits. I called them intangible benefits. They are the social costs; the costs of death, disability, pain, grief, etc. One can try, if one likes, to put a price on those in pounds sterling, as some planners of highway systems do in comparing road and rail systems, but in general I do not see the doctors doing it.

J. S. Cameron (London): Dr Cattell has raised an important point. What happens next is that shortage of dialysis places makes transplantation appear cheaper than it really is, and this situation is probably no longer true. Since policy is determined by the sort of calculations that we have to do right now, it is important to look at the implications of this. What has probably happened in the past is that because of a shortage of dialysis places, people were not put back on dialysis after graft failure and therefore died. Death – we have already agreed – is cheap. Secondly, the transplanters and their physician colleagues pushed too hard on treatment to save failing grafts and patients died of all the horrible complications with which we are only too familiar, whereas adequate dialysis provision would allow these patients to be treated, and would allow them to return to dialysis. The cost of the failed graft does not appear in most of the analyses that are done and, until recently, the sort of mortality rate Dr Parkin showed in the graph was usual. I believe that the Australians first showed that the mortality of the patient, even when 50% of cadaver grafts were failing in the average population treated, could be pushed to less than 10% – into single figures over 5 years following the graft, even though one, two, or even three grafts were done during that time. The implications for this on the costs of transplantation and the number of dialysis places needed, given that our mortality is now down to single figures, are enormous, which reinforces further earlier statements about the need for more

dialysis places and more dialysis units to support the transplant programmes.

Boulton-Jones (Glasgow): Can I return to Dr Parkin's interesting slide
showing the correlation between numbers treated per million against the
national income. The correlation shown was most reassuring to administrators because it means that we are being zealous in apportioning the
funds. However, he has also said that there is a high percentage of transplantation and a high percentage of home dialysis patients; both of them
cheaper forms of treatment. That means that we should be well above the
line on the graph if we are allotting the same amount of money.

Parkin: So that the proportion of our GNP spent on dialysis and on renal
disease is probably less than it should be. That is probably right.

C. P. Swainson (Edinburgh): Dr Parkin has shown very nicely how the kind
of analysis he has described can help us, and can help doctors in general,
to decide between different modes of treatment of the same illness. But
how does he, as a health planner, begin to approach the problem of deciding
the allocation of resources between similar forms of chronic illness? For
example, take nephrology's main rival, heart disease.

Parkin: That is why I tentatively suggested using cost-benefit, because that
is the only objective way of doing it, illogical as it is. There is no other
objective way of doing it. Otherwise it is purely subjective.
    We do take the financial considerations into account. Cost-benefit can
be rejected as crude for looking at life-years saved and the benefits in terms
of how much someone would earn. But other criteria, such as the age of
patients, or whether they are diabetic, or for example the 92-year-old
patient with a stroke, have to be considered in cost benefit. We do it
intuitively, whether we like it or not.

Miss S. Taber: Should we not be looking at the available kidneys? Dr
Parkin has said that these are limited. Perhaps we should be putting
more money into improving the supply of cadaver kidneys. In the US they
have a system using a transplant coordinator, run by a business organization, and they have available the numbers of kidneys that they want. More
of our finances in the UK should be put to trying to improve the supply of
cadaver kidneys.

Parkin: I should have thought that that was a logical conclusion. I am no
expert in renal disease, but having spent some time reading through the

statistics that seems to be the most obvious – apart from increasing the number of centres. I have said that there is only one centre per million, but we do very well on that. That is not to say that we do not need more. Apart from that, we should be sorting out the supply of cadaver kidneys. It should be relatively simple.

Cameron: We have no need to go to the US for this information. We should be looking harder – as Dr Cattell did in the survey which he did for the Renal Association – at the variations in service provided both in terms of dialysis and in terms of transplantation throughout the different regions of Great Britain and Northern Ireland. These variations are very large.

One of the questions which the health planners might answer is how much of the variation resides with the different structure of medical care in those areas and how much is the direct result of financial deprivation. This is capable of analysis. Some regions, including our own South-East Metropolitan Region, are already treating 38 patients per million of population per year. If we can do this because we have more cash than other regions, then there are implications for planning.

Parkin: A comparison of those areas that are doing well or are doing badly in terms of dialysis within the UK shows that they correspond quite well to the analysis of whether they are plus or minus 50% over the amount of funding. There is no doubt about that.

5

The practicalities of limited care

The need to reconsider forms of treatment for patients on long-term haemodialysis

Helen Rosenthal

5.1   INTRODUCTION

Ever since regular haemodialysis for chronic renal failure became an accepted form of treatment rather than sheer adventurism, the debate around the relative merits of home dialysis, hospital dialysis, limited care and transplantation has flourished around the world. According to the pre-occupations and prejudices of each renal unit, the superiority of one form of treatment over another is demonstrated by the degree of patient rehabilitation, or the expressed preferences of the patient, by cost-benefit analyses or patient survival statistics. It is salutary to view this debate in the wider setting under which health care is delivered in a particular country. Differing health care systems subject to different forces and pressures can play determining roles in making available particular forms of treatment. If those determining forces and pressures continue to prevail, our need to justify the form of treatment which we offer may blind us to the changing needs of that most important person – the patient. Nowhere can this be seen so dramatically as in high-cost, high-technology, highly specialized treatments like chronic haemodialysis.

The UK has consistently led the field in home dialysis. While the European average of patients on home dialysis as a percentage of all patients on regular dialysis was 19.2% in 1975, the figure was 66% for the UK. Over the preceding 5 years, the UK regularly had the highest percentage of home dialysis patients. By contrast, in the USA, there was a rapid decrease in home dialysis over the 3 years 1972–75, from 42% to 24%. This was accompanied by a simultaneous increase in the number of patients using limited-care facilities. This more than compensated numerically for the drop in numbers of home dialysis patients[1].

Why should there have been a sustained prevalence of home dialysis in the UK, but not in the rest of Europe to anything like the same extent? Why is limited care apparently replacing home dialysis in the USA?

In the UK, our socialized system of health care has undoubtedly played an important part in promoting home dialysis, despite the initial tardy response of the then Ministry of Health to demands for funding for this form of treatment. The existence of the National Health Service has encouraged people to expect and demand health care as a right. This meant that a vociferous demand for dialysis for patients with kidney failure could be expected, and free treatment at that. Expectations were fulfilled. A key question was to be how to provide this extremely expensive form of treatment for as many patients as possible.

The National Health Service had an inheritance of specialist and non-specialist hospitals housed typically in cramped Victorian buildings in inner-city areas without physical space for expansion. Health care was not high amongst the Government's priorities for spending, and the rate of spending on health care as a percentage of our gross national product was steadily slowing down[2]. Thus the climate was not ripe for the rapid growth of highly specialized new units. Home dialysis was apparently the only way that the demand for treatment could begin to be met. It was the only way that the small numbers of medical, nursing and technical staff skilled in dialysis techniques could hope to support a steadily growing population of patients. Luckily there was and is substantial evidence that the rehabilitation of home dialysis patients was more successful than that of hospital-based patients, and that the risk of hepatitis amongst patients and staff was dramatically reduced. And so was born the British taste for home dialysis.

In the USA, with its free-market system of health care and health insurance, another influence is felt in the development of patterns of treatment – that of financial incentives and disincentives. It has been suggested that the falling off of home dialysis during the years 1972–75 was as a result of the increase in limited-care units[1]. But what were the reasons for that growth? It is likely that it has been caused by the financial disincentive to the patient to dialyse at home (health insurance does not cover the entire cost of treatment), and by the financial advantage to the physician to have the patient dialyse in the limited care unit or hospital setting.

In neither the UK nor the USA can the needs of the patient at the time be said to be the prime consideration in determining the forms of treatment to be offered.

The economic good sense of putting resources primarily into home dialysis in the UK has been amply reinforced by evidence of the many practical advantages to the dialysis patient and his or her family. The relatively small number of renal units meant that the catchment area of each unit was wide. After their initial period of training, patients no longer had to travel long distances for treatment. They could dialyse as and when they liked, and could return to full-time work.

5.2 SOME PLANNING CONSIDERATIONS

Home dialysis has thus continued to be the main form of treatment offered in the UK as a matter of expediency. The staff of individual renal units have been encouraged by all the evidence suggesting the success of home dialysis, as far as the patients treated are concerned. But there has been little serious reference to the unmet regional and national need for dialysis. There has been little attempt to address in a practical way the problem of inequalities of distribution of dialysis facilities amongst different regions.

There has been little serious consideration of the changing needs of our existing population of patients already established on home dialysis.

In planning for future needs, it is essential that these three considerations are linked together since they have a circular relationship (Figure 5.1). The

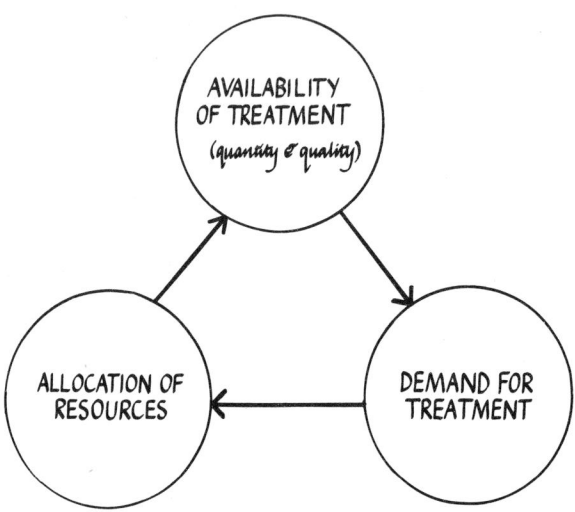

Figure 5.1   Planning considerations

demand for treatment is created by the current availability of treatment[3], i.e. local doctors are less likely to refer patients to hospitals with dialysis facilities if they feel that dialysis will not be available because of limited resources. But resources for the future are allocated all too often according to the existing demand. For example, the City and East London Area Health Authority plan for 1977–78 rightly describes the allocation by the North-East Thames Regional Health Authority for dialysis in the AHA as arbitrary[4]. The capital allocation for dialysis for 1977–78 of £150 000 was the same as it had been the previous year, without regard even for inflation – a cut in real terms of 17%!

If current availability, demand and allocation of resources are linked in this way, then it should be possible to use pressure for change in one area as a tool for influencing the other areas in a planned way. It is in this light that the need for and practicalities of a limited-care unit in Essex is examined starting with a survey of dialysis patients at the St. Leonard's/St. Bartholomew's Regional Renal Unit in Hackney in East London.

5.3   A SURVEY OF PATIENTS LIVING IN ESSEX

The patients at the St. Leonard's/St. Bartholomew's Renal Unit come from all over the North-East Thames Health Region, but are mainly concentrated in east London and south-east Essex. A few come from outside the Region. Currently there is a total of 72 patients established on home dialysis. The proportion of patients referred annually from Essex has increased from 33% in 1968 to 50% in 1976. A total of 40 patients from Essex has been established on home dialysis since 1968. The survey focuses on the experience of these 40 patients.

The renal unit offers a joint home dialysis and transplantation programme, but offers no facilities for regular limited-care or hospital-based dialysis. It is becoming increasingly clear that these facilities are inadequate to meet the changing needs of our patients.

As we gain confidence in our ability to train patients for home dialysis, so we develop a more catholic attitude towards patient selection. Patients now come on to the home dialysis programme who in earlier days would have been turned down because of their social, psychological or economic situation. We now have single patients who have no partner, and who dialyse entirely on their own. We have patients who are separated or divorced and patients who are single parents. We have immigrant patients who speak limited English and patients who have difficulty in reading.

Hand-in-hand with less stringent selection comes a galaxy of practical problems, the chief of which is bad housing, closely followed by low income, unemployment, and unstable family relationships.

5.4   HOUSING AND HOME DIALYSIS

East London and south-east Essex have a high density of local authority and Greater London Council housing. Council houses are allocated according to family size, and so council tenants will almost by definition not have a spare room. The St. Leonard's/St. Bartholomew's Renal Unit has always operated a policy of using only a spare room for dialysis, for reasons of hygiene (easier to keep clean), and for psychological reasons (easier to close the door and forget about dialysis). With the wider use of disposable artificial kidneys, automatic supply units with built-in washing-through mechanisms, and shorter hours of dialysis, this policy could change. However, the need for rehousing would not decrease dramatically, as rooms in many council houses and flats are cramped and dialysis in the sitting room or bedroom would still be unacceptable in many cases.

Of our 40 Essex patients, only 15 had rooms in their houses which were

TABLE 5.1   Home dialysis arrangements for 40 patients from Essex

Suitable room for conversion	15
Elaborate conversion, extension or portable cabin	9
Rehoused	15
No permanent solution	1
Total	40

suitable for conversion into dialysis treatment rooms (Table 5.1). Nine had expensive portable cabins, extensions to their houses, or elaborate conversions. Fifteen had to be rehoused by the local authority or Greater London Council. For one patient, an owner-occupier, there was no solution as his house was under planning blight because of a road scheme. Council housing was refused, and the patient is temporarily receiving what is rather inadequate dialysis on a portable dialysis machine.

Thus the solution for ten patients was extremely costly in initial capital outlay. Fifteen other patients had to endure the considerable domestic upheaval and worry of moving house, and frequently moving to a new neighbourhood, while travelling to the renal unit three times weekly for dialysis. Financial assistance with moving is only automatically forthcoming for patients claiming Supplementary Benefit – another hidden cost of NHS 'free' dialysis. Some patients have felt pressured by the renal unit into accepting larger council accommodation which they did not like, so that there would be no delay in starting home dialysis. This may have contributed to domestic and dialysis-related problems which occurred later.

5.5   LENGTH OF TIME BEFORE HOME DIALYSIS

Another factor worthy of consideration is the length of time it takes from the first dialysis at the renal unit to the first home dialysis. This is determined by two factors; the time taken to adapt the patient's home, and the patient's ability to dialyse. Adapting the home involves drawing up plans, seeking estimates, and carrying out the building work. The time taken will depend on the efficiency of the various public authorities involved, and the amount of bureaucratic red tape deemed necessary. The patient's ability to dialyse depends on having an adequate fistula, adequately controlled weight gains and blood pressure, a lack of other medical problems, competence in dialysis technique, and confidence in his or her own ability to dialyse. Competence and confidence will in turn be influenced by the staffing of the renal unit. At the same time as increasing numbers of patients are being accepted for dialysis each year (made possible by recycling of capital equipment), staffing levels are being frozen because of financial cutbacks. A lower staff/patient ratio leads to less concentrated teaching. Strain on the staff leads to rapid staff turnover, and patients cannot depend on having their accustomed teacher.

Table 5.2   Average length of time between first hospital dialysis and first home dialysis of 40 patients from Essex, according to home dialysis arrangement

Suitable room for conversion	7–8 months
Elaborate conversion, extension or portable cabin	8–9 months
Rehoused	10–11 months

Looking at the length of time between the first hospital and first home dialysis in the 40 Essex patients, there has been a general trend for this time to increase slightly between 1968 and 1976 (Table 5.2). If broken down according to whether the patient had to be rehoused or not, it can be seen that rehousing tends to prolong the time by 2–4 months.

5.6   THE CHANGING NEEDS

If the capital expense to the National Health Service, the expense to the patient in moving house, and inconvenience and expense of travelling anything up to 60 miles to the renal unit during training were the happy end of the story, our policy of home dialysis alone would be easily justified. But the happiest end to the story for many patients is successful kidney transplantation, and the removal of dialysis equipment from their homes. For patients who are not transplanted and are ageing, there may be increasing difficulty with access sites and additional medical complications, which will limit the possibility of continued home dialysis. The cumulative stress of home dialysis may cause social or psychological problems, which will also make home dialysis impossible. From these patients there will be an increasing demand for frequent and possibly permanent unit-based dialysis.

Table 5.3 shows how the circumstances of 17 patients have changed

TABLE 5.3   Changes in circumstances of 40 home dialysis patients in Essex

Successful transplants	7
Failed/failing transplants	4
Return to unit-based dialysis	3
Deaths	3
Unchanged	23
Total	40

since they were established on home dialysis. It is clear that for a sizable minority of patients, home dialysis cannot be a permanent solution.

5.7 THE NEED FOR LIMITED-CARE DIALYSIS

Taking into account the changing needs of our patients and the catchment area of the St. Leonard's/St. Bartholomew's Renal Unit, the evidence suggests a considerable and immediate need for an additional satellite dialysis unit in Essex, offering limited-care dialysis. Furthermore, the St. Leonard's/St. Bartholomew's Renal Unit does not have the monopoly of patients with chronic renal failure in Essex. The catchment area of The London Hospital Renal Unit is identical. The Royal Free Hospital Renal Unit is also in the North-East Thames Health Region and maintains some patients in Essex. The needs of these two units should also be taken into account, thus creating a regional facility for limited care.

Training in dialysis for the patient needs to take place at the parent-unit where there is medical and out-patient back-up. But once a patient has been trained, there is no reason why he or she should not dialyse in a limited-care setting, if home dialysis is not possible for some reason. Limited care would mean that the patient could either be totally autonomous, or could receive assistance from staff in certain clearly defined areas, e.g. needling, machine preparation and clearing up.

A limited-care unit would offer a flexible solution to changing problems. Patients could use it in a variety of different situations. It could be the permanent base of those few Essex patients who are at present dialysing long-term or permanently in the hospital. It could be used as an interim measure for patients requiring rehousing or who suffer long delays in the completion of their home dialysis adaptations, but are otherwise self-sufficient in their treatment. This would save the patient money as well as time, since travelling expenses are only automatically refunded to patients who claim Supplementary Benefits. This can cause considerable hardship to patients who are at work or claiming other benefits. It might be used occasionally as a long-term solution for patients whose homes are particularly difficult to convert and who may be good candidates for transplantation. Patients who had temporarily or permanently lost confidence in their ability to dialyse at home could use it. It could be used to give patients on 'holiday' a break from dialysing at home on their own.

The St. Leonard's/St. Bartholomew's Unit already offers this facility to home patients, but not one of the 11 patients who came into the Unit in 1977 for holiday dialysis came from Essex. Presumably, the distance, travelling time and expense involved cancel out the benefit for patients who live some distance away. It is probable therefore that there would be a considerable demand for holiday dialysis in an Essex limited-care unit.

5.8 SITING AND STRUCTURE

The flexible usage of such a unit should be reflected in its physical structure. A system of linked prefabricated units would be cheap and would allow for future expansion. The conversion of an existing disused building might also be considered. The siting of the unit would depend on the geographical distribution of the patients of all the renal units concerned, and should take carefully into account the question of ease of access by public transport. The Essex patients from the St. Leonard's/St. Bartholomew's Unit come mainly from south Essex, in the triangle formed between Basildon, Chelmsford and Southend-on-Sea (Figure 5.2). Since the smaller number of patients from north Essex travel the greatest distances, the siting of a limited-care unit in Chelmsford would seem practical.

The use of disposable dialysers and automatic supply units with built-in washing-through mechanisms would obviate the need for separate 'dirty' and 'clean' areas. It would also simplify the plumbing and drainage arrange-

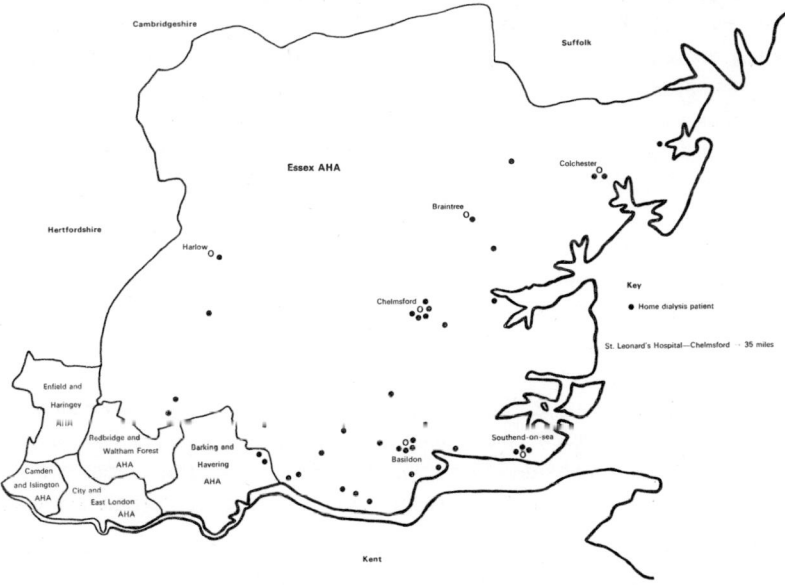

Figure 5.2   Distribution of home dialysis patients from St. Leonard's RDU living in Essex

ments. Armchairs rather than beds would allow a greater number of patients to dialyse in a smaller space, and would help discourage the patient from feeling that he or she was an invalid. Patients who had formerly dialysed at home might be especially prone to this.

The number of dialysis stations would depend finally on the projected regional need for limited-care dialysis. Four dialysis stations would allow 16 patients thrice-weekly dialysis, dialysing for 6-hour sessions, during the day and evening. The number of patients would increase to 24 if an over-night shift were included. Staffing considerations would also play a part in determining the size of the unit.

Besides the dialysis area, there should be space for storage of supplies and cleaning equipment, and WC, washing and changing facilities of a minimal kind. A living-room area with a small cooker where patients could prepare snacks could also serve as a staff room.

5.9   STAFFING AND WORKING HOURS

A unit with four dialysis stations could be staffed by Artificial Kidney Assistants (AKA), with one AKA in attendance at any one time. AKAs might staff the unit on a rotational basis from the parent units to prevent over-dependence on any one AKA, and prevent that AKA from becoming isolated. Technical back-up would come from the parent units. Technicians would do routine servicing and emergency call-outs as they do for home dialysis patients. Cleaning would be done by local domestic staff.

Patients would have to be responsible for their own drugs as if they were dialysing at home, to avoid the legal complications of the administration of drugs by AKAs. Patients would also keep their own dialysis records, and would attend the parent unit for routine medical examinations, unless facilities were developed for a renal out-patient clinic at a local hospital. The same would apply for routine urea and electrolyte blood tests, and hepatitis B antigen tests. The monitoring of patients and staff for hepatitis would need to be carefully organized, and a code of practice laid down for the unit.

A limited-care unit set up on this basis would represent a considerable challenge to the present piecemeal development of services for chronic renal failure. The considerations will be different in rural areas, but the same considerations could be readily applied to other urban areas of Britain.

5.10 CONCLUSION

When the National Health Service was reorganized in 1974, part of the aim was to provide regional budgets out of which comprehensive health services could be developed[5]. But there is little evidence that this is taking place either within individual regions, or amongst different regions. The policy of the Resource Allocation Working Party of redistribution of resources away from the four London regions and Merseyside serves only to spread the jam more thinly in a time of economic recession and cutbacks in public spending. The North-East Thames Regional Health Authority is the best served in the country as far as numbers of patients on long-term dialysis and numbers of weekly sessions by nephrologists are concerned. Yet even in this region, we are nowhere near treating the 33–40 patients per million population per year that it is estimated could benefit from long-term dialysis[6].

The setting up of a Regional Limited-Care Dialysis Unit would encourage local renal units to overcome their tendency to be isolated and insular. It would demand a serious attempt to assess the problem of the unmet need for dialysis. The presence of such a unit would encourage local doctors to refer patients with chronic renal failure to hospitals with dialysis facilities. Patients who today are dying because of doubts that the facility to treat them exists could be offered treatment. It would encourage the establishment of local renal out-patient clinics. Finally it would offer an important new type of care that would widen the spectrum of treatment available, to offer a more flexible and comprehensive service to people with chronic renal failure.

The correctness of asking for more resources in a field of medicine that already swallows up a large slice of the cake may be questioned, especially in a time of economic restraint. But conversely, if renal services are to be 'rationalized', it is our responsibility to make known the real needs of our patients. If we fail to, we will find ourselves not only with inadequate but inappropriate facilities.

References

1. Gurland, H. J., Brunner, F. P., Chantler, C., Jacobs, C., Schärer, K., Selwood, N. H., Spies, G. and Wing, A. J. (1976). Combined report on regular dialysis and transplantation in Europe, VI, 1975. *Transpl. Assoc.*, **13**, 3
2. Central Statistical Office Annual Abstract of Statistics (1975). No. 112
3. Abel-Smith, B. (1976). *Value for Money in the Health Services.* Ch. 7 (London: Heinemann)

4. Area Plan 1977–78, The City and East London Area Health Authority (Teaching)
5. National Health Service Reorganisation Act (1973). Section 47 (London: HMSO)
6. Report of the Executive Committee of the Renal Association (1976). Distribution of nephrological services for adults in Great Britain. *Br. Med. J.*, 2, 903

DISCUSSION

Miss S. Taber: I would be interested in what members of the audience would feel about a limited-care unit without the nursing staff.

Mrs Deirdre E. Jones (London): One is very conditioned by what one is used to. It is the middleman between home dialysis and the hospital, which is the problem. We are very happy to let the patients do everything at home and to leave the responsibility to relatives. It is hard to visualize this in-between area. Why should a well-trained properly-educated Artificial Kidney Assistant (AKA) not manage such a situation? One gets concerned as much for the AKA's welfare as for the patients' in the situation when something goes wrong. It is a question of how much responsibility can be put on to the patient, and how much, possibly, on to the AKA. It is an area that has not been clearly defined. It is disheartening that nothing has come from the DHSS symposium on this. Hopefully the RCN group will come up with something. However, we have discussed this kind of area for years, and nothing really concrete is coming forward as guidelines.

Taber: What came out of the DHSS symposium was that we are to go back to the guidelines that were issued in 1966, or so the RCN delegation that went to the Department of Health was told. So we are back on the 1966 guidelines.

B. H. B. Robinson (Birmingham): We have been planning a similar unit and we would aim to get patients trained to a home dialysis standard, running their own dialysis, perhaps with the help of their relatives. All that the attendant would do would be to make sure that they clear up after themselves. If we look too much at guidelines and at who shall be responsible for what we shall rapidly find that we are running another hospital-type set up.

J. M. Bone (Liverpool): We are at the bottom of the league table as regards resources and the provision of facilities and we have no official hospital dialysis unit where we can support patients awaiting transplantation. We have been looking at limited care to support patients, primarily for transplantation in the first instance. If the transplant fails the patients will be back to limited care, or we might be able to arrange home haemodialysis. For the moment we have taken our proposals as far as we can. In the present financial climate the draught blows quite cold and there has been a call for savings of a million pounds in the District, so it is likely that we are in something of a limbo. Hopefully things might improve in the next financial year, and we might have the resources.

A. C. Kennedy (Glasgow): What thought has been given to the precise siting of the proposed unit? Would it be in the grounds of a hospital, or not?

Miss Rosenthal: It could be, but that is not necessary.

Kennedy: If it is in the grounds of a hospital, it will be difficult to get the Authority to stand back and not impose responsibilities, such as insisting on a qualified nurse being in attendance.

Rosenthal: It would be a matter of weighing up the advantages and the disadvantages. An existing but disused building in the grounds of a hospital might be available for conversion

Kennedy: But, with respect, that would become a part of that hospital.

Miss Mary E. Selsby (London): I could not agree more with Professor Kennedy. I do not think that such a unit should be in the hospital grounds. That could only lead to problems.

I can see problems in using such a unit for patients who are waiting to be rehoused. Patients who have been in hospital for any length of time often lose the incentive to undertake home haemodialysis and I can see similar dangers arising with limited care.

Rosenthal: I can see the point, but in my own experience most patients want to get home. They do not enjoy being in a hospital setting. If the general atmosphere was superior to a hospital that might make a difference.

W. R. Cattell (London): Limited care has to be *limited* care. The patients must be self-sufficient dialysers and it then becomes a question of whether they dialyse in the unit or at home. I do not think that that really matters.

I would not be too unhappy about an individual who was permanently on self-supervised dialysis in a satellite limited-care unit if that was what he elected to do.

We ought to have some flexibility about this. The patient who requires treatment and who is capable of self-treatment could be treated in his own home, if suitable, or in a truly limited-care setting.

Selsby: But then such a unit would not be used for the patient awaiting rehousing.

Cattell: It might, but then the patient elects to have a house prepared. If there is any doubt about him waiting one would not waste the money.

6

Experience in self-care and limited-care haemodialysis in 340 patients
A. W. Siemsen

6.1   INTRODUCTION

Good preventive medical programmes and increased ability to resolve acute medical problems have resulted in a longer life expectancy and an increased incidence of chronic medical illness. The rate of dying varies from one person to another but is basically a function of the ageing process and superimposed disease. As part of the ageing process, there are concerns of adaptation to loneliness and various physical and mental infirmities[1]. In this setting the patient may have additional problems such as hypertension, coronary artery disease, cerebral vascular disease, diabetes mellitus or malignant processes.

The new technologies of haemodialysis and transplantation have made it possible to sustain life past the point where it would have normally ended. However, there remains a degree of uncertainty about their long-term effects on the body and the burdens which they place on families and societies. We have little understanding of the nature of uraemic toxins, which characteristically produce neuro-behavioural manifestations. Because of multifaceted patient and societal concerns created by increasing chronic medical illness and the new technologies, we must carefully evaluate all of the alternate treatment programmes so that the most reasonable course of action may be determined by patient and physician.

Patient selection to determine who will benefit from these treatment modalities can probably only be morally and legally justified if all patients with equal degrees of medical illness are chosen at random, such as by a lottery[2]. We have never practised patient selection because we have been unable to predict which patients will do well on dialysis and which will have serious medical and emotional problems. Flipping a coin would have been as accurate as our predictions.

To make an informed, competent decision of method and modality of care, the uraemic patient must be removed from his uraemic environment by dialysis or transplantation, have an opportunity to experience the nature of the treatment programmes, and have any emotional or adjustment problems evaluated and treated. Thus, nearly all patients not moribund from non-uraemic causes should be dialysed for a trial period so that they might adequately evaluate the situation themselves.

Our patients were offered: (*a*) living related transplantation if a suitable donor was available, (*b*) self-care dialysis at home or in an outpatient facility as near their home as possible or (*c*) limited-care dialysis in an outpatient facility near a hospital. If cadaveric transplantation was desired, the patient was placed on the waiting list. All self-dialysis patients entered a special teaching programme. Language barriers were not a contraindication to self-dialysis training. Home patients were required to have a back-up member who was taught by the patient. Re-use of the dialyser was routinely taught although some home patients subsequently discontinued this practice. The staff-to-patient ratio in the self-care facility was 1:5, as not all patients were totally independent. However, most were able to set up the dialyser, perform their dialysis and clean the dialyser. Many required assistance in placing the fistula needles. Re-use of the dialyser was utilized in all self-care facilities. The self-care facilities were commonly used by home patients when the back-up member desired a holiday. They were also used as an intermediate facility for home patients to gain confidence away from the centre before dialysis was actually done at home. This seemed to be particularly important in more remote areas. The ratio of staff to patients in the limited-care facilities was 1:3, as total care was provided by nurses or technicians. In Hawaii there are dialysis facilities located on three neighbour islands, as well as on Oahu in the State of Hawaii and in Majuro and Guam in Micronesia. Home patients were located on islands throughout the State and in Tahiti.

6.2 STATUS OF SELF-DIALYSIS TEACHING

Of the 349 patients admitted to our programme between 1 October 1968 and 30 November 1976, nine chose immediate living related transplantation or expired with less than one month of dialysis. The remaining 340 patients were retrospectively divided into three groups based on the age at initiation of dialysis: (a) 7–44 years (mean age 30.8 years), (b) 45–59 years (mean age 52.4 years), and (c) 60–80 years (mean age 66.5 years). Table 6.1 shows that 241 patients entered the self-dialysis teaching programme (SDTP) and the remainder were treated in the limited-care facilities (LCF). In the entire programme, 70.9% entered the self-dialysis teaching programme. This ranged from 79.1% in the younger age groups to 58.6% in the older age group. With advancing age a greater percentage entered the limited-care facilities.

TABLE 6.1   Status of self-dialysis teaching, 1 October 1968 – 30 November 1976

Age (years)	Number of patients		Total
	Entered LCF	Entered SDTP	
7–44	31 (20.9%)	117 (79.1%)	148
45–59	39 (32.0%)	83 (68.0%)	122
60–80	29 (41.4%)	41 (58.6%)	70
Entire programme	99 (29.1%)	241 (70.9%)	340

LCF – Limited care facility
SDTP – Self-dialysis teaching programme

TABLE 6.2   Status of self-dialysis teaching, 1 October 1968 – 30 November 1976

| Age (years) | % Male | | |
	Entered LCF	Entered SDTP	Entire age group
7–44	61.3%	53.8%	55.4%
45–59	76.9%	57.8%	63.9%
60–80	69.0%	75.6%	72.9%
Entire programme	69.7%	58.9%	62.0%

Table 6.2 characterizes these groups by the percentage that were males. It can be noted that the percentage of males in each group increased from 55.4% in the youngest age group to 72.9% in the older age group with 62% of the entire dialysis population being male. The percentage of males entering the teaching programme tended to parallel the increased percentage of males in each age group. Nevertheless, more males were treated by limited-care dialysis (69.7%) than entered the teaching programme (58.9%). Thus, females tended to be more interested in self-dialysis than males.

TABLE 6.3   Status of self-dialysis teaching, 1 October 1968 – 30 November 1976

| Age (years) | % Diabetics | | |
	Entered LCF	Entered SDTP	Entire age group
7–44	19.4%	8.5%	10.8%
45–59	46.2%	25.3%	32.0%
60–80	75.9%	24.4%	45.7%
Entire programme	46.5%	17.0%	25.6%

The incidence of diabetes mellitus in each group is depicted in Table 6.3. The diagnosis of diabetes mellitus was made in 25.6% of those in the entire dialysis population. The frequency of this diagnosis increased with advancing age from 10.8% in the youngest group to 45.7% in the oldest age group. There was clearly a greater percentage of diabetics who required care in the limited-care programmes (46.5%) as compared with those entering the self-dialysis teaching programme (17%). This was explainable by the greater incidence of medical complications, including severe cerebral and coronary vascular disease, as well as blindness, in the limited-care group.

6.3 INITIAL MODALITY OF SELF-DIALYSIS

Table 6.4 subdivides the ultimate destination of those who entered the self-dialysis teaching programme into home and self-care facilities (SCF). This group does not total 241, the number entering the teaching programme, because of transplantation, deaths and those remaining in the teaching unit

TABLE 6.4   Initial modality of self-dialysis

Age (years)	Number of patients		
	Home	SCF	Total
7–44	59 (50.9%)	57 (49.1%)	116
45–59	43 (52.4%)	39 (47.6%)	82
60–80	12 (40.0%)	18 (60.0%)	30
Entire programme	114 (50.0%)	114 (50.0%)	228

as of 30 November 1976. In analysing the same three age groups, it was found that 50.9% of the younger age group went home; whereas this was only accomplished in 40% of the older group. Of the total group entering the teaching programme, 50% went home and 50% were treated in a self-care facility. The usual reasons a patient did not go home were lack of a back-up member, unstable psychological problems at home or inadequate housing. Thus, our initial experience (Tables 6.1 and 6.4) suggests that 30% of the patients on chronic maintenance dialysis would require limited-care dialysis while 35% could be treated at home and 35% in a self-care facility. These numbers are slightly biased as there is no home dialysis in Micronesia.

The percentage of males in each of the self-dialysis teaching age groups is summarized in Table 6.5. In general, and particularly in the middle age

TABLE 6.5   Initial modality of self-dialysis

Age (years)	% Males		Entire age group
	Home	SCF	
7–44	50.8%	56.1%	53.4%
45–59	46.5%	69.2%	57.3%
60–80	75.0%	72.2%	73.3%
Entire programme	51.8%	63.2%	57.4%

TABLE 6.6   Initial modality of self-dialysis

| Age (years) | % Diabetic | | |
	Home	SCF	Entire age group
7–44	8.5%	8.8%	8.6%
45–59	18.6%	25.6%	22.0%
60–80	33.3%	22.2%	26.7%
Entire programme	14.9%	16.7%	15.8%

group, a greater percentage of females were dialysing at home than males. Table 6.6 demonstrates that the diabetics who entered the self-dialysis teaching programme were eventually divided equally between the home and self-care programmes.

It is important to consider transfers from the initial programmes which the patients entered. Table 6.7 shows that 14.5% of those taught self-dialysis eventually entered other programmes. The highest rate of transfer occurred in the older age group. The usual transfer of a home-care patient was to a self-care facility although, before the 21 home patients transferred, they had accumulated 357 patient-months of experience at home. The most common cause of transfer was the magnitude of the emotional burden on the back-up member in the family. Multiple back-up members clearly aided successful home dialysis. When the back-up member was the husband, there were more transfers than when the back-up member was the wife.

The transfers from self-care facilities were generally to a limited-care facility, although two patients eventually went home. However, before the eight patients transferred, they had experienced 90 patient-months in self-care dialysis. The usual cause of the self-care transfers was increasing medical complications which had arisen on dialysis, such as poor cardiac output, serious cardiac arrhythmia and cerebral vascular accidents.

TABLE 6.7   Self-dialysis transfers

| Age (years) | Number of patients | | | % of those taught for age group |
	Home	SCF	SDTP	
7–44	13	0	0	11.1%
45–59	6	2	0	9.6%
60–80	2	6	6	34.1%
Entire programme	21	8	6	14.5%

There were six patients (2.5%) who were unable to complete the self-dialysis teaching programme and had to be transferred to a limited-care facility. These patients were all in the older age group. Of the 35 patient transfers, 31.4% were diabetic, as compared with 17% entering the teaching programme, and 62.8% were male, as compared with 58.9% entering the teaching programme.

6.4 MORBIDITY AND MORTALITY

Any treatment programme must initially be evaluated from the perspective of morbidity and mortality. Table 6.8 shows that our data is based on 7824 patient-months or 652 patient-years of experience. The largest experience

TABLE 6.8   Patient-months of experience, 1 October 1968 – 30 November 1976

Age (years)	LCF	SDT	Home	SCF	Entire age group
7–44	965	107	1669	1379	4120
45–59	686	114	1128	572	2500
60–80	702	48	182	272	1204
Entire programme	2353	269	2979	2223	7824

of 2979 patient-months was accumulated in home dialysis. The younger age group with 4120 patient-months was larger than the other two age groups. The index of morbidity chosen was number of hospital days. This data is presented in Table 6.9. This was corrected to hospital days per 1000 patient-months of experience so that the various treatment modalities and age groups could be compared.

TABLE 6.9   Hospital days per 1000 patient-months of experience

Age (years)	LCF	SDT	Home	SCF	Entire age group
7–44	3258	1878	747	1004	1451
45–59	4729	1316	1007	1420	2137
60–80	4199	938	1582	2412	3270
Entire programme	3968	1472	897	1283	1950

In the entire dialysis programme, our patients had been hospitalized 1950 days per 1000 patient-months of dialysis, or these patients were in the hospital for 1 day out of every 15.4 days on dialysis. Home patients had the lowest number of inpatient days with 1 per 33.4 days on dialysis and limited-care, the highest with 1 day out of 7.6 days on dialysis. The lowest incidence of hospitalization was in the younger age group on home dialysis with 1 hospital day out of every 40.2 days on dialysis. There were increasing hospital days associated with advancing age. The most common cause of hospitalization was related to vascular access.

The number of hospital days per admission are shown in Table 6.10. This averaged 10.1 days for the entire programme and increased with advancing age.

TABLE 6.10   Hospital days per admission

Age (years)	LCF	SDT	Home	SCF	Entire age group
7–44	9.1	6.9	7.7	8.3	8.5
45–59	12.5	6.8	9.5	8.8	10.8
60–80	12.2	5.6	9.9	15.6	12.3
Entire programme	11.0	6.7	8.6	9.5	10.1

The cumulative survival curves for diabetics and non-diabetics is given in Table 6.11. The non-diabetic survival curve in our experience was intermediate between living related and cadaveric transplantation. A more

TABLE 6.11   Haemodialysis cumulative survival

Years	Non-diabetic (%) ($n = 253$)	Diabetic (%) ($n = 87$)
0.25	93.9	98.8
0.5	91.6	88.7
1.0	87.5	74.3
2.0	80.6	53.8
3.0	70.8	33.5
4.0	61.2	23.2
5.0	59.1	
6.0	51.7	

sensitive index of mortality is the number of deaths per 1000 patient-months of experience. Table 6.12 shows that the mortality for the entire programme was 12.8 deaths per 1000 patient-months of experience. The mortality was 14.0 for males and 10.8 for females per 1000 patient-months of experience. Like morbidity, mortality increased with advancing age and was highest in the limited-care group.

TABLE 6.12   Mortality per 1000 patient-months of experience

Age (years)	LCF	SDT	Home	SCF	Entire age group
7–44	12.4	—	6.0	3.6	6.6
45–59	29.2	—	12.4	12.2	16.4
60–80	32.8	20.8	22.0	14.7	26.6
Entire group	23.4	3.7	9.4	7.2	12.8

If one analyses the data for morbidity (Table 6.9), it can be noted that the number of hospital days for limited-care patients was 3.1–4.4 times greater than for self-care or home patients. If one analyses the data for mortality (Table 6.12), it is apparent that deaths for the limited-care patients were 2.5–3.2 times greater than for home or self-care patients. These comparisons should not lead to a conclusion that limited-care dialysis is adverse. The limited-care patients are older, have a higher incidence of diabetes mellitus and other medical complications, and reflect a life-plan in which many patients, initially treated at home or in a self-care programme, eventually required total patient care.

6.5   RECENT TRENDS

The data presented was a total experience over the past 8 years. There are some important recent trends to be considered. Table 6.13 shows that the percentage of home patients progressively rose through 30 June 1973. In July of 1973, the 92nd Congress enacted Public Law 92–603 which substantially relieved the financial burden of end-stage renal disease patients; however, it contained several disincentives to home dialysis. It can be noted that the percentage of patients at home has progressively decreased since that time. The absolute number of patients going home is shown in

TABLE 6.13   Modality of dialysis

Date	Home (%)	SCF (%)	LCF (%)
30/6/71	40	18	42
30/6/72	40	24	36
30/6/73	49	21	30
30/6/74*	46	26	28
30/6/75	39	35	26
30/6/76	25	46	29

* Date funding acted against home dialysis

TABLE 6.14   Absolute number of new patients entering a programme

Date	Home	SCF	LCF
30/6/71	12	7	2
30/6/72	12	9	2
30/6/73	15	10	5
30/6/74*	7	29	11
30/6/75	8	24	14
30/6/76	3	47	21

* Date funding acted against home dialysis

Table 6.14. The absolute number of patients going home rose until enactment of the legislation and has since progressively decreased. In this programme, where there has been no change in the number of diabetics or medically more complicated patients accepted, it suggests that other factors such as loss of incentives or family burdens may be operational. The percentage and absolute number of patients entering self-care facilities has dramatically increased. The upward changes in the limited-care programme are less marked.

6.6   SOCIETAL CONCERNS

Through our advancing technology we can now prolong the life of a patient with end-stage renal disease. The new technology carries with it degrees of uncertainty and risk. It may produce severe emotional, physical and financial burdens on the patients and their families. The dissipation of tremendous resources causes society to debate the degree of benefit conferred on one group as compared to the burdens borne by another. Each society must make value judgements based on its goals and allocate resources appropriately to such things as building roads, subsidizing symphonies, combating unemployment, fighting wars, supporting end-stage renal disease, etc. If these resources are infinite, we could dialyse patients in posh surroundings with maximum services and conveniences. If resources are limited, as they are in our programme, we must consider more efficient forms of dialysis at home or in self-care facilities where cost, in our experience, can be reduced by 70% and 40% respectively. These reductions in cost ignore payment of the back-up member at home and require dialyser re-use. There may be patients who desire transfer out of home dialysis because of emotional stresses and burdens on the family, or patients in self-care facilities who develop medical complications which require limited-care dialysis. As the technology continues to advance and the societal constraints increase, we will probably develop an inverse relationship between scientific medicine and freedom of therapeutic choice[3].

Our self-care facility at Majuro in the Marshall Islands has dialysed 10 patients for three years at a location 2400 miles from Honolulu. This unit is operated only by nurses without a nephrologist in attendance. Wireless communication usually takes 24 hours or longer. The morbidity and mortality of this facility has been no different from our closer units. A nephrologist does visit the atoll every 4–5 months to evaluate the progress of patients. Complications occurring on dialysis are managed in Honolulu. Further cost reduction can be obtained by increased utilization of our nursing staff.

The public and our nursing personnel are well aware of the recent medical advances. We must constantly evaluate them as to the nature of chronic illness. We must dispel the notion that going to a doctor automatically offers the potential of a restored optimal state of health[4]. Patients on dialysis are not restored to their usual state of health which existed prior to the onset of uraemia. This frequently leads to frustration on the part of the nursing staff because there may be no dramatic improvement in the patient from one dialysis to another. A psychiatric nurse clinician plays a vital role in helping the staff to become more aware of their own feelings and that of their patients.

The major emerging moral, legal and medical concern is under what circumstances can dialysis be discontinued. The role of the informed competent adult and the guardian in the decision-making process requires further study.

Thus, with increasing chronic illness and advancing technology, we must constantly examine two spheres of interaction: medical and societal. How much of the burden should be borne by the patient and how much by society? We should tailor the dialysis to the patient needs in so far as possible within the limits of the burdens tolerated by society. We must examine all of the alternative solutions for the patients, their families and their society. Only in this way can we come up with the most reasonable course of action. The confidence of our patients and our society depends on our ability to handle them correctly.

References

1. Williams, R. H. (1969). Our role in the generation, modification and termination of life. *Arch. Intern. Med.*, **124**, 215
2. Dukeminier, J. and Sanders, D. (1971). Legal problems in allocation of scarce medical resources. *Arch. Inter. Med.*, **127**, 1133
3. Kountz, S. L. (1975). The effect of bioscience and technological momentum on the surgical treatment of chronic illness. *Surgery*, **77**, 735
4. Teschan, P. E. (1970). On the pathogenesis of uremia. *Am. J. Med.*, **48**, 671

DISCUSSION

A. M. Martin (Sunderland): Given Dr Siemsen's large experience with haemodialysis in diabetics, does he agree with the suggestion that heparinization accelerates the onset of blindness?

Siemsen: To give a scientific answer to that question I would need records going back over a period of time and I do not have that information. We have no peritoneal experience at this point; we are starting. We are starting largely because in diabetics there are problems of access, and at that point in time we shall start that study.

However, I believe that there is a consensus of opinion among nephrologists in the US today that heparin does aggravate failing vision in diabetics.

R. J. Winney (Edinburgh): Dr Siemsen seems to have a high incidence of diabetics. Were they all insulin-dependent diabetics since this may affect the complication rates?

Siemsen: They were not all insulin-requiring diabetics. However, I should point out that in Hawaii, and particularly in the Pacific Basin, there is an increased incidence of diabetes. The best statistics on this are obtainable from the Atomic Energy Commission. They have carried out a study and there is a higher incidence of diabetes.

Mrs Deirdre E. Jones (London): May we have a brief rundown on how the home training is approached.

Siemsen: We have a language problem and almost all the teaching is done by illustration. Most people can be taught to read numbers and we put numbers on all the switches. A great deal is 'watch monkey, do monkey' and a lot of teaching is done that way, with some of it done conventionally, where the subject is suitable, using illustrations, and the nurse doing the teaching. It is all on a one-to-one basis.

Jones: With how much relative involvement?

Siemsen: The patient is first taught to dialyse himself, and the patient then teaches the back-up member. The patient should be the prime mover.

A. C. Kennedy (Glasgow): I was interested to hear Dr Siemsen say that he considered that he had limited financial resources. All things are relative!

Siemsen: It took us two years of heavy lobbying to get funds from the State. It took an immense amount of time and energy before we were eventually successful. We have a pact with the legislature that we will keep the costs down and they will keep the patients alive, but they do watch it closely.

Kennedy: Given Dr Siemsen's experience of dialysing patients of 75, 80, 84 years of age, with many other physical problems, has he any doubts about the wisdom of doing this?

Siemsen: No, not at all. The gravest question that arises in my mind is because of the complications of diabetes. With vascular access problems, prolonged hospitalization, pain for the patient from repeated vascular procedures, loss of extremities unrelated to the vascular procedures, and disease, one must ask oneself how meaningful this life is.

Kennedy: Which is what I am asking.

Siemsen: But it is meaningful to that patient. Physicians might ask themselves whether it is meaningful to them, but it is meaningful to that patient and it is meaningful to that family.

J. M. Bone (Liverpool): One comment on the use of terms. Problems will arise in the future when we relate limited-care facilities to self-care facilities as there are at least two other terms on the horizon, one of them minimal-care, which is a slightly different aspect. However, Dr Siemsen uses the term 'limited-care' for what we would call hospital dialysis and he uses 'self-care' for what we would probably call limited-care dialysis. There is a spectrum of care between the hospital and the home and very different patients will require to be slotted into it depending on their circumstances.

Our use of limited-care, or our intended use of limited-care, will be for transplant support with a high turnover, and in these circumstances a staff ratio of five to one is probably adequate. But the patient who had a rejected kidney, who was rehabilitated and was back on self-care dialysis could probably go out to the periphery, not necessarily to his home, but perhaps to a health centre or to a facility nearby to a district general hospital, which would be total self-care.

There is a problem with terms.

Siemsen: When the original paper was presented in 1972, the term 'limited-care' was used for what would now be called self-care. Where we have acute renal failure and a critically ill patient, the ratio is usually one to one. Limited-care is the next step down, the stable maintenance patient, where we can use the ratio of one to three. That is limited, and not what it was. We then have a teaching programme to do self-care, either at home, or in a special self-care facility, where we try to get the patients as near totally independent as is possible.

That is how we are now defining it.

Unidentified speaker: I believe that Dr Siemsen said that he took people on to dialysis for a trial period and that they could withdraw. In the total number of cases, how many have asked to withdraw?

Siemsen: None. However, I believe the time is coming when someone will walk in and say that they are tired of the regime, that the burden is getting too great, and that they want to stop.

We have had problems making decisions, not where the patient wanted out, but where the patient was stroked out, deeply comatose, still had brainwaves but was not opening his eyes or responding, still had reflexes, and my inclination was to discontinue dialysis. In that one particular set of circumstances I was threatened with a law suit. Under such circumstances there should be ways to stop dialysis.

Our biggest area of concern now is how we are to stop.

W. R. Cattell (London): The implication earlier was that we must move towards less skilled people being available to deliver the care, and that doctors are not needed, probably nurses are not needed, and so on. This raises implications of medico-legal responsibility. I do not know about Honolulu, but in the US there are certainly problems with people suing the doctor on hand. In the limited-care situation, how would medical personnel cover themselves against being sued?

Siemsen: Most patients want to go home, or to be near their homes, and they are grateful for the opportunity to have what they are doing thoroughly explained to them.

Apart from that, I believe that one has to be a Martin Luther King and take a chance.

Cattell: Is there any legal indemnity, some kind of process for protection of those involved? Do the patients give some undertaking?

Siemsen: The limited-care facilities are all located in hospital grounds, but that is because back-up would then be on hand. We do not yet provide self-care, i.e. like at home, although that will have to come.

A. L. G. Moss (Nottingham): As a social worker I probably see things from a slightly different perspective. I was most interested in the description of the social and non-medical problems which are most important, and I tried to relate to something said by an earlier speaker to what we have been saying about limited-care. For several of the patients whom I come across their main need is to be able to dialyse in another situation apart from their own home, and in the UK it is too expensive for them to do it in hospital. I would see limited-care fulfilling that need. I maintain, and many of the patients maintain, that we ask too much of them to cope with the burden of home dialysis. It is a small percentage, but it is very important to that small percentage.

Siemsen: How many cases has Mr Moss seen where dialysis has driven a couple to divorce?

Moss: Not many personally, but I have come across cases that are on the brink, and my colleagues have also come across such cases.

Siemsen: In such circumstances it is probably best to bring the patient out of self-care facilities and to try to preserve that marriage.

Moss: Which is what I am suggesting. My point is that in the UK patients are asked to take on the burden of home dialysis. I grant that that is mainly because there is no other alternative, but patients are told that they must dialyse at home, and there is an assumption that patients and their relatives must accept that regardless. I am suggesting that that assumption is wrong.

Siemsen: I would say that too.

SECTION THREE

Some Clinical Problems
Chairman:
J. S. Cameron

7

Hypertension
J. D. Briggs

7.1 MECHANISM OF HYPERTENSION

Blood pressure commonly rises as chronic renal failure advances to the point where regular dialysis is needed to maintain life[1]. Sodium and renin have often been invoked in the pathogenesis of hypertension, and once dialysis has been initiated, it is possible to influence these two factors independently, the former by dialysis and the latter by bilateral neph-

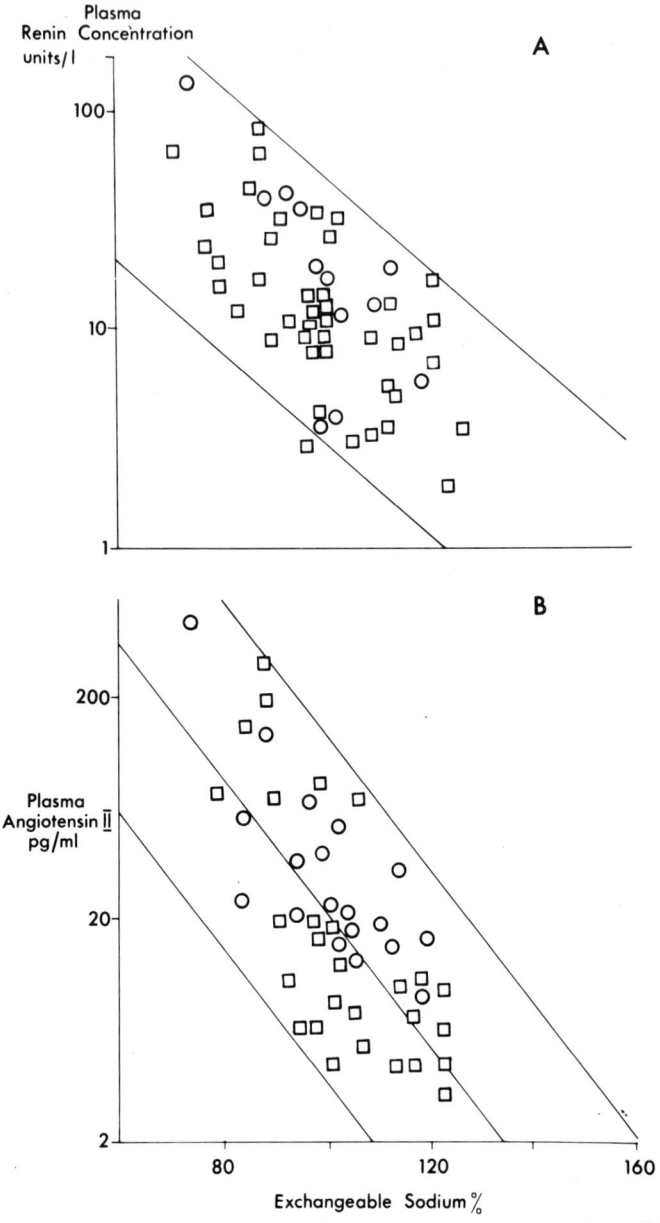

Figure 7.1 Relationship of exchangeable sodium to plasma renin (A) and to plasma angiotensin II (B) in normotensive patients with (O) and without (□) chronic renal failure

rectomy. The ability to do this has led to intensive study of hypertension in this situation.

Although excess sodium can raise blood pressure, the effect is variable and a consistent relationship between blood pressure and the level of exchangeable or plasma sodium is not commonly found in hypertensive patients[2]. Renin has a pressor effect through its active product, angiotensin II. There is, however, no close relationship between blood pressure and plasma renin in most types of hypertension[2]. By contrast, if one examines sodium and renin together, some positive relationships emerge and one cannot consider a role for sodium in hypertension in isolation from a role

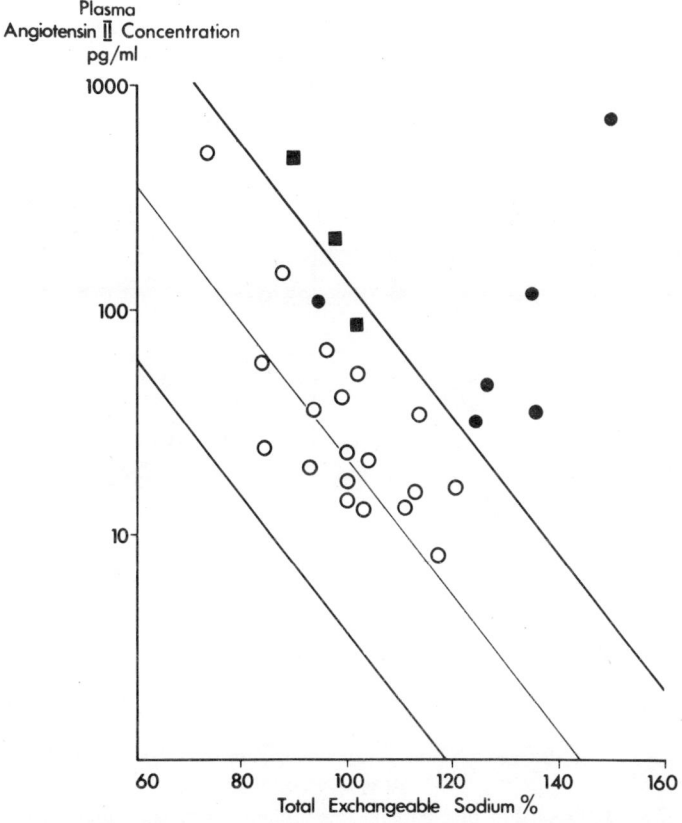

Figure 7.2 Relationship of exchangeable sodium to plasma angiotensin II in chronic renal failure patients with normal (○) and elevated (●) blood pressure. Also shown is the relationship for patients with malignant hypertension without renal failure (■)

for renin or vice versa. Figure 7.1 demonstrates the inverse relationship which exists between exchangeable sodium and both plasma renin and angiotensin II in normotensive patients with and without renal failure. As plasma renin and angiotensin II levels correlate very well in this situation, the inverse relationship with exchangeable sodium is virtually identical for each. In contrast to normotensive patients, those with hypertension and renal failure have high plasma angiotensin II levels in relation to exchangeable sodium (Figure 7.2). If the blood pressure can be restored to normal either by dialysis or bilateral nephrectomy, the abnormally high plasma angiotensin II levels will fall back to within the range in relation to exchangeable sodium which is seen in normotensive patients (Figure 7.3). Patients who are normotensive before treatment have plasma angiotensin II levels which are initially within the normal range in relation to exchangeable sodium and which remains in this range following dialysis or bilateral nephrectomy (Figure 7.3).

It is generally agreed that there are two forms of hypertension in chronic

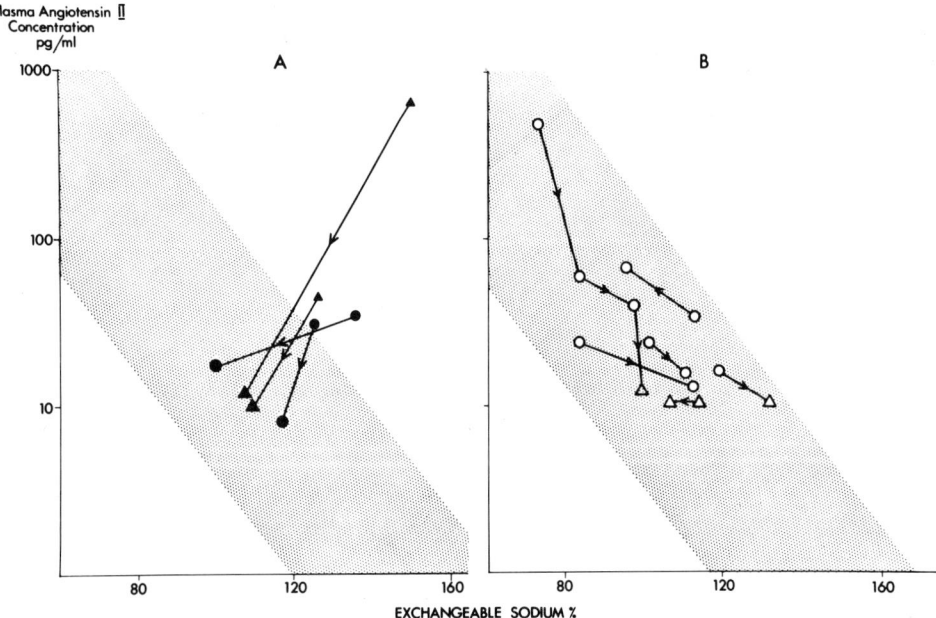

Figure 7.3   Relationship of exchangeable sodium to plasma angiotensin II. In panel A are four patients with chronic renal failure and hypertension before and after restoration of blood pressure to normal by dialysis (●) or bilateral nephrectomy (▲). In panel B are five patients with chronic renal failure without hypertension before and after dialysis (○) or bilateral nephrectomy (△)

renal failure, the more common controllable by dialysis, and an infrequent form which is unresponsive to dialysis[3]. In the former type, the relationship between plasma renin and exchangeable sodium is more horizontal than in normotensive subjects[3], as illustrated diagrammatically in Figure 7.4. This

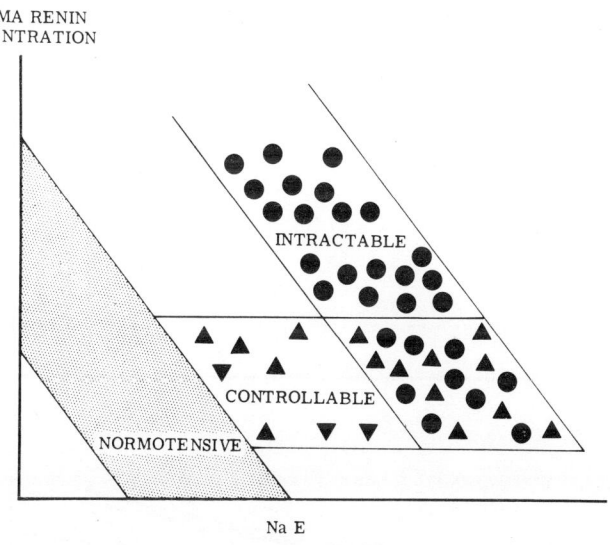

Figure 7.4 Diagrammatic representation of the relationship of exchangeable sodium (NaE) to plasma renin in chronic renal failure patients with controllable (▲) and intractable (●) hypertension

form of hypertension could arise if renin release were unresponsive to changes in sodium balance. There is supporting evidence for this in that the rise of plasma renin in patients of this type is relatively small during deprivation of dietary sodium or during sodium and water depleting dialysis treatments[4]. By contrast, in the intractable form of hypertension, plasma renin is abnormally raised in relation to exchangeable sodium, and remains so at all levels of exchangeable sodium (Figure 7.4). In these patients one would expect that an attempt to reduce blood pressure by sodium depletion would lead to a marked rise in plasma renin and such changes have in fact been demonstrated[4]. Figure 7.5 clearly illustrates the difference in renin response to dialysis in the two groups of patients. In the five patients with intractable hypertension, plasma renin rose in response

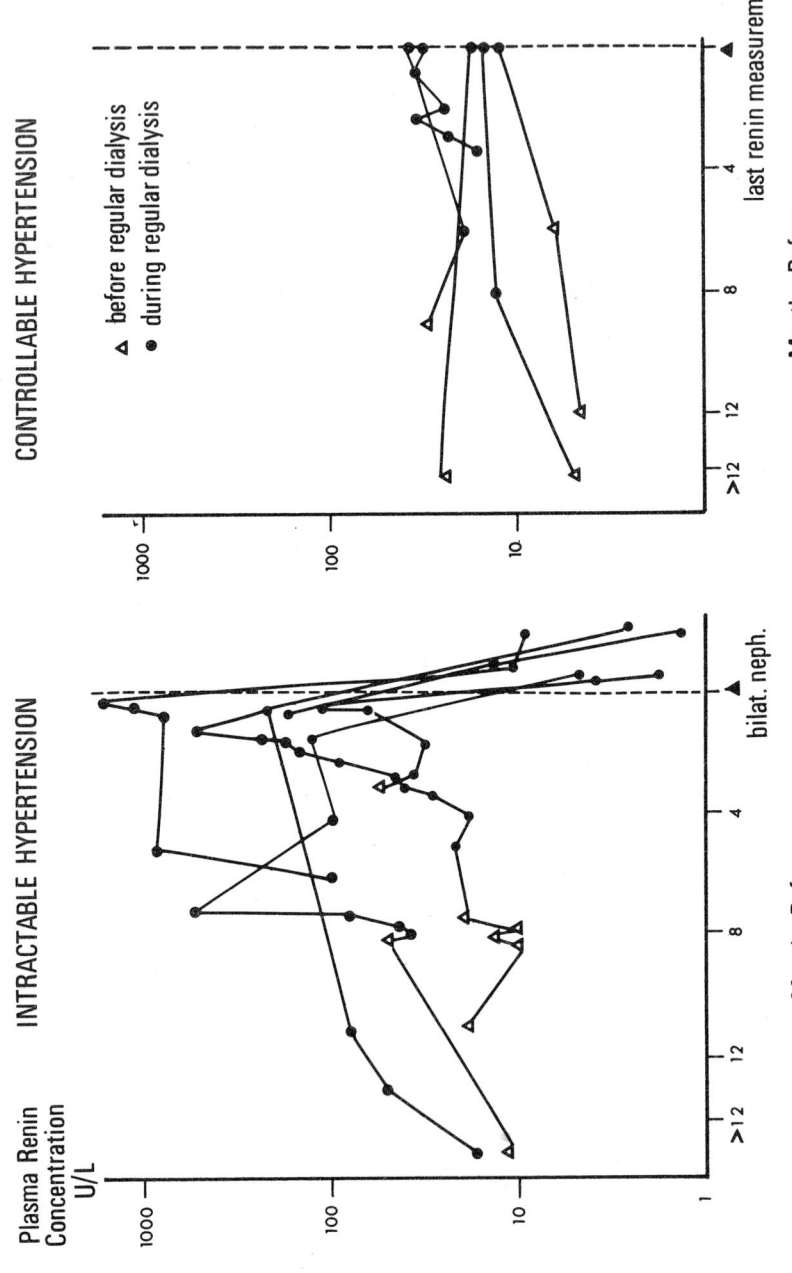

Figure 7.5 Plasma renin in chronic renal failure patients with hypertension before ($\triangle$) and during ($\bullet$) regular dialysis. On the left are five patients with intractable hypertension and on the right five patients with hypertension which was controlled by dialysis

to sodium depletion during dialysis. Following bilateral nephrectomy there was a dramatic fall in plasma renin levels. The five patients whose blood pressure was controlled by sodium removal had plasma renin levels which were within the normal range or only slightly elevated, with no significant rise in response to sodium removal by dialysis.

Thus the hypertension found in the majority of regular dialysis patients is sodium dependent and the blood pressure can be controlled by removal of sodium and water during dialysis. In the few remaining patients, plasma renin levels are high, blood pressure cannot be controlled by sodium removal, and bilateral nephrectomy may be required.

7.2 MANAGEMENT OF HYPERTENSION

The pattern illustrated diagrammatically in Figure 7.6 is a familiar one. In patients with progressive chronic renal failure, renal function will deteriorate slowly with the passage of time. This is often associated with a

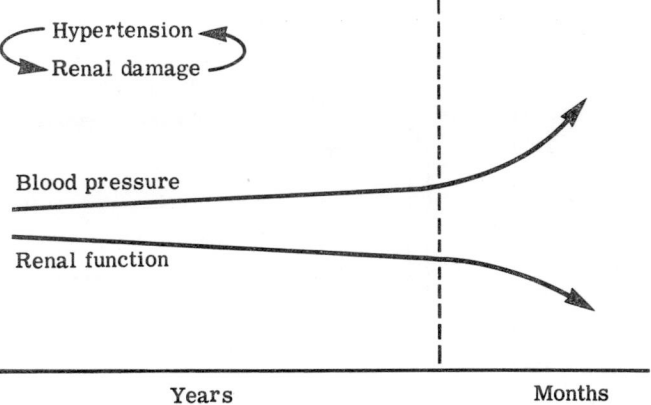

Figure 7.6   Diagrammatic representation of relationship between blood pressure and renal function in chronic renal failure.

slow rise in blood pressure, but a stage may be reached when the hypertension suddenly enters an accelerated or malignant phase. This is commonly accompanied by a much more rapid decline in renal function. Thus, good blood pressure control is essential if unnecessarily rapid deterioration in renal function is to be avoided. Several drugs are available for the control of hypertension. Of those routinely available, there is no one drug or combination of drugs which has been shown to be markedly superior to the remainder. β-Adrenergic blocking drugs have been shown to inhibit the effect of renin[5] and therefore in theory should be useful in states of 'high renin' hypertension. Our experience is that while they may be effective in this situation they are by no means invariably so. Hydralazine, which has a direct relaxant effect on vascular smooth muscle, is a useful drug and is probably best used in combination with β-blockade. Thiazide diuretics, methyl dopa, clonidine and prazosin all have a place either on their own or in combination. Bethanidine is a less satisfactory drug than those just mentioned in view of the undesirable degree of postural hypotension which it often produces.

Finally minoxidil (6-imino-1,2-dihydro-1-hydroxy-2-imino-4-piperidinopyrimidine) has been shown to be a potent antihypertensive in patients with renal and other forms of hypertension[6,7]. Minoxidil has a direct relaxant effect on vascular smooth muscle and in addition has two other almost invariable effects, an increase in heart rate and sodium retention[8]. To counteract these two effects it should be given with a β-adrenergic blocking drug and with a diuretic. Forty-four patients, half of whom had impaired renal function, have been treated with minoxidil in the Glasgow

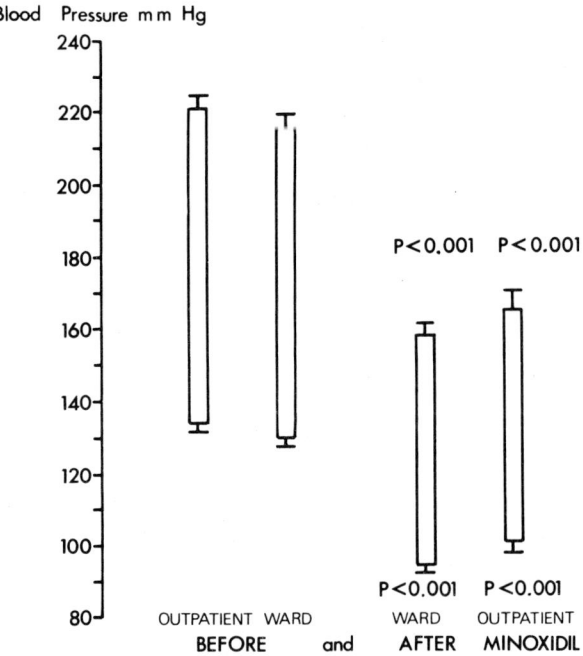

Figure 7.7   Mean supine blood pressure in 44 patients, 22 of whom had impaired renal function, before and after the administration of minoxidil

Blood Pressure Clinic. All were refractory to the commonly used anti-hypertensive drugs with diastolic blood pressure levels greater than 120 mmHg despite treatment. Figure 7.7 shows that blood pressure control with minoxidil was excellent both in the ward and later under out-patient conditions. Side-effects in these 44 patients consisted of fluid retention with left ventricular failure in three patients, gynaecomastia in three patients and invariable hirsutism. While not of undue consequence in the male, the degree of hirsutism in the female patients was disfiguring, but could be markedly improved by the use of a depilating cream.

7.3 HYPERTENSION IN PATIENTS UNDERGOING REGULAR HAEMODIALYSIS

In the majority of patients blood pressure can be controlled by removal of sodium and water during dialysis. Using changes in body weight as an index of alteration in body water and salt content, Figure 7.8 shows how

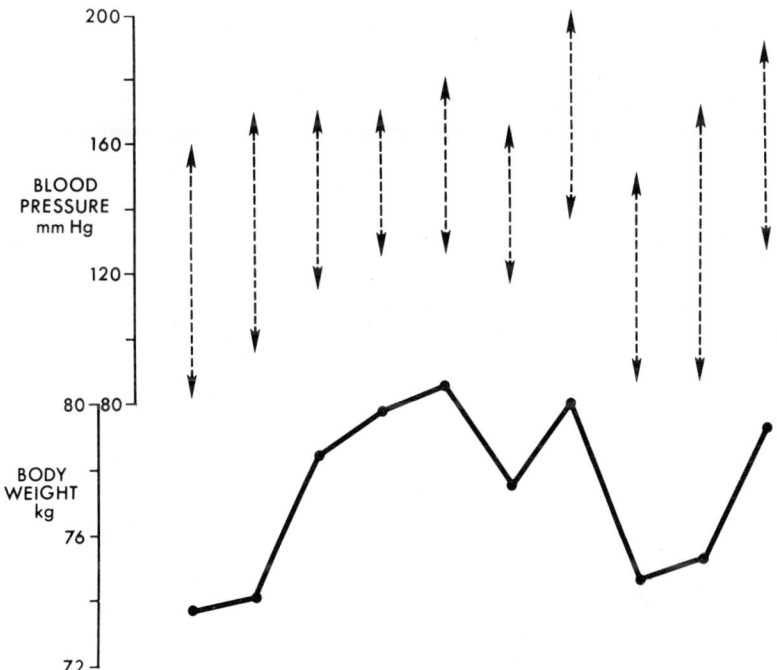

Figure 7.8 Serial supine blood pressure and body weight measurements in a regular dialysis patient showing the close relationship between blood pressure and body weight

these correlate closely with blood pressure. The proportion of patients whose blood pressure can be controlled by dialysis alone varies between centres, but the usual proportion is in the range 70–80%[9,10]. In most of the remaining patients, adequate blood-pressure control can be achieved by the use of antihypertensive drugs, but a small group of patients remain whose blood pressure is refractory to both dialysis and drugs. In the Western Infirmary, 8% of dialysis patients have been in this third group and in several cases, bilateral nephrectomy has had to be performed as an emergency because of the severity of the hypertension. Although in our experience the blood-pressure response to bilateral nephrectomy has almost always been excellent[11], there is a significant morbidity. Of the 12 patients nephrectomized in the Western Infirmary because of intractable hypertension, five developed major post-operative complications, and one of these died. A further two patients developed minor complications. In addition to the immediate post-operative morbidity, a fall in haemoglobin invariably occurred, leading to a reduced quality of health and sometimes the need for regular blood transfusion.

Because of the undesirable effects of bilateral nephrectomy, patients should be carefully assessed before the decision is taken to proceed with

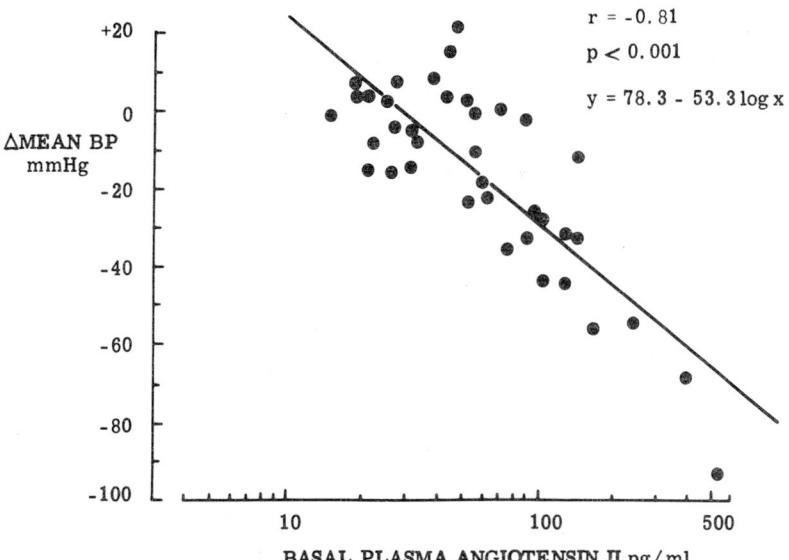

Figure 7.9   Basal plasma angiotensin II plotted against the change in mean blood pressure during the infusion of saralasin in 38 patients with various types of hypertension

this operation. Three criteria can be used. Firstly in all cases the patient should have hypertension which is refractory to dialysis and drugs. Secondly, the plasma renin or angiotensin II level should be significantly elevated or thirdly, as an alternative, the blood pressure should fall during the infusion of saralasin.

Saralasin is an octapeptide with six of its amino acid constituents identical to those of angiotensin II. Only the two terminal amino acids differ, saralasin containing sarcosine and alanine while angiotensin II contains asparagine and phenylalanine. As a consequence of its chemical similarity, saralasin acts as a competitive inhibitor to the action of angiotensin II. A saralasin infusion will therefore lower the blood pressure in patients with high plasma angiotensin II levels. Figure 7.9 shows the good

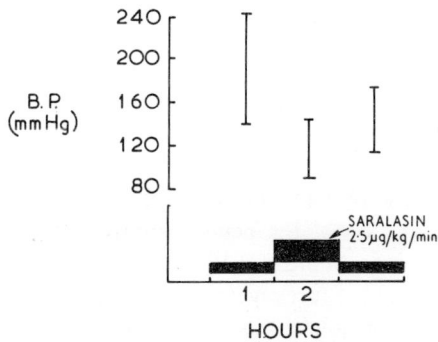

Figure 7.10   Supine blood pressure before, during and after the infusion of saralasin in a regular dialysis patient with intractable hypertension

correlation which exists between the degree of blood pressure fall during a saralasin infusion and the plasma angiotensin II levels. The figure was compiled with results from patients with a variety of types of hypertension. Most of the dialysis patients with severe hypertension are represented by circles in the bottom right-hand corner as they have much higher plasma angiotensin II levels than most other hypertensive patients. Figure 7.10 shows an example of the blood-pressure lowering effect of a saralasin infusion in a dialysis patient with intractable hypertension. This patient subsequently had an excellent blood-pressure response to bilateral nephrectomy. A saralasin infusion can therefore predict whether hypertension is likely to benefit from bilateral nephrectomy and provides useful confirmation of the significance of a high plasma angiotensin II level. It can also provide sufficient information on its own should plasma renin or angiotensin II measurements not be available.

Treatment policy in the Western Infirmary for dialysis patients with intractable hypertension is currently changing for two reasons. Firstly there is concern with regard to the morbidity associated with bilateral nephrectomy. Secondly the availability of minoxidil, with its markedly superior effect to previously available antihypertensives, has reduced the need for nephrectomy.

We have treated with minoxidil three dialysis patients whose blood pressure was resistant to dialysis and conventional antihypertensive drugs. The mean lying blood pressure on conventional drug therapy was 198/124. At 2–4 months after starting minoxidil the mean lying blood pressure had fallen to 148/89. This blood-pressure response was not associated with any side-effects nor was it due to any concomitant reduction in body weight.

7.4   BLOOD PRESSURE FOLLOWING RENAL TRANSPLANTATION

Forty-one patients were picked at random from those followed up for at least 2 years after successful transplantation. Twenty-two of these patients were on antihypertensive therapy at this time. Fourteen of the 41 patients had, for various reasons, had bilateral nephrectomy performed prior to transplantation. Only 7% of the nephrectomized patients were receiving antihypertensive therapy compared to 78% of those not previously nephrectomized. Very similar figures were reported by Cohen in a series of 81 patients[12]. Thus pre-transplant bilateral nephrectomy, irrespective of the indication for its performance, undoubtedly has a beneficial effect on blood pressure following transplantation. Curtis *et al.* showed that additional factors favouring a normal blood pressure were good graft function, the use of living related, as against cadaver donors, and alternate-day steroid therapy[13].

7.5   CONCLUSIONS

Blood pressure can be controlled in most regular haemodialysis patients by a combination of a low sodium intake and removal of excess sodium by dialysis. Some patients, however, require antihypertensive drugs as well. In a small number, 5–10% in most series, blood-pressure control is poor and our policy until now has been bilateral nephrectomy in these patients. In the future, the use of minoxidil will reduce though not eliminate the need for nephrectomy. Care is required to ensure that a reduction in the incidence of nephrectomy does not lead to the presence of too many severely hypertensive patients following transplantation. It could be argued that the operative morbidity of nephrectomy would be lower in transplanted compared to dialysis patients and the disadvantage of a further fall in haemoglobin would not apply. While this is probably true, it is very difficult following transplantation to determine if the elevated blood pressure is due to ischaemia of the transplant or to the patient's own kidneys. Thus there remains a definite place for pre-transplant bilateral nephrectomy in the patient with intractable hypertension although the frequency with which this operation will be performed in the future will be less than in the past.

References

1. Brown, J. J., Dusterdieck, G. O., Fraser, R., Lever, A. F., Robertson, J. I. S., Tree, M. and Weir, R. J. (1971). Hypertension and chronic renal failure. *Br. Med. Bull.*, 27, 128

2. Davies, D. L., Beevers, D. G., Brown, J. J., Fraser, R., Ferriss, J. B., Lever, A. F., Medina, A., Morton, J. J. and Robertson, J. I. S. (1973). Sodium and the renin-angiotensin system in patients with hypertension. *Proc. IVth Int. Congr. Endocrinol.*

3. Schelekamp, M. A., Beevers, D. G., Briggs, J. D., Brown, J. J., Davies, D. L., Fraser, R., Lebel, M., Lever, A. F., Medina, A., Morton, J. J., Robertson, J. I. S. and Tree, M. (1973). Hypertension in chronic renal failure: an abnormal relation between sodium and the renin–angiotensin system. *Am. J. Med.*, 55, 379

4. Brown, J. J., Curtis, J. R., Lever, A. F., Robertson, J. I. S., De Wardener, H. E. and Wing, A. J. (1969). Plasma renin concentration and the control of blood pressure in patients on maintenance haemodialysis. *Nephron*, 6, 329

5. Bühler, F. R., Laragh, J. H., Baer, L., Vaughan, E. D. and Brunner, H. R. (1972). Propranolol inhibition of renin secretion. *N. Engl. J. Med.*, 287, 1209

6. Gottlieb, T. B., Katz, F. H. and Chidsey, C. A. (1972). Combined therapy with vasodilator drugs and beta-adrenergic blockade. *Circulation*, 45, 571

7. Limas, C. J. and Freis, E. D. (1973). Minoxidil in severe hypertension with renal failure. *Am. J. Cardiol.*, 31, 355

8. Gilmore, E., Weil, J. and Chidsey, C. (1970). Treatment of essential hypertension with a new vasodilator in combination with beta-adrenergic blockade. *N. Engl. J. Med.*, 282, 521

9. Chrysanthakopoulos, S. G., Kastagir, B. K., Jubiz, W. and Kolff, W. J. (1972). Hypertension in patients on maintenance hemodialysis: evaluation of peripheral renin activity and bilateral nephrectomy. *Am. J. Med. Sci.*, 264, 9

10. Hull, A. R., Long, D. L., Prati, R. C., Pettinger, W. A. and Parker III, T. F. (1975). The control of hypertension in patients undergoing regular maintenance dialysis. *Kidney Int.*, 7, (Suppl. 2), 184

11. Medina, A., Bell, P. R. F., Briggs, J. D., Brown, J. J., Fine, A., Lever, A. F., Morton, J. J., Paton, A. M., Robertson, J. I. S., Tree, M., Waite, M. A., Weir, R. and Winchester, J. (1972). Changes of blood pressure, renin and angiotensin after bilateral nephrectomy in patients with chronic renal failure. *Br. Med. J.*, 4, 694

12. Cohen, S. L. (1973). Hypertension in renal transplant recipients: role of bilateral nephrectomy. *Br. Med. J.*, 3, 78
13. Curtis, J. J., Galla, J. H., Kotchen, T. A., Lucas, B., McRoberts, J. W. and Luke, R. G. (1976). Prevalence of hypertension in a renal transplant population on alternate-day steroid therapy. *Clin. Nephrol.*, 5, 123

DISCUSSION

Unidentified speaker: When groups of antihypertensives were used, did several of the patients develop postural hypotension on or off dialysis?

Briggs: It was not a major problem. We have tended recently to concentrate on β-blockers and this has not been a problem with them. It is with some of the other hypertensives. Bethanidine is obviously a good example of a drug which would never be used nowadays.

Unidentified speaker: Has there been any evidence of patients presenting with so-called 'rigid vessels', and postural dropping whilst dialysing?

Briggs: We have had no trouble with that. Our policy is slightly different from average in that our patients tend to have relatively small weight gains between dialysis. They tend to put on less weight, perhaps 1 kg or 1.5 kg between dialysis, which is less than in many centres.

Unidentified speaker: How long between dialysis?

Briggs: Thrice a week.

J. A. Kanis (Oxford): I find the interrelationships between measurements such as vascular volume, renin and blood pressure, which all seem to be interdependent, difficult to understand. I wonder whether partial correlations between them have been studied in an attempt to identify causal relationships. It is difficult to infer causal influences from correlations.

I ask this because Dr Briggs mentioned that the effects of saralasin might provide the basis for a test to decide whether a patient's hypotension might respond to bilateral nephrectomy. It seems possible that the response of any hypertensive patient might be augmented by volume depletion and that volume status should be taken into account before the saralasin effect can be interpreted.

Secondly, what is the evidence that hypertension in patients with disturbed renal function has any deleterious effect on their renal tissue?

Briggs: The first point is very valid. When a saralasin test is done it is necessary to make sure that one is not dealing with a volume-depleted or sodium-depleted patient, because that would give different results. We, as a standard, always do the saralasin test immediately prior to dialysis so that we are dealing with a relatively salt-repleted patient.

There is an anecdotal impression that hypertension does destroy renal tissue. I have seen several patients whose function has deteriorated rapidly when they have entered an accelerated hypertensive phase. I am not too well up in the literature in terms of careful and full studies but it is certainly my impression, and I think that it is a fairly general impression.

J. S. Cameron: I was interested in exactly this question in patients with glomerular disease and I hunted the literature high and low to find any evidence of whether this widespread impression was indeed true. I came up with only one paper[1], a combined university/clinic 19-centre retrospective survey from Germany published in German. Retrospective data had been analysed out in terms of blood pressure, correcting out for the type of histology with and without hypertension. Hypertension had an undoubted deleterious effect in this retrospective survey – which is one of the problems with data of that kind.

As far as I am aware it is the only evidence, and there is no other prospective study, controlled or uncontrolled.

Kanis: I bring this up because we have been looking at the rate of fall of creatinine as the reciprocal of function and we have been rather impressed to find that in some patients who have started off with normotension and who have developed hypertension, the slope has not changed when they have become quite markedly hypertensive, and has, further, not changed when that hypertension has been treated.

Briggs: Possibly there is a difference where there is severe hypertension.

R. Ahmad (Liverpool): What does Dr Briggs consider to be the optimum concentration of sodium in the dialysis solution? It amazes me that the dialysis solution supplied to NHS hospitals should vary between 120 and 145 mmol.

Briggs: It is not necessary to control hypertension by running with a low dialysate sodium.

We ourselves have not tried to run at a relatively high level. I know of experiments running at 141. We run at a sodium concentration of 137 mmol/l which seems fairly average.

Reference

1. Sarre, H. *et al.* 1971. Nephrotisches Syndrom des Erwachsenenalters. *Deutsche Med. Wochenschr.*, **96**, 225

8

Dialysis encephalopathy
M. K. Ward and
T. G. Feest

8.1   INTRODUCTION

Efficient dialysis brings about a rapid reversal of the neurological syndromes seen with 'end-stage uraemia'. Sensorial clouding, perceptual errors, hallucinations, asterixis, myoclonus, focal and grand mal seizures, decerebrate and decorticate postures are all improved by adequate haemodialysis (see Raskin and Fisherman for review)[1, 2]. However patients whose lives have been prolonged by intermittent dialysis may develop other encephalopathic features. Before discussing 'dialysis encephalopathy' the differential diagnosis must be considered.

8.2   DIFFERENTIAL DIAGNOSIS

Neurological signs and symptoms are frequently seen in patients maintained on regular dialysis and have many causes. Patients may develop neurological sequelae of their primary disease process, such as hypertension or disseminated lupus erythematosis. Clouding of consciousness, delirium and hallucinations may accompany intercurrent infection, septicaemia, meningitis or encephalitis.

The metabolism and excretion of many drugs or their metabolites are altered by impaired renal function[3]. Dementia-like syndromes with or without speech disorders have been described with hypnotics, sedatives, tranquillizers, anti-parkinsonian drugs and antiepileptic therapy[4]. The benzodiazepines (flurazepam and diazepam) have been shown to produce encephalopathic syndromes[5]. Little is known about the effects of long-term administration of these drugs in dialysis patients or the possible potentiation with other drugs in uraemic man. Intermittent heparinization or continued anticoagulation exposes haemodialysis patients to the risk of subdural haematoma[6].

Because we rely on a mechanical device to maintain 'normal' levels of sodium, potassium, calcium and magnesium during dialysis there is a potential danger that acute or chronic alterations in the concentration of the dialysate due to mal-functioning proportioning units (despite so-called fail-safe devices) can lead to syndromes presenting as alteration of neurological function. Sodium and water depletion in hot weather and anaemia can present as neurological syndromes. Headache, nausea, vomiting, delirium, convulsions and obtundation are associated with fluid and electrolyte shifts produced by haemodialysis (disequilibrium syndrome)[2] and have been attributed to changes in osmotic pressure and pH within the brain and CSF[7]. Because the semi-permeable membrane is a passive device essential substances as well as 'toxins' can transfer out of or into the patient during haemodialysis. An encephalopathic syndrome attributed to thiamine deficiency has been described[8]. Acute copper intoxication has been described due to rapid transfer of copper from dialysate to blood showing that dialysate contaminated with trace elements can cause toxic symptoms[9].

8.3   DIALYSIS ENCEPHALOPATHY SYNDROME

8.3.1   Introduction

First described by Alfrey[10] in 1972 this neurological syndrome has become well documented in Europe (150 cases recorded at EDTA, Helsinki, 1977), Japan[11], Australia[12] and centres in the USA[13,14], and has been a significant cause of death in dialysis populations.

8.3.2   Clinical description of neurological syndrome (Newcastle-upon-Tyne)

Between 1970 and May 1977, 17 patients on haemodialysis were seen with this neurological syndrome. Fifteen presented with a distinctive inter-mittent slurring of speech towards the end of dialysis or within a few minutes of the termination of dialysis. This was often first noted by rela-tives or nursing staff. Two patients presented with fits 6 months before their speech disorder became apparent. Patients deteriorated over a period of 5 to 17 months to a stage where they were unable to speak or talk intelligibly. All patients developed intellectual impairment progressing in nine to global dementia and death. Disordered motor function varied from myoclonic jerks of facial muscles and limbs to widespread muscular spasms involving the whole of the body. These were often precipitated by attempted speech, lifting limbs against gravity or walking. Personality changes, depression, aggressive outbursts and emotional lability were prominent features in five of the patients. Six patients developed a cere-bellar syndrome characterized by incoordination of limbs or speech associated with a fatigue phenomenon, accurate limb movements and speech becoming disorganized after a few minutes' effort which improved after a period of rest.

The most useful diagnostic test was an electroencephalogram which showed a distinctive pattern with an increase in slow wave activity associ-ated with spike and slow wave bursts[14, 15].

We have been impressed with the close association of this syndrome and the osteomalacic type of renal ostedystrophy seen in patients on intermittent haemodialysis in the Northern Region[16]. Fifteen of the 17 patients had evidence of bone pain or myopathy and 14 out of 15 patients who had bone biopsies showed the picture commonly seen in Newcastle of osteomalacia with little or no osteitis fibrosa. Platts[17], Flendrig[18] and Alfrey[19] have also noted this association of the encephalopathic syndrome with renal osteodystrophy.

8.3.3   Therapy

No successful therapy has been reported. Attempts with levodopa, dimercaprol, penicillamine, rubidium, dexamethasone, physostigmine, vitamins[11] and bromocryptine[40] have all failed. Myoclonic jerks and grand mal seizures can be controlled with intermittent diazepam or clonazepam. Three of our patients remained static with little progression of encephalopathy over 3–9 months when phosphate binders were discontinued and they were transferred to a deionized water supply. Improvement has been seen in two patients who had successful renal transplantation[20], although five other patients reported from the same unit showed progressive deterioration after renal transplantation despite good renal function. This experience of the failure of transplantation to affect the progression of the neurological disease is the more commonly reported outcome[16, 17]. In fact, Platts[17] reported the presentation of the syndrome following successful renal transplantation. Improvement has been reported in one case following parathyroidectomy and hypercalcaemia was thought to be a contributing factor only[21].

8.3.4   Histopathology

No gross macroscopic abnormalities in the brain have been reported. The documented abnormalities were histopathological. Features noted included astrocyte proliferation with neuronal loss in the cortex, and purkinge cell loss with Bergman gliosis in the cerebellum[11, 16]. This lack of specific histological and macroscopic abnormalities suggest that the aetiology is probably a toxic metabolic encephalopathy[11].

8.4   AETIOLOGY OF DIALYSIS ENCEPHALOPATHY

8.4.1   Introduction

There are no histological features that suggest either known bacteriological or virus infection as the aetiological agent. A 'slow' virus is an alternative hypothesis but to date no animal passage experiments performed either in the USA or in the UK have reproduced the encephalopathic syndrome.

Maintenance haemodialysis exposes patients to the risk of a 'deficiency syndrome' or the accumulation of a 'toxic substance'. It seems unlikely that the distinct geographical distribution of this syndrome can be accounted for by minor differences in dialysis technique, or by a deficiency syndrome produced by dialysis. It seems more likely that the distinct geographical distribution supports the hypothesis that it is an accumulation of one or more toxic substances.

8.4.2   Evidence for aluminium as the possible 'toxin'

Aluminium is the most plentiful metal in the earth's crust and is only exceeded in abundance by silica and oxygen. Unlike other metals no biological functions have been demonstrated for aluminium and there is no evidence that it is a major coenzyme factor in man[22]. Although exposure of man to aluminium is inevitable there are very few reports of illness in workers working in the production and processing of aluminium which has been directly attributed to aluminium toxicity. The commonest problem encountered is that of pulmonary fibrosis in workers exposed to pulverised aluminium metal[23]. However McLaughlin and co-workers[24] described one man working in a ball mill using aluminium flake powder who developed a strikingly similar encephalopathic syndrome to that described in our dialysis patients. Tissue aluminium levels in this patient were found to be extremely high.

A recent review of studies in laboratory animals with orally administered aluminium compounds documents the conflicting results obtained[22]. It appears that if hypophosphataemia is avoided then there is little evidence of aluminium being toxic when given orally, although there is inconclusive evidence that aluminium-loaded animals may have a disturbance of phosphate metabolism even when hypophosphataemia is avoided[25].

However, the direct application of aluminium-containing compounds to nervous tissue in animal models was first shown to be toxic more than 30 years ago[26].

8.4.3   Accumulation of aluminium in man

The total body burden of aluminium may be increased by absorption from the gastrintestinal tract or by direct parenteral administration. Clarkson and colleagues[27] performed balanced studies on patients with chronic renal failure receiving aluminium-containing phosphate binders which showed that they could easily be placed in a positive aluminium balance. Kaehny and colleagues[28] showed a rise in plasma aluminium levels and urinary excretion of aluminium in normal subjects taking aluminium-containing compounds. A recent survey[29] showed that ingestion of aluminium-containing compounds among haemodialysis patients in Europe did not correlate with the encephalopathic syndrome. If aluminium accumulation is the cause of dementia this suggests that the gastrointestinal tract may not be the major source of aluminium in patients maintained on intermittent haemodialysis or the prescribed dose was not ingested by the patients. However, we have seen one patient with chronic renal failue not on intermittent haemodialysis who was given aluminium hydroxide 80–100 ml daily for 12 months and regular monthly estimations of serum phosphate showed that she never became hypophosphataemic. This patient developed myopathy, bone pain and dementia. Histopathology showed that her bone lesion was predominantly osteomalacia with little osteitis fibrosa, a similar picture to that seen in patients on haemodialysis in Newcastle-upon-Tyne[30].

The major source of aluminium appears to be the water supply used in the preparation of dialysate for haemodialysis. Flendrig, Krus and Das[18] reported the appearance of the encephalopathic syndrome associated with myopathy and fractured bones in patients dialysed in his unit which used the same water supply as another unit where the syndrome was not seen. It was found that aluminium electrodes placed in the water supply to his dialysis unit had dissolved and that the water supply had become contaminated with aluminium. The other dialysis unit had not used the same aluminium electrode system. There was a striking increase in the tissue level of aluminium in the patients dying of encephalopathy in his dialysis unit compared to patients dying with normal renal function, patients dying with chronic renal failure and patients with chronic renal failure who were dialysed in other centres in Holland.

This is the nearest to a double-blind control trial of intravenously administered aluminium compounds that is ever likely to be carried out in man. Previously, Alfrey and associates[31] had studied a considerable number of trace metals in the tissues of patients dying of chronic uraemia and dialysis encephalopathy (Cu, Fe, Zn, As, Se, Br, Rb, Si, Mo, Cd, Sn, Pb and Al). They found a strikingly significant elevation in the aluminium content of the tissues of patients dying with encephalopathy when compared with patients dying with normal renal function and dialysis patients dying of other causes. Table 8.1 documents the tissue aluminium content of dialysed uraemic patients who died of other causes (DO) compared to those who died with encephalopathy (DE) and a control group who died

TABLE 8.1   Tissue aluminium in dialysed uraemic patients who died of other causes (DO) compared to those who died with encephalopathy (DE) and a control group who died with normal renal function (C)

Author	Method	C	DO	DE
(A) Brain (mg/kg)				
Flendrig 1976[18]	NA	11.9 (2)*	12.1 (2)	90.8 (4)
Alfrey 1976[19]	FAAS	1.3 (6)†	7.63 (6)	24.98 (6) (grey matter)
Ward 1976[16]	FAAS	9.5 (4)†	—	26.5 (4) (grey matter)
(B) Liver (mg/kg)				
Flendrig 1976[18]	NA	15.8 (7)*	32.9 (5)	610.2 (4)
Alfrey 1976[19]	FAAS	4.3 (11)†	182.0 (6)	381.0 (14)
(C) Bone (mg/kg)				
Flendrig 1976[18]	NA	10.6 (4)*	23.5 (5)	272.0 (2)
Alfrey 1976[19]	FAAS	2.4 (7)†	104.0 (28)	251.0 (12)

NA = Neutron activation
FAAS = Flameless atomic absorption spectrophotometry
* Dry tissue
† Dry defatted tissue
( ) = Numer of studies

with normal renal function (C). It has been known since 1971[32] that patients in Newcastle have had a high aluminium content in their bones, and in four patients with dialysis encephalopathy frontal lobe grey matter had elevated aluminium levels when compared with a control group[16]. Four dialysis units in the United Kingdom account for 70% of the case reports of patients with the encephalopathic syndrome (Plymouth, Leeds, Sheffield, Newcastle)[33]. In all these areas there is either naturally high aluminium content in the water or alum precipitation is used as a method of water treatment (range of aluminium level is 30–1200 μg/l)[34]. Among 12 renal units in the London area dialysis encephalopathy is rare and 'Newcastle bone disease' uncommon. The water supply to the renal units in London is from supplies that do not normally use alum coagulation and do not have a high natural aluminium content to the water (aluminium level usually less than 50 μg/l)[34].

Aluminium is not removed efficiently by water softeners or by a weak based deionizer which is nearing regeneration. Aluminium appears to be most efficiently removed by reverse osmosis with or without polishing deionization depending on the reverse osmosis unit used providing the unit and membrane are intact[35].

8.5   PREVENTION BY ADEQUATE WATER TREATMENT

The failure to treat effectively the encephalopathic syndrome and the osteo-malacic type of bone disease suggests that the metabolic inhibitor or inhibitors causes irreversible alteration to the metabolic mechanisms effected or is so well bound within the body that it is not easily removed. It has been shown[36-38] that prevention by adequate water treatment from the initiation of haemodialysis is the most effective treatment for severe osteomalacic bone disease. No patients treated for the whole of their dialysis history on deionized water in Newcastle have developed encephalopathy.

The correlation of tissue aluminium content with duration of dialysis[19] may suggest that the accumulation is passive and the metal inert. Cartier[39] found high tissue levels in dialysed patients with or without the encephalopathic syndrome. The dose and rate of aluminium accumulation and individual patient differences to increased total body aluminium have not been studied in man. It is possible that aluminium needs another factor or is a marker and these water supplies have an unassociated but as yet undetermined toxin.

8.6   CONCLUSIONS

1. Neurological syndromes presenting in patients on haemodialysis are not uncommon and may be due to a variety of factors.
2. Dialysis encephalopathy syndrome is a distinct neurological syndrome, usually associated with myopathy and bone disease, characterized by osteomalacia with little or no osteitis fibrosa.
3. Higher tissue aluminium levels have been demonstrated in patients dying with the dialysis encephalopathy syndrome than dialysis patients dying of other causes in Europe, Australia and the USA.
4. The geographical distribution of the encephalopathic syndrome within the UK is associated with areas known to have a high natural aluminim content of the water or where alum precipitation is used in the water treatment.
5. Aluminium is not removed efficiently by water softeners, the most commonly used water treatment for haemodialysis in the UK.
6. The above evidence is highly suggestive that aluminium is toxic to uraemic man maintained on intermittent haemodialysis though the mechanism is not understood.
7. Adequate water treatment from the initiation of dialysis appears to prevent the development of dialysis encephalopathy and the associated osteomalacic type of renal osteodystrophy.

ACKNOWLEDGEMENTS

We are indebted to Professor D. N. S. Kerr for unending help and encouragement, to Professor D. A. S. Shaw and members of the Department of Neurology, Professor B. Tomlinson and Dr R. Perry of the Department of Neuropathology and the Scientific Services of the Regional Water Authorities for providing data on the aluminium content of the water supplies.

References

1. Raskin, M. M. and Fishman, A. R. (1976). Neurological disorders in renal failure (Part I). *N. Engl. J. Med.*, **294**, 3, 143
2. Raskin, M. M. and Fishman, A. R. (1976). Neurological disorders in renal failure (Part II). *N. Engl. J. Med.*, **294**
3. Kerr, D. N. S., Dettli, L., Rawlins, M., Leber, H. W. and Maddocks, J. (1976). Drug metabolism in uraemic renal failure. *Proc. ED.T.A.*, **13**, 597 (London: Pitman Medical)
4. McCelland, M. A. (1977). Psychiatric Disorders. In O. M. Davis (ed.). *Textbook of Adverse Drug Reactions*, pp. 335–349 (Oxford: Oxford University Press)
5. Taclob, L. and Needle, M. (1976). Drug induced encephalopathy in patients on maintenance haemodialysis. *Lancet*, **ii**, 704
6. Leonard, A. and Shapiro, F. L. (1975). Subdural haematoma in regularly haemodialysed patients. *Ann. Intern. Med.*, **82**, 650
7. Arieff, A. Z., Massiz, S. G. and Bonientos, A. (1973). Brain water and electrolyte metabolism in uraemia, effects of slow and rapid haemodialysis. *Kidney Int.*, **4**, 177
8. Lopez, R. I. and Collins, G. K. (1968). Wernicke's encephalopathy: a complication of chronic haemodialysis. *Arch. Neurol.*, **18**, 248
9. Lyle, H. I., Payton, J. E. and Hui, M. (1976). Haemodialysis and copper fever. *Lancet*, **i**, 1324
10. Alfrey, A. C., Mischell, J. M., Barks, J. S., Coniguglia, S. R., Rudolph, M., Lewine E. and Holmes, J. M. (1977). Syndrome of praxia and multifocal seizures associated with haemodialysis. *Trans. Am. Soc. Artif. Intern. Organs*, **18**, 257
11. Barks, J. S., Alfrey, A. C., Huddlestone, J., Norenberg, M. D. and Lewine, E. (1976). A fatal encephalopathy in chronic haemdialysis patients, *Lancet*, **ii**, 764
12. Barratt, L. J. and Lawrence, J. R. (1975). Dialysis associated dementia. *Aust. N. Z. J. Med.*, **5**, 62
13. Mahurkar, S. D., Dhar, S. R., Saltra, R., Meyers, L., Smith, E. C. and Dunea, G. (1973). Dialysis dementia, *Lancet*, **1**, 1412
14. Chokroverty, S., Bruetman, M. E., Berger, V. and Reyes, M. G. (1976). Progressive dialytic encephalopathy. *J. Neurol., Neurosurg. Psychiat.*, **39**, 411
15. Nodel, A. M., Wilson, W. P. (1976). Dialysis encephalopathy: a possible seizure disorder. *Neurology*, **26**, 1130

16. Ward, M. K., Pierides, A. M., Fawcett, P., Shaw, D. A., Perry, A. M., Tomlinson, B. E. and Kerr, D. N. S. (1976). Dialysis encephalopathy syndrome. *Proc. E.D.T.A.*, **13**, 348 (London: Pitman Medical)

17. Platts, M. M., Moorehead, P. J. and Greech (1973). Dialysis dementia. *Lancet*, ii, 159

18. Flendrig, J. A., Krus, H. and Das, H. A. (1976). Aluminium intoxication: the cause of dialysis dementia? *Proc. E.D.T.A.*, **13**, 355 (London: Pitman Medical)

19. Alfrey, A. C., Le Grendrere, G. R. and Kaehny, W. P. (1976). The dialysis encephalopathy syndrome. *N. Engl. J. Med.*, **294**, 184

20. Silke, B., Fitzgerald, G. R., Hanson, S., Carmody, M. and O'Dwyer, W. F. (1977). Treatment of dialysis dementia by renal transplantation, Abstract *E.D.T.A.*, Helsinki, p. 266

21. Ball, J. M., Barkas, D. E. and Madison, D. S. (1977). Effect of subtotal parathyroidectomy on dialysis dementia. *Nephron*, **18**, 151

22. Sorenson, J. R. J., Campbell, R. I., Tepper, L. B. and Limgg, R. D. (1974). Aluminium in the environment and human health. *Environ. Hlth Perspect.*, **8**, 3

23. Jordan, J. W. (1961). Pulmonary fibrosis in a worker using aluminium powder, *Br. J. Indust. Med.*, **18**, 21.

24. McLaughlin, A. F. G., Kazantizis, G., King, E., Teare, D., Porter, R. J. and Owen, R. (1962). Pulmonary fibrosis and encephalopathy associated with inhalation of aluminium dust. *Br. J. Indust. Med.*, **19**, 253

25. Ondreicka, R., Kortus, J. and Ginter, E. (1971). Aluminium: its absorption, distribution and effects on phosphorous metabolism. In S. C. Skorgra and D. Waldron-Edward (eds.). *Intestinal Absorption of Metal Ions, Trace Elements and Radio Nuclides*, p. 293 (Oxford: Pergamon Press)

26. Faeth, W. M. (1955). Threshold studies on production of experimental epilepsy with alumina cream. *Proc. Soc. Exp. Biol. Med.*, **88**, 329

27. Clarkson, E. M., Lucks, V. A., Hynson, W. V., Bailey, R. R., Eastwood, J. B., Woodhead, J. S., Clements, V. R., O'Riordan, L. H. and De Warden, H. E. (1972). The effect of aluminium hydroxide on calcium, phosphorous and aluminium balances, the serum parathyroid hormone concentration and the aluminium content of bone in patients with chronic renal failure. *Clin. Sci.*, **43**, 519

28. Kaehny, W. D., Hegg, A. P. and Alfrey, A. C. (1977). Gastrointestinal absorption of aluminium from aluminium containing antacids. *N. Engl. J. Med.*, **296**, 1389

29. Jacobs, C., Brunner, F. P., Chantler, C., Donckerwolcke, R. A., Gurland, H. J., Hathway, R. A., Selwood, N. H. and Wing, A. J. (1977). Combined report on intermittent dialysis and renal transplantation in Europe, VII, 1976. *Proc. E.D.T.A.*, **14**, 3. (London: Pitman)

30. Ellis, H. A. and Peart, K. M. (1973). Azotaemia renal osteodystrophy: a quantitative study on iliac bone. *J. Clin. Pathol.*, **26**, 83

31. Alfrey, A. C., Smythe, W. R., Ibels, I. S. and Mannelly, L. L. (1976). Trace element abnormalities in chronic uraemia. *Second Annual Progress Report* (University of Colorado)

32. Parsons, V., Davis, C., Goode, C., Ogg, C. and Siddiqui, J. (1971). The aluminium content of bone in patients on haemodialysis. *Br. Med. J.*, **4**, 273

33. Ward, M. K. (1977). Survey of United Kingdom Dialysis Units. (In preparation)
34. Scientific Services of the United Kingdom Water Authorities
35. Strong, A., Ward, M. K., Parkinson, I. and the Scientific Services (Wear Division), Northumbria Water Authority. (In preparation)
36. Posen, G. A., Gray, D. G., Jaworsky, R., Couture, R. and Rashid, A. (1972). Comparison of renal osteodystrophy in patients dialysed with deionised and non-deionised water. *Trans. Am. Soc. Artif. Intern. Organs.*, **18**, 405
37. Leather, H. (1975). Dialysis bone disease in Plymouth. Presented at *Dialysis Symposium 1975* (Elga Publication)
38. Kerr, D. N. S. (1977). Renal osteodystrophy (The Osmond Lecture). Presented at the Renal Association
39. Cartier, F., Allain, P., Peckers, G. J. and Garre, M. (1977). Comparative study of patients with and without encephalopathy syndrome, Abstract *E.D.T.A.*, Helsinki, p. 186
40. Ward, M. K. (1976). Unpublished observation

DISCUSSION

B. Silke (Dublin): In the 3-year period 1972–75 we had 15 cases of dialysis dementia, but unlike the Newcastle group we have had no evidence whatsoever of mineral bone disease occurring in association with this syndrome. Perhaps this reflects a local bone problem in Newcastle. None of our patients had significant osteomalacia or hypophosphataemia.

In our experience transplantation proved the only effective treatment and two patients showed significant improvement as evidenced by a reversal of clinical and EEG parameters.

However, what is important is that in an 18-month period we have seen no new cases, despite no alterations in treatment or dialysis technique. We are therefore doubtful of the aluminium intoxication theory or the significance of the various phosphate binders. We believe that this is a disease that came, and is perhaps on the wane. We are happy to see it go away because we were not able to do anything that had any effect on it. Could this syndrome be getting less, or is it just a localized phenomenon?

Ward: I do not think that it is getting less in the UK. A survey is in progress to discover whether there have been any new cases since the regional survey was completed in 1975.

At least half of our patients were on home dialysis. They used different dialysers and different types of proportionating units and we do not think that the dialyser makes any difference.

Aluminium intoxication has not been excluded. Unless the aluminium content of the water supply and the patient is known it is not possible to prove that it is not due to aluminium intoxication. We were fooled by this for a while. In fact, the aluminium in the water supply goes up and down like a yo-yo, and it can be anything from 50 μg to 1.5 mg/l in the same water supply over a period of time, and without following it regularly one can have no idea of the cumulative mean aluminium content that these patients are exposed to. Dr Silke did not say whether they measured the aluminium content in the water supply, or in the brain. I am glad to hear of the success with transplantation and that this syndrome is apparently on the wane.

We have some evidence that the aluminium content in one geographical area in the UK appeared to be satisfactory for 9 months to a year, and suddenly mean levels rose towards the end of 1976. If the experiments in animals can be extrapolated to man, then there is a delay period between the accumulation of aluminium and the clinical syndrome. Cases of dementia may be seen within the next 6–9 months. Animal experiments have shown that there is a delay before the syndrome develops once the aluminium has been given to the animals.

I do not know why aluminium is toxic. In Newcastle we are convinced that it is something in the water, and we have been suspicious of this for about 8 years. We compared ourselves with East Birmingham to see whether there was any connection with fluoride, and were unable to find any (both Newcastle and East Birmingham have fluoridated water). East Birmingham has no bone disease, and no dementia – and nor is it on an aluminium containing water supply! The aluminium-containing water supply areas are Plymouth, where there are cases of dementia and bone disease; the Leeds area, where cases of dementia and bone disease occur; Sheffield, where there are cases of dementia and bone disease, and Glasgow. I am not so sure about Glasgow. The water supply has a small amount of aluminium in it, but most of the cases in Glasgow come from the Highlands, and we hope to be able to measure the content of aluminium in the Highland water.

In the non-alum water treatment areas, London and the Thames Basin, where aluminium coagulation is not used for water treatment, there is virtually no histological Newcastle bone disease, and no dementia. Therefore the evidence epidemiologically is extremely strong.

J. A. Kanis (Oxford): That there is no clinical evidence of osteomalacia would not necessarily mean that there is no histological evidence of osteomalacia. I have certainly been impressed by the association of dialysis dementia with the histological appearance of osteomalacia. There is no proof that aluminium and dialysis dementia are causally related and the aluminium may be a marker for another compound.

Ward: I accept that, though it is difficult to interpret Dr Flendrig's data unless there is more than one toxin.

Kanis: In view of Dr Ward's comments on the possible effects of calcium phosphate transport this may be meaningful.

I read an interesting abstract – I cannot remember where – on the effects of parathyroidectomy on dialysis dementia. Would Dr Ward comment on that?

Ward: That patient was extremely hypercalcaemic, and this may have been contributing to the syndrome, but I cannot interpret that completely.

R. Ahmad (Liverpool): We must be sure to classify dementia into two categories, reversible dementia and irreversible dementia. We must be sure that we are not removing something from the patients. The artificial kidney does not perform like a normal kidney. It may be that for patients on a restricted protein diet something essential is being removed and that that, and not the aluminium, is the cause of the problem.

Ward: I entirely agree that we do not know what we are removing from our patients. We have tried to exclude the phosphate problem. We know that thiamine can cause a dementia-like syndrome. Earlier in the Paper I outlined some of the things that must be excluded – thiamine and other problems and drugs. The 'removal theory' does not explain the geographical distribution. We are now so convinced that it is a water-born toxin that we have decreed that no patient may go home unless he is on a de-ionizer, or on some form of water therapy that will remove whatever is in the water supply. I agree that aluminium may still be a marker and could accumulate in the brain as a secondary phenomenon, but I would subscribe to the view that the more likely explanation is that which I have already given, that somehow the aluminium is the toxic agent, or its metabolic influence on uraemic man is the toxic influence.

If patients continue to be dialysed on aluminium-containing water supplies I would be very interested, because in 2 or 3 years' time we would be able to compare the Newcastle group with that group and see whether we have solved the problems and they have not.

9

Anaemia in patients with chronic renal failure treated by intermittent haemodialysis – aetiology and treatment
R. J. Winney and
J. S. Robson

9.1   INTRODUCTION

In recent years understanding of the pathogenesis of the anaemia associated with chronic renal failure has increased more slowly than knowledge of bone disease. As a result progress in the treatment of anaemia has been overshadowed by the more dramatic success of the synthetic vitamin D metabolites in the treatment of renal osteodystrophy. Nevertheless progress has been made and anaemia should not now severely restrict the activities of the majority of haemodialysis patients.

9.2   PATHOGENESIS OF ANAEMIA IN CHRONIC RENAL FAILURE[1-3]

The two main factors responsible for the anaemia of chronic renal failure are haemolysis and impaired erythropoiesis. The reduction in red blood cell survival correlates with the degree of uraemia[4] and results from a toxic effect of uraemia, although the mechanism is not clear. However, since the degree of haemolysis should be easily compensated for by a normally functioning marrow depressed erythropoiesis limiting production of red blood cells is probably the main mechanism[5]. Until recently the decreased erythropoiesis was believed to be due to an inhibitory effect of uraemia on bone marrow but, although the severity of anaemia parallels the degree of uraemia, this relationship varies widely from patient to patient[6]. It is now recognized that insufficient production of erythropoietin is an important, and possibly the main factor resulting in depressed erythropoiesis in chronic renal failure. Table 9.1 summarizes current knowledge concerning this hormone. The importance of erythropoietin deficiency in the patho-

TABLE 9.1   Erythropoietin – summary of current knowledge

1. Erythropoietin is a glycoprotein of M.W. 46 000

2. *Sites of production*
    (*a*) renal – *either* kidney synthesizes erythropoietin
            – *or* kidney synthesizes an enzyme, erythrogen, which reacts with a
            plasma-borne substrate, produced in the liver, to generate bio-
            logically active erythropoietin
    (*b*) extrarenal – ? liver, ? spleen

3. *Control of production* – mediated by oxygen supply relative to rate of oxygen
    consumption

4. *Substances known to stimulate erythropoietin production:*
    – androgens
    – cobalt chloride

genesis of renal anaemia is supported by the finding of low plasma levels of erythropoietin in these patients compared to high levels in anaemic patients without renal disease[7]. However, it is likely that the diseased kidney does have some residual erythropoietin secretion since anephric patients on haemodialysis are more severely anaemic than patients on haemodialysis with kidneys *in situ*[8]. While the low plasma levels of erythropoietin in patients with chronic renal failure are likely to result mainly from destruction of renal tissue, an erythropoietin inhibitory effect of uraemic plasma has also been reported[9]. The evidence to date points to erythropoietin deficiency as the main reason for depressed erythropoiesis in chronic renal failure. That uraemia is also a factor in the depressed erythropoiesis is suggested by the observations that a uraemic environment has an inhibitory effect on marrow cultures[10] and that erythropoiesis improves in haemodialysis patients without any rise in plasma erythropoietin[11].

The therapeutic role of erythropoietin in renal anaemia must await further developments in the assay and purification of this hormone. However, a number of substances have been shown to influence erythropoietin secretion and they might have important therapeutic implications in patients with chronic renal failure; two such substances, androgens[12] and cobalt chloride[13], are referred to in Sections 9.6 and 9.7.

9.3   EFFECT OF HAEMODIALYSIS ON PATHOGENETIC MECHANISMS

With regular haemodialysis haemolysis may improve slightly[1] but red blood cell survival does not return to normal[11]. Some improvement in erythropoiesis also occurs resulting in a tendency for the anaemia to improve slowly[6, 11], the degree of improvement being related to frequency and duration of haemodialysis[1]. The observation that the improvement in erythropoiesis occurs without any rise in plasma erythropoietin suggests that it results from improved control of uraemia[11, 14]. However, improved nutrition from an increase in protein intake may also be a factor improving erythropoiesis in haemodialysis patients[15]. Figure 9.1 shows that in our

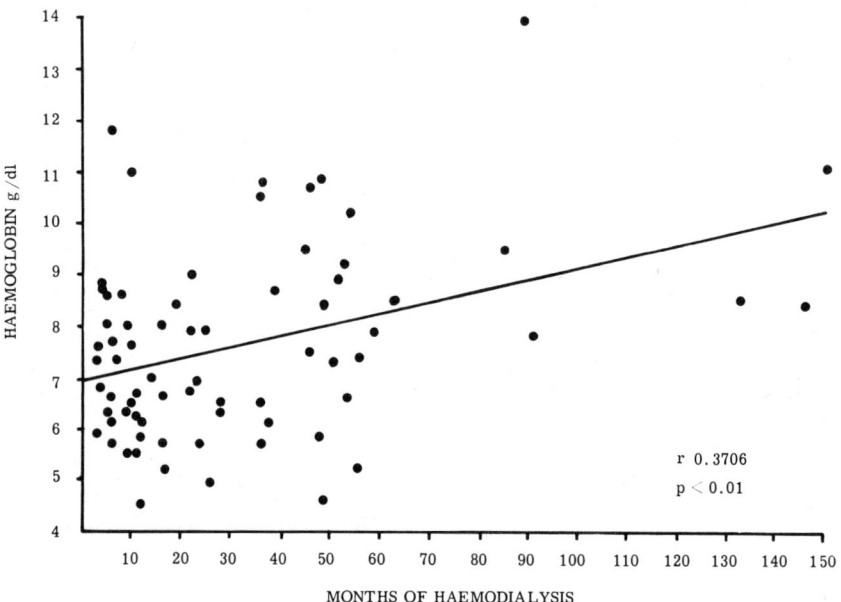

Figure 9.1   Relationship of haemoglobin to duration of haemodialysis in patients on haemodialysis

haemodialysis patients there is a tendency for the haemoglobin to rise very slowly with increasing duration of haemodialysis but there is a marked variation in the degree of anaemia at any one time. There was also no relationship in these patients between the degree of anaemia and the plasma creatinine concentration. Thus it seems likely that variation in residual erythropoietin secretion or other factors have an important role in determining the degree of anaemia in haemodialysis patients.

Although haemodialysis may lead to some improvement in anaemia, in other ways it can aggravate the anaemia, and potential improvement may thus be masked.

Chloramines, a substance used for drinking water purification all over the world, may further reduce red cell survival in patients treated by haemodialysis. Return to normal red blood cell survival has been reported using chloramine-free dialysate[16]. In addition, in some areas with a particularly high chloramine content in tap water, a significant improvement in anaemia has been described following the addition of ascorbic acid, a reducing agent, to the dialysis fluid[17].

Haemodialysis may also adversely affect erythropoiesis in two ways. Firstly, water-soluble vitamins are lost in the dialysis fluid and the loss of folic acid in particular may lead to megaloblastic erythropoiesis[18]. The regular administration of oral supplements of water-soluble vitamins prevents this potential complication. Secondly, and probably most important, haemodialysis by its very nature is associated with chronic blood loss[19-21]. Table 9.2 lists the most important reasons for this blood loss. With advances in technology blood loss during haemodialysis has been considerably reduced but a patient on regular haemodialysis treatment still loses a minimum of 3 l annually (Table 9.2). This represents a daily loss of 2 mg of

TABLE 9.2   Annual blood loss in haemodialysis patients

	Hospital dialysis twice weekly	Home dialysis thrice weekly
Blood sampling	1150 ml	300 ml
Cannulation of fistula	728 ml	1092 ml
Residual loss in dialyser	1040 ml	1560 ml
Total	2918 ml	2952 ml

iron assuming a haemoglobin of 7 g/dl and is likely to be more than this in some patients. With accurate measurements an iron loss of 5–6 mg of iron has been estimated[1]. Haemodialysis patients may therefore develop iron deficiency unless they are given iron supplements. Thus whereas iron deficiency is a minor factor in the anaemia of chronic renal failure it might become an important factor further impairing erythropoiesis in patients treated by haemodialysis.

9.4   IRON DEFICIENCY IN HAEMODIALYSIS PATIENTS

9.4.1   Incidence

In the early days of haemodialysis blood transfusion was given regularly to treat the anaemia of patients on haemodialysis. This more than compensated for blood loss and there was a real risk of iron overload[22]. However, since the risk of contracting hepatitis has been recognized blood

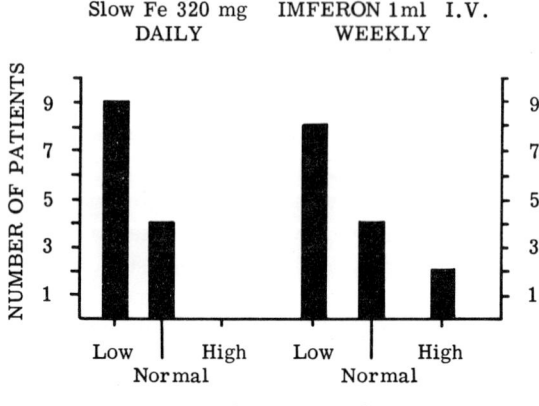

Figure 9.2   Marrow iron stores in patients on haemodialysis before treatment with oral and intravenous iron

transfusion has been restricted and many studies now reveal a high incidence of depleted iron stores in haemodialysis patients who are not taking iron supplements[23, 24]. Figure 9.2 shows the sternal marrow iron stores in two groups of patients in Edinburgh before treatment with either oral or intravenous iron. In all patients blood transfusion was used only if there was severe symptomatic anaemia or to replace major acute blood loss. Most of the patients had depleted marrow iron stores although 25% of patients had normal iron stores while in a minority the stores were high; these findings confirm previous observations. Although in the majority of patients whom we studied the plasma iron was below normal and the percentage saturation of the total iron binding capacity was low, there was a very poor correlation between both of these measurements and marrow iron stores, an observation made previously[25, 26]. Thus neither plasma iron nor percentage saturation is a reliable guide to the state of iron stores or to the need for iron supplements. Serum ferritin levels, however, correlate well with marrow iron stores in haemodialysis patients[27]. Since the measurement of serum ferritin is less disturbing to the patient than assessment of marrow iron stores it is likely to become a useful means of monitoring iron stores in haemodialysis patients.

9.4.2   Effect of iron therapy on anaemia in haemodialysis patients

Figure 9.3 shows the effect of oral and intravenous iron supplements on the haemoglobin in patients on haemodialysis. The marrow iron stores in

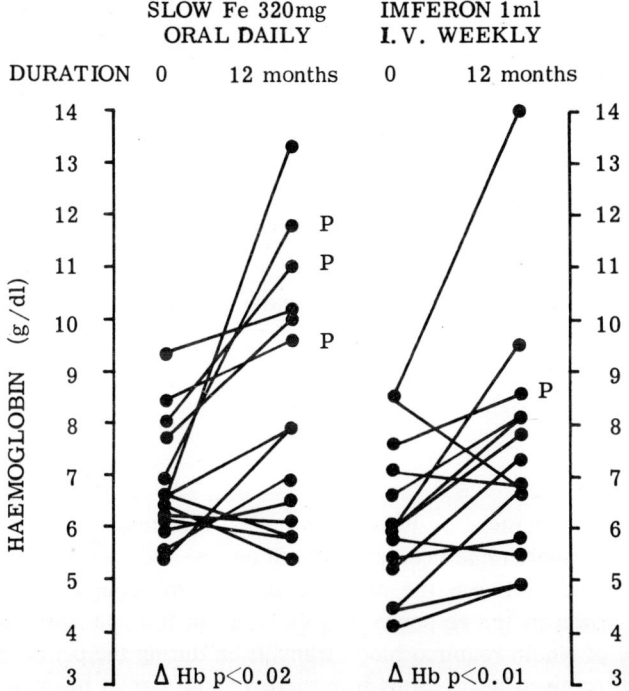

Figure 9.3   Haemoglobin before and after treatment with oral and intravenous iron in patients on haemodialysis. Values of haemoglobin for each patient before and after treatment with iron are indicated by closed circles, the two values being joined by a line. The significance of the change in haemoglobin with iron is shown for each group. P indicates patients with polycystic kidney disease

these patients before iron theapy are shown in Figure 9.2. In the majority of patients iron was given for 12 months before reassessment but some patients were reassessed earlier if other aspects of treatment altered. The patients were all treated by haemodialysis for 8 h twice weekly and were randomly allocated to one of the two treatment groups, there being 14 patients in each group. Details of these patients are shown in Table 9.3. The majority of patients were established on haemodialysis before this study but three of the patients given oral iron and one of the patients given intravenous iron commenced haemodialysis at the onset of the study. The dietary protein in all patients was 70 g daily providing 12–20 mg of elemental iron and all patients took oral supplements of a vitamin B complex tablet, ascorbic acid and folic acid. The oral iron was given as a slow release oral iron preparation (Slow Fe), in a dose of 320 mg daily before breakfast providing 100 mg of elemental iron daily. The intravenous iron was given as Imferon, 1 ml weekly providing 50 mg of elemental iron; the Imferon being given during dialysis through the venous chamber of the venous return line from the dialyser. The haemoglobin in the two groups

TABLE 9.3   Details of haemodialysis patients treated with oral and intravenous iron supplements

Treatment	Number of patients	Age (years) mean ± SEM	Duration haemodialysis (months) mean ± SEM
Slow Fe 320 mg daily (100 mg Fe)	14 (9M, 5F)	35 ± 2.9	10.5 ± 7.1
Imferon 1 ml i.v. weekly (50 mg Fe)	14 (11M, 3F)	39 ± 3.3	23.5 ± 7.4

did not differ significantly before treatment. After treatment a significant rise in haemoglobin had occurred in both groups and there was no significant difference between the response in the two groups. In individual patients however, the response was variable. In four patients given oral iron, one of whom required blood transfusion during the period of study, and in three given intravenous iron there was no rise in haemoglobin. In addition two patients given intravenous iron, in whom there was a negligible rise in haemoglobin with iron, required blood transfusion for symptomatic anaemia. At the other extreme one patient in each group, neither of whom had polycystic kidney disease, attained a normal haemoglobin in response to iron. The response to iron could not be related to the type of renal disease except that a rise in haemoglobin occurred in all patients with polycystic kidney disease; however, even in these patients the response was very variable. There was no correlation between the change in haemoglobin in response to iron therapy and either the duration of haemodialysis or the marrow iron stores. Thus patients with normal marrow iron stores were as likely to show a good response to iron as patients with low stores. No factor could be identified which was clearly associated with lack of improvement in anaemia although more severe blood loss could not be excluded as a cause since blood loss was not recorded accurately. Figure 9.4 shows the response to iron supplements in a female with polycystic kidney disease and illustrates the marked improvement in anaemia which is achieved in some patients. Prior to the onset of haemodialysis the haemoglobin was 11 g/dl and fell progressively to 6 g/dl after 28 weeks of haemodialysis, there being no major blood loss in this period. After treat-

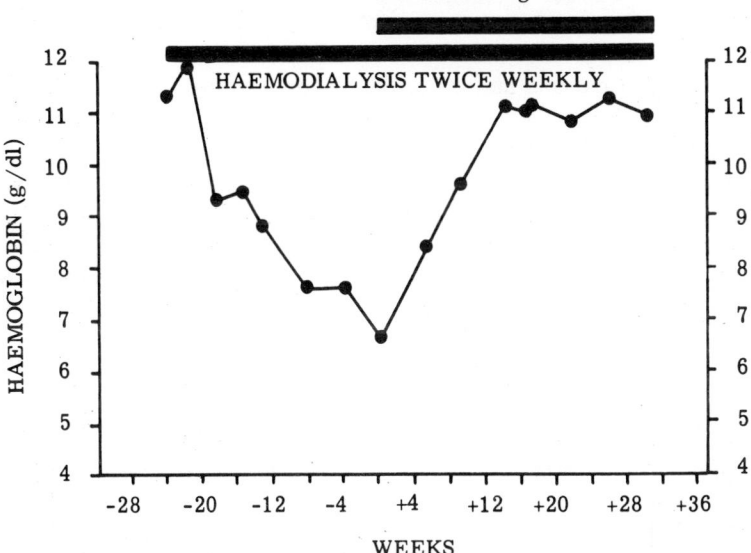

Figure 9.4   Response of anaemia to oral iron therapy in a female patient with polycystic kidney disease on haemodialysis

ment with oral iron, and without any alteration in dialysis regime, the haemoglobin rose progressively to 11 g/dl over the next 20 weeks.

These results confirm previous observations that a significant rise in haemoglobin in haemodialysis patients occurs following both oral[23, 28, 29] and intravenous iron supplements[25, 30-33] and as a result blood transfusion can be minimized – only three of the 28 patients in the study required blood transfusion during the 12-month period of iron therapy. In addition the results indicate that oral iron supplements are as effective as intravenous iron supplements, an important observation since in the past there has been controversy regarding the efficiency of iron absorption in chronic renal failure[24, 34, 35]. However, more recent studies indicate that iron absorption in chronic renal failure is normal and is regulated by the state of iron balance[36].

It is likely that the improvement in anaemia in response to iron is mainly due to correction of iron deficiency. However, in contrast to some previous observations[23, 25] there was a marked variation in the response irrespective of the initial iron status. The failure to predict the response of anaemia to iron therapy from the initial iron status may reflect both the limitations of the methods used to assess iron status and marked variation in blood loss. However, other factors may be involved in determining the response to iron in addition to iron status. In view of the known chronic blood loss in haemodialysis patients and, since the response to iron may be difficult to predict from the iron status, iron supplements should be given routinely to all haemodialysis patients.

When advocating long-term therapy the risk of iron overload must be considered. Marrow iron stores were reassessed in seven of our patients given oral iron and in nine given intravenous iron; after 12 months of treatment none developed high iron stores. Increased iron stores as indicated by serum ferritin have, however, been found after treatment with

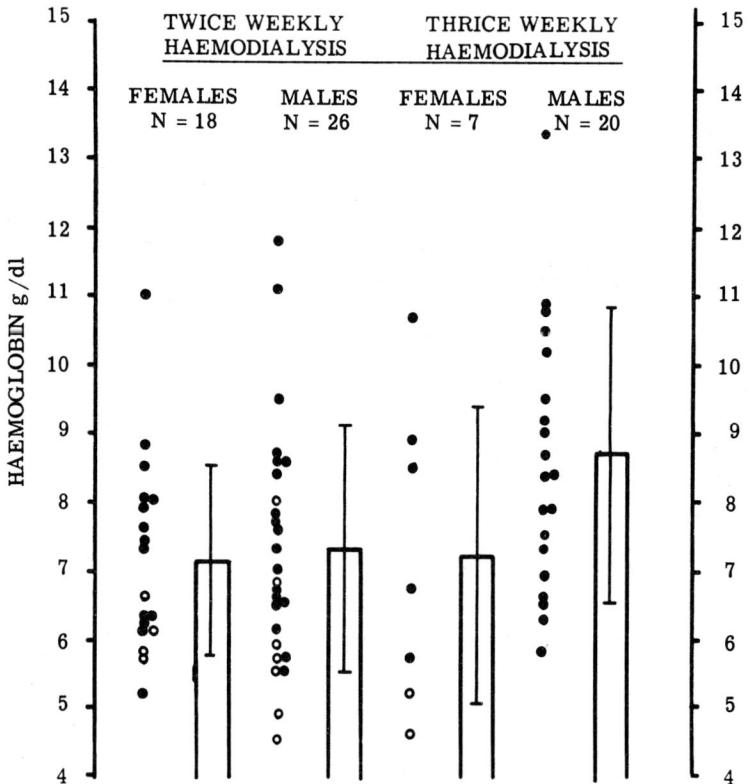

Figure 9.5   Effect of sex and frequency of haemodialysis on anaemia in haemodialysis patients. Closed circles indicate haemoglobin values for non transfused patients and open circles indicate values for patients who required blood transfusion in the previous year. The mean haemoglobin (± 1 SD) for each group is indicated by the column

intravenous iron for a longer period[27]. As the theoretical risk of inducing iron overload may be greater with intravenous than with oral iron the use of oral iron supplements may be safer on a long-term basis.

9.5 OTHER FACTORS INFLUENCING THE DEGREE OF ANAEMIA IN HAEMODIALYSIS PATIENTS

Sex, frequency of dialysis, the nature of the underlying renal disease and bilateral nephrectomy have all been reported to influence the degree of anaemia in haemodialysis patients.

9.5.1 Sex and frequency of dialysis

Figure 9.5 shows the haemoglobin in patients treated by haemodialysis twice and three times weekly according to sex. With haemodialysis for 6–8 h twice weekly there is no difference in haemoglobin in males compared to females and the proportion of patients requiring blood transfusion in each group is similar. In contrast in male patients treated by haemodialysis for 6 h three times weekly the haemoglobin is significantly higher than that both in males ($p < 0.02$) and females ($p < 0.02$) treated by haemodialysis twice weekly, and no patient required blood transfusion. In the limited number of females treated by haemodialysis for 6 h three times weekly the haemoglobin is in general no better than in those treated twice weekly. It has previously been suggested that anaemia is more severe in females than in males[1]. These results suggest that sex is not an important factor influencing anaemia on twice weekly haemodialysis. Improvement in anaemia with increased frequency of haemodialysis is well recognized[1]. However, our results suggest that increasing the frequency of haemodialysis produces a greater improvement in anaemia in males than females. That increasing the frequency of dialysis is of value in improving anaemia is confirmed when one looks at the change in haemoglobin in individual patients moving from twice to three times weekly haemodialysis (Figure 9.6). For the group as a whole there was a significant rise in haemoglobin with increasing frequency of dialysis. In individual patients the response was variable but a significant number of patients showed a beneficial rise in haemoglobin and this occurred in some females as well as males.

9.5.2 Nature of renal disease

Figure 9.7 shows the haemoglobin in our haemodialysis patients according to type of renal disease. Anaemia was least severe in patients with poly-

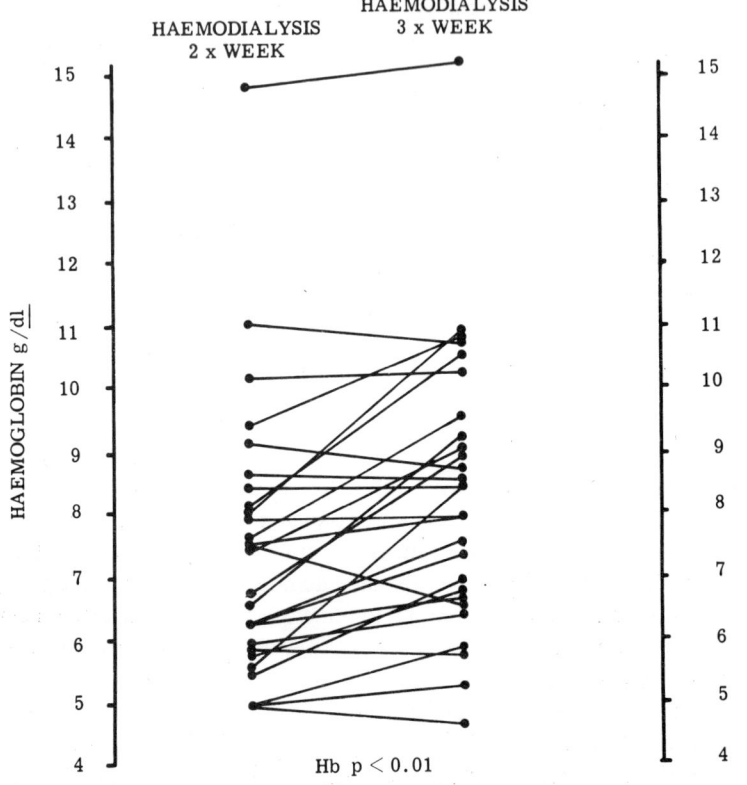

Figure 9.6   Change in haemoglobin in haemodialysis patients with increased frequency of haemodialysis. Haemoglobin values in individual patients on twice and thrice weekly haemodialysis are indicated by the closed circles, the two values being joined by a line

cystic kidney disease, the haemoglobin in this group being significantly higher than in patients with glomerulonephritis, pyelonephritis or hypertensive renal disease ($p < 0.001$) and this confirms previous similar findings[37]. Surprisingly, patients with congenital renal disease other than polycystic kidney disease had the next best haemoglobin although this was only significantly higher than that in patients with glomerulonephritis ($p < 0.05$). It has previously been suggested that patients with pyelonephritis and hypertensive renal disease are more severely anaemic than other patients[1]. However, we found no difference in the degree of anaemia in pyelonephritis compared to glomerulonephritis. Although the haemoglobin in patients with hypertensive renal disease was not significantly different to that in glomerulonephritis or pyelonephritis these patients

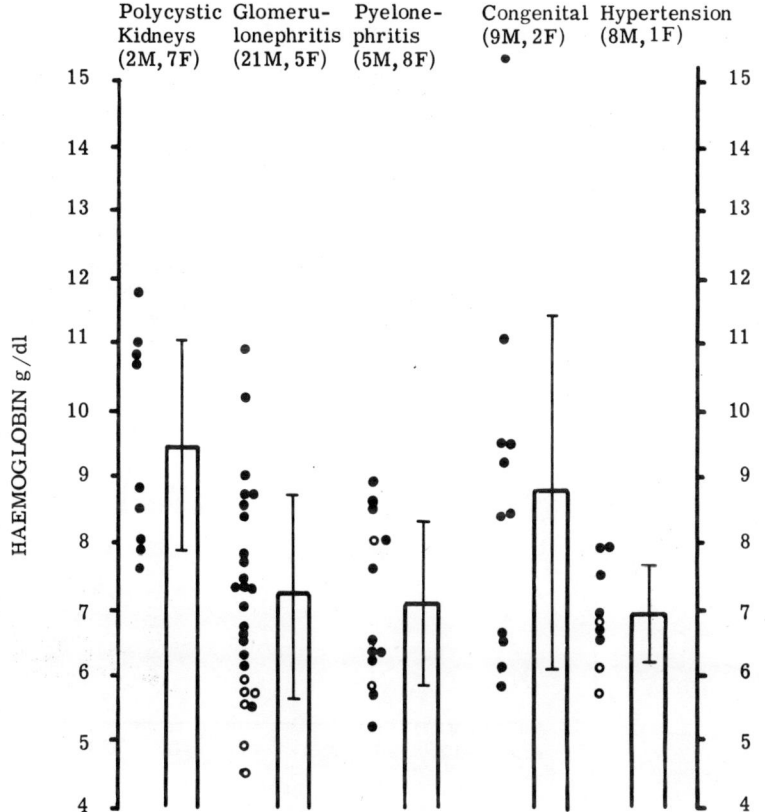

Figure 9.7 Haemoglobin in haemodialysis patients according to type of renal disease. Closed circles indicate haemoglobin values for non transfused patients and open circles indicate values for patients who required blood transfusion in the previous year. The mean haemoglobin (± 1 SD) for each group is indicated by the column

seemed less capable of achieving more normal haemoglobin values. Thus the nature of the underlying renal disease may have some influence on the degree of anaemia and this could be related to residual erythropoietin secretion. In each disease type the range of haemoglobin values is wide so that residual erythropoietin secretion must vary widely within any disease type or there must be other factors involved.

9.5.3   Effect of bilateral nephrectomy

The deleterious effect of bilateral nephrectomy on anaemia in haemodialysis patients is well recognized, nephrectomized patients requiring
twice the rate of blood transfusion as patients with intact renal tissue[8].
Figure 9.8 illustrates the catastrophic effect of bilateral nephrectomy on

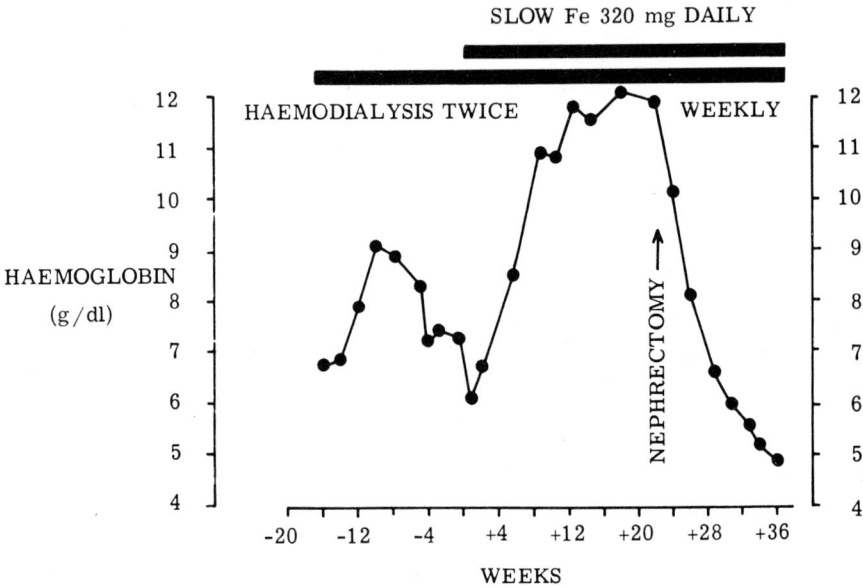

Figure 9.8   Effect of bilateral nephrectomy on anaemia in a male patient with
polycystic kidney disease on haemodialysis

anaemia in a patient with polycystic kidney disease. Although this patient
was anaemic following the commencement of regular haemodialysis the
haemoglobin rose progressively towards normal after treatment with oral
iron supplements. At this point bilateral nephrectomy was performed in
preparation for renal transplantation and the haemoglobin thereafter fell
progressively to 5 g/dl over 10 weeks and for the first time blood transfusion was required for symptomatic anaemia. The response in this patient
stresses the role which damaged renal tissue plays in determining the
degree of anaemia. Because of the resultant morbidity bilateral nephrectomy should never be performed in haemodialysis patients without very
clear indications.

9.6 EFFECT OF ANDROGENS ON ANAEMIA IN HAEMODIALYSIS PATIENTS

The use of androgens in the treatment of renal anaemia has a good theoretical basis as is shown in Table 9.4[3]. A number of studies have demonstrated a significant improvement in anaemia in haemodialysis patients in response to parenteral androgens[38-41] the oral preparations having a less

TABLE 9.4   Effects of androgens on erythropoiesis

1.	Stimulates endogenous production of erythropoietin by the kidney and possibly by extrarenal sources
2.	Increases responsiveness of bone marrow to erythropoietin
3.	Stimulates erythropoiesis *in vitro*

consistent effect[42, 43]. In some studies the irregular administration of parenteral iron may have influenced the results[38, 39] and one controlled study failed to show a significant benefit from androgen therapy[44]. More recently Von Hartitzsch and Kerr[32] have shown that the improvement in anaemia in response to androgens is no greater than that achieved with parenteral iron therapy. They also found that use of both together produced no greater effect than either used alone. There must, therefore, be doubt about the place of androgens in the treatment of anaemia in haemodialysis patients particularly since they may give rise to a number of adverse effects (Table 9.5) some of which are disturbing, especially to female patients. Figure 9.5 shows that the majority of haemodialysis patients given iron supplements can be maintained asymptomatic without severe anaemia and without the need for blood transfusion; it therefore seems unreasonable to subject these patients to the risk of troublesome effects of androgens. It has been suggested that androgens should be restricted to the small proportion of patients who, despite adequate dialysis and iron supplements, have persisting severe anaemia necessitating blood transfusion[1]. Included in this category are patients with refractory anaemia following bilateral nephrectomy. A significant improvement in anaemia

TABLE 9.5   Adverse effects of androgens

Virilization in females
Acne
Hyperlipidaemia
Priapism in males
Cholestatic jaundice

with reduction in blood transfusion requirements has been reported following treatment of anephric haemodialysis patients with androgens[38]. However, in general the response is less marked than in patients with intact
kidneys and the results of treatment in some studies have been disappointing[32, 44].

9.7   COBALT CHLORIDE AS A TREATMENT OF REFRACTORY ANAEMIA FOLLOWING BILATERAL NEPHRECTOMY

Experimentally cobalt chloride stimulates erythropoietin secretion[13] and
therefore might be of value in the treatment of anaemia in haemodialysis
patients. In haemodialysis patients with refractory anaemia following bilateral nephrectomy a significant improvement in anaemia with reduction
in blood transfusion requirements has been reported following treatment
with cobalt chloride[45]. However, a number of side effects, some potentially
serious, may occur during therapy[45] and the role of cobalt in the treatment
of refractory anaemia is not clear.

9.8   BLOOD TRANSFUSION REQUIREMENTS IN HAEMODIALYSIS PATIENTS

Since 1970 we have restricted blood transfusion to a minimum, blood
transfusion being given only for severe symptomatic anaemia or to replace
major acute blood loss. Since 1972 all haemodialysis patients in Edinburgh
have taken regular oral iron supplements. Table 9.6 shows the blood
transfusion rate in our dialysis unit over the past 2 years. In both periods,
approximately one third of patients treated by haemodialysis required

TABLE 9.6   Blood transfusion requirements in haemodialysis patients in
Edinburgh

---

1.   *August 1975 to August 1976*
     – 50 patients treated for 329 patient months
     – 16 patients (32%) required blood transfusion
     – total blood transfused 55 units
     Transfusion rate 0.12 units/ patient month

2.   *August 1976 to April 1977*
     – 60 patients treated for 401 patient months
     – 21 patients (35%) required blood transfusion
     – total blood transfused 78 units
     Transfusion rate 0.17 units/ patient month

TABLE 9.7 Indications for blood transfusion in haemodialysis patients in Edinburgh. August 1976 to April 1977

1. Symptomatic Anaemia: 43 units given to 11 patients
   – 8 patients given 2 units or less
   – 3 patients given more than 2 units

2. *Replacement of blood loss during dialysis:* 2 units in 1 patient

3. *Medical and surgical complications:* 33 units given to 8 patients
   – post transplant rejection 4 units
   – pericardial effusion 8 units
   – bilateral nephrectomy (2 patients) 13 units
   – transplant nephrectomy 2 units
   – splenectomy 2 units
   – bleeding peptic ulcer 4 units

blood transfusion and the overall transfusion rate was only 0.1 unit per patient month.

Table 9.7 shows the indications for blood transfusion during the last year. Only 50% of the blood used in this period was given as treatment of symptomatic anaemia, and of the 11 patients in this category eight required 2 units or less while the remainder of the blood was required by the other three patients. Thus very few patients require regular blood transfusion for symptomatic anaemia. Only one patient required blood transfusion to replace acute blood loss during haemodialysis and this stresses the marked reduction in acute blood loss during haemodialysis in recent years. The remainder of the blood given in this period was required because of medical and surgical complications and this could not have been prevented.

As is illustrated in Figure 9.5, in the majority of haemodialysis patients, who are given a high protein intake with oral supplements of water soluble vitamins and iron, the haemoglobin can be maintained at a reasonable level without the need for blood transfusion, in a few patients the haemoglobin can be maintained at a nearly normal level while only in a small proportion is regular blood transfusion necessary.

References

1. Koch, K. M., Patyna, W. D., Shaldon, S. and Werner, E. (1974). Anaemia of the regular haemodialysis patient and its treatment. *Nephron*, 12, 405
2. Fried, W. (1975). Erythropoietin and the kidney. *Nephron*, 15, 327
3. Naets, J. P. (1975). Haematological disorders in renal failure. *Nephron*, 14, 181
4. Shaw, A. B. (1967). Haemolysis in chronic renal failure. *Br. Med. J.*, 2, 213

5. Desforges, J. F. and Dawson, J. P. (1958). The anemia of renal failure. *Arch. Intern. Med.*, **101**, 326

6. Eschbach, J. W., Adamson, J. W. and Cook, J. D. (1970). Disorders of red blood cell production in uremia. *Arch. Intern. Med.*, **126**, 812

7. Naets, J. P. and Heuse, A. F. (1962). Measurement of erythropoietin stimulating factor in anemic patients with and without renal lesions. *J. Lab. Clin. Med.*, **60**, 365

8. Van Ypersele de Strihou, C. and Stragier, A. (1969). Effect of bilateral nephrectomy on transfusion requirements of patients undergoing chronic dialysis. *Lancet*, **ii**, 705

9. Fisher, J. W., Hatch, F. E., Roh, B. L., Allan, R. C. and Kelley, B. J. (1968). Erythropoietin inhibitor in kidney and plasma from anemic uremic human subjects. *Blood*, **31**, 440

10. Markson, J. L. and Rennie, J. B. (1956). The anaemia of chronic renal insufficiency. The effect of serum from azotaemic patients on the maturation of normoblasts in suspension cultures. *Scot. Med. J.*, **1**, 320

11. Eschbach, J. W. Jr., Funk, D., Adamson, J., Kuhn, I., Scribner, B. H. and Finch, C. A. (1967). Erythropoiesis in patients with renal failure undergoing chronic dialysis. *N. Engl. J. Med.*, **276**, 653

12. Fried, W., Marver, D., Large, R. D. and Gurney, C. W. (1966). Studies on the erythropoietin stimulating factor in the plasma of mice after receiving testosterone. *J. Lab. Clin. Med.*, **68**, 947

13. Goldwasser, E., Jacobson, L. O., Fried, W. and Plzak, L. (1958). Studies on erythropoiesis: V The effect of cobalt on the production of erythropoietin. *Blood*, **13**, 55

14. Mann, D. L., Donati, R. M. and Gallagher, N. I. (1964). Erythropoietin assay and ferrokinetic measurements in anemic uremic patients. *J. Am. Med. Assoc.*, **194**, 1321

15. Giordano, C., De Santo, N. G., Rinaldi, S., Acone, D., Eposito, R. and Gallo, B. (1973). Histidine for the treatment of uraemic anaemia. *Br. Med. J.*, **4**, 716

16. Hartitzsch, B. Von, Carr, D., Kjellstrand, C. M. and Kerr, D. N. S. (1973). Normal red cell survival in well dialysed patients. *Trans. Am. Soc. Artif. Intern. Organs*, **19**, 471

17. Botella, J., Traver, J. A., Sanz-Guajardo, D., Torres, M. T., Sanjuan, I. and Zabala, P. (1977). Chloramines, an aggravating factor in the anaemia of patients on regular dialysis treatment. *Proc. E.D.T.A.*, **14**, 192 (London: Pitman

18. Hampers, C. L., Streiff, R., Nathan, D. G., Snyder, D. and Merrill, J. P. (1967). Megaloblastic hematopoiesis in uremia and in patients on long-term hemodialysis. *N. Engl. J. Med.*, **276**, 551

19. Lindsay, R. M. and Burton, J. A. (1972). Blood loss from cannulation sites during haemodialysis. *Scot. Med. J.*, **17**, 266

20. Hocken, A. G. and Marwah, P. K. (1971). Iatrogenic contribution to anaemia of chronic renal failure. *Lancet*, **i**, 164

21. Lindsay, R. M. and Kennedy, A. C. (1972). Dialysers and blood loss in regular dialysis therapy. *Proc. E.D.T.A.*, **9**, 437 (London: Pitman Medical)

22. Curtis, J. R., Eastwood, J. B., Smith, E. K. M., Storey, J. M., Verroust, P. J., De Wardener, H. E., Wing, A. J. and Wolfson, E. M. (1969). Maintenance haemodialysis. *Q. J. Med.*, **61**, 49

23. Baker, L. R. I., Cattell, W. R., Child, J. A. and Saudie, E. (1975). Iron therapy in maintenance haemodialysis. *Clin. Sci.*, **48**, 529

24. Eschbach, J. W., Cook, J. D. and Finch, C. A. (1970). Iron absorption in chronic renal disease. *Clin. Sci.*, **38**, 191

25. Morgan, T. (1972). The effect of intravenous iron on the haematocrit of patients on maintenance haemodialysis. *Med. J. Aust.*, **1**, 852

26. Beutler, E., Robson, M. J. and Buttenwieser, E. (1958). A comparison of the plasma iron, iron-binding capacity, sternal marrow iron and other methods in the clinical evaluation of iron stores. *Ann. Intern. Med.*, **48**, 60

27. Hussein, S., Priesto, J., O'Shea, M., Hoffbrand, A. V., Baillod, R. A. and Moorhead, J. F. (1975). Serum ferritin assay and iron status in chronic renal failure and haemodialysis. *Br. Med. J.*, **1**, 546

28. Wallace, M. R. (1971). The effect of oral iron on the anaemia of patients on maintenance haemodialysis. *N.Z. Med. J.*, **74**, 167

29. Strickland, I. D., Chaput de Saintonge, D. M., Boulton, F. E., Brain, A. J. S., Goodwin, F. J., Marsh, F. P. and Zychova, Z. (1974). A trial of oral iron in dialysis patients. *Clin. Nephrol.*, **21**, 13

30. Carter, R. A., Hawkins, J. B. and Robinson, B. H. B. (1969). Iron metabolism in the anaemia of chronic renal failure. Effects of dialysis and of parenteral iron. *Br. Med. J.*, **3**, 206

31. Stewart, W. K., Fleming, L. W. and Shepherd, A. M. M. (1976). Haemoglobin and serum iron responses to periodic intravenous iron-dextran infusions during maintenance dialysis. *Nephron*, **17**, 121

32. Hartitzsch, B. Von and Kerr, D. N. S. (1976). Response to parenteral iron with and without androgen therapy in patients undergoing regular haemodialysis. *Nephron*, **17**, 430

33. Wright, F. K., Goldsmith, H. J. and Hall, S. M. (1968). Iron responsive anaemia in repeated dialysis treatment without routine blood transfusion. *Proc. E.D.T.A.*, **5**, 179 (Amsterdam: Excerpta Medica Foundation)

34. Brozovich, B., Cattell, W. R., Cottrall, M. F., Gwyther, M. M., McMillan, J. M., Malpas, J. S., Salsbury, A. and Trott, N. G. (1971). Iron metabolism in patients undergoing regular dialysis therapy. *Br. Med. J.*, **1**, 695

35. Lawson, D. H., Boddy, K., King, P. C., Lenton, A. L. and Will, G. (1971). Iron metabolism in patients with chronic renal failure on regular dialysis treatment. *Clin. Sci.*, **41**, 345

36. Milman, N. and Larsen, L. (1976). Iron absorption in patients with chronic uraemia undergoing regular haemodialysis. *Acta Med. Scand.*, **199**, 113

37. Maggiore, Q., Navelesi, R., Biagini, M., Balestre, P. L. and Giagnoni, P. (1967). Comparative studies of uraemic anaemia in polycystic kidney disease and in other renal diseases. *Proc. E.D.T.A.*, **4**, 264 (Amsterdam: Excerpta Medica Foundation)

38. Shaldon, S., Koch, K. M., Oppermann, F., Patyna, W. D. and Schoeppe, W. (1971). Testosterone therapy for anaemia in maintenance haemodialysis. *Br. Med. J.*, **3**, 212

39. Hendler, E. D., Goffinet, J. A., Ross, S., Longnecker, R. E. and Bakovic, V. (1974). Controlled study of androgen therapy in anemia of patients on maintenance hemodialysis. *N. Engl. J. Med.*, **291**, 1046

40. Williams, J. S., Stein, J. H. and Ferris, T. M. (1974). Nandrolone Deconate therapy for patients receiving hemodialysis. *Arch. Intern. Med.*, **134**, 289

41. Hartitzbch, B. Von, Kerr, D. N. S., Morley, G. and Marks, B. (1977). Androgens in the anaemia of chronic renal failure. *Nephron*, **18**, 13

42. Davies, M., Muckle, T. J., Cassells-Smith, A., Webster, D. and Kerr, D. N. S. (1972). Oxymethalone in the treatment of anaemia in chronic renal failure. *Br. J. Urol.*, **44**, 387

43. Lindholm, D. D., Fisher, J. W., Vieira, J. A., Dombeck, D. H., Bernal, G. and Lerthora, J. (1973). Clinical effects of oral fluoxymesterone in patients with dialysis-controlled uremia. *Trans. Am. Soc. Artif. Intern. Organs*, **19**, 475

44. Ball, J. H., Lowrie, E. G., Hampers, C. L. and Merrill, J. P. (1975). Testosterone therapy in hemodialysis patients. *Clin. Nephrol.*, **4**, 91

45. Duckham, J. M. and Lee, H. A. (1976). The treatment of refractory anaemia of chronic renal failure with cobalt chloride. *Q. J. Med.*, **69**, 277

DISCUSSION

A. W. Siemsen (Honolulu): Were Winney's patients taken off antacids?

Winney: No, they were not.

Siemsen: There is considerable evidence that antacids do bind oral iron. There have been several studies that showed that it does not respond quite so well, and one reason was that the patients were on oral antacid.

Winney: Our patients also took ascorbic acid, and that may have had some effect on the absorption of iron. They do take them, and we did get a response, but whether there is a variation in response is something that could be looked at further.
   They were taking their antacids.

J. S. Cameron: And what about oral vitamins, including pyrodixine?

Winney: Yes.

C. P. Swainson (Edinburgh): There is a relationship with the time of day when they are taken. Vitamins and similar substances are usually taken fasting, before breakfast, whereas aluminium binders and phosphate binders are usually taken before meals. There might be an effect from that.

R. Gabriel (London): How were haemoglobin measurements standardized, and were red cell masses done in these people.

Winney: I cannot answer the point on standardization of haemoglobin without asking the haematologist. Red cell masses were not done.

B. H. B. Robinson (Birmingham): We did some work a few years back on red cell masses and we measured the haemoglobin in dialysis patients and we were surprised to find how well they correlated in that the haemoglobin really did seem to relate to changes in red cell mass.

Since it now looks as though it will be mandatory upon us to transfuse the patients who are to have transplants, how will this affect our approach to the management of renal anaemia?

Winney: From the point of view of the patients, in terms of their own management, particularly those with polycystic kidneys, it would be unethical to give them blood transfusions and prevent them from achieving a normal haemoglobin level from their own marrow. Regular transfusions have been shown to be one of the factors depressing readings in these patients. I find that very difficult.

Robinson: But there are a number of people who would consider it unethical to transplant somebody who had not had a transfusion.

J. S. Robson (Edinburgh): The number of transfusions required to achieve the immunological advantage is very small so it might not affect the overall haematological position very much.

10

Mineral metabolism in chronic renal failure
J. A. Kanis

10.1   INTRODUCTION

Since the advent of dialysis and renal transplantation, patients with end-stage chronic renal disease are surviving for long periods of time, whereas formerly they would have died. Of the many disorders that affect such survivors, much attention has been directed to disturbances in mineral metabolism. Advances in the past few years, particularly in the field of vitamin D metabolism, have led to an understanding of some of the pathogenic processes which give rise to these disorders. The 'spin-off' has been that, despite the complexity of the disorders, the objectives of treatment and the ways in which these objectives might be realized, have become clearer.

This report considers mainly the problems which are encountered in advanced renal failure. For a wider appraisal of the subject the reader is referred to a number of reviews[1-4].

10.2   DEFINITION AND PREVALENCE OF RENAL BONE DISEASE

The skeletal disorders which are found in chronic renal failure (Table 10.1) may occur singly or in various combinations. None of these disorders is however unique to renal disease and none is specific to a particular population of patients such as those managed conservatively, those on haemodialysis or indeed transplanted patients. There are, however, differences in the prevalence of the various abnormalities not only within these population sub-groups but also between renal units[5-7]. Some of these differences reflect the use of differing criteria for the diagnosis of bone disease.

Bone disease is frequently a major clinical problem in the young[8], particularly at the time of skeletal maturity, when requirements for vitamin

TABLE 10.1   Features of renal bone disease. Metastatic calcification may be the result of disturbed mineral metabolism but cannot be considered a skeletal disorder except in the ectopic calcification of cartilage (e.g. pseudogout) and osteoid

---

Retardation of growth
Osteomalacia and rickets
Osteitis fibrosa
Osteosclerosis
Periosteal new bone formation
Osteoporosis
Osteonecrosis
Metastatic calcification

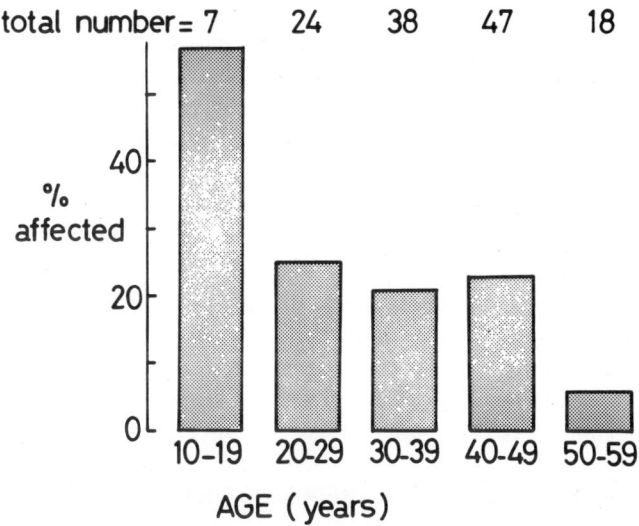

Figure 10.1   Prevalence of subperiosteal erosions on x-ray examination in 134 patients about to start treatment with haemodialysis

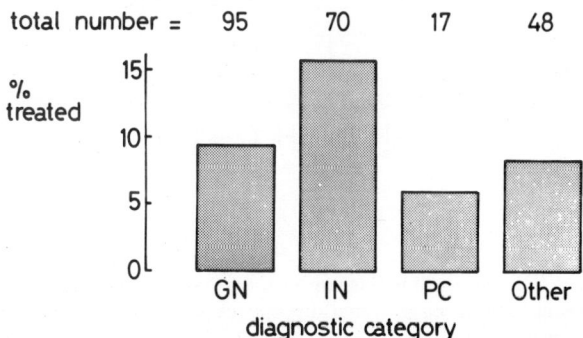

Figure 10.2   Prevalence of osteitis fibrosa associated with bone pain in 230 patients established on dialysis treatment. Patients were subdivided according to the nature of their renal disorder (GN, glomerulonephritis; IN, interstitial nephropathy, i.e. chronic pyelonephritis and analgesic nephropathy; PC, polycystic disease; the term 'other' includes patients in whom the diagnosis was doubtful). Affected patients were selected for treatment with D-metabolites. A greater proportion of patients with interstitial nephropathy required treatment than was necessary in patients with other renal diseases

D may be the greatest. The prevalence of osteitis fibrosa at end-stage renal disease is highest in this age group and decreases progressively with age (Figure 10.1). Patients with interstitial forms of renal disease may also be more susceptible[9,10] (Figure 10.2) which might reflect a comparatively longer duration of uraemia compared to patients with other forms of renal disease. An alternative explanation might be that damage to interstitial tissue destroys tubular sites responsible for the production of vitamin D metabolites or for the degradation of parathyroid hormone. Other factors which affect the incidence of renal bone disease include geographical variation and environmental factors[5-7, 11, 12], but the mechanisms by which these factors cause bone disease are obscure. Recent advances in our understanding of the disturbances in metabolism that occur in chronic renal failure have resulted in the proposal that several 'pathophysiological pathways' may be of prime importance.

10.3   PATHOGENESIS OF RENAL BONE DISEASE

Two of the concepts of the pathogenesis of renal bone disease have been popularized in recent years. The first holds that hyperparathyroidism and

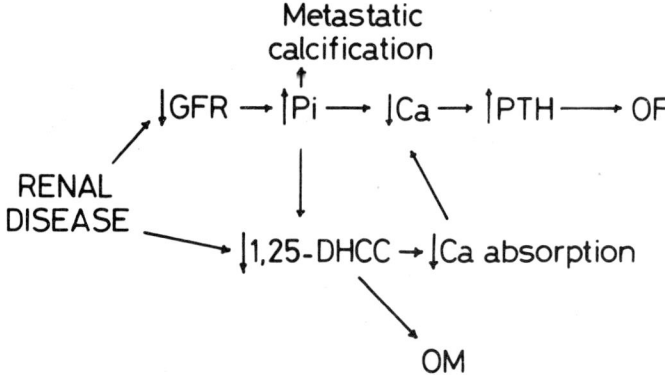

Figure 10.3.   Schematic flow diagram to show current hypotheses for the pathogenesis of renal bone disease. Renal disease results in progressive decrements in glomerular filtration rate (GFR) and in the ability to synthesize 1,25-dihydroxy-cholecalciferol (1,25-DHCC). An increase in plasma phosphate (Pi), due to a fall in GFR, stimulates the secretion of parathyroid hormone (PTH) indirectly by decreasing plasma levels of calcium (Ca). Because of the biological effects of PTH, plasma levels of Ca and Pi tend toward normal at the expense of increased secretion of PTH and osteitis fibrosa (OF) until the decrease in GFR outstrips the compensatory capabilities of PTH. Hyperphosphataemia may further inhibit synthesis of 1,25-DHCC. Malabsorption of calcium may contribute to secondary hyperparathyroidism, and a deficiency of D induce osteomalacia (OM)

its skeletal consequences (osteitis fibrosa) is the result of phosphate retention. The other proposes that defective production of 1,25-dihydroxy-cholecalciferol by the kidney results in malabsorption of calcium and defective mineralization of bone (osteomalacia). These hypotheses are not mutually exclusive (Figure 10.3).

10.3.1 Phosphate metabolism

Elegant animal experiments[13,14] have demonstrated that incremental restriction of dietary phosphate, in proportion to decrements induced in glomerular filtration rate, may abolish the secondary stimulation of secretion of parathyroid hormone. The hypothesis derived from these experiments holds that a rise in plasma phosphate due to impaired renal function, results in a decrease in the ionized fraction of plasma calcium and thus stimulates the secretion of parathyroid hormone. The increase in circulating parathyroid hormone so induced, reduces the renal tubular reabsorption of phosphate, so that any increase in plasma levels of phosphate due to chronic renal failure is minimized. The maintenance of a near normal plasma level of phosphate, together with the calcaemic effects of parathyroid hormone (increased bone resorption and renal tubular reabsorption of calcium), mean that disturbances in the ionized fraction of plasma calcium are also minimal. Thus, during the course of progressive renal failure, plasma levels of calcium and phosphate remain relatively normal but at the expense of an ever-increasing secretion rate of parathyroid hormone. When the decrement in filtration is too great to be compensated by the renal effects of parathyroid hormone, hyperphosphataemia and hypocalcaemia accompany high levels of parathyroid hormone.

The importance of this pathogenic mechanism in man is perhaps supported by finding increased circulating levels of parathyroid hormone and an inverse relationship between plasma calcium and phosphate in patients in the early stages of chronic renal failure[15,16]. In addition, the administration of phosphate to healthy subjects may reduce plasma calcium levels and increase those of parathyroid hormone. There is however conflicting evidence as to the effects of chronic manipulation of plasma phosphate on the secretion of parathyroid hormone in man[16-18]. Moreover, in chronic renal failure, raised plasma levels of parathyroid hormone might be due to its impaired degradation by the kidney. Irrespective of the mechanisms by which levels of parathyroid hormone are increased, it is not certain whether the hormone is circulating in an active form, since measurements made using radioimmunoassay might not reflect biological activity.

Phosphate is also an important factor in the mineralization of bone.

There is a striking negative correlation between prevailing levels of plasma phosphate and the amount of non-mineralized osteoid in patients with chronic renal failure and in patients with normal renal function[5,19,20]. This relationship is not necessarily dependent on vitamin D status or on renal function since the correlation is observed in dialysis patients (Figure 10.4);

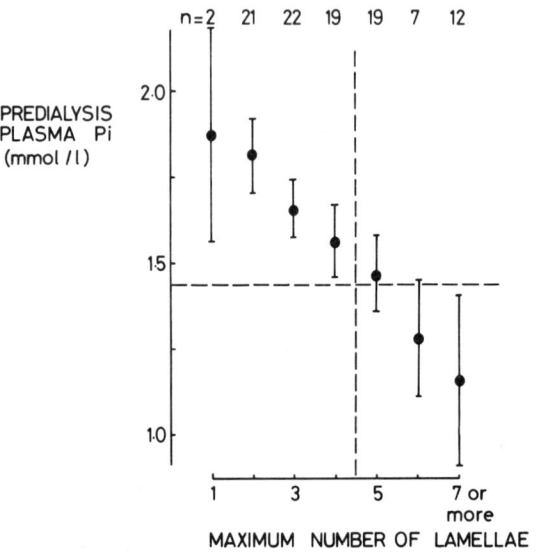

Figure 10.4   Relationship between plasma phosphate (mean of values taken immediately before a dialysis treatment $\pm$ SEM) and the number of osteoid lamellae seen in histological sections. Osteomalacia (five or more lamellae) was uncommon in patients with high levels of plasma phosphate. Evidence of osteomalacia was commonly noted in patients whose plasma phosphate lay below the upper limit for the normal range (horizontal dashed line). (From Kanis et al.[5])

and in Pagetic patients, it exists independently of circulating levels of 25-hydroxy-vitamin D_3. The causal significance of this relationship is suggested by observations in patients with or without renal disease that phosphate restriction may induce and phosphate repletion may cure defective mineralization of bone[11,21]. The levels of plasma phosphate in patients with chronic renal failure below which osteomalacia may be induced are considerably higher than those associated with defective mineralization in patients with normal renal function.

10.3.2   Vitamin D metabolism

Disturbed metabolism of vitamin D may be an important additional factor
in the pathogenesis of osteomalacia and hyperparathyroidism in chronic
renal failure. It is well recognized that large but unphysiological doses of
vitamin D_2 or D_3 may increase the intestinal absorption of calcium and
improve osteomalacia and osteitis fibrosa in such patients[22]. This resistance to vitamin D (in the sense that doses of vitamin required to effect a
biological response are much greater than the physiological requirements
necessary to maintain the integrity of the normal skeleton) is thought to
be due to defective metabolism of vitamin D. The kidney may be the
major site of synthesis of dihydroxylated metabolites of vitamin D (1,25-
dihydroxycholecalciferol   and   24,25-dihydroxycholecalciferol)[23-25].   The
development of bone disease and D-resistance of patients with chronic
renal disease may result in part from impaired endogenous production of
these hormones[23-26]. Production of 1,25-dihydroxycholecalciferol is defective in patients with advanced chronic renal disease, and the absence of
this hormonal form of vitamin D has been considered to contribute in
large measure to the D-resistance and bone disease of such patients. However, long-term administration of $l\alpha$-hydroxylated metabolites of vitamin
D does not always result in an improvement in bone disease, and apparently favourable biochemical responses may be associated with de-
mineralization and occasionally with deterioration of pre-existing bone
disease[10,27,28]. Patients with severe renal impairment, including anephric
patients, do not necessarily have bone disease nor does this inevitably
develop with time[5]. These observations suggest that factors, other than
defective renal production of 1,25-dihydroxy vitamin D_3 may be at least as
important. Preliminary studies showing effects of 24,25-dihydroxychole-
calciferol on retention of calcium, mineralization, and cartilage metabolism
suggest that deficiency of this hormone in chronic renal failure may also be
important in the production of bone disease.

10.3.3   Other factors

Renal failure is associated with the retention of potential toxins such as
indoles, guanidines, phenols, aliphatic amines and other 'middle molecules'
which are yet to be identified[29,30]. Substances normally found in trace
amounts such as fluoride[12], aluminium[31], vitamin A[32,33] and cadmium[34]
may also accumulate and contribute to disordered mineral metabolism.
Disturbances in acid-base balance[35-36] and in the metabolism of hormones
other than parathyroid hormone and vitamin D occur in chronic renal

failure. Affected hormones include calcitonin, growth hormone, sex hormones, prolactin and thyroid hormone, all of which may variously affect skeletal tissue itself or the metabolism of its regulating hormones[37-41]. The relative importance of these factors is controversial and, at present, their relevance in modifying approaches to treatment is uncertain.

10.4 PATHOGENESIS OF ECTOPIC CALCIFICATION

Though collagen promotes the precipitation of calcium and phosphate *in vitro*, the physiological mechanisms which initiate the formation and growth of mineral crystals and the factors which inhibit these processes in various connective tissues are unknown. In chronic renal failure the additional factors controlling soft-tissue calcification are also unclear,

TABLE 10.2   Clinical manifestations of disturbed mineral metabolism in chronic renal failure

	Disorders	*Clinical consequences*
1.	Hyperparathyroidism and osteitis fibrosa	Skeletal deformity Bone pain Pruritis
2.	Osteomalacia and decreased availability of vitamin D and phosphate	Skeletal deformity Bone pain Pathological fracture Proximal myopathy Haemolytic anaemia
3.	Osteoporosis	Pathological fracture Skeletal deformity
4.	Osteonecrosis	Joint pain Osteoarthrosis
5.	Osteosclerosis and periosteal new bone formation	None known
6.	Ectopic calcification	
	(*a*) Periarticular	Joint pain and limitation of movement
	(*b*) Skin and eye	Pruritis, red eye syndrome, corneal calcification
	(*c*) Vascular	Limitation of vascular access sites (including those required for transplantation). Vascular insufficiency of skin and muscle. ? Atheroma
	(*d*) Visceral	Heart block, cardiac failure, respiratory failure

though disturbed metabolism of collagen, pyrophosphate and magnesium may be important. From clinical observation[4,42] it is clear that the availability of calcium and phosphate are of direct importance, which is hardly surprising since they are invariable constituents of ectopic deposits. Ectopic calcification may be induced by the use of dialysate solutions rich in calcium or by increasing the intestinal absorption of calcium with vitamin D[43,44]. Fluctuations in plasma phosphate are generally greater than those seen in calcium[4], and changes in the availability of phosphate must be quantitatively more important than those of calcium.

Symptoms of ectopic calcification depend upon the tissues which are involved (Table 10.2). Symptoms and the deposits themselves may improve following restriction of dietary phosphate, or measures which reduce the balance of calcium. The possible importance of parathyroid hormone is suggested by the improvements in pruritis, periarticular or vascular calcification which may follow parathyroidectomy[4], though it is difficult to dissociate effects attributable to removal of parathyroid hormone itself from consequential changes in mineral metabolism.

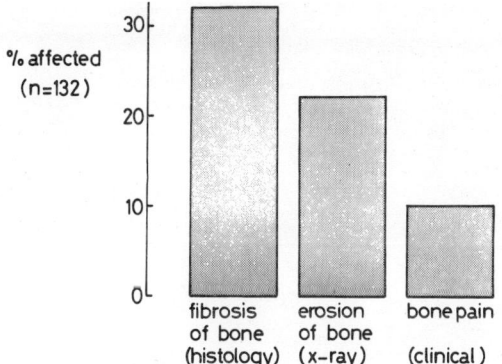

Figure 10.5   The prevalence of hyperparathyroidism in 132 patients with end-stage chronic renal failure about to start treatment with long-term haemodialysis. The prevalence depends upon the diagnostic criteria used and the methods of assessment. Histological abnormalities (marrow fibrosis) are more frequent than radiographic abnormalities. Symptoms occur in a minority.

10.5 FEATURES OF RENAL BONE DISEASE

Though renal bone disease is common, symptoms arising directly from skeletal disease itself are unusual[4] (Figure 10.5). But underlying biochemical disorders giving rise to bone disease may also express themselves clinically (Table 10.2).

10.5.1   Osteitis fibrosa

Histological features include the deposition of excessive amounts of fibrous tissue in the marrow spaces. This is associated with an increase in the numbers of active looking bone cells (osteoclasts and osteoblasts). Plasma levels of parathyroid hormone, alkaline phosphatase, and hydroxy-proline are higher than those found in patients without fibrosis and provide useful biochemical markers of disease activity[45]. Subperiosteal resorption of bone is the characteristic radiographic feature, but is less commonly seen than abnormalities in histology of bone (Figure 10.5). In some instances, particularly in children, erosions may give rise to skeletal deformities (Figure 10.6). Bone pain is uncommon (Figure 10.5).

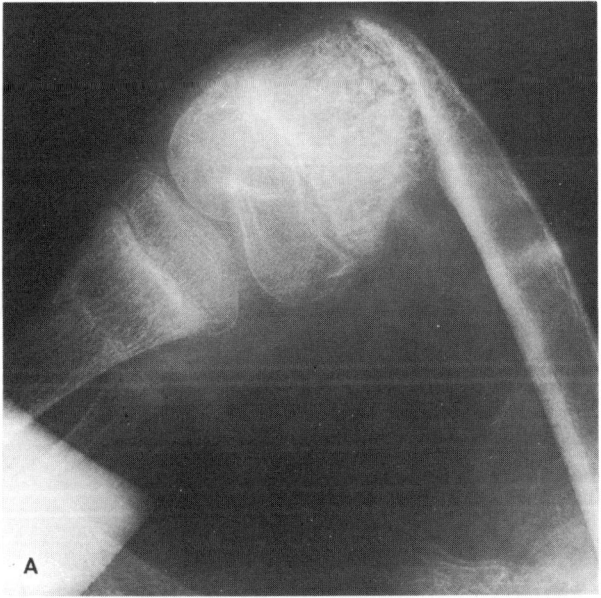

Figure 10.6   Radiographic features of renal bone disease. (A) Subperiosteal bone resorption in a child with renal failure. Resorption has caused deformity of the femur (from Kanis *et al.*[45])

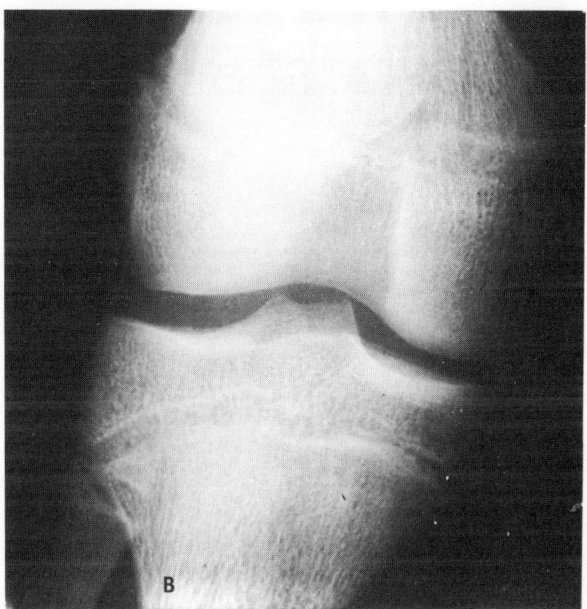

Figure 10.6 (B) Appearances similar to rickets in the tibia of a child with untreated renal bone disease (from Kanis *et al.*[45])

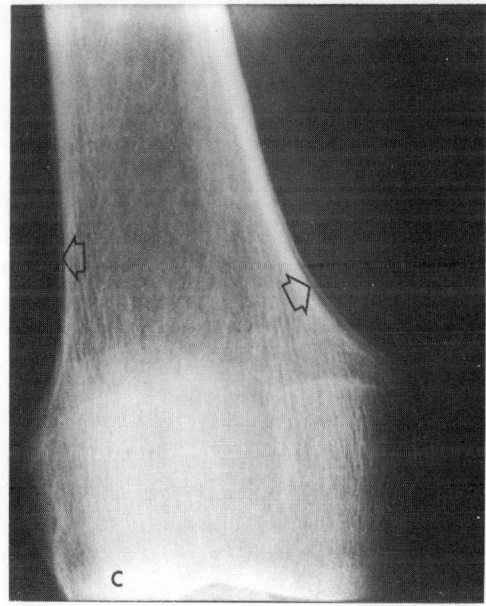

Figure 10.6 (C) Periosteal new bone formation. The periosteal separation from the mineralized cortex of the femur is shown by the arrows

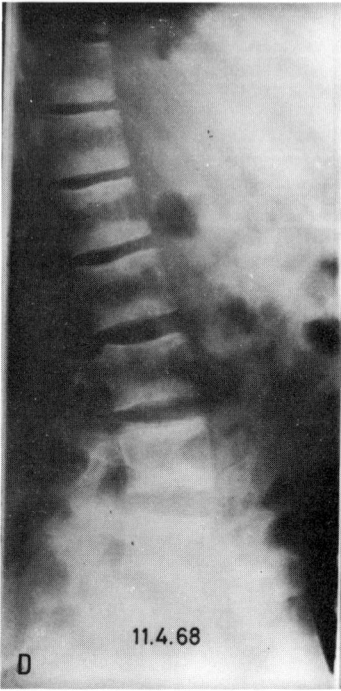

11.4.68

D

Figure 10.6   (D) Osteosclerosis of the spine. Alternate bands of sclerosis give rise
to a 'rugger jersey' appearance

10.5.2   Osteomalacia

In chronic renal disease an increase in the amount of unmineralized bone
(osteoid) may reflect its increased formation, defective mineralization or
both. The incidence of osteomalacia varies enormously between renal
units. In Oxford its incidence is low and does not increase with the duration of dialysis treatment even in anephric patients[5] which suggests that
defective production of metabolites of vitamin D may not be the major
factor in the pathogenesis of osteomalacia.

Bone cell counts, in the absence of osteitis fibrosa, are commonly low
and, unlike nutritional rickets, plasma levels of alkaline phosphatase may
be normal[46]. In some cases osteoblast function may be suppressed by low
levels of plasma phosphate induced by over-zealous administration of
phosphate binding agents or by the accumulation of aluminium. Radiographic abnormalities, similar to those found in D-deficient disorders
(Figure 10.6) are relatively uncommon and bone biopsy, rather than

x-rays or plasma measurements, may be the most powerful diagnostic aid. *In vivo* neutron activation analysis to measure total body or spinal calcium may provide a sensitive indirect index of response to treatment[27], but this technique is not widely available.

10.5.3 Osteosclerosis and periosteal new bone formation

These disorders are due to an increase in bone matrix either below the periosteal surface or in trabecular bone. These disorders are usually diagnosed by their characteristic x-ray appearances (Figure 10.6)[47] since they do not give rise to clinical problems. Osteosclerosis and periosteal new bone formation may be induced in experimental animals by the infusion of high doses of parathyroid hormone[48] but in patients with chronic renal failure they may be associated more with osteomalacia, where levels of parathyroid hormone are characteristically lower[49] than with osteitis fibrosa. Osteosclerosis may be seen for the first time on x-ray when osteomalacia is effectively treated with vitamin D.

10.5.4 Osteoporosis

A reduction in bone mass is commonly observed in chronic renal disease but is associated with abnormalities in bone matrix[1]. For this reason the term osteopaenia is sometimes used to distinguish the disorder from osteoporosis which by definition presupposes normality of collagen matrix. Osteoporosis is commonly progressive in patients on dialysis treatment[50] and the rate of bone loss may be accelerated for a short time after transplantation[51]. Its aetiology is unknown but factors of possible importance include the level of calcium used in the dialysis fluid, the administration of drugs which include steroids, cytotoxic agents and heparin as well as alterations in the metabolism of vitamin D[51, 52].

10.5.5 Avascular necrosis

Avascular necrosis occurs most commonly when steroids are used in the treatment of the underlying renal disorder (especially transplantation). It is likely that the combination of steroids and chronic renal failure are additive risk factors, since its occurrence is uncommon in steroid-treated patients without chronic renal failure or rarely noted in patients with renal impairment who are untreated with steroids. The pathogenesis of avascular necrosis is unknown and this is reflected by the increasing number of causative factors which have been invoked[53]. The disorder may be symptomless but pain is frequently present, which is presumably due to progressive necrosis, collapse of bone and secondary osteoarthrosis.

10.5.6 Metastatic calcification

The prevalence and effects of metastatic calcification are aspects of mineral metabolism that have been less well studied than others. This is due to the difficulties with which it is diagnosed in its early stages and its uncertain contribution to mortality and morbidity. In patients with florid ectopic calcification, it may give rise to serious disability and death (Table 10.2), but more frequently it presents as an incidental finding on radiographs and cannot be directly implicated in the morbidity of affected patients. It is however possible that calcification in blood vessels, even to an extent which is undetectable by x-ray techniques, may have important clinical consequences. For example, in patients with chronic renal failure, the risk of death and morbidity from atherosclerotic vascular disease may be greater than that of the healthy population[54]. Whilst risk factors such as hyperlipidaemia and hypertension may be important in this respect, the role of disturbed mineral metabolism might also be important in the regulation of platelet function or in the growth of atherosclerotic plaques. Observations that the diphosphonates, inhibitors, of mineralization and crystal growth, may prevent the induction of atheroma in animals fed atherogenic diets, give some credence to this view.

The factors which operate to give rise to calcification at various non-skeletal sites may well differ since periarticular lesions are commonly improved by restriction of dietary phosphate or by parathyroidectomy[4], but their effects on vascular, ectodermal and visceral calcification are less predictable (Figure 10.7).

10.6 TREATMENT

Treatment strategy should be based not only on the nature of the skeletal disorder but also on a careful assessment of the biochemical abnormalities by which the disorder arose. The likely management of the chronic renal disease itself should also be considered since, for example, therapeutic approaches may depend on the probability of subsequent transplantation.

10.6.1 Prophylaxis

There are a number of preventative measures which should be considered in all patients with advanced renal impairment. It is probable that the

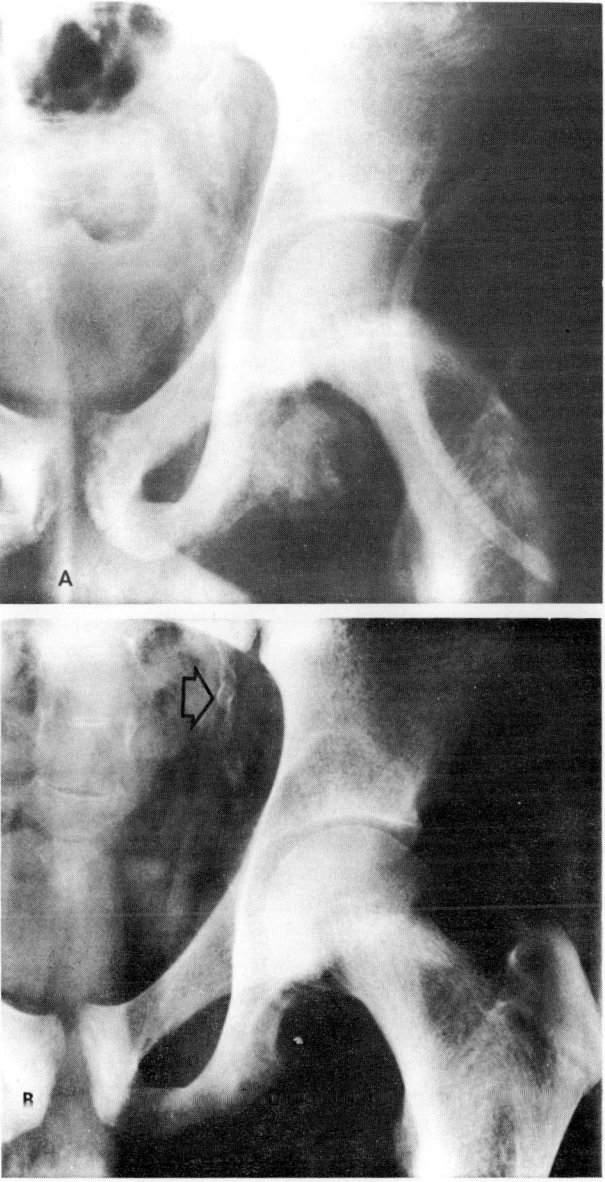

Figure 10.7 Metastatic (periatricular and vascular) calcification and erosions of bone in a patient treated by intermittent haemodialysis (A). X-rays taken 6 months after subtotal parathyroidectomy (B) show regression of erosions and soft tissue deposits but persistence of vascular calcification (arrow)

restriction of dietary intake of protein, as currently practised, is a greater factor in the induction of morbidity than it is in achieving beneficial effects. With respect to mineral metabolism, protein deficient diets tend to restrict the intake of vitamin C and pyridoxine[55,56] which both act as essential co-factors in the formation and maturation of collagen. These factors should be given as dietary supplements. In contrast, vitamin A accumulates, at least in the plasma of patients with chronic renal failure[55]. Vitamin A may cause bone resorption *in vitro* and augment the release of parathyroid hormone. Overdose with vitamin A *in vivo* may induce bone disease and hypercalcaemia, and supplements containing this vitamin should therefore be avoided.

Unlike the experimental models developed in the dog, there is at present no evidence that restriction of dietary phosphate in proportion to the degree of renal insufficiency, will prevent the secondary stimulation of parathyroid hormone. It is not practical to limit the dietary intake of phosphate but decreased availability of phosphate for absorption can be achieved with the use of phosphate-binding agents. These should be given to avoid the risks of metastatic calcification. In view of the association between osteomalacia and low plasma levels of phosphate, the amount of phosphate-binding drugs given should be regulated according to their effects on plasma phosphate. The level of predialysis plasma phosphate that best balances the risks of metastatic calcification and osteomalacia is unknown but probably lies between 1.6 and 2.2 mmol/l in dialysis patients (Figure 10.4).

Unlike the net intestinal absorption of phosphate which is largely dependent on the dietary load, the net absorption of calcium is more critically dependent on the presence of the vitamin D metabolites. It is thought that deficiency of 1,25-dihydroxycholecalciferol, which results from damage to renal tissue and from hyperphosphataemia, is the cause for the calcium malabsorption found in uraemia. But in some patients, especially those not yet on dialysis treatment, deficiency of this metabolite may also be due to low plasma levels of 25-hydroxycholecalciferol[57] induced by dietary restriction of vitamin D, imposed either by the patient or the physician. This can easily be remedied. The use of drugs which interfere with the metabolism or action of vitamin D, such as steroids, phenytoin and barbiturates[58] should, where possible, be avoided. In patients with end-stage renal disease, in whom the dietary intake of vitamin D is adequate, defective renal production of 1,25-dihydroxycholecalciferol probably accounts, in large measure, for the malabsorption of calcium. In such cases net absorption of calcium can be augmented by increases in the dietary intake but massive doses are required[59]. Unless the diet is deficient in calcium, increases in absorption are more readily induced with the use of vitamin D. Vitamin D and its metabolites will increase intestinal absorption of calcium and increase the plasma concentration. At present, the prophylactic use of these agents in preventing defective mineralization or secondary hyperparathyroidism is not established, though they may be effective in the prevention of osteopaenia or in the treatment of established bone disease.

The dialysis membrane provides a site for the loss or the incorporation of calcium into the body. The net transfer is dependent on shifts in plasma pH and protein levels, and on the respective calcium concentrations of plasma and dialysis fluid. The use of a low dialysate calcium (1.25 mmol/l) may aggravate osteopaenia but might also decrease the risk of metastatic calcification[52]. The use of calcium rich dialysis fluids (2.00 mmol/l) is not advised, despite reports of decreased secretion of parathyroid hormone[60], since metastatic calcification may be accentuated and the skeletal response disappointing[43]. As in the case of optimum levels of plasma phosphate, the ideal calcium concentration of dialysis fluid is unknown. Observations using a variety of techniques suggest that osteopaenia does not follow the use of dialysis fluids with a calcium level of 1.63 to 1.75 mmol/l[52,61].

10.6.2   Established bone disease

The administration of vitamin D, 25-hydroxy-, 1α-hydroxy- and 1,25-dihydroxy vitamin D may all increase plasma calcium, augment the balance and intestinal absorption of calcium and phosphate, and suppress the secretion of parathyroid hormone[10,22,45] (Figure 10.8). The rationale for their use in bone disease is based on the supposition that a decrease in the secretion of parathyroid hormone will reverse osteitis fibrosa and that the effects of the vitamin itself on target tissues will directly or indirectly induce normal mineralization. In practice, symptoms regress in the majority of patients but histological improvements are less consistently seen[10,28]. It is not yet known whether patients who fail to respond to vitamin D_2 or D_3 will respond more favourably to 1α-hydroxylated metabolites. The factors that may affect the outcome of treatment with the metabolites of D_3 include the severity of bone disease and the prevailing plasma level of calcium[10,62], which in turn may reflect the degree of parathyroid autonomy. Patients with high levels of plasma calcium respond poorly and the risks of inducing hypercalcaemia and soft tissue calcification are proportionately greater. The use of these agents, however, does not appear to aggravate vascular or corneal deposits, provided that plasma phosphate is controlled and prolonged hypercalcaemia is avoided. In

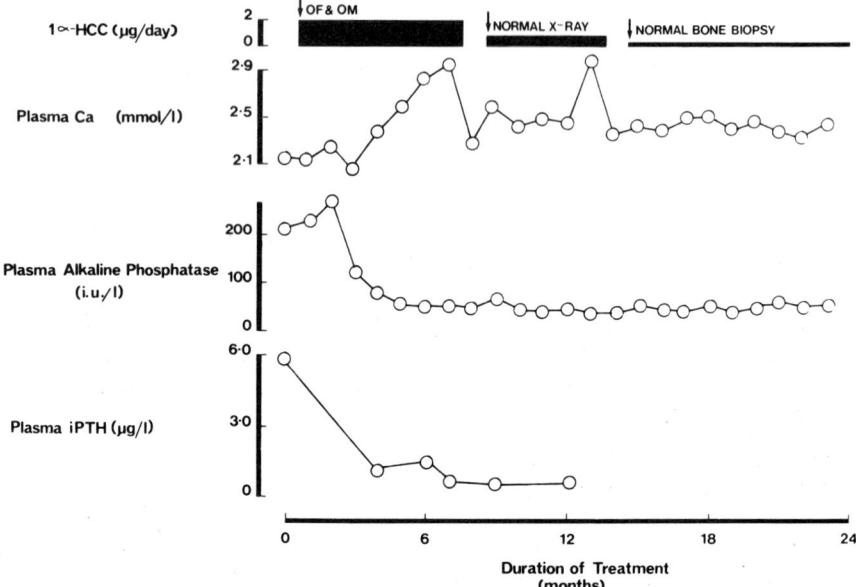

Figure 10.8   Long-term treatment of renal bone disease with lα-hydroxychole-calciferol (lα-HCC) in a dialysis-treated patient with renal bone disease. Healing of osteitis fibrosa (OF) and osteomalacia (OM) occurred within 15 months. Episodes of hypercalcaemia occurred suddenly and the dose of lα-HCC tolerated decreased when plasma alkaline phosphatase had fallen to normal levels (from Kanis *et al.*[58])

patients with severe metastatic calcification, parathyroidectomy or trans-plantation should be considered.

A potential advantage in the use of a metabolite whose production is impaired is that a decreased dose range may be required compared with the parent vitamin. However, in patients with osteitis fibrosa or osteo-malacia, the dose needed of lα-hydroxy metabolites may also change abruptly over an 8-fold range at various stages of treatment[58]. In general, the dose tolerated (in order to avoid hypercalcaemia) decreases with time (Figure 10.8). The greatest risk of hypercalcaemia occurs at the start of treatment and later when biochemical responses are nearing completion[62]. Plasma calcium should be monitored frequently during those risk periods. Currently, there is no evidence that the metabolites of vitamin D exert therapeutic effects in any way different from the parent compound. How-ever, in the case of 1,25-dihydroxycholecalciferol and its synthetic ana-logue, lα-hydroxycholecalciferol, their rapid onset and reversal of bio-logical activity confer significant advantages over other preparations

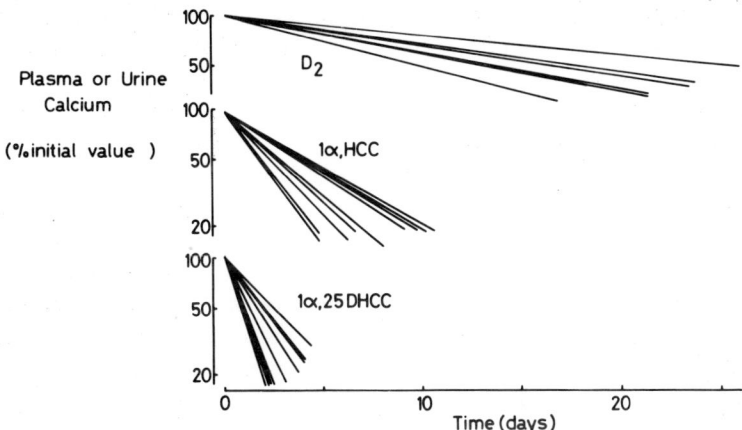

Plasma or Urine Calcium

(%initial value)

Figure 10.9   Rate of reversal of biological effects after stopping vitamin D₂ and the 1α-hydroxylated derivatives. The fall of plasma or urine calcium (observed minus asymptotic value) is shown on a logarithmic scale and expressed as a percentage of the initial value. (From Kanis and Russell[63])

(Figure 10.9)[63]. The dose may be more easily and rapidly titrated against requirements and inadvertent overdose more rapidly corrected with the 1α-hydroxylated metabolites than with vitamin D_3, D_2, dihydrotachysterol, or 25-hydroxycholecalciferol.

It might be expected that the widespread use of the vitamin D metabolites might eventually decrease the need for parathyroidectomy. At present there is still a need for parathyroidectomy where medical management has failed to improve bone disease or where metastatic calcification and hypercalcaemia are present. In patients with severe bone disease, especially in children where complications may develop rapidly, urgent parathyroidectomy may be considered. However, even in severe and rapidly progressive bone disease, a trial of medical treatment is well worthwhile and serves a dual purpose: if bone disease is rapidly controlled the need for parathyroidectomy may be avoided; if, on the other hand, there remains the need for surgery, the prior treatment with 1α-hydroxylated metabolites of D_3 will considerably decrease the post-operative complications of parathyroidectomy[64] (hypocalcaemia, hungry bones syndrome).

Total parathyroidectomy has been advocated on the grounds that the stimulus for the secretion of parathyroid hormone persists post-operatively and parathyroid hyperplasia will recur[65]. Developments in recent years allow this view to be challenged with increasing confidence. Though parathyroidectomy may be followed by rapid and striking improvements in osteitis fibrosa, pruritis and ectopic calcification[4] (Figure 10.7), patients may be left with persistent osteomalacia, refractory to treatment with vitamin D or its metabolites when total excision is performed. Subtotal parathyroidectomy might also be preferred if the patient is to be transplanted. Finally, if expectations of the ability of the D metabolites to suppress parathyroid gland stimulation are realized by long-term experience, then the use of these metabolites after partial parathyroidectomy may prevent recurrent hyperplasia.

Successful kidney transplantation may rapidly modify renal bone disease. Metastatic calcification and osteitis fibrosa usually regress though healing of bone may take a considerable period of time. Transplantation is, however, associated with an increased incidence of some of the disorders of mineral metabolism, particularly osteopaenia and avascular necrosis[51,53]. Post-transplant hypercalcaemia may give rise to the occasional need for parathyroidectomy[66].

ACKNOWLEDGEMENTS

I am grateful to the Wellcome Trust, the National Kidney Research Fund and the Peel Medical Research Trust for their support in various aspects of this work.

References

1. Avioli, L. V. and Teitelbaum, S. L. (1976). The renal osteodystrophies. In B. M. Brenner and F. C. Rector (eds.). *The Kidney*. pp. 1542–1591. (Philadelphia: W. B. Saunders Company)

2. De Luca, H. F. (1976). Recent advances in our understanding of the vitamin D endocrine system. *J. Lab. Clin. Med.*, **87**, 7

3. Coburn, J. W., Hartenbower, D. L. and Norman, A. W. (1974). Metabolism and action of the hormone vitamin D – Its relation to diseases of calcium homeostasis. *West. J. Med.*, **121**, 22

4. Katz, A. I., Hampers, C. L. and Merrill, J. P. (1969). Secondary hyperparathyroidism and renal osteodystrophy in chronic renal failure. *Medicine*, **48**, 333

5. Kanis, J. A., Adams, N. D., Earnshaw, M., Heynen, G., Ledingham, J. G. G., Russell, R. G. G. and Woods, C. G. (1977). Vitamin D, osteomalacia and chronic renal failure. In A. W. Norman, K. Shaefer, J. W. Coburn, H. F. DeLuca, D. Fraser, H. G. Grigoleit and D. v. Herrath (eds.). *Vitamin D. Biochemical, Chemical and Clinical Aspects Related to Calcium Metabolism*. pp. 671–673. (Berlin: de Gruyter)

6. Kerr, D. N. S., Walls, J., Ellis, D. H., Simpson, W., Uldall, P. R. and Ward, M. K. (1969). Bone disease in patients undergoing regular haemodialysis. *J. Bone Joint Surg.*, **51B**, 587

7. Eastwood, J. B. and De Wardener, H. E. (1975). Renal osteodystrophy. In N. F. Jones (ed.). *Recent Advances in Renal Disease*, **1**, 177

8. Mehls, O., Krempien, B., Ritz, E., Scharer, K. and Schuller, H. W. (1973). Renal osteodystrophy in children on maintenance haemodialysis. *Proc. E.D.T.A.*, **10**, 197

9. Henderson, R. G., Ledingham, J. G. G. and Woods, C. G. (1974). Renal osteodystrophy in relation to the cause of renal failure. *Kidney Int.*, **6**, 62

10. Coburn, J. W., Brickman, A. S., Sherrard, D. J., Singer, F. R., Baylink, D. J., Wong, E. G. C., Massry, S. G. and Norman, A. W. (1977). Clinical efficacy of 1,25-dihydroxy-vitamin D_3 in renal osteodystrophy. In A. W. Norman, K. Shaefer, J. W. Coburn, H. F. DeLuca, D. Fraser, H. G. Grigoleit and D. v. Herrath (eds.). *Vitamin D. Biochemical, Chemical and Clinical Aspects Related to Calcium Metabolism.* pp. 657–666. (Berlin: de Gruyter)

11. Dent, C. E. and Winter, C. S. (1974). Osteomalacia due to phosphate depletion from excessive aluminium hydroxide ingestion. *Br. Med. J.*, **1**, 551

12. Rao, T. K. S. and Friedman, E. A. (1975). Fluoride and bone disease in uremia. *Kidney Int.*, **7**, 125

13. Slatopolsky, E., Calgar, S., Gradowska, L., Canterbury, J., Reiss, E. and Bricker, N. S. (1972). On the prevention of secondary hyperparathyroidism in experimental chronic renal disease using 'proportional reduction' of dietary phosphorus intake. *Kidney Int.*, **2**, 147

14. Bricker, N. S. (1972). On the pathogenesis of the uremic state. *N. Engl. J. Med.*, **286**, 1093

15. Reiss, E., Canterbury, J. M. and Kanter, A. (1969). Circulating parathyroid hormone concentration in chronic renal insufficiency. *Arch. Intern. Med.*, **124**, 417

16. Coburn, J. W., Popovtzer, M. M., Massry, S. G. and Kleeman, C. R. (1969). The physiochemical state and renal handling of divalent ions in chronic renal failure. *Arch. Intern. Med.*, **124**, 302

17. Reiss, E., Canterbury, J. M., Bercovitz, M. A. and Kaplan, E. L. (1970). The role of phosphate in the secretion of parathyroid hormone in man. *J. Clin. Invest.*, **49**, 2146

18. Walton, R. J., Russell, R. G. G., Smith, R., Kanis, J. A. and Woodhead, J. S. (1976). The effects of a diphosphonate on phosphate transport in man. In L. Avioli, P. Bordier, H. Fleisch, S. Massry and E. Slatopolsky (eds.). *Phosphate Metabolism, Kidney and Bone.* pp. 329–343. (Toulouse: Nouvelle Imprimerie Fournié)

19. Walton, R. J., Woods, C. G., Russell, R. G. G., Kanis, J. A. and Clark, M. (1976). Histological measurements in Paget's disease of bone and their response to EHDP. *Calc. Tiss. Res.*, **22** (suppl.), 295

20. Bishop, M. C. (1973). Plasma biochemistry in haemodialysed patients. *Lancet*, ii, 1328

21. Baker, L. R. I., Ackrill, P., Cattell, W. R., Stamp, T. C. B. and Watson, L. (1974). Iatrogenic osteomalacia and myopathy due to phosphate depletion. *Br Med. J.*, **3**, 150

22. Stanbury, S. W. and Lumb, G. A. (1962). Metabolic studies of renal osteo-dystrophy. *Medicine*, **41**, 1

23. Fraser, D. R. and Kodicek, E. (1970). Unique biosynthesis by kidney of a biologically active vitamin D metabolite. *Nature* (London), **228**, 764

24. Mawer, E. B., Backhouse, J., Taylor, C. M., Lumb, G. A. and Stanbury, S. W. (1973). Evidence for failure of formation of 1,25-dihydroxycholecalciferol in chronic renal failure. *Lancet*, i, 626

25. Taylor, C. M. (1977). The measurement of 24,25-dihydroxycholecalciferol in human serum. In A. W. Norman, K. Shaefer, J. W. Coburn, H. F. DeLuca, D. Fraser, H. G. Grigoleit and D. v. Herrath (eds.). *Vitamin D. Biochemical, Chemical and Clinical Aspects Related to Calcium Metabolism.* pp. 541–543. (Berlin: de Gruyter)

26. Kanis, J. A., Heynen, G., Russell, R. G. G., Smith, R., Walton, R. J. and Warner, G. T. (1977). Biological effects of 24,25-dihydroxycholecalciferol in man. In A. W. Norman, K. Shaefer, J. W. Coburn, H. F. DeLuca, D. Fraser, H. G. Grigoleit and D. v. Herrath (eds.). *Vitamin D. Biochemical, chemical and clinical aspects related to calcium metabolism.* pp. 793–795. (Berlin: de Gruyter)

27. Naik, R., Gosling, P., Price, C., Robinson, B. H. B., Dabek, J. T., James, H. M., Kanis, J. A. and Smith, R. (1976). Whole body *in vivo* neutron activation analysis in assessing treatment of renal osteodystrophy with 1α-hydroxycholecalciferol. *Br. Med. J.*, 2, 79

28. Kanis, J. A., Earnshaw, M., Henderson, R. G., Heynen, G., Ledingham, J. G. G., Naik, R., Oliver, D. O., Russell, R. G. G., Smith, R., Wilkinson, R. H. and Woods, C. G. (1977). Correlation of clinical, biochemical and skeletal responses to 1α-hydroxycholecalciferol in renal bone disease. *Clin. Endocrinol.*, 7, 45s

29. DeFronzo, R. A., Andres, R., Edgar, P. and Walker, W. G. (1973). Carbohydrate metabolism in uremia: A review. *Medicine*, 52, 469

30. Gitelman, H. G. (1970). Uremic toxins and mineral metabolism. *Arch. Intern. Med.*, 126, 793

31. Parsons, V., Davies, C., Goode, C., Ogg, C. and Siddiqui, J. (1971). Aluminium in bone from patients with renal failure. *Br. Med. J.*, 4, 273

32. Smith, F. R. and Goodman, D. S. (1971). The effects of disease of the liver and kidneys on the transport of vitamin A in human plasma. *J. Clin. Invest.*, 50, 2426

33. Chertwo, B. S., Williams, G. A., Kiani, R., Stewart, K. L., Hargis, G. K. and Flayter, R. L. (1974). The interactions between vitamin A, vinblastine and cytochalasin B in parathyroid hormone secretion. *Proc. Soc. Exp. Biol. Med.*, 147, 16

34. Feldman, S. L. and Cousins, R. J. (1973). Influence of cadmium on the metabolism of 25-hydroxycholecalciferol in chicks. *Nutr. Rep. Int.*, 8, 4

35. Goodman, A. D., Leman, J., Lennon, E. J. and Relman, A. S. (1965). Production, excretion and net balance of fixed acid in patients with renal acidosis. *J. Clin. Invest.*, 44, 495

36. Pellegrino, E. D. and Biltz, B. S. (1965). The composition of human bone in uremia. *Medicine*, 44, 397

37. MacIntyre, I. (1977). Comparative aspects of the biochemistry of the regulation of vitamin D metabolism. In A. W. Norman, K. Shaefer, J. W. Coburn, H. F. DeLuca, D. Fraser, H. G. Grigoleit and D. v. Herrath (eds.). *Vitamin D. Biochemical, Chemical and Clinical Aspects Related to Calcium Metabolism.* pp. 155–164. (Berlin: de Gruyter)

38. Lancer, S. R., Bowser, E. N., Hargis, G. K. and Williams, G. A. (1976).

The effect of growth hormone on parathyroid function in rats. *Endocrinology*, **98**, 1289

39. Barbour, G. L. and Sevier, B. R. (1974). Adrenal responsiveness in chronic hemodialysis. *N. Engl. J. Med.*, **290**, 1258

40. Heynen, G., Kanis, J. A., Ledingham, J. G. G., Oliver, D. O. and Russell, R. G. G. (1976). Evidence that endogenous calcitonin protects against renal bone disease. *Lancet*, **ii**, 1322

41. Kanis, J. A., Earnshaw, M., Heynen, G., Ledingham, J. G. G., Oliver, D. O., Russell, R. G. G., Woods, C. G., Franchimont, P. and Gaspar, S. (1977). Changes in histologic and biochemical indexes of bone turnover after bilateral nephrectomy in patients on hemodialysis. *N. Engl. J. Med.*, **296**, 1073

42. Parfitt, A. M. (1969). Soft tissue calcification in uremia. *Arch. Intern. Med.*, **124**, 544

43. Mirahmadi, K. S., Duffy, B. S., Shinaberger, J. H., Jowsey, J., Massry, S. G. and Coburn, J. W. (1971). A controlled evaluation of clinical and metabolic effects of dialysate calcium levels during regular hemodialysis. *Trans. Am. Soc. Artif. Intern. Organs*, **17**, 118

44. Henderson, R. G., Kanis, J. A., Ledingham, J. G. G., Oliver, D. O., Russell, R. G. G., Smith, R. and Walton, R. G. G. (1976). Comparative effects of 1α-hydroxycholecalciferol in children and adults with renal glomerular osteodystrophy. In S. P. Nielsen and E. Hjorting-Hansen (eds.). *Calcified Tissues 1975*. pp. 221–225. (Copenhagen: FADL's Forlag)

45. Kanis, J. A., Henderson, R. G., Heynen, G., Ledingham, J. G. G., Russell, R. G. G., Smith, R. and Walton, R. J. (1977). Renal osteodystrophy in non-dialysed adolescents: long-term treatment with 1α-hydroxycholecalciferol. *Arch. Dis. Childh.*, **52**, 473

46. Bishop, M. C., Smith, R., Ledingham, J. G. G. and Oliver, D. O. (1971). Biochemical markers in renal bone disease. *Proc. E.D.T.A.*, **8**, 122

47. Rabinovich, S., Meema, H. E. and Oreopoulos, D. G. (1976). Histological observations of periosteal new bone formation in renal osteodystrophy. In Z. E. G. Zaworski (ed.). *Proceedings of the First Workshop on Histomorphometry*. p. 117. (Ottawa: University Press)

48. Kalu, D. N., Doyle, F. H., Pennock, J. and Foster, G. V. (1970). Parathyroid hormone and experimental osteosclerosis. *Lancet*, **i**, 1363

49. Simpson, W., Ellis, H. A., Kerr, D. N. S., McElroy, M., McNay, R. A. and Peart, K. N. (1976). Bone disease in long-term haemodialysis: the association of radiological with histological abnormalities. *Br. J. Radiol.*, **49**, 105

50. Stanbury, S. W. (1972). Azotemic renal osteodystrophy. In I. MacIntyre (ed.) *Clinics in Endocrinology and Metabolism*. p. 267. (Philadelphia: W. B. Saunders)

51. Atkinson, P. J., Hancock, D. A., Acharya, V. N., Parsons, F. M., Prockor, E. A. and Reed, G. W. (1973). Changes in skeletal mineral in patients on prolonged maintenance dialysis. *Br. Med. J.*, **4**, 519

52. Bone, J. M., Davison, A. M. and Robson, J. S. (1972). Role of dialysate calcium concentration in osteoporosis in patients on haemodialysis. *Lancet*, **i**, 1047

53. Briggs, W. A., Hampers, C. L., Merrill, J. P., Hager, E. B., Wilson, R. E., Birtch, A. G. and Murray, J. E. (1972). Aseptic necrosis in the femur after renal transplantation. *Ann. Surg.*, **175**, 282

54. Ibels, L. S., Stewart, J. H., Mahoney, J. F., Neale, F. C. and Sheil, A. G. R. (1977). Occlusive arterial disease in uraemic and haemodialysis patients and renal transplant recipients. *Q. J. Med.*, **46**, 197

55. Kopple, J. D. and Swendseid, M. E. (1975). Vitamin nutrition in patients undergoing maintenance hemodialysis. *Kidney Int.*, **7**, 79S

56. Sullivan, J. F. and Eisenstein, A. B. (1970). Ascorbic acid depletion in patients undergoing chronic hemodialysis. *Am. J. Clin. Nutr.*, **23**, 1339

57. Eastwood, J. B., Harris, E., Stamp, T. C. B. and DeWardener, H. E. (1976). Vitamin-D deficiency in the osteomalacia of chronic renal failure. *Lancet*, ii, 1209

58. Kanis, J. A., Russell, R. G. G. and Smith, R. (1977). Physiological and therapeutic differences between vitamin D, its metabolites and analogues. *Clin. Endocrinol.*, **7**, 191s

59. Clarkson, E. M., Durrant, C., Phillips, M. E., Gower, P. E., Jewkes, R. F. and De Wardener, H. E. (1970). The effect of a high intake of calcium and phosphate in normal subjects and patients with chronic renal failure. *Clin. Sci.*, **39**, 693

60. Goldsmith, R. S., Furszyfer, J., Johnson, W. J., Fournier, A. E. and Arnaud, C. D. (1971). Control of secondary hyperparathyroidism during long term hemodialysis. *Am. J. Med.*, **50**, 692

61. Naik, R. B., Dabek, J. T., Heynen, G., James, H. M., Kanis, J. A., Robertson, P. W., Robinson, B. H. B. and Woods, C. G. (1977). Measurement of whole body calcium in chronic renal failure: effects of 1α-hydroxycholecaciferol and parathyroidectomy. *Clin. Endocrinol.*, **7**, 139s

62. Kanis, J. A., Russell, R. G. G., Naik, R. B., Earnshaw, M., Smith, R., Heynen, G. and Woods, C. G. (1977). Factors influencing the response to 1α-hydroxycholecalciferol in patients with renal bone disease. *Clin. Endocrinol.*, **7**, 51s

63. Kanis, J. A. and Russell, R. G. G. (1977). Rate of reversal of hypercalcaemia and hypercalciuria induced by vitamin D and its 1α-hydroxylated derivatives. *Br. Med. J.*, **1**, 78

64. Boyle, I. T., Fogelman, L., Boyce, B., Thomson, J. E., Beastall, G. H., McIntosh, I. and McLennan, I. (1977). 1α-hydroxy vitamin D_3 in primary hyperparathyroidism. *Clin. Endocrinol.*, **7**, 215s

65. Ogg, C. S. (1967). Total parathyroidectomy in treatment of secondary (renal) hyperparathyroidism. *Br. Med. J.*, **4**, 331

66. Grimelius, L., Johansson, H., Lindquist, B. and Wibell, L. (1972). Tertiary hyperparathyroidism occurring during a renal transplantation programme: report and discussion of three cases. *J. Pathol.*, **108**, 23

DISCUSSION

B. Silke (Dublin): Is there any evidence to suggest that any of the newer analogues are superior to AT 10 in the treatment of renal bone disease?

Cameron: AT 10 is also known as DHT – dihydrotachysterol; it is one preparation of it.

Kanis: There are a number of reports which suggest that there are quite large differences between the various vitamin D-like compounds in their effects upon target tissues. Whether these differences are important in the treatment of renal bone disease is unknown, and there is no convincing evidence, to date, which might suggest that the way in which a therapeutic effect was achieved with one compound differs significantly from the effects of the various other vitamin D-like compounds. However, there is one real advantage in the use of the 1α-hydroxylated metabolites of vitamin D in that their onset and reversal of action is more rapid than that of the other compounds. This means that the dose can be readily titrated according to requirements, and should the patient inadvertently be poisoned, hypercalcaemia may be reversed very rapidly.

Cameron: I can endorse that.

J. S. Robson (Edinburgh): When we think of renal bone disease, we think of the cumulative distortions which have occurred over the previous 5–10 years and there are a number of things that can be unravelled.
  Taking Dr Kanis's three methods of treatment, at what stage should they be applied? What does he think about starting at a very early stage long before there is any clinical evidence, and possibly minimal chemical or bone histological evidence, with the idea of preventing renal bone disease? Would one start before there is any gross architectural distortion that we know to be associated with it?

Kanis: I sympathize with the sentiment that prevention is better than cure. It is certainly possible to modify the natural history of established renal bone disease in some affected patients, but I am not sure whether this use of these agents is pharmacological or physiological, since I am not convinced that the major component of renal bone disease is due to a defective production of 1α-hydroxylated metabolites. Their prophylactic use may not, therefore, be analogous to endocrine replacement therapy.

It is a little early to say with any confidence that renal bone disease could be prevented, although I sympathize with the idea.

Robson: Has anyone tried?

Kanis: A number of trials are currently underway to examine the prophylactic effects of 1,25-dihydroxycholecalciferol and 1α-hydroxycholecalciferol.

R. Ward (Newcastle-upon-Tyne): One of the hallmarks of Newcastle bone disease is that it is unresponsive to D_2, D_3, 1α, 1,25, and DHT, and that it moves on relentlessly.

Has Dr Kanis any comment or experience on this?

Kanis: I hinted briefly that there are large geographical differences in the nature of bone disease seen in various units. 'Newcastle bone disease' is characterized by excessive amounts of osteoid, very few numbers of cells on the osteoid surfaces, and a relatively low level of plasma alkaline phosphatase. It seems to be a kind of osteoblast poisoning which might be due to aluminium, for example in the dialysis fluid or the enthusiastic use of phosphate binders in the past. We do see this type of bone disease, but it occurs in perhaps 2% of our dialysis population and, unlike that of Newcastle, its incidence does not increase with time on dialysis. It is very much more common in Newcastle, but it does occur elsewhere.

F. M. Parsons (Leeds): There is another method by which calcium loss occurs during dialysis, which has been largely ignored. We all know that there is decreased absorption of dietary calcium in renal failure but in addition each time a patient is dialysed about 60 to 100 mg of calcium is removed by ultrafiltration. Further loss occurs when blood is washed back from the dialyser with saline for calcium is not 'reverse dialysed' from dialysate to blood compartment to give a normal diffusible level in the saline. In total a patient can lose anything up to 1700 mg of calcium per week either from the gastrointestinal tract or during dialysis. There will be considerable variation from patient to patient. Some will remain in relatively reasonable calcium balance for they may have better absorption of calcium.

It is all very well talking about the use of vitamin D metabolites or analogues but we must really prevent the negative calcium balance that can be induced by dialysis.

Kanis: Metabolic balance studies are extremely difficult to do on dialysis patients. Dr Bishop in our unit has tried to measure calcium balance in the past, but the techniques used incurred too great an error to provide accurate information.

Parsons: Not the dialysis inaccuracies, surely, for during dialysis there is usually a loss of weight which means that calcium is lost from patient to dialysis fluid.

Kanis: Losses of calcium during dialysis depends on a variety of factors. They depend on the changes in pH, protein concentration and on the duration of dialysis. Perhaps of greatest importance, they depend on the level of calcium that is used in the dialysis fluid. The optimum level of dialysate calcium is not precisely known, but there are data, derived from the rather elegant technique of total body neutron activation analysis, which can give an estimate of calcium balance over a prolonged period of time. The use of dialysate calcium of about 1.65 mmol/l seems to prevent bone loss.

The use of higher concentrations of calcium in the dialysis fluid (up to 2 mmol/l) has been advocated to suppress parathyroid activity but the results are rather disappointing in terms of reversing histologial abnormalities or of decreasing the secretion of parathyroid hormone over the long term. Such procedures also incur the risks of increasing the incidence of metastatic calcification.

We are not neglecting the problem. It is a difficult area to investigate and the successes that have been achieved in that area have been relatively limited.

Cameron: Dr Parsons would like to see the trial with all the regimens that have been mentioned using calcium containing wash-back fluid at the end of the dialysis rather than manipulation of the calcium concentration in the dialysis fluid.

Parsons. As one of the many aspects.

B. H. B. Robinson (Birmingham): Unless one uses excessive volumes, most wash-back fluid does not get into the patient. Most of the blood in the dialyser returns into the patient. I do not think that aspect of technique is very significant in relation to calcium. A few mmols of calcium that will be lost by ultrafiltration will be more than compensated for by using a bath calcium above the level of plasma ultrafilterable calcium. *In vivo* neutron activation studies from our department show that very nearly all patients on dialysis are in positive calcium balance.

Kanis: Various data, using a variety of other techniques, have shown that calcium levels in the dialysis fluid from about 1.63 to 1.75 mmol/l are perhaps the optimum in terms of preventing bone loss and minimizing metastatic calcification.

Parsons: Many other investigations have suggested that it is necessary to have 1.75–2.0 mmol/l of calcium in the dialysis fluid to correct both the ultrafiltration deficit, and also the negative gastrointestinal balance. It is not just the technique of dialysis that leads to a negative balance, but the inability of the intestinal tract to absorb calcium. In fact body calcium is lost into the gastrointestinal tract, and this is where it becomes even more difficult to undertake routine measurements.

Kanis: This is where the technique of whole body *in vivo* neutron activation is ideal, because repeated measurements provide an overall balance measurement. Certainly bone loss during dialysis can be largely prevented.

SECTION FOUR

**Psychological and
Personal Aspects**
Chairman:
M. Carmody

SECTION FOUR

11

Psychological problems of the paediatric haemodialysis patient
D. S. James

11.1   PROBLEMS REFERRED TO IN THE LITERATURE

1.1.1   Mental defence mechanisms

Many papers refer to DENIAL[1-3] which shields a person from facing the severity of his problem and its apparent consequences. In some situations this is an adaptive process, especially in the early stages of a disorder as it may prevent a more serious and complete breakdown. Later it may become maladaptive because if the condition is not accepted, the patient may be prevented from making the right manoeuvres to cope with it. Sand *et al.*[4] say that people do best who discuss their anxieties openly and make no use of mental defence mechanisms which may make them inaccessible to such discussion. Villard[5] found that adults under stress from dialysis polarize into two types. Some become passive and submissive while others over-compensate with optimism or euphoria.

11.1.2   Depression

Abram[6] mentioned four stages of adaptation to dialysis. At first the patient is uraemic, low and depressed for biological reasons. He then begins dialysis and feels an improvement in health but is anxious about the technicalities and fears mechanical failure. In the third stage a reactive depression is likely to occur when the problems of dependency and long-term adaptation to the handicap have to be faced. When this is coped with he enters the fourth phase of rehabilitation. Abram[2] refers to a series of

3478 dialysis patients of whom 166 hastened their death either actively or by passive non-compliance with their treatment regimens.

With children in the early stages of dialysis one finds it difficult to decide to what extent the depressions may be 'biological' and to what extent they are reactive. The mood is sometimes labile on dialysis and can vary markedly from day to day. The use of tricyclic antidepressants in uraemia has been discussed[7] but in children it is often more appropriate to look at ways of adding extra support and helping those caring for the child at home and in hospital to 'tune in' to the patient's distress until the depressive phase passes.

11.1.3   Effects on the family

The spouses of patients undergoing dialysis may require extra support because of the emotional stresses of the situation[8], and in vulnerable families, persons other than the dialysis patient may become mentally ill[9]. A secure marriage not surprisingly suggests that rehabilitation will be successful but unstable marriages may be broken apart. Two papers concerning children undergoing dialysis make similar points. Bernstein[10] reviewed 12 children who were dialysed and then transplanted. Stress symptoms during dialysis often reflected the child's pre-morbid emotional state. The child with previous adjustment problems will find that his maladjustment becomes exacerbated with the added stress of dialysis. The importance of good parental management as a prognostic factor for satisfactory adjustment is also mentioned. Ten of Bernstein's children adapted reasonably well, showing some defences of denial and fantasy, but two broke down with severe depressions and regressive episodes.

Forty-seven children on a dialysis/transplant programme were reviewed from Los Angeles[11] and two distinct problem groups were seen. One group began to withdraw, sleep and turn away and another group became increasingly attention seeking, demanding and dependent. Again the potentiation of family disruption was seen. Where the parents' marriage was vulnerable its break-up was hastened, whereas close caring relationships between the parents caused the family to tighten up into an even more cohesive group.

11.2   THE GLASGOW CHILDREN ON DIALYSIS

11.2.1   Psychiatric assessment

The Renal Unit in the Royal Hospital for Sick Children in Glasgow is just for children. It is an attractive compact ward and communications are good. There have now been 17 children on dialysis aged between 6 and 14 years on arrival. An initial psychiatric interview is done when dialysis is contemplated, along with a psychological assessment giving information about the child's attainments and intelligence. The parents are seen by the psychiatrist to screen them for mental illness and abnormal attitudes, while the psychiatric social worker overlaps and establishes social difficulties and problems in the family pattern of relationships.

11.2.2   The importance of a settled marriage and a settled mother

The data shown in Tables 11.1 and 11.2 is only based on rating scales and opinions, although such soft data sometimes conveys more meaning than more objective tests which may not measure quite what is intended.

Table 11.1 concerns the relationship between psycho-social problems experienced in the family during the child's dialysis and the quality of the parents' marriage rated at the first interview. The marriages were rated on a four point scale: 1. Satisfactory; 2. Stresses contained; 3. Severe stresses and 4. Broken up. In Table 11.1, ratings 1 and 2 are labelled 'marriage satisfactory' and marriages rated 3 or 4 are included under the title 'severe stress or separation'.

TABLE 11.1   Psycho-social problems experienced during dialysis and quality of the parents' marriage at the onset of treatment

Marriage at onset	During dialysis	
	Family cope	Psycho-social problems
Marriage satisfactory	5	0
Severe stress or separation	3	8
Association of problems during dialysis and marital stress before treatment		$P < 0.05$ (Fisher test)

Some of the psycho-social problems encountered included heavy drinking, poor mental health, financial troubles and other manifestations of not coping with the situation.

Although the data is 'soft' there is a significant association between the families that experienced problems during the child's dialysis and those which were under marital stress before the treatment began.

The three misfits in Table 11.1 are all atypical. One family which had

TABLE 11.2 Child's adjustment to dialysis and the mother's mental state at the onset of treatment

Mother's mental state at onset	During dialysis	
	Child copes	Child has symptoms
Mother all right	5	0
Mother; psychiatric problem or mother absent	2	10
Association of child's adjustment problems and impairment of mothering by poor mental health or separation		$P < 0.25$ (Fisher test)

been separated was reunited, in another, there had been a divorce but the mother was about to remarry, and in the third, a very caring grandmother had taken over.

Table 11.2 is concerned with the relationship between the mother's mental state at the onset of the dialysis and the child's subsequent adjustment to the situation. Although two-thirds of the mothers were rated as showing some impairment, it is not implied that they were sufficiently unwell to merit admission to a psychiatric hospital. These mothers were showing some symptoms of anxiety or depression, were often taking psychotropic drugs and were prone to use the interview situation to discuss their own emotional needs. Where the children had adjustment problems these were likely to be withdrawal, regression, depression or attention demanding. Table 11.2 shows that the child copes best when the mother is in good mental health. The link between neurosis in the mother and symptoms in the child is an important piece of child psychiatry and was highlighted by Professor Rutter in 1966[12].

11.2.3 Intelligence of the children

The measured intelligence quotients ranged from 74 to 142, that is from borderline defective to very bright. Inspection of our data does not yet show intelligence to be related to prognosis for good dialysis. One of our dull children manages very well on home dialysis and the very bright one is doing splendidly as well.

11.2.4 The long-term effects of home dialysis on the family

We have five surviving children who have been on home haemodialysis for several months. In three families the interpersonal relationships are *status quo*. One family shows stress, partly because of social and financial problems resulting from the need to move house and one family has reunited from a previous separation because of the dialysis situation.

11.3 HOW DOES THE FAMILY COPE?

11.3.1 The parental responses

These are some of the ways that enable families to cope with the impact of learning that they have a child with a kidney disorder that will need long-term dialysis. The same principles apply where the child is found to be diabetic, mentally retarded or to be suffering from leukaemia. These reactions are described in textbooks of child psychiatry[13] and are usefully discussed by Steinhauer *et al.*[14].

11.3.1.1 *Denial*

This occurs where the loss of function has not been accepted and if the prognosis is felt to be pessimistic or even incorrect by the parents they may take the child away for another opinion just as treatment is being planned. The same mental mechanism may prevent realistic expectations of the child's limitations and lead to friction between the doctor and the parents. The extent of denial is not a factor of intelligence. Where there is serious illness there is often apparent lack of judgement shown by relatives until they can accept the situation realistically.

11.3.1.2 *Anger*

Sometimes parents will be quite aggressive to medical and nursing staff. This results from a normal grief about the child's loss of function. People can become upset and angry about a fault developing in their car and blame the manufacturer or the garage quite forcibly. The chronic failure of a child's kidney is even more serious and often there is a need to blame someone. Parents may become bitter with their friends but are more likely to find fault with their family doctor or the hospital staff.

11.3.1.3 *Guilt*

Frequently the angry feelings turn inwards as in bereavement reactions and this intra-punitive anger becomes guilt. The parents blame themselves. Perhaps they should have gone to the doctor earlier. Perhaps they should have pushed for a hospital appointment sooner or given better information. 'If only I had not sent him out in the rain and been nicer to him this wouldn't have happened.' Parents may feel to be victims of fate or see the child's disorder as proof of their own inadequacy.

11.3.1.4   Depression

If the guilt is not coped with it can precipitate depression and the mood becomes increasingly flat with morbid thoughts, tearfulness and suicidal ideas. Biological symptoms include sleep disturbance, appetite loss and weight changes.

11.3.1.5   Marital stresses

Parents faced with a sick child may both want extra emotional support but have little to give. Fathers may escape into working long hours rather than face the demands for support in the home. One parent may adopt a pathological attitude towards the sick child and the other may challenge this with inevitable increasing friction.

11.3.1.6   The siblings

Further tension may occur because of the focus onto the sick child who needs to visit the hospital for three days per week. The other children may be somewhat deprived of their usual parental interest but unable to show their displeasure because 'who can be jealous of his sick brother'. The bottled up ill feeling presents in other ways, perhaps as a falling off in school performance, as psychogenic pain or even by joining an antisocial peer group.

11.3.1.7   Abnormal attitudes

Although many parents accept the situation and help the child to feel valued, some show *rejection* in various ways. The child may be poorly clad in comparison to his siblings or there may be repeated requests for re-admissions to hospital. A more subtle kind of rejection is shown by parents who initially give the impression that they are very caring. During successive interviews it is noticed that they are dissatisfied with the child's achievements and medical progress, which causes the child to be undermined. They are trying to say 'look what good parents we are, we are doing everything to get him right and still he won't be well'. This is a rejecting attitude masked by an apparent overprotection. The more straightforward *overprotection* is also damaging to the child and occurs where the parents are excessively anxious.

11.3.2   The child's responses

11.3.2.1   *Denial*

As previously mentioned, this mechanism enables the child to exclude stressful situations from his thoughts. The resulting behaviour may appear detached and inconsistent towards the demands of treatment, for example, refusal of a diet which he feels to be unnecessary.

11.3.2.2   *Reaction formation*

This is shown by the child who needs to appear tough and to dominate his friends. From under this defence, frequently emerges a child who is anxious, brittle and eventually discloses a poor self-opinion. A disability requiring dependence on repeated medical treatment is prone to generate this response.

11.3.2.3   *Regression*

This is shown by many children under stress when they become more dependent and infantile. They may crave undivided adult attention, wish to be fed, request medications and make heavy demands on nursing staff.

11.3.2.4   *Obsessions*

Some children indulge in magical thinking. 'If I tap the medicine three times it won't go wrong.' The resulting rituals and unnecessary attention to irrelevant detail may irritate the nursing staff and exhaust the child.

11.3.2.5   *Fantasy*

Younger children may shut out the unpleasant reality world by becoming lost in the more acceptable world of make believe. Much of children's literature and media programmes assume high levels of fantasy.

The above are 'coping mechanisms' which enable the child to remain in reasonable mental health. Where these mechanisms give inadequate protection or where the stresses become too severe the child may break down into illness needing more specialized psychiatric help. The common illnesses are:

11.3.2.6 *Massive withdrawal*

Occurs with blatant lack of cooperation and motivation. A child has been observed where his dialyser became disconnected and he made no effort to raise alarm as the blood poured onto the floor.

11.3.2.7 *Anxiety neurosis*

This may occur with obsessional thinking, feelings of impending doom, tension symptoms and inability to cope.

11.3.2.8 *Depression*

This is also seen with psychogenic pain, sleep disturbance, anorexia, poor concentration, fears and morbid guilty thoughts. Depressed children are clingy to parents and staff and the cheerful approach often lacks empathy and hence fails to alleviate the distress. Much of the above maladaptive behaviour can be averted by attention to the following points.

11.4 HOW TO AVERT PSYCHOLOGICAL PROBLEMS

The emotional impact of a child on long-term dialysis *effects the whole family* either directly or indirectly through the reaction of another family member.

It takes time for those involved to work through the defences and reach a *realistic acceptance* of the situation. The nephrologist should share the details and prognosis with parents at an early stage and enable further discussion time to clarify points which have not been heard (denial) and also show that there are no ill feelings from the parents' initial responses which may have been anger.

Marital stress can be minimized by *seeing both parents together* so that the information is not moulded into armaments for disagreements. *Frequent appointments* should be offered where pathological attitudes develop and the handling of these situations may be passed to an experienced social worker.

Children on dialysis should be encouraged to talk out their fantasy. The conspiracy of silence should be avoided. Children may have gross misconceptions about their kidneys or the dialysis. One child thought he had to go inside the machine to have his blood washed.

The child's *school attainments* should be monitored. Much time can be lost before dialysis and from days off attending the unit. The child feels lost and can 'give up'. Our own unit has a teacher and the education authorities can usually provide extra help if the problem is made clear to them. These children will rely on non-physical jobs when they grow into adult life and education is especially important. Staff working in renal units should *not bear hostility personally*. Reasons for parental anger and non-cooperation from children have been discussed. To turn against one's clients in confrontation will play into the psychopathology.

The team approach can be helpful in dealing with psycho-social problems and community links including the child's school. Regular case conferences involving nephrologist, nurses, dietician, teacher, play leader, social worker, psychologist and psychiatrist can ensure good communications between those involved. The team should not however encroach on the medical management decisions and the team leader should be the nephrologist in charge.

Nursing staff should not rival with the parents. The dependency of the child meets a vocational emotional need in a caring nurse. Parents may resent the child's attachment to nursing staff and it is easy to undermine a parent with social problems, which may increase the child's distress and cause the family to find fault with the unit. Nevertheless the nurse or doctor will get to know the dialysis children intimately, and like the good parent, they *must set limits* on the child's behaviour. It is caring to enforce diet, treatment and reasonable conduct but this should be done with a positive relationship so that the patient does not feel disliked. It is this trusting relationship that is the major defence against the emergence of psychopathology.

References

1. Glassman, B. M. and Siegel, A. (1970). Personality correlates of survival in a long-term hemodialysis program. *Arch. Gen. Psychiat.*, 22, 566
2. Abram, H. S. (1970). Survival by machine: the psychological stress of chronic hemodialysis. *Psychiat. Med.*, 1, 37
3. Short, M. J. and Wilson, W. P. (1969). Roles of denial in chronic hemo-dialysis. *Arch. Gen. Psychiat.*, 20, 433
4. Sand, P., Livingston, G. and Wright, R. G. (1966). Psychological assessment of candidates for a hemodialysis program. *Ann. Intern. Med.*, 64, 602
5. Villard, H. P. (1969). The psychiatric consultant in the renal dialysis and transplant unit. *Un. Med. Canada*, 98, 233
6. Abram, H. S. (1969). The psychiatrist, the treatment of chronic renal failure and the prolongation of life. *Am. J. Psychiat.*, 126, 157
7. Neary, D. (1976). Neuropsychiatric sequelae of renal failure. *Br. J. Hosp. Med.*, 15, 122
8. Shambaugh, P. W. and Kanter, S. S. (1969). Spouses under stress: group meetings with spouses of patients on hemodialysis. *Am. J. Psychiat.*, 125, 928

9. Cramond, W. A. (1971). Renal transplantations – experiences with recipients and donors. *Sem. Psychiat.*, **3**, 116

10. Bernstein, D. M. (1970). Emotional reactions of children and adolescents to renal transplantation. *Chld. Psychiat. Hum. Devel.*, **1**, 102

11. Korsch, B. M., Fine, R. N., Grushkin, C. M. and Negrete, V. F. (1971). Experiences with children and their families during extended hemodialysis and kidney transplantation. *Pediat. Clin. N. Am.*, **18**, 625

12. Rutter, M. (1966). Children of sick parents; an environmental and psychiatric study. *Maudsley Monogr. no. 16.* Oxford University Press

13. Kanner, L. (1957) *Child Psychiatry*, 3rd edn. (Springfield, Ill.: Charles C. Thomas)

14. Steinhauer, P. D., Mushin, D. N. and Rae-Grant, Q. (1974). Psychological aspects of chronic illness. *Pediat. Clin. N. Am.*, **21**, 825

12

Social and psychological problems of the adult haemodialysis patient
Kirsty M. Marshall and
T. Walmsley

12.1   INTRODUCTION

In this paper we will describe the process of adjustment to treatment on dialysis, giving some attention to significant problems of adaptation, with examples. Chronic illness is recognized to be a family problem, and we will describe briefly some of the family demands and adjustments which are necessary for successful dialysis; and we shall discuss the importance of inter-disciplinary involvement in helping patients with the psycho-social problems of their treatment.

12.2   THE PATIENT

12.2.1   Emotional stresses

It has long been recognized that patients on chronic dialysis are faced with a variety of emotional stresses as a result of their illness and treatment.[1] Briefly, some of these problems are: fear of dying, and of frequent sub-jections to pain and illness; fear of loss of job and income; uncertainty about the future; changes in life-style, family and social status.

The most important step in assessing the patient's eventual response to the onset of renal failure is to observe his reaction to the illness in its initial stages. The degree of acceptance which each person and his family achieves dictates much to his ultimate well-being and successful adaptation.

12.2.2   Grief reaction

It is usual for people to approach severe physical loss through a process of realization which is akin to grief.[2] 'The reaction to loss of a limb, and for that matter to loss of function of a vital part is grief and depression'[3]. The patient moves from denial of the loss towards a gradual acceptance. Patients who have been told of the nature and severity of their illness may deny the information, even when this has been most carefully and explicitly shared. Such denial is a mechanism for coping with initial shock and for avoiding overwhelming anxiety and seems to be necessary for many people before the full implication of the illness can be recognized.

12.2.3   Anxiety

As realization dawns, denial may be replaced by acute anxiety, when the patient comes to depend very heavily on the support and understanding of hospital staff, and needs the comfort of relatives and friends. Reassurance is inadequate at this stage. It is important that the patient should be helped to express feelings of anxiety which assist him in moving towards greater self-assertiveness.

It is well established that many patients become preoccupied with events leading up to the onset of illness which is paralleled by the 'regret' of bereavement. Some patients single out particular events which, to them, appear significant, even if apparently unrelated to the disease. A patient told us in all seriousness that his health had begun to deteriorate following an accident at work. He was a railwayman who some years before becoming ill had his foot crushed by a train. He was convinced that his renal failure in some way was provoked by this event.

Anger may be directed towards doctors or other people who could have prevented the onset of illness and the patient may bitterly regret some action of his own. Some patients fail to move beyond the stage of feeling bitter and angry about the injustice of illness. This is wasteful of the emotional energy which should be directed towards effective rehabilitation. One patient, a miner, spent all his dialysis life 'fighting for his cause' in bitter recriminations against doctors and his local community to the extent that he was quite unable to return to any kind of positive existence at home or at work.

12.2.4 Sexual problems

Concern about 'loss of self' or mutilation is paramount for most patients, fears of 'never being the same again', of being changed and damaged. Such feelings reflect the importance of self-image and maintenance of self-esteem. Sexual problems are probably related to interference with body-image, and patterns of sexual functioning amongst renal patients are very variable. Some patients remain sexually active, despite other physical limitations from the illness, while others may be impotent. Potency seems to relate more to emotional well-being and self-esteem than to the degree of physical disability. Here too, it is important to examine pre-dialysis behaviour. A man who had considerable dependency needs and always 'enjoyed ill health', was described by his wife as having 'everything he ever wanted' once he started dialysis, whilst another, who was previously very concerned with schemes for improving his physical fitness, was unable to tolerate what seemed like the personal and physical assault of renal failure.

12.2.5 Importance of assessment

In establishing a programme of support for dialysis patients and their families, it has been useful to recognize the similarities with the process of bereavement. It is possible to identify and prevent reactions which complicate progress towards healthy adaptation. Difficulties arise from distortion of this process, from unresolved anger and depression. Dependent patients may find the life-supporting equipment terrifying and lapse into an attitude of helpless invalidism. Over-assertive patients may adopt a defence of denial which collapses catastrophically later in treatment. A depressive state frequently centres on ruminations of loss; loss of kidney function, of health and well-being, of previous occupational and social adjustment.

12.2.6   Symptoms of stress

During the training phase of treatment, psychiatric problems may be manifest as non-verbal cues. Lateness in arrival for hospital dialysis, difficulties in cannulation, refusal to look at the dialysis machine and an increase in non-specific symptoms may mark unspoken ambiguities of feeling towards the continuation of treatment. Occasionally frank neurotic states such as phobias or dissociation may supervene in the patient or his spouse. The patient on home dialysis may feel deserted by the hospital team and behave with hostility or indifference at out-patient attendances. Dialysis may become irregular and be accompanied by manipulative and attention-seeking behaviour. Repeated admissions with metabolic embarrassment or dietary indiscretion and associated weight gain are often the hallmark of such patients with separation anxiety. Here, the family around the patient is of key importance.

12.3   THE FAMILY

Successful dialysis depends on the support of the family, and its members may experience considerable stress in coping with treatment over a protracted period of time. Much depends on established patterns of family and marital behaviour prior to the onset of treatment. The continuous crisis of regular dialysis may lead to polarization of behaviour, sometimes aggravating an existing family problem, although previously poor relationships may sometimes be improved. For example, a patient whose renal failure had developed insidiously over some years, had severe marital problems by the time she was referred for treatment. It was an immense relief to both her and her husband to discover another explanation for her behaviour, and the shared experience of home dialysis was constructive in re-establishing a positive relationship.

The unrelenting nature of the illness and constant climate of uncertainty is difficult for many couples, who describe the need to readjust their values in learning to live from day to day and to limit expectations for the future. This can be positive as well as negative, but attitudes depend on individual aspirations and achievements. An older patient who is married and a father has valued the extra life granted to him by dialysis and can enjoy, at secondhand, the accomplishments of his children. A young single man has limited investment in dialysis because of curtailed opportunities for fulfilling hopes and ambitions.

Every family is faced by the challenge of adjustment. It is not only that the machine makes extra demands, but that responsibilities are shared differently. So much energy goes into maintaining basic tasks of living and working that other matters assume lower priority. This may include management of the children as well as decision making and financial responsibilities. It seems that where the whole family can be involved in recognizing and accepting the changes which are inevitable — where children, for example, can be helped to contribute in a positive way to the family's tasks — the effect can be to unify all the members.

For some families the demands of dialysis have been met by quite major role changes. These may be reasonable and healthy for particular family needs, even if bizarre to others. It is important to assess each individual family's functioning, and to help the members to achieve their own answers for coming to terms with dialysis treatment. This demands a high level of understanding of individual needs and difficulties by all members of the care team.

12.4 TEAM MEETINGS

Experience in the Medical Renal Unit in Edinburgh suggests that considerable morbidity in chronic patients can be avoided by the institution of regular team meetings. These occur weekly and last 1 hour. Face-to-face contact is regarded as essential and there is no agenda. All team members are encouraged to bring up any contemporary difficulties in patient management. As the meetings proceed such difficulties frequently bring to light differences in staff attitudes which can be squarely faced. Confrontation in the presence of a disinterested third party frequently permits a reformulation and resolution of the difficulty. There is a clear conclusion here: patient morbidity often reflects conflict among the staff. Some staff may be over-protective of a particular patient while others are covertly rejecting[4]. Bringing such a difference to the surface improves the care of the patient and increases the cohesiveness of the unit staff.

12.5 CONCLUSION

Chronic dialysis is usefully regarded as a non-specific stress to which certain personalities are peculiarly vulnerable. At the inception of treatment, anxiety should be regarded as the norm. Terror, hostility or bland acceptance may signal chronic psychological instability and require psychiatric exploration. The main bulk of psychiatric morbidity in dialysis patients consists of neurotic illness and the reactions of abnormal personalities. Acute confusional states and transient paranoid psychoses are occasional hazards of treatment; chronic organic psychosis is rare.

In the care of the patient on chronic haemodialysis two groups are usually involved. The patient's family have to make considerable adjustment and often require professional help to do so. The dialysis team is a second group which often reflects the conflicts of the first and which by deliberate recognition of its psycho-social problems can better serve its patients and increase its future effectiveness.

References

1. Cramond, W. A., Knight, P. R. and Lawrence, J. R. The psychiatric contribution to a renal unit undertaking chronic haemodialysis and renal homotransplantation. *Br. J. Psychiat.*, 113, 1201
2. Parkes, C. M. (1972). *Bereavement: Studies of Grief in Adult Life.* (London: Tavistock Publications)
3. Fisher, S. H. (1960). Psychiatric conditions of hand disability. *Arch. Phys. Med. Rehab.*, 41, 62
4. Kaplan De-Nour, A. and Czaczkes, J. W. (1968). Emotional problems and reactions of the medical team in a chronic haemodialysis unit. *Lancet*, ii, 987

DISCUSSION

Miss H. Rosenthal (London): Has either of the speakers any experience of working with groups of dialysis patients?

Miss K. M. Marshall: Not groups of patients, but we do have a spouse group in Edinburgh which has been running for almost 4 years. Patients sometimes reject that kind of contact with each other. In Edinburgh they will meet informally in the unit, but they have often avoided any other kind of contact. Individual patients have tried to institute this, but it has not been successful.

The spouse group have given each other a tremendous amount of support and they have been able to acknowledge some of their fears, fears about death of the partner and so on, quite directly with each other.

D. S. James (Glasgow): We have purposefully had no group for the children. There is a big scatter of age and intelligence. Some patients are at a much more advanced stage of understanding and coping with the mechanisms than others, and a group would not gel.

In addition to that, most of the patients come into the unit for 3 days a week, and if they were to get together in a group a number of them would have to come in for an extra day. Ours is a regional centre and some of them come a long way and they would not want to come another day.

We have been talking about a parent group. We feel that it is something we should perhaps venture to establish, and now that the unit has been running for 4 years it is probably time we did something about it.

A. L. G. Moss (Nottingham): May I endorse what Miss Marshall said about groups. In our own unit we have experimented with a group for spouses. At the beginning we did think about providing something for the patients, but we decided that the real need wasn't there, it was for the spouses, and that was borne out by the work we have done with them since. If it can be accomplished, then I would recommend that way of working for renal units. The same must go for parents of child patients. The spin-offs are fantastic. The kind of inter-reaction achieved in that type

207

of group situation in terms of mutual support and people being able to air what they really feel about things is much greater than would be achieved on an individual one-to-one basis. A further benefit that we have had has been a patients' association which grew from the first of our groups and which has been able to make a large contribution to the work of the unit in the City.

Mrs J. A. Lipman (London): If there is no children's group as such, how do the children react within the unit?

James: The children on dialysis are usually in separate cubicles, which reduces the amount of contact. There is one room where two children are dialysed together, and usually the television is on, although there are pairs that communicate fairly openly with each other.

We have a play leader and a teacher, and in term time there is one-to-one assistance going for a bit of the time where they would otherwise be interacting.

I am sure that there is a lot of informal contact, but there is no great fostering of a group feeling.

A. Murphy (Glasgow): In general, contact is good, but it has positive and negative effects. The child who is self-cannulating can produce a positive or a negative effect on the non-cannulating child opposite. By and large we feel that it is good to keep the children together and in contact. In our situation two are in contact and one is on his own and we move them around. The children get on well with each other. Outside the hospital they are beginning to see each other socially.

Mackenzie (Canada): Our diagnostic guidelines are probably at an adequate stage to recommend that just as a particular physical finding, e.g. blood pressure, is monitored regularly, we could monitor psychological dimensions. For example, the degree of denial, the amount of regression, the amount of assumption of personal control over dialysis events, and so on. Perhaps it would be useful to think of including as a regular monitoring dimension psychological attributes along with physiological ones. That would help to sharpen up our application of sometimes woolly behavioural ideas, particularly for staff who are not particularly trained in psychiatric terminology.

Miss Marshall mentioned impotence as being a fairly common problem. In my own experience in our unit there is often a general diminution of interest in sexual function during a dialysis period, but in a number of patients, probably one third to one half – and I believe that this is reflected in other units – after transplant impotence becomes a major problem. This seems to be regardless of physiological findings and it is certainly not related to other evidence of peripheral neuropathy, and it presumably has a psychological component. Many of the cases I have seen have otherwise seemed to have quite satisfactory psychological adaptations, and I am at a bit of a loss to explain the discrepancy. Perhaps there is some symbolic significance of having a foreign object in the pelvic area. I do not know the reason, but the experience is shared in other units.

James: On the question of whether to monitor the mental mechanisms in a more systematic way, we re-assess our children from time to time but I have some misgivings about it. I do not know that too much intrusion of psychiatry and psychology in the formal way of testing is particularly helpful to people who already have a damaged self-esteem. One would hope that if a unit is functioning properly – and I think that I can say this of the Glasgow unit – that the nursing staff, the dietician, the play leader and the nephrologist are sufficiently in contact to be able to monitor these things almost intuitively, which in many ways is a better measure than a test.

In any case, although I have shown that there are marital problems and difficulties in families with coping and that some of the children throw off some of these defence mechanisms, at the end of the day I am not sure. The children on home dialysis still have their dialysis irrespective of these factors. If I had been allowed my head, then the first two children, who are fairly successfully managing at home, would have been over-protected and not allowed that chance, because I would have said that it was too difficult. The medical and paediatric approach which optimistically assumes that they will cope has paid off. I must therefore have some anxieties about how intrusive the psychiatrist becomes.

Mackenzie: If I might respond to that. We routinely use problem-oriented records and I can see nothing wrong with self-care, for example, or ability to learn, as being an item on a problem list.

C. Burdett (Leicester): We have heard something of the problem of stress resulting in a person becoming less able to cope with the situation. I would suggest that a model of the person under stress is the person on the machine. I would also suggest that the various defence mechanisms are merely reflections of stimulus avoidance. We should be working towards diminishing fear response by graded exposures of the patients towards the fear.

James: Modelling is very important. There are two principles involved in the interactions between parents and their children. The behavioural approach with the consistency of reward and punishment, modelling and learning is one. The other has to do with the more analytical approach and the relationship between the two.

When dealing with neuroses in childhood, the parent becomes depressed and the child no longer has his needs provided. The mother becomes irascible, complains of being made ill, of being given a headache. She tells the child to go away and that they cannot go out. At other times she will feel guilty because she is depressed and she will try to make up to the child. This is clearly seen in the school phobic situation where the mother will lose her temper one day because the doctor says the child is all right. Then the next day she will be all over him because he has been sent home from school. She feels she is a bad mother, and wonders if the child is all right. Given this subtle sharing of a neurosis which usually begins with the parent and then involves the child, the modelling explanation is much too simple, and in these situations we are seeing both principles. If there is a long-standing conduct disorder, or a personality disorder, then modelling is very important. If it is a middle-class well-put-together biddable over-protective family, then sometimes the analytical or psychotherapy model may get one further in putting in the necessary corrective counselling.

13

Haemodialysis – a personal viewpoint
J. C. Baillie

I developed a renal problem in December 1973 and I spent most of 1974 on an in-patient and out-patient basis at the Royal Infirmary of Edinburgh.

My introduction to the 'Kidney Machine' is rather hazy as I was very ill at the time and I did not appreciate the gravity of the situation. When I did realize what was happening to me I was very frightened and insecure.

In due course I was discharged from hospital and attended the Medical Renal Unit twice a week for dialysis. These were 10-hour sessions every Wednesday and Sunday. I was often unwell during and after dialysis. The next day was also often uncomfortable, with stomach cramp and sickness.

It was about this time that I realized this was to be a permanent situation and if I were to stay alive I would have to learn to live with it. I went through a period of depression when problems seemed insurmountable and coping with life was difficult and tiresome. I dreaded the hospital dialysis days and was thankful that there were only two per week.

The staff in the Medical Renal Unit began to educate me in the basic principles of dialysis and in the necessary physiological adaptations which would be required for this procedure to work.

As an in-patient I had a Teflon shunt implanted in my leg, providing a connection for the machine. This first shunt and a subsequent one in the other leg proved unsatisfactory for long-term dialysis and I had to undergo

211

another minor operation so that a permanent Cimino fistula could be constructed in my arm. This ensured entry and exit points for the blood during dialysis. This part of haemodialysis is still an unpleasant operation, as a needle wrongly placed can cause a blood flow problem and running repairs are necessary.

I now had to consider returning to business and was greatly helped by a sympathetic company who were most helpful in adjusting my gradual return to work. At this time I occasionally felt unwell and often collapsed, even in the street. I made a concentrated effort to play a useful and profitable part in the commercial world again and I think that this, along with quiet encouragement from my family, helped me to accept the situation in which I found myself.

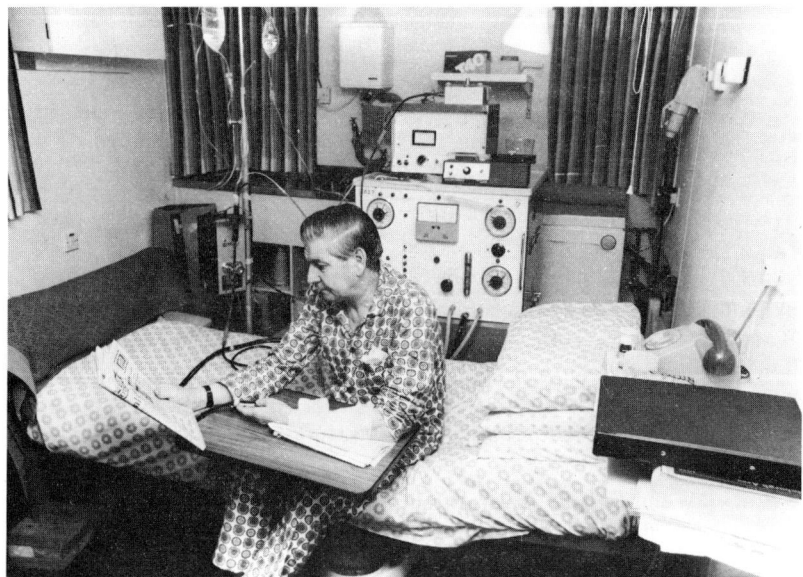

Figure 13.1   Interior of Portakabin

Regular dialysis and a strict low sodium diet slowly improved my health. The lack of salt in food makes the diet boring and tasteless, but I firmly believe that adhering to the diet makes the difference between being well and unwell (although I would never admit this to my dietitian). Compensation is round the corner, as I can have a meal of my choice while dialysing. Fluid intake is limited to 600 ml per day and my party piece about this is that if I am only allowed 600 ml of fluid a day, I would rather have it as whisky!

Once it had been proved that I was a successful dialysis patient, home dialysis was suggested to me. Treatment three times a week would be beneficial and I had the necessary facilities in my garden for a Portakabin. I also had an attendant, my wife, to help operate and maintain the Portakabin and its contents. Home dialysis appealed to my wife and myself from the start. Hospital dialysis had been a very time-consuming operation, involving 10–12 hours per treatment and often terminating at 2 or 3 o'clock in the morning. After this I had to drive home feeling unwell and unable to sleep. Also, we hoped to make a routine which would least affect the family and my work.

Just over a year after I had my first dialysis, a Portakabin was placed in my garden by the local authority and the necessary equipment was installed. This placed the responsibility of working the machine with my wife and myself. It was with some apprehension that we prepared for our first dialysis, but a nurse from the Medical Renal Unit guided us through our first week. Then we were on our own. An efficient back-up service of technicians and administrators were, however, only a 'phone call' away.

Even at home, dialysis is still a time-consuming operation. Dialysing for 6 hours three times a week and preparing the machine, etc. I spend 27 hours a week in the Portakabin. In addition to this, my wife has to clean the floor and all surfaces after each dialysis. Businesswise, I have the same problem – time. I should be more mobile in my job than I am, although I did manage a quick trip to Finland last autumn.

Home dialysis has improved my health immensely and the benefit of dialysing three times a week has become apparent as I have returned to my normal weight and to a feeling of physical well-being. In general, I find that I can cope much better with life. The machine is no longer the MONSTER it was and the unit is now referrred to by the family as 'THE SLAMMER'. Holidays are a big problem as far as the family are concerned and I miss my 3 weeks' fishing holiday in the Western Highlands in the summer.

A kidney transplant, I suppose, has always been in my mind, but I realize that as a successful dialysis patient I am a low priority for transplantation. If I were offered a transplant I would have to consider it very carefully, as I now keep in very good health and I know that my machine will not reject. It may hiccup occasionally, but that is all.

So what have we got to look forward to? We look forward to new and improved equipment which will cut down dialysis time and perhaps to the use of a mobile unit for holidays and perhaps to a MIRACLE.

14

Haemodialysis and transplantation – a personal experience
J. A. Henry

A previous speaker at this symposium gave us food for thought when he posed the question, 'how meaningful is this life?'. And he gave us an answer when he told us that not one of 350 patients, once given a trial of haemodialysis, refused to continue. Each case history represents the story of an individual and his will to live.

Very often the doctor can only attempt a guess at the real feelings and the difficulties that his patient is experiencing. As a doctor who has been through chronic renal failure, 7 years of haemodialysis and a renal transplant, I would like to comment on some aspects of the experience I have undergone. After 8 years of chronic glomerulonephritis from 1961 to 1969, I was started on home haemodialysis following 2 months of hospital dialysis. At that time I dialysed on my own for three 10-hour sessions each week. Life on haemodialysis was often not easy, but I managed to stay at work regularly and to fulfil the long hours demanded of a house physician. In the beginning I was so pleased to be alive and able to work that I did not seriously consider renal transplantation.

Once a patient is established on haemodialysis the prognosis is good, But the really long-term figures, of the order of 10 years, are still insufficient to draw reliable conclusions, particularly as many of the patients who form the basis for these figures were among the very first patients to be dialysed. I think I could be considered as one of the 'second generation' of haemodialysis patients – I was not moribund at the start, I was on home haemodialysis, my blood pressure was always well controlled and I was never transfused for chronic anaemia. Consequently, I viewed my prognosis on haemodialysis as excellent.

Many informed and educated patients once established on haemodialysis are very reluctant to put their names forward for transplantation, because of the risk it represents, even though it may liberate them from all the difficulties that accompany dialysis. Spending about 30 hours per week preparing, or being attached to, or clearing up after using a kidney machine, is a big limitation. On top of that are the restrictions in diet and fluid intake with the social difficulties entailed. Chronic tiredness, job difficulties, family tensions, dependence on a machine, and many other aspects of the enforced change in lifestyle makes dialysis an experience which requires considerable adaptation and a lot of effort.

Being a doctor made it even more difficult for me in the beginning, because I understood all the risks and complications of the various aspects of my treatment right from the start. Later on, I think it became an advantage, because I was able to manage my health more carefully. My relationships with the medical staff in charge of my case were always good. I often had strong ideas about my management and put my case forcibly at times but I always followed their advice faithfully. On only one occasion – which I shall mention later – did I deliberately mislead them.

In the background, however, was the constant dream of leading a dialysis-free life. I longed for a way of life away from the stresses of dialysis, from which there is no break, no holiday. And the only way to this was through a renal transplant. I knew the risks; the main ones that concerned me were the mortality, together with the morbidity – from the operation, with all its technical complications, and also from rejection, infection, malignant disease and osteoporosis. Cadaver transplantation has a mortality of around 25% over the first 2 years, with a further 25% of patients returning to dialysis. The figures improve considerably with a living related donor, and are probably better if the patient is healthy and managing well on dialysis, but they remain daunting. I have several friends who intend to remain on dialysis because they do not see transplantation as an acceptable alternative[1]. The gamble of a one in four mortality is not lightly undertaken, particularly when there is no guarantee for the survivor that his quality of life will necessarily be better after transplantation.

An acid test is to ask the people who know all the arguments. I have made a point of asking a number of nephrologists the telling question, 'Would you, if you were established on dialysis, choose to have a renal transplant?' The invariable answer is 'I would stay on dialysis'. These same doctors recommend renal transplantation to their patients. I can perfectly understand their attitude; by offering transplantation they are able to do more good to more patients with the available resources. Their moral dilemma is a very real one. Dialysis, apart from being a far from ideal treatment, is a luxury that cannot be provided in an unlimited way, although it undoubtedly offers the best chance of survival. The ideal solution is to have a functioning transplant without the hazards of con-ventional immunosuppressive therapy, but that is clearly a long way off.

At the time, I never really considered the ethics of my initial refusal to be transplanted, or whether other patients were being denied a place on a dialysis programme because of it. Looking back, I believe from an ethical standpoint that individual freedom takes precedence in these matters.

For $4\frac{1}{2}$ years I refused even to allow my blood to be taken for tissue typing. I was keeping reasonably well and was pushing ahead with a career in hospital medicine. Transplantation is an open-ended commitment; with all its uncertainties and its considerable morbidity I might no longer be able to plan my life or to remain at work so predictably.

However, as time went on, I gave more and more serious consideration to transplantation, and added weight was given to my thoughts by the occurrence of painful Looser's zones in my ribs and stress fractures of the metatarsals due to prolonged therapy with aluminium hydroxide. However, it had its desired effect, because there was no trace of ectopic calcification after 7 years on dialysis, and in fact the bony complications all healed rapidly with reduction in the dose of aluminium hydroxide.

In 1974, I was attending hospital for a routine check, when a technician came to take blood for tissue typing. I let her go ahead. If I had been asked in advance, I think I would have refused. The result was then entered in the computer system of the National Organ Matching and Distribution Service. This provoked further thoughts on transplantation, and I began to think about a living related donor kidney. I had my blood tissue typed at a hospital other than my own. The result was stuck on the wall of my dialysis room for several months before I took any action. Eventually I asked my parents to be tissue typed. Both had acceptable ABO groups and each had two out of four antigens. Both my sisters were also tissue typed. Neither of them was HLA identical; they were both quite disappointed.

I was still slowly pondering the problem, but taking no positive steps, till just a year ago, when my arm was forced by a telephone call which said, 'HLA identical kidney for you in Liverpool'. A four antigen – 'full house' –

match is too rare an opportunity to refuse. Any misgivings were thrown overboard, and I fell for the bait with a sense of elation. If it had been anything less than identical I do not think I would have accepted it. I went immediately to the hospital and had the necessary x-rays and microbiological investigations. I dialysed that night. The following day I went to hospital to work as usual; the promise of a transplant was not yet confirmed. However, during the day I had a cryptic message telling me to 'starve'. I knew what it meant and went to hospital for the operation.

The first week after transplantation is still very hazy. I was told afterwards of a number of visitors that I had spoken to, but I have no recollection to this day of their having visited me. I do remember my fascinated delight at seeing *my* urine collecting in a bag by the bedside, having been produced by someone else's kidney. The intensive care, with monitor and intravenous infusions, I took very much for granted. The pain was considerable, bladder spasms were trying and the wound was quite sore, but I was able to sit up and walk quite quickly.

My first excursion outside the hospital was 9 days after the operation, and I left the hospital for lunch with friends on the 10th day. By the 11th day I considered my rehabilitation complete when I went to a local hostelry for a pint of beer. I remember my surpise when I felt the call of nature and had to ask the way to the convenience. I had had many gin-and-tonics in the same pub but had never used their facilities until then. It was a further 10 days before I was discharged from hospital, still on large doses of corticosteroids and immunosuppressive therapy. I had had no rejection episodes. The most worrying problem was that the donor of my kidney was found to have a small adenocarcinoma of the bronchus on post mortem examination. The consultant in charge of the unit came along a few days after the operation to tell me about this unexpected finding, and said that while he thought that the risk of there being a secondary deposit in the transplanted kidney was very small, the decision was up to me. He said, 'You're in the life and death business, you're used to making decisions and taking the risks'. I decided to keep the kidney, though an article in the *British Medical Journal* one week later about the transplantation of a kidney containing malignant disease which caused the death of the recipient[2] almost made me go back on the decision.

The other problems were routine compared with that. I accepted the dyspepsia from the high steroid dosage, though I was disturbed by the muscle wasting and weakness also due to steroid therapy. I also put up with the nocturia which was accentuated by a minute bladder capacity — after being virtually anuric for 7 years it takes time for bladder capacity to return to full size, and I recall marking out with joy when I could retain

150 ml, later 200 ml and so on. I never have to get up at night to pass urine now.

Another problem during the post-operative period was the possibility of rejection. I was warned to watch out for an increase in the size of the kidney, or tenderness, or an unexpected rise in my temperature. After 11 days I drew my transplant surgeon's attention to an increase in the size of the kidney. He examined it and laughed, commenting that this was the expected physiological hypertrophy. It is very consoling when you know that your transplant has started to grow. However, the increase in size as I became more mobile was difficult to put up with – having a strange object down in my right iliac fossa made walking difficult and totally altered my gait, so much so that my right hip began to ache. I know that the complication of avascular necrosis of the femoral head is more common on the same side as the transplant, and that this has been ascribed to alteration in vascular supply, but I wonder if the stress of walking in a different way is a more important factor.

After discharge from hospital I was taking a pleasant holiday when I began to feel very tired and exhausted, but I did not relate it to the kidney, as there were no other symptoms at the time. After attending for a routine check, I was called back because my plasma creatinine level had risen considerably. I was readmitted – 5 weeks after the operation – and treated for a rejection episode with bolus therapy of high dose methylprednisolone and also radiotherapy to the kidney which was considerably enlarged, firm and slightly tender.

As the episode subsided I suddenly began to spike a high temperature each evening. After 3 days I was certain that I had a viral infection and announced the fact, but was disbelieved. I was subjected to a large series of investigations including sigmoidoscopy and even re-exploration of the kidney after ultrasound had shown a small space behind the kidney which could have contained pus, but in fact did not. My liver was found to be just palpable, but I denied that it was tender since I knew that this would lead to a liver biopsy. The pyrexia continued for several weeks and only subsided on reduction of my immunosuppressie therapy. All the acute investigations were negative although immune complexes were found in the blood, and retrospective investigations of sera which had been collected showed rising titres of Ebstein-Barr virus dating back to the time of the operation, which was presumably due to blood transfusion or to a recrudescence of latent infection, though there was a third, much more remote possibility which I almost completely discarded.

By a strange coincidence, Dr Carmody – the Chairman of this session of the symposium – was in charge of the patient who received the partner kidney from the same donor. I was fascinated to hear that his patient also had a pyrexial illness after transplantation, for which no cause was found. It is interesting to speculate that the infection may have come from the donor; we intend to look further into the story. He also told me last night of the concern that they had about the possibility of malignancy in their recipient; the medical team decided against removal of the kidney without consulting their patient. He still has it, without signs of malignancy.

My main feeling towards the end of my hospital stay was one of relief now that the long period of hesitation and doubt was over. Transplantation itself had resolved the dilemma of whether to have a transplant or not, but it left in its wake a different set of uncertainties which were largely out of my control. By far the main one was the possibility of rejection. The anxiety of the first few weeks gradually receded as the kidney showed signs of taking up permanent residence. Perhaps the strangest feeling of all was the mixed emotion on going back to my treatment room and looking at the machine which, despite any of the moments when I hated it, had been my constant and reliable companion for 7 years.

Later on, when I was back at work, a renal unit technician phoned me asking if they could remove the kidney machine that morning. I told him to go ahead. That evening when I got home, the room looked very bare without the machine and other pieces of equipment. I really felt on my own, rather like someone who has always swum inside his depth, and then goes into deep water where he cannot feel the bottom any more. I also felt more confident then that there was a new future ahead.

Because of the added complications I was off work for just 3 months. I had been warned that my work record (two days off work in 7 years while on haemodialysis) would be much less reliable after renal transplantation due to morbidity from at least some of the complications which so often occur. However, I have been back at work full-time, without missing a day since then, on quite a small dose of the standard therapy (prednisolone 8 mg and azathioprine 100 mg daily) and no other drugs, with good renal function. My latest endogenous creatinine clearance was 52.7 ml/min. I am normotensive, with a haemoglobin which rose to normal within 2 months of operation.

The only continuing complication is of recurrent renal stones, which is a rather unusual problem post-transplantation and possibly under-recognized since symptoms are minimal. There is no sensation of renal colic, because the transplanted kidney and ureter have no nerve supply.

The future now looks good, though I am still concerned about the long-term complications of permanent drug therapy. As a small preventative measure, I have started playing squash regularly in order to minimize the chances of developing osteoporosis. At this distance – just over a year – I am glad to have had my renal transplant. I do not need to tell you that the quality of life is incomparably better; more I think than the rather arbitrary figure of 25% which has been quoted[3].

I took a gamble that has paid off. Apart from quality of life I feel that after 1 year a patient with a functioning transplant who is on a low dose of immunosuppressive therapy probably has a comparable prognosis to that if he had remained on dialysis. If I should have the misfortune to return to dialysis, I would again go through the misgivings I have described, but I would view a further renal transplant with less reluctance.

Many people have said to me, referring to life on haemodialysis, 'I could never go through that kind of experience, I just would never be able to put up with it'. My reply to them all is that if they were actually faced with it, they would manage very well, since there are immense reserves in each of us which often lie dormant until a challenge appears. When such a challenge comes it can be accepted and coped with, particularly if one has faith, the support and affection of family and friends, and a strong sense of purpose in life. In fact, like many of life's misfortunes, the experience of living with renal failure can be character-forming, and can even enrich a person's life.

References

1. Eady, R. A. J. (1973). Why I have not had a kidney transplant after nine and one-half years as a haemodialysis patient. *Transpl. Proc.*, **5**, 1115
2. Barnes, A. D. and Fox, M. (1976). Transplantation of tumour with a kidney graft. *Br. Med. J.*, **1**, 1442
3. Klarman, H. E., Francis, J. O. and Rosenthal, G. D. (1968). Cost effectiveness analysis applied to the treatment of chronic renal disease. *Med. Care*, **6**, 48

15

Some problems of staff stress in dialysis-transplantation units
Mary Brown

15.1   INTRODUCTION

This paper will describe some of the stresses encountered by the staff and patients of a renal dialysis and transplant unit.

The stress is mainly brought about by the type of illness treated, the techniques involved and the isolation of the renal unit from the rest of the hospital.

Staff roles come under conflict if the problems are not brought to frequent and constructive discussion.

Stress itself results in agitation, frustration, sensitivity and resentment. The emotions involved are provoked by occurrences in everyday life. Stress is a part of every working person's life and is certainly not alien to hospitals and renal transplant units. There are, however, some aspects of stress which are more apparent in this speciality than in others.

15.2   SPECIAL PROBLEMS OF PATIENTS

All patients admitted to haemodialysis/transplant units come to be treated for an incurable disease. They are aware that their condition can be treated by haemodialysis, peritoneal dialysis or transplantation along with the necessary adherance to fluid and dietary restrictions, drugs and changes in social and employment habits. Although these patients know that treatment is possible, they are aware that they cannot be cured. Having been informed of their condition, they regard dialysis or transplantation as their last hope. Both patients and relatives are under a great deal of stress, which puts an added strain on their nursing management[1].

The patient who is to be treated by haemodialysis must learn all the technical skills necessary for this procedure, as well as becoming familiar with the required diet, drugs and fluid. He must learn this from the staff of the renal unit, with whom he is going to be closely associated for some years.

The patient who is being treated by transplantation has to undergo surgery and be educated in the use of immunosuppressive drugs and steroid treatment. He has the constant fear of rejection, which may cause him to be agitated and unsure of himself. This has a profound effect on the patient's family. If the transplant is successful, he will not have such close links with the staff of the unit as the dialysis patient does. He must, however, discipline himself to regular checkups at the clinic.

Both dialysis and transplant patients are under a great deal of stress, particularly at the commencement of their treatment. The staff of the renal unit must be educated to appreciate and alleviate the adjustment problems which the patients face.

The main difference between the renal dialysis and transplant unit and other units of the hospital is that here the patient is not just treated with understanding and help in all possible ways, but is also actively involved as a part of the team. He must be included in the decisions concerning his future. Other members to be included in the team are the patient's family, who will be closely concerned in the actual treatment.

15.3 SPECIAL PROBLEMS OF STAFF

Bearing in mind that the patient is automatically included, let us turn to the other members of the team, i.e. the staff of the dialysis/transplant unit.

15.3.1 Team work

The patient comes into contact with the staff from the time that a diagnosis is made. The physician in charge of the patient's diminishing renal function must keep the patient informed of all the possibilities of treatment and truthfully discuss the advantages and disadvantages of each. At the same time he must assess the type of treatment most suitable. The nursing staff may meet the patient while he is in consultation with his physician and have the opportunity to offer an opinion on which course of treatment would best suit him. During this preliminary assessment, all members of the team who are invited to discuss the case are under stress, as the responsibility of a wrong decision regarding treatment at this stage could do irreversible damage to the patient's physical and psychological state. Close contact must be kept with the patient's social worker, who shares the responsibility of helping with the choice of treatment and rehabilitation.

Once the type of treatment has been decided upon, the success of its maintenance depends on the team, including the patient and his family. 'Several disciplines working together do not make a team. Effective team-work requires attention to the process of working together as well as the technical skills each practitioner brings'[2].

As the patient's treatment necessitates a long-term connection with the unit, any inter-staff stress will soon become apparent to him and will affect his relationship with the team.

15.3.2 Nursing staff

The dialysis/transplant unit is staffed by qualified nurses who have a keen interest in the work they do and who have a genuine concern for all the problems the patient comes up against.

Qualified nurses working together have problems amongst themselves, quite apart from the personality clashes which occur in any field of work. Resentment towards each other regarding degrees of responsibility may occur and must be curtailed quickly by group discussion which must be truthful but not hurtful. This problem must be dealt with by the nurse in charge and as many of the team as can be helpful towards establishing priorities for the smooth running of the unit. All helpful opinions must be discussed and, if possible, a satisfactory conclusion reached so tasks are shared in a way that will benefit the whole team.

The nurse in charge of the unit nursing team has many problems. She must diagnose staff stress before it becomes disruptive. Hopefully she can rely on her staff to discuss their problems with her. To enable her to do this, she needs a mature and calm outlook even when the unit is very busy and other matters are awaiting her attention. Even in particularly busy circumstances, she must be available to deal with staff problems, or the result could be detrimental to the care of the patient. The nurse in charge must have the ability to delegate tasks fairly and in return the nurses must be grateful to learn from her example. The nurses working on a dialysis/transplant unit must remember that all final decisions lie with the nurse in charge. As they are familiar with the work of the unit, some with several years' experience, they must help by making suggestions towards any form of treatment or administration known, to their superior. Once the pros and cons of such a suggestion have been considered and a decision made, they must abide by it without bearing any resentment towards another member of staff if they disagree with the final outcome.

The nurse in charge may have help from her Nursing Administrator. In many cases, on the other hand, the Nursing Administrator is inexperienced in this specialization and cannot have a full understanding of the problems involved. This leaves the nurses without senior nursing support. This is not an unfamiliar problem on any specialized unit but it is an added stress.

Team problems do not occur only among nursing personnel. There may well be a disagreement between physician and surgeon or between dietitian and nurse. Again, open discussion can lead to a positive and constructive result and the patient's treatment will continue to be of benefit, hopefully without his realizing there was a conflict. A patient should be included in discussion where two parties have helpful suggestions to make, e.g. regarding diet. For obvious reasons he must be excluded if there is a lack of discipline in the differing personnel.

15.3.3   Medical staff

Team disagreement may be related to a communication gap between the medical staff and the nurses. In all matters of treatment nurses who have high standards and expectations but who do not receive the support of their medical staff will become discontented. In this situation, one of two results may ensue:

(1) The nurses work hard and try to maintain their high standards of care but essentially become frustrated by the lack of involvement of the medical staff. They try not to let their stress affect the patient, but if the situation continues, inevitable breakdown of the team will occur.

(2) They give up the fight. They do not expect too much of their patients. Discipline becomes minimal and the high standard of care will drop. This leads to disillusionment as the nurses know they could do better.

Medical and surgical staff can contribute greatly to the team's success by including all members of nursing staff in decisions regarding treatment. The experienced nurse may have contributory reports to make on a patient's progress which cannot be known to a doctor who visits the patient once or twice a day. The inexperienced nurse will always have something to learn by joining in discussion about her patient. It can be most disheartening to care for a patient for many hours, only to be excluded from any decision about his treatment. Communication between the doctor, the bedside nurse and the patient is most important in this respect.

The experienced dialysis nurse at times has difficulty working with new junior members of the medical team. For the moment, her practical knowledge of dialysis is superior to his. She may have to make a quick decision in an acute case without waiting for his diagnosis. This can cause friction. The consultant in charge will find that this may be solved if new members of the medical staff are educated to respect the experience of the dialysis nurse.

15.3.4   Technical staff

Communications between the technical staff of the unit and the rest of the team must have no barriers. Lack of patient orientation by a technician may result in poor treatment. Alternatively, the rest of the staff must respect the technician's knowledge of his subject and not meddle in this field without consulting him. It is too easy in this situation to end up doing each other's work inefficiently, which is obstructive to the team goal and causes unnecessary friction. 'An important part of nursing on the renal unit is to relieve tension for patients used to living under constant strain'[1].

The staff try to create a relaxed environment for the sake of the patient. An informal atmosphere is encouraged, although difficulty may be encountered trying to maintain mutual respect. New staff and patients may try to take advantage of this informal situation and take some time to adjust to it. This informality may be regarded as unusual by the nursing administration of the hospital and the unit staff may come under criticism. It is difficult to convince the nursing administration that basic nursing standards are maintained even though the nurses are on first name terms with each other and with the patients. Hopefully, it will be realized that the staff are trying to construct a relaxed though respectful relationship with each other and their patients.

15.3.5   Close staff–patient relationships

The staff of the unit come to know the patients and their relatives closely. This is good and the patients trust them with all their problems – medical, social and emotional. In this relationship, the team motive must not be disregarded. A patient and member of staff trying to iron out a problem on a one-to-one basis may be unable to solve it. The member of staff will feel she has failed her patient and the patient still has his problem. Thus two people are under added strain that could be alleviated if the problem had been shared with the team. 'Information must be freely shared. The concept of confidentiality must be altered to include the team, or it will not serve to protect the patient, but to constrict effective teamwork'[3].

Because the staff and patients know each other throughout a period of time they do become friendly, sometimes on a social basis. Staff would not be human if they were not involved with their patients. The death of a patient is upsetting, particularly if the patient has been treated by the unit for some time and is regarded as a friend. The only solution is to be of as much help as possible to the bereaved relatives and try to give some comfort to the other patients on the unit who have been friendly with the deceased. Trying to boost the morale of the other patients and give them renewed confidence in themselves and their treatments brings the team back together again.

A similar stress for patients and staff arises after transplantation. A patient may be discharged from hospital full of health and hope for the future, only to be readmitted in acute rejection. It can be very difficult to hide the staff's disappointment from the patient.

15.3.6   Hepatitis

Dialysis units have the added stress of a possible outbreak of hepatitis at any time. Those who have worked in the speciality for some time will be acutely aware of the possible outcome. The responsibility of controlling the tests for Hepatitis B Antigen on staff, patients and visitors is most important.

15.3.7   Isolation

Visitors to the unit must be restricted, so it functions as an isolated part of the hospital. This is not always good for the morale of the staff. Although they enjoy specializing, there is a danger of forgetting that other parts of the hospital exist, to the extent that new members of staff may only mix socially with those of their own team. This social isolation is not to be encouraged.

15.4   TEACHING AND TRAINING

In the general running of the unit, the staff must become teachers in three areas:

(1) The home-dialysis training scheme.
(2) The training of members of staff.
(3) The education of lay-people with an interest in this field.

Education is an area in which many members of staff are not trained and some find it very difficult.

The training of patients for home-dialysis is rewarding for the most part. However, some patients do not learn quickly and need a great deal of time, patience and understanding. Sometimes a patient does not reach the expected standard despite intensive teaching. The staff do not forget him when he is placed in the home. He is a constant worry, needing many domiciliary visits and many re-calls to clinic for checkups.

Other patients admitted for home-training come to be regarded as unsatisfactory and they must remain on hospital dialysis. The staff, who have tried to train the patient to the best of their ability, feel they have failed and the patient feels disappointed. The staff–patient relationship has to be reassessed before satisfactory hospital dialysis can commence.

15.5 SUMMARY

In summary, though stress does exist in dialysis/transplant units, it is at times more apparent than others. The staff and patients, by striving to be active members of the team, can overcome the problems which arise.

References

1. Richards, G. M. (1974). The emotional aspects of nursing in a renal transplant unit. *Proc. Europ. Dial. Transpl. Nurses Ass.*, 2, 47
2. Kress, H. and Nason, F. (1976). A perspective: the interdisciplinary approach to patients with chronic disease (teaming). *J. Am. Ass. Nephrol. Nurses and Tech.*, 3, no. 1
3. Hayot, M., Kaplan-Nour, A. and Czaczkes, J. W. (1975). Inter-team relationship in a renal unit. *Proc. Europ. Dial. Transpl. Nurses Ass.*, 2, 52

DISCUSSION

B. H. B. Robinson (Birmingham): Dr Henry made an important point about having a purpose in life. In the current unemployment situation with social security provision such that many of the patients who have less well-paid jobs are better off not working than working, there are real problems. However, the effect on morale for patients who are not at work can be quite disastrous and we should perhaps encourage our patients to find something to do.

Carmody: It is important that they do not just stay at home all day.

Robinson: It is obvious that we have not done enough work on what influences patients' lifestyles. I do not know enough about what they can and cannot do.

Henry: It is very difficult to define. It has to be assessed in each individual case. Some will have a virtual 100% rehabilitation and others, for whatever reason, may never get around to being able to work.

F. M. Parsons (Leeds): The EDTA Registry would suggest that evening/ night dialysis gives a better chance for rehabilitation. Perhaps this is one of the advantages of home dialysis versus hospital dialysis. In providing hospital dialysis are we offering our facilities at the right time of day?

Baillie: I looked on time away from work as something temporary, and it was being able to work that really led me to accept the situation. Dr Henry told me that he was able to dialyse through the night, and that he was even able to go to sleep. I could never do that, and I do not think that there are many patients who could plug in and go off to sleep. I found that any movement on the arm would cause blood flow problems.

Henry: I would not have been able to carry out my job if I had not been dialysing at night. At the beginning, when I had an old-fashioned dialyser, we were recommended to dialyse 10 hours, and that takes 12 hours out of the day so I had to sleep on dialysis if I was to work for even 5 days a week.

Parsons: Should day dialysis at hospitals perhaps be shut down?

Henry: It might have an important place for the housewife with a family who wants to be at home in the evening, but for someone who wants to work every day it is better to dialyse late in the evening or overnight.

Baillie: Where one can dialyse late in the evening there is not much of a problem. It does not affect the working day too much.

Parsons: So we are providing a pretty lousy dialysis service in the hospitals?

Henry: There is so much more to be said for home dialysis in terms of independence and mobility in the sense that one can choose when to dialyse, and which nights one wants to dialyse.

A. C. Kennedy (Glasgow): The duration of dialysis is a further pertinent factor. When our unit reduced from two 10-hour spells a week for each patient to three 5-hour spells the number of patients at work increased substantially.

C. Burdett (Leicester): There is evidence that patients on home dialysis seem to return to work more effectively. Perhaps because they have learnt to control their own situations and their own dialysis problems there is greater personal control over everything in life.

Mrs Deirdre E. Jones (London): Is there any way to help relieve the stresses of patients that is not being carried out at the moment?

Mrs M. Brown: Some patients, although we do get them on to home dialysis, do need extra help. They need several domiciliary visits, and this highlights one possible need for 'in-centre' dialysis. A lot of general practitioner medical centres seem to have been built, with clinics for babies and clinics for all kinds of things, and I can see no reason why such centres should not include three or four dialysis rooms where patients could go in and dialyse, and there would be a nurse in the building, and a doctor on the premises in the event of a cardiac arrest. That is all that is needed, and all the support that the patients want. They want to know that there is some-body medical nearer than a hundred miles who knows vaguely what they are doing. This would bring in the community services. I do not know what others in the profession think about bringing the community services into dialysis.

Ms Jennifer Wedderburn (Nottingham): What about rotating staff from the renal unit out into the field? The renal unit tends to be rather isolated, and one tends to forget that there is another part of the hospital. I some-times wonder whether rotating the staff out of the unit for a period of 6 months might help in some way. In other countries, e.g. America, staff do move out.

Brown: It probably would help. However, with the work situation being what it is and the staff situation being what it is, the unit cannot afford to lose staff for six months of the year.

Wedderburn: And there would be a problem of retraining experienced staff for the renal unit. However, it is a shame that it cannot be considered.

A. W. Siemsen (Honolulu): Here again the self-care unit is very important. Our own self-care units run two shifts a day and they will soon be open all 24 hours and patients can come and dialyse at any time that they want.

   That also answers the question just asked. Our staff do rotate from limited care to self-care to acute care. There is a variety of patients and it does give some relief.

SECTION FIVE

Practical Management
Chairman:
A. C. Kennedy

16

Evaluation of four disposable dialysers
Kathleen Nicholson

16.1 INTRODUCTION

In 1965 the number of regular dialysis patients notified to the EDTA for the whole of Europe was 160. By 1971 this number had risen to 7000 and by 1975 it exceeded 22 000. This dramatic rise has led to logistic and financial problems which have been tackled with varying degrees of success in the different European countries.

By 1975 the budget for regular dialysis in the United Kingdom had risen to £12 million per annum and by now will be much higher. The current period of financial restrictions imposed on the National Health Service has aggravated the situation.

In this setting the introduction of financial savings, even of limited degree, would be helpful. Such savings, however, should not interfere with the efficiency of dialysis to the individual patient as the quality of life in many cases is already sub-optimal.

In the early days of regular dialysis the Kiil dialyser was widely used but was recognized to have several disadvantages. It required space for building and storage and employment of extra personnel. Its use also heightened the risk of cross infection.

In recent years there has been a move towards the use of disposable dialysers, mainly for greater convenience and to lessen the risk of spread of hepatitis. This move has, of course, imposed a greater cost burden with which many Health Authorities have difficulty in coping.

The purpose of this paper is to briefly review the use of three disposable hollow fibre dialysers and one of the disposable Kiil type. Five aspects were examined, namely ease of use, urea and creatinine clearance, ultra-filtration and the cost and efficiency of re-use. Details of the four dialysers are shown in Table 16.1. The Travenol, Nephros (Organon) and Cordis Dow are all hollow fibre kidneys while the Gambro is a disposable Kiil type.

TABLE 16.1   Details of the four dialysers

Manufacturer	Model	Surface area (m^2)	Cost (per dialyser)
Cordis Dow	Mark 4	1.3	£17
Travenol HF	SM1786	1.5	£18
Organon	Nephros 16F.160	1.6	£23
Gambro	Lundia Optima 17 micron	1.0	£15

The Cordis Dow is the only one sterilized by formalin and this has the disadvantage of requiring more complete flushing out by saline prior to use. The burst rate was zero in all cases. This represents a considerable advantage over some earlier dialysers. The volume of saline required to

TABLE 16.2   Washback volume and residual blood volume*

	Cordis Dow	Travenol HF	Nephros	Gambro
Washback volume (ml)	210	300	450	320
Residual blood volume (ml)	2.5	2.5	3.7	3.3

* The figures for washback volume are the mean of six measurements in each case. The values for residual blood volume are those measured by the Newcastle Renal Unit using haemoglobinometry.

virtually clear the dialyser and venous line at end of dialysis is shown in Table 16.2. The Cordis Dow comes out of this comparison best and the Nephros worst with the Travenol and Gambro in an intermediate position. Also shown in Table 16.2 is the residual blood volume which is acceptably low in all cases.

The clearance of urea and creatinine was measured using the standard formula:

$$C = \frac{Q_b(C_a - C_v)}{C_a}$$

C = clearance
Q_b = blood flow (ml per min)
C_a = arterial blood concentration
C_v = venous blood concentration

Figure 16.1 shows the urea clearance of the four kidneys. The Travenol and Gambro are more efficient than the Nephros and Cordis. The creatinine clearance (Figure 16.2) similarly shows the Tavenol and Gambro to

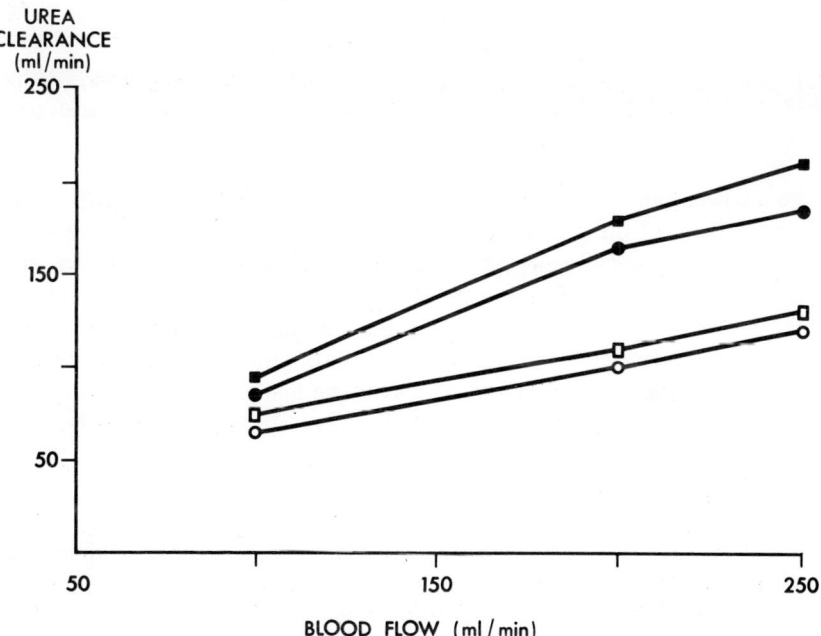

Figure 16.1   Urea clearance at blood flow rates of 100, 200 and 250 ml/min of the Travenol (■), Gambro (●), Nephros (○) and Cordis Dow (□) dialysers. Each value is the mean of six experiments.

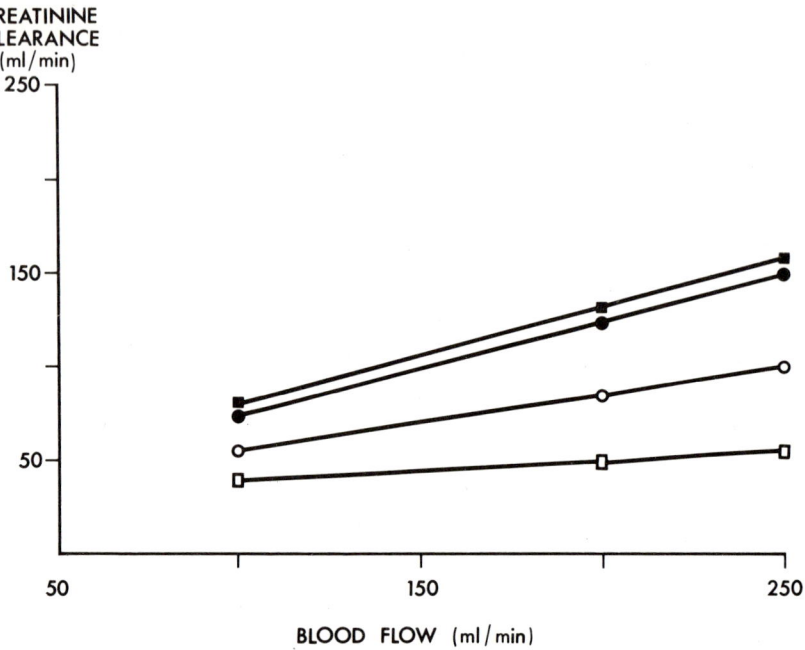

Figure 16.2   Creatinine clearance at blood flow rates of 100, 200 and 250 ml/min of the Travenol (■), Gambro (●), Nephros (○) and Cordis Dow (□) dialysers. Each value is the mean of six experiments

be the best, but in this case the Nephros was superior to the Cordis Dow. Comparison of the ultrafiltration characteristics is shown in Figure 16.3. The highest rate was achieved by the Nephros, with the Travenol next. The rate for the Gambro came next, being much lower than the Travenol at the higher transmembrane pressure, though slightly higher at the lower pressure. These figures relate to the Gambro with 17 micron membrane thickness while it is the 13 micron membrane that is used in most dialysis units. The kidney with the lowest ultrafiltration rate was the Cordis Dow.

16.2   RE-USE OF DIALYSERS

Table 16.3 shows the cost per dialysis related to the number of times the dialyser is re-used. These figures relate only to the dialyser and do not include the lines or other items. Although there is a fairly large variation in cost between the four dialysers, this difference becomes much smaller and therefore less important with re-use.

Also there is little benefit in extending the number of uses beyond six, as

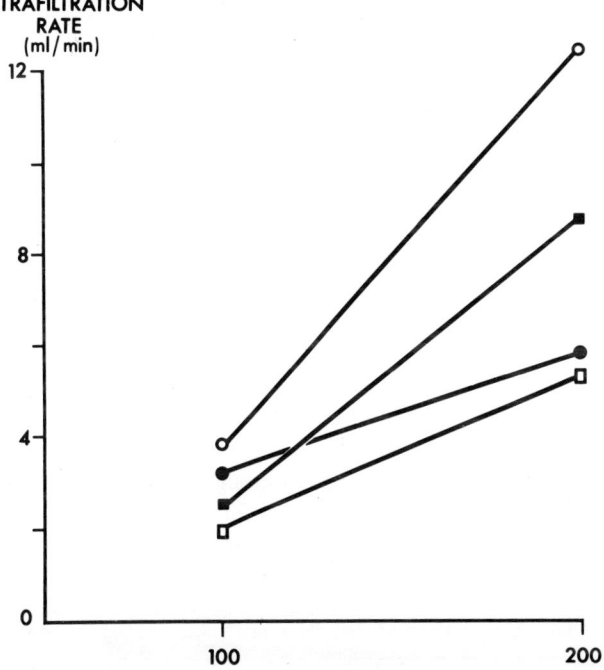

Figure 16.3 Ultrafiltration rate at transmembrane pressures of 100 and 200 mmHg, of the Travenol (■), Gambro (●), Nephros (○) and Cordis Dow (□) dialysers. Each value is the mean of six experiments. The blood flow rate was 100 ml/min

the financial saving per dialysis thereafter becomes small. Taking our unit as an example with 25 patients on thrice weekly dialysis, the annual cost of dialysers when used only once is approximately £71 000. This figure was derived by using the mean of the cost of the four types of dialysers under evaluation. If one used each dialyser six times, the annual cost would

TABLE 16.3 Cost of the dialysers for single, three and six uses

	Single use	Three uses	Six uses
Cordis Dow	£17.00	£5.67	£2.83
Travenol HF	£18.00	£6.00	£3.00
Nephros	£23.00	£7.67	£3.83
Gambro	£15.00	£5.00	£2.50

be less than £12 000, giving rise to a saving each year of £59 000. This saving does not take into account the additional labour costs of re-use but this item is small in relation to the sum saved.

Numerous techniques have been described for re-use. Our method has consisted of flushing out the dialysate compartment with tap water at a pressure of 1000 mmHg (about 20 lb/in^2) and by a form of reverse osmosis this clears the residual blood from the hollow fibres very efficiently. This method cannot be applied to the Gambro and we have not so far re-used this type of dialyser. It should, however, be emphasized that Gambro dialysers are satisfactorily re-used in a number of dialysis units. The use of dialysate to flush out the kidney has been shown to be superior to water and we intend to adopt this method in the future. Following the flushing out, which takes approximately 20 min, the volume of the blood compartment can be measured and this compartment is then filled with 2.5% formaldehyde until the next use (see discussion).

It is important to determine if the efficiency of the dialyser decreases with re-use and our results in relation to this are shown in Table 16.4. One can see that there is no significant decrease in efficiency as measured by urea and creatinine clearances with up to six uses.

TABLE 16.4   Urea and creatinine clearance values during first use and re-use*

	Urea clearance (ml/min)		Creatinine clearance (ml/min)	
	First use	Re-use	First use	Re-use
Travenol HF	210	203 (6)	155	145 (6)
Nephros	124	149 (5)	104	109 (5)
Cordis Dow	128	118 (4)	54	56 (4)

* Each figure is the mean of six experiments. The figures in brackets refer to the number of times each dialyser was re-used. The fact that the Cordis Dow dialyser was used four times in comparison to six times for the Travenol dialyser arose by chance and not design. The blood flow rate for all experiments was 250 ml/min.

16.3   CONCLUSION

Table 16.5 summarizes, using a simple plus system, the relative merits of the four types of dialyser. The Travenol HF and Gambro are best with regard to cost, ease of use and efficiency, but the Travenol HF is much easier to re-use. The Nephros is the least satisfactory in most respects while the Cordis Dow occupies an intermediate position.

To summarize, the currently available hollow fibre dialysers are efficient and easy to use. In addition, their design allows re-use on several occasions without a significant decrease in efficiency. In view of the considerable financial saving, there is a powerful argument for the introduction of re-use in all dialysis units using hollow fibre dialysers.

TABLE 16.5 Summary of the comparative merits of the four types of dialysers

	Ease of use	Cost	Urea clearance	Re-use
Cordis Dow	++	++	++	+
Travenol HF	+++	++	+++	+++
Nephros	++	+	++	+
Gambro	+++	+++	+++	

Key: + Mediocre, + + Satisfactory, + + + Good

DISCUSSION

R. Ahmad (Liverpool): Re-use of the dialyser adds to the time needed for dialysis. The patient who dialyses for 6 hours three times a week will have to put in extra time. What is needed are automatic dialyser washout devices.

A second point. We have had no direction from the DHSS as to where the legal responsibility lies if anything should happen to the patient because the dialyser is re-used. We have been re-using dialysers with considerable success in the case of Travenol and we have also had success in re-using Gambro, and it is all done by automatic re-use devices.

Miss K. Nicholson: We have no automatic re-use machine, although I am aware that they exist.

Ahmad: My patients are re-using dialysers at home, and by using an automatic machine the dialyser can be cleaned and sterilized for re-use in 15 minutes.

Nicholson: The main motive for re-using the kidneys is to save money and that saving can probably be used to employ an additional orderly.

Ahmad: Re-use can even save time.

A. C. Kennedy (Glasgow): Miss Nicholson and Dr Ahmad are really in agreement but the tenor of Dr Ahmad's point should be addressed to a 'Man from the Ministry'. Is there one here?

R. M. Melville (Edinburgh): I am not from the Ministry, but from the Home and Health Department.

Dr Ahmad's point about the responsibility if anything should go wrong because of the re-use of dialysers is a difficult one. I understand from colleagues in the DHSS that having taken bacteriological advice, the general feeling is that the Department cannot recommend the re-use of these disposable dialysers.

Kennedy: If they do not recommend it, can they tolerate it?

Melville: We are not over aware that it is happening.

F. M. Parsons (Leeds): In re-use of dialysers have any pyrexial reactions occurred?

Nicholson: We have not had any.

Parsons: Miss Nicholson said that the dialysers were re-sterilized with $2\frac{1}{2}$% formalin. It should be $2\frac{1}{2}$% formaldehyde. A solution of $2\frac{1}{2}$% formalin is 1% formaldehyde. It is crucial to get the percentages right and there is a difference in terminology between formalin and formaldehyde.

R. J. Winney (Edinburgh): The Cordis Dow is no longer formalin sterilized and is now available in a dry form.
    Secondly, when comparing costs of dialysers, should the variable ultra-filtration rate be taken into account? In some patients this requires replacement with as much as 3 litres of saline, which costs money, and this should be taken into account in comparing the costs of the various dialysers.

Nicholson: I know that Cordis Dow are now dry, but when the paper was prepared we were still using the old Cordis Dow.
    Secondly, while we have been ultrafiltrating our patients, they have not in fact required saline.

J. S. Robson (Edinburgh): Miss Nicholson gave the Travenol three stars for re-use. What characteristic justifies that? Is it ease, or cost, or clearance?

Nicholson: Clearance. We can re-use the Travenol more times than we can re-use the Cordis or the Nephros.

Ahmad: The Travenol is cheaper than the Cordis and has slightly higher clearances for creatinine and urea. I have re-used dialysers as many as 12 times with no trouble, but the point should be made that if a dialyser is re-used more than six times then the amount of money saved is minimal compared to the effort which must be put in it.

Ms Briony Furlong (London): Why has Miss Nicholson not re-used the Gambro? Were there any specific difficulties?

Nicholson: To begin with we did have some difficulty in re-using the Gambro, and we decided to leave it to a later date and to try to re-use it again.

Mrs Deirdre E. Jones (London): Would Miss Nicholson define her methodology of re-use.

Nicholson: Briefly. When the patient comes off dialysis the technicians flush out the dialyser with saline. Residual blood volume is measured, and on that will depend whether it is re-used again. It is then flushed out clear and filled with formaldehyde $2\frac{1}{2}\%$.

Wallace (Glasgow): One of the reported complications of re-using dialysers is that the patients may develop an anti-N, an antibody to the red cell antigens. There have been reports from Australia and from America, and so far it would seem that this complication only occurs where formalin is used for sterilisation. The point was considered in Glasgow before Miss Nicholson started to re-use dialysers.

Does anybody know whether this complication has been observed in Britain?

J. D. Briggs (Glasgow): We ourselves have not re-used enough to measure these antibodies before and after so we have no direct experience. I am not aware of any figures from British units. There seems to have been some debate on this and a Paper was read at EDTA a couple of years back which referred to these antibodies being found after even a single use. I do not know whether it is at all certain how much part re-use plays in the production of these antibodies. There has been some concern about it in relation to possible effects in such patients should they be transplanted. However, we do not know the answer.

I believe that we could get round it. It is a cold antibody, and if one was careful not to transplant a kidney without first warming it up that would probably avoid any risk.

A. W. Siemsen (Honolulu): Our series on measuring antibodies in coil re-use was published in 1976[1] and it clearly demonstrated that the incidence was already high in patients with higher serum creatinines. It was a function of the uraemic process, or something else, but not the re-use. There was no difference between those patients whose dialysers were re-used and those whose dialysers were not re-used. It was already high in people that had creatinines of 10, 11 and 12 but were never dialysed, and there was no difference between patients on peritoneal dialysis and haemo-dialysis. I know of no clinical significance to anti-M.

M. Ward (Newcastle): We have seen anti-M and anti-N antibodies in formalin re-used Meltec multipoint dialysers, which is what we use routinely in our patients. So far we have seen no problems clinically after transplantation.

Ms Jennifer Wedderburn (Nottingham): How many times after re-use is the maximum effective clearance, comparable with the first time used?

Briggs: We have not re-used kidneys excessively. As Dr Ahmad pointed out earlier, the financial saving does not make it worth re-using more than six times. We did re-use a few of the kidneys seven or eight times, but we stopped because it did not seem worth going on. Our figures show no significant fall-off in performance if they are used six times.

There is perhaps some variance with the Newcastle figures.

Ward: We are suprised that people can produce such good clearances after multiple re-use. it may be that their control of heparinization is very much better than we practise in Newcastle. We have had trouble with the Cordis Dow 4's and 5's. They have shown a tremendous drop off in clearance after re-use, even one, two, or three times.

We did re-use the Travenol. To be fair we found that this was the best one to re-use and the clearances were high, but there was still a drop off. We have only re-used them three times. We are financed by the Department and they are not that interested in trying to save money. We are trying to persevere and we may test some of the automatic re-use equipment if we can get our hands on it.

Reference

1. Nolph, K. D., Husted, F. C., Sharp, G. C. and Siemsen, A. W. (1976). Antibodies to nuclear antigens in patients undergoing long-term haemodialysis. *Am. J. Med.*, **60**, 673

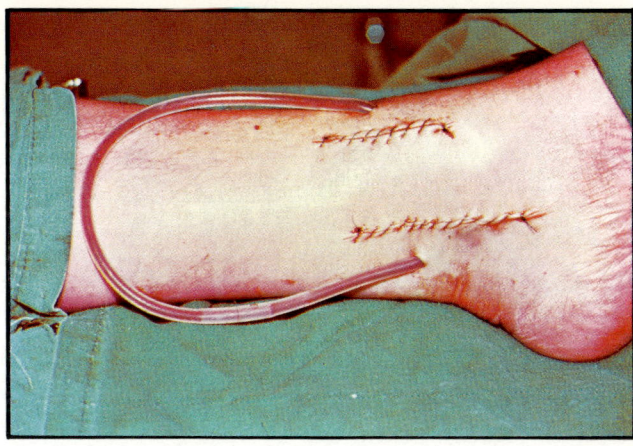

Figure 17.1
Teflon–Silastic
shunt at ankle

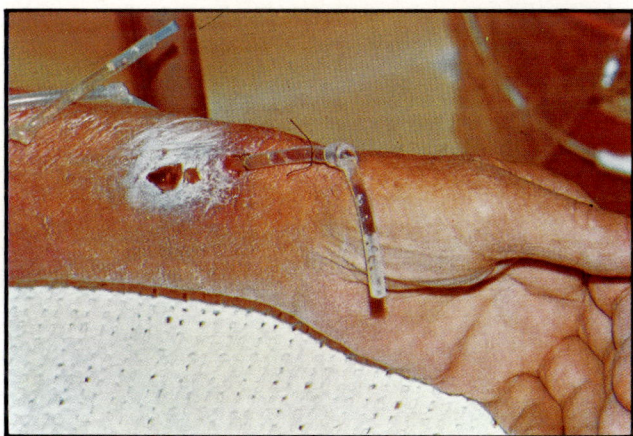

Figure 17.2
Teflon–Silastic shunt with
overlying skin necrosis

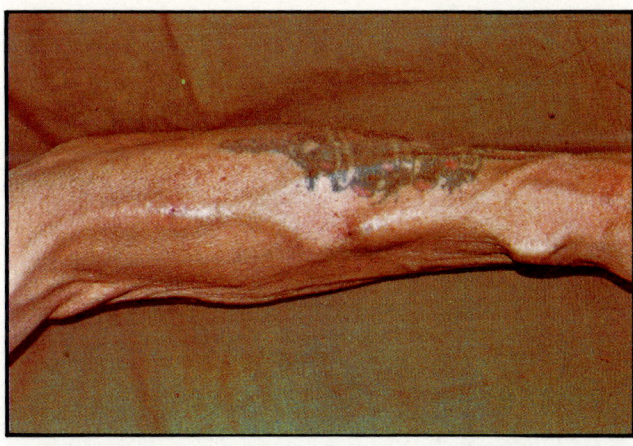

Figure 17.3
Forearm veins in mature
radiocephalic fistula

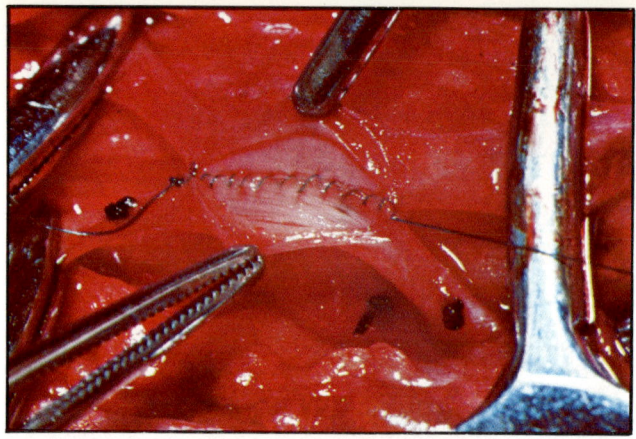

Figure 17.4
Side-to-side anastomosis
between radial artery and
cephalic vein

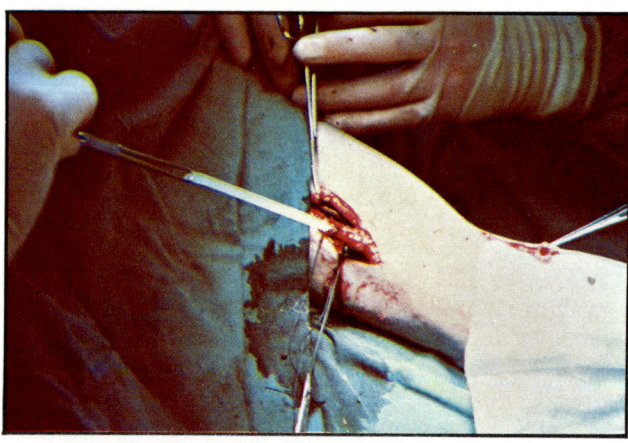

Figure 17.5
Removal of core from
mature Sparks mandril

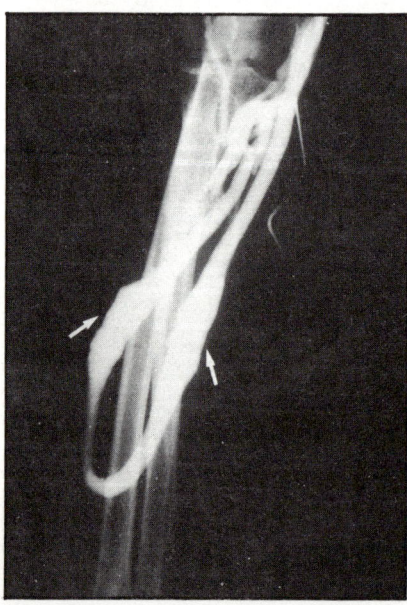

Figure 17.6
Aneurysmal dilatation (arrowed) produced
by conventional dialysis cannulae in a
Sparks mandril

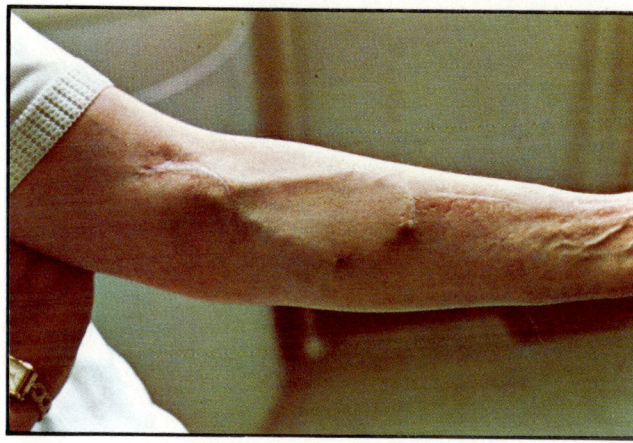

Figure 17.7
Mature forearm saphenous
vein graft loop

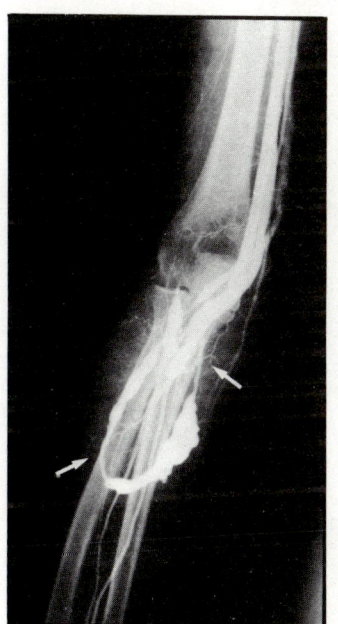

Figure 17.8   Angiogram showing two stenotic
segments (arrowed) produced by
cannulation in a forearm saphenous
vein graft loop

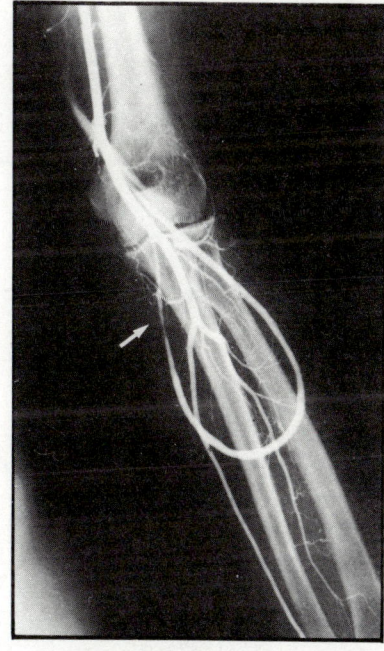

Figure 17.9
Angiogram showing diffuse stenosis
(arrowed) in a forearm saphenous
vein graft loop

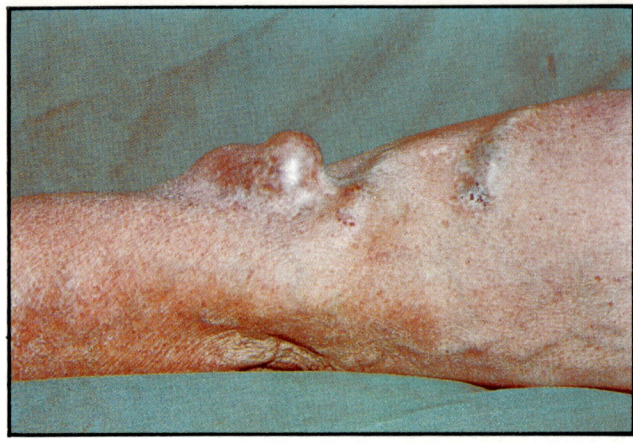

Figure 17.10
Aneurysmal dilatation of
a vein graft

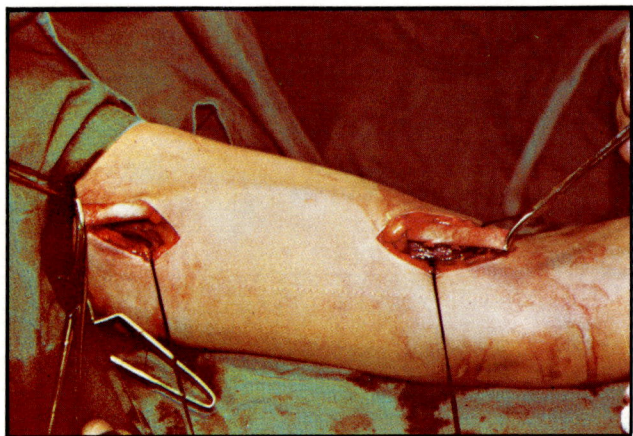

Figure 17.11
Subcutaneous positioning
of an upper arm bovine
heterograft

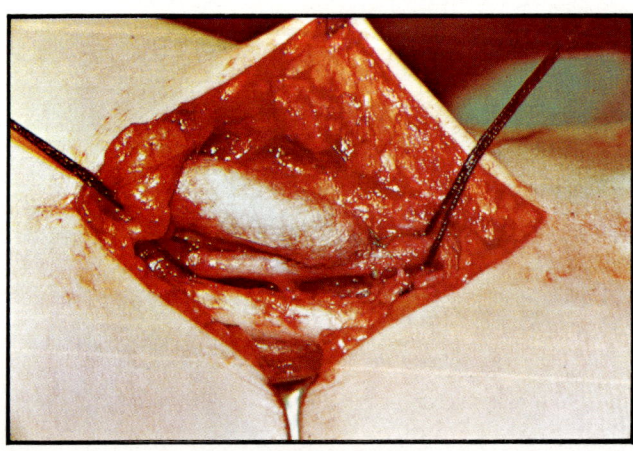

Figure 17.12
Anastomosis of bovine
heterograft to the brachial
artery

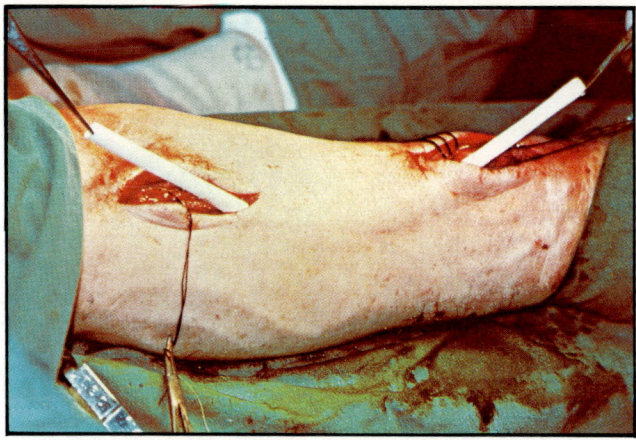

Figure 17.13
Subcutaneous positioning of
a straight forearm expanded
PTFE graft

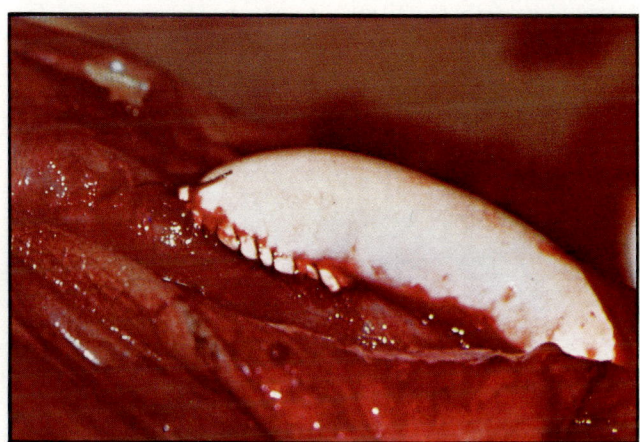

Figure 17.14
Arterial anastomosis of an
expanded PTFE graft

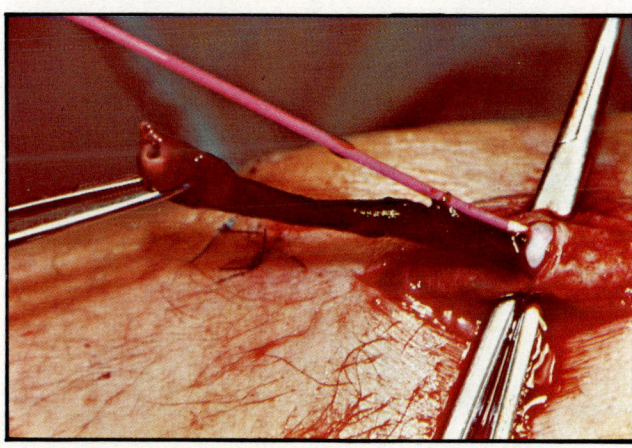

Figure 17.15
Thrombectomy by balloon
catheter of an occluded
expanded PTFE graft

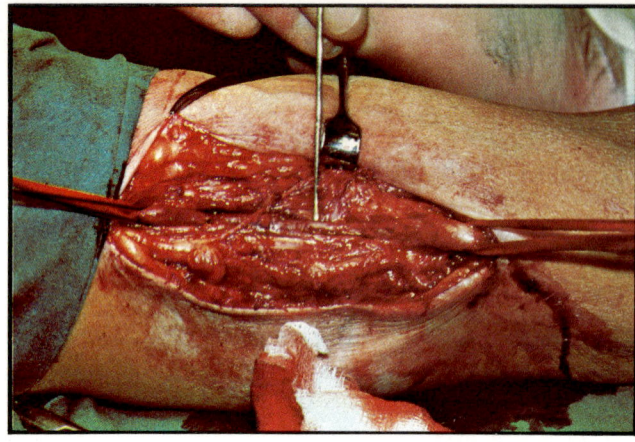

Figure 17.16
Operative appearance of
venous stenosis (at pointer)
between expanded PTFE
graft anastomosis (taped on
right) and normal draining
vein (taped on left)

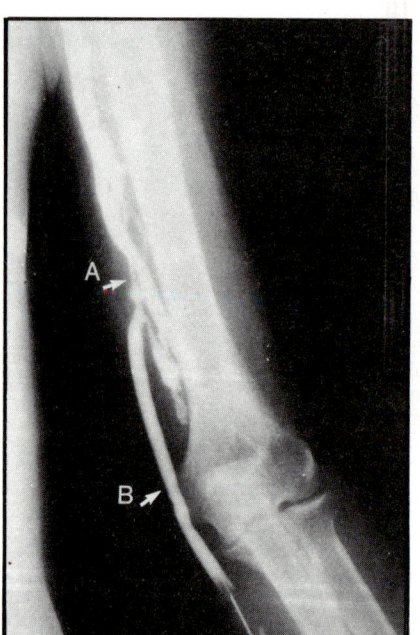

Figure 17.17
Angiogram showing stenosis (A) of
run-off vein adjacent to anastomosis
of expanded PTFE graft (B)

A

B

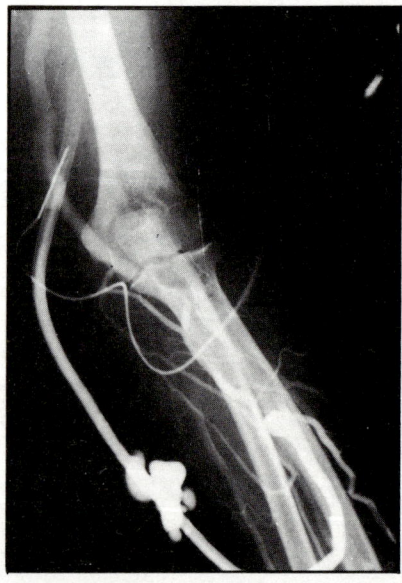

Figure 17.18
Cannulation aneurysm
in a PTFE graft

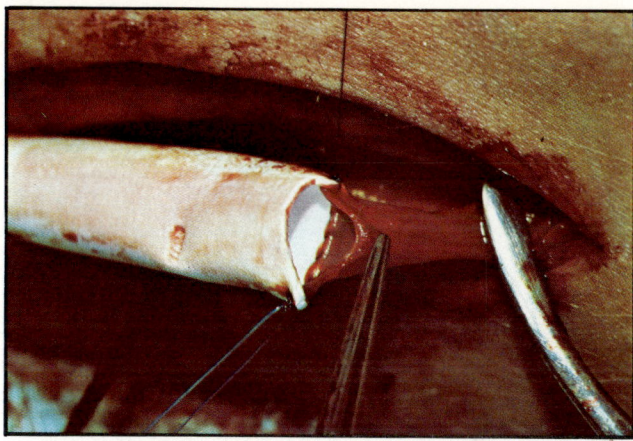

Figure 17.19
End-to-end anastomosis of
expanded PTFE graft

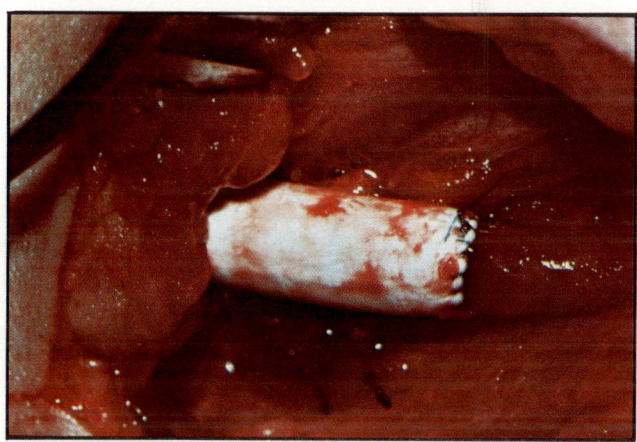

Figure 17.20
Completed anastomosis
between expanded PTFE
graft and axillary vein

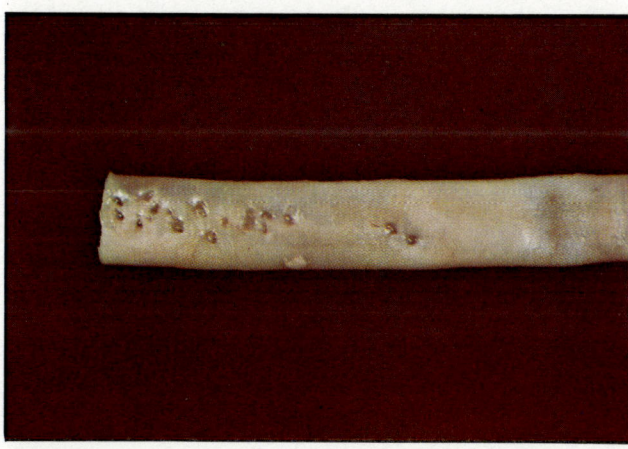

Figure 17.21
Dialysis needle holes in
excised expanded PTFE graft

17

Developments in vascular access
A. McL. Jenkins

17.1 INTRODUCTION

In the last decade there has been considerable progress in techniques of secondary vascular access. The primary methods, which include the Quinton–Scribner Teflon shunt and the Brescia–Cimino arteriovenous fistula at the wrist, are applicable to most patients requiring haemodialysis with intact peripheral vessels. However, many dialysis units have increasing numbers of patients with failed primary access or who have absent peripheral vessels owing to arterial or venous occlusive disease. More patients in this group are being encountered as dialysis units relax their criteria of acceptance regarding age and conditions such as diabetes.

The secondary forms of access include alternative positioning of Teflon shunts and arteriovenous fistulae but recently much attention has been focused on vascular conduits used as subcutaneous grafts. Autologous, homologous and heterologous conduits have been used and lately there has been renewed interest in pure prosthetic materials with some encouraging clinical reports.

Whereas in past years the patient who was coming to the end of his 'shunt life' was an accepted entity, the numerous techniques now available ensure that some form of reasonably safe and reliable vascular access can be instituted.

17.2 FORMULATION OF AN ACCESS POLICY

Whatever form of long-term access is selected the patient's individual needs must be considered. Of basic importance is to place the access at a site convenient for use by the dominant hand. When end-stage renal failure can be anticipated a wrist arteriovenous fistula is the simplest and best form of vascular access. Its timely formation may make a Teflon shunt with its attendant complications unnecessary. However, if dialysis is urgent an ankle Teflon shunt usually proves satisfactory until an arterio-venous fistula becomes usable.

In certain categories of patient one or both of the two primary forms of access may not be possible. These include patients with (a) Occluded arteries and veins at ankle and wrist due to previous failed vascular access or obliterative vascular disease. (b) Weak pulses at ankle or wrist. Poor flow and occlusion is likely to occur if such vessels are used. (c) Heavily calcified vessels. Such vessels may be difficult to suture and rarely develop good flow. They are commonly seen in diabetics. (d) Unsuitable anatomical configuration of forearm veins. The veins may lie deeply in subcutaneous tissue or may be multiple. This usually becomes evident on failure of a wrist arteriovenous fistula to mature and is commonest in women.

In these situations some form of secondary access will be required. It is preferable to attempt a simple secondary procedure in the first instance such as a brachial arteriovenous fistula before embarking on the more major operation of insertion of a vascular conduit.

Patients who have functioning conduits should be reviewed at intervals because of the well known tendency for stenosis to develop in association with some types. It is better to diagnose such lesions either clinically or angiographically in time to carry out corrective surgery rather than lose an irreversibly clotted graft.

17.3 COMPLICATIONS OF VASCULAR ACCESS PROCEDURES

Access operations on blood vessels are attended by most of the risks inherent in vascular surgery. In addition there are certain special complications relating to arteriovenous shunting of blood and to the use of dialysis cannulae.

17.3.1 Infection

Infection in association with vascular access operations is potentially of serious significance. If introduced at the time of operation it is difficult to eradicate, especially when vascular prostheses are involved, and secondary haemorrhage may occur from anastomoses. Removal of the prosthesis is likely to be necessary. Local infection at cannulation sites is a moderately common complication. It often responds to conservative treatment but can also result in severe haemorrhage.

17.3.2 Aneurysms

Aneurysmal dilatation of veins adjacent to an arteriovenous fistula is comparatively common but is not often attended by serious complications. Dilatation of saphenous vein grafts occurs especially if the veins were initially varicose.

False aneurysms may result from cannulation of vascular grafts too soon after implantation before the subcutaneous tissues have become adherent to the outer surface of the graft.

17.3.3 Graft stenosis and thrombosis

Occlusion of a graft in the early postoperative period is likely to be due to faulty technique or selection of vessels with poor flow. Occlusion of a well established graft may be caused by stenosis in the graft itself or in the draining vein. Outflow stenosis results in an excessively turgid graft with an exaggerated pulse. Marked bleeding also tends to occur on removal of cannulae from such grafts at the end of dialysis.

17.3.4   High output cardiac failure

Shunts and arteriovenous fistulae inevitably reduce peripheral resistance and in susceptible patients cardiac failure may occur[1]. However, this is comparatively uncommon and we have not so far seen it in our own patients. Limitation of the size and number of fistulae is probably important in prevention.

17.3.5   Limb ischaemia

This is commonest in association with more proximal limb fistulae[2] but also occurs with fistulae at wrist level[3]. Vascular disease in diabetes may exacerbate ischaemia distal to a fistula and has been described by Buselmeier[4]. In diabetics who have concomitant distal vascular disease the radial artery beyond the fistula should therefore be ligated to prevent retrograde flow of arterial blood from the hand to the fistula.

17.3.6   Hand swelling

This occurs comparatively frequently and is due to retrograde arterialization of a vein. It is occasionally marked and in our own series one patient with retrograde arterialization from a wrist arteriovenous fistula developed gross swelling and ulceration of the fingers. Ligation of the affected vein resolved the symptoms.

17.4   VASCULAR ACCESS TECHNIQUES

17.4.1   The Teflon shunt

The technique described by Quinton, Dillard and Scribner[5] in 1960 made long-term haemodialysis possible and was a major advance in treatment of renal failure. The principle is familiar to all dialysis units as are the associated complications leading to shunt failure. The shunt with its external Silastic tubing and Teflon vascular tips is usually inserted into the posterior tibial artery and long saphenous vein at the ankle (Figure 17.1). Numerous other sites are possible but the wrist is avoided if long-term dialysis is likely in order to save the vessels for a radiocephalic arterio-venous fistula. Insertion into the brachial artery gives good flow but spoils distal arteries for future use. Other sites have been described including the inferior epigastric artery and vein[6]. To avoid necessity of arterial ligation around the shunt tip a short segment vein graft can be anastomosed to the side of an artery and used to contain the tip so preserving arterial con-tinuity. This technique has been described with the femoral artery[7], and the brachial artery[8].

Precise surgical technique is essential for good shunt function. Forcing a too large tip into an artery strips up a cuff of intima leading to throm-bosis whereas a 'temperamental' shunt is often caused by vessel tip angu-lation. Unless the Silastic tubing is well buried in subcutaneous tissue skin necrosis may occur while a haematoma round the tubing encourages infection (Figure 17.2).

In spite of good operative technique most of these shunts fail in 3–6 months. The usual causes are stenosis leading to thrombosis in the vein adjacent to the vessel tip and infection, which occurs in a range of 17–50% of patients[9].

17.4.2   Arteriovenous fistulae

The standard side-to-side radiocephalic anastomosis at the wrist was described by Brescia et al.[10], and is the procedure of choice for long-term haemodialysis (Figures 17.3, 17.4). Anastomosis end of vein to side of artery is used by some to prevent distal arterialization of the veins of the hand which on occasion produces severe swelling[11]. Numerous variations of the technique have been described along with alternative sites. One of the most useful when the forearm vessels are unsuitable is the brachio-cephalic fistula[12,13].

17.4.3   Sparks mandril

This device was originally designed for peripheral vascular surgery but has been used subsequently for vascular access[14]. It consists of a solid Silastic rod covered with a double layer of loosely knitted Dacron and provides a method of 'growing' an artificial blood conduit in situ. The mandril is buried subcutaneously in the desired position and becomes incorporated into the tissues, the ends being placed near a previously located artery and vein. Six weeks after implantation the ends are mobilized and the Silastic rod is withdrawn, leaving a smoothly lined conduit (Figure 17.5). The mature mandril is then anastomosed to the vessels and can then be used for haemodialysis cannulation.

The obvious disadvantage of the mandril is the 6-week growing period, which is always inconvenient, and two operations are needed. We have found that it is not always technically simple to anastomose the rather bulky ends to smallish limb vessels. We have used conventional cutting dialysis needles and have noted consistent development of aneurysms of the conduits in the areas penetrated (Figure 17.6). Anastomotic aneurysms have also developed in those longstanding mandrils which have had to be re-anastomosed to bypass dilations caused by needling.

Others have found the patency rate among mandrils to be inferior to autogenous vein grafts[15] and this means of access is now used less frequently.

17.4.4   Vein grafts

Since the original description of a forearm loop constructed from the long saphenous vein[16] numerous other forms of the graft have been used. Autogenous grafts are most commonly employed but others have shown that preserved homografts also function[17, 18].

The suitability of various veins has been described by Bell and Calman[19]. The long saphenous vein in the thigh is consistently the best for use as a graft though occasionally the distended diameter is poor and if less than 5 mm we employ other means of access. The cephalic vein in the upper arm is also a good graft source but the obvious scarring and discomfort which follow its removal discourage its frequent use. The external jugular veins are also a possible source of graft material.

17.4.4.1   *Graft configurations*

(a) *Forearm grafts* – The most commonly employed forearm grafts are loops arising from the brachial artery near the elbow with return to an adjacent vein (Figure 17.7). They usually function well, but straight forms between the brachial artery and a distal vein are also satisfactory[20]. In our experience the loop types have better patency. Artery to artery grafts have been described between the brachial and radial artery[11].

(b) *Upper arm grafts* – Upper arm grafts are less convenient from the patient's point of view but this form between the brachial artery distally and basilic vein proximally (or vice versa) develop very high flow rates. Such grafts should arch anteriorly to overlie the biceps. Proximity to the neurovascular bundle may result in nerve damage from faulty cannulation and in our experience with various conduits in this position severe local discomfort can occur during dialysis presumably from pressure of the needles on the nerve trunks.

(c) *Lower limb grafts* – Self cannulation of lower limb grafts is easy as both of the patient's hands are free. Transection of the saphenous vein distally in the thigh with anastomosis of the proximal cut end to the femoral artery near the groin results in a high flow loop[21]. It has the technical advantage that an arterial anastomosis only is required.

17.4.4.2   Complications of vein grafts

(a) *Thrombosis* – The incidence of thrombosis of vein grafts is probably lower than with other types of conduit. In our own recent series of 27 vein grafts, of which most were forearm types, there were four occlusions and on each occasion the graft was lost (Table 17.1). We now carry out intermittent check angiograms to identify correctable lesions which might cause

TABLE 17.1   27 Autogenous saphenous vein grafts for vascular access. Thrombotic loss (follow-up 2 months to 2 years)

Graft form	No. inserted	No. occlusions	No. lost (weeks)
Forearm straight	5	1	1 (12)
Forearm loop	19	3	3 (20; 36; 57)
Upper arm straight	2	0	0
Thigh loop	1	0	0
Totals	27	4	4

thrombosis and have demonstrated two types of stenosis. One occurs adjacent to the needling sites giving two localized stenotic segments in a graft (Figure 17.8). The other is a diffuse stenosis with no clear termination point situated in a part of the graft not used for needle insertion (Figure 17.9). The former in some degree was present in the majority of the longstanding grafts, but the diffuse type was seen in two of the 27.

In our experience thrombosis may also develop when a faulty technique is used for removing needles. If excess digital pressure is used to stop bleeding graft flow ceases entirely and clotting results if this is maintained. This applies to all vascular access grafts but does not seem to ocur with arteriovenous fistulae possibly because communicating veins maintain some flow. Patients whose access has been changed from a fistula to a conduit should be appropriately warned.

(b) *Aneurysmal dilation* – Aneurysmal dilation has occurred in some grafts in our own series but has produced surprisingly little disturbance to graft function (Figure 17.10). There seems little danger of severe haemorrhage from the dilated areas and unsightliness may be the main indication for repair or alteration in the means of access.

(c) *Haemorrhage* – Severe haemorrhage may result if an infected focus develops at a cannula puncture site. This occurred with one patient in our series who repeatedly cannulated the same spot. Dramatic haemorrhage necessitated ligation of the segment but access function was preserved by means of a local bypass graft.

17.4.5   Bovine artery heterograft

In 1970 Rosenberg[22] described the use of modified bovine carotid arteries in arterial surgery and since then many others have used this graft for vascular access[23-28]. The results were reviewed by Rosenberg[29]. The grafts which are treated with ficin and with glutaraldehyde tanning are not significantly antigenic[30]. When implanted they incite a fibroblastic reaction unlike the cellular inflammatory response of untreated heterografts. They can be obtained in diameters suitable for vascular access, though the smallest easily obtainable diameter (7 mm) is on the large side for distal limb grafting.

Straight forms between an artery and vein or artery and artery[31] appear to give a higher patency rate than loops. Haimov[27] found that three of four loops clotted soon after surgery. Favourable sites are in the thigh and upper arm though forearm straight forms may also be acceptable[23]. We have used these grafts in a small number of patients in the upper arm and have had no complications over a period of $2\frac{1}{2}$ years (Figures 17.11, 17.12). In some centres the bovine graft is considered to be the best means of secondary vascular access provided that loop forms are avoided[24,26,32].

Bovine and Dacron grafts have been shown to be equally susceptible to experimental infection with *Staphylococcus aureus* but anastomotic disruption occurred more frequently with bovine material[33]. Several workers have reported infected foci at needling sites[24,32], and there is a risk of formation of false aneurysms. There is some evidence to suggest that bovine grafts should not be used for three weeks from the time of insertion as the incidence of aneurysms may thereby be increased.

17.4.6 Expanded polytetrafluoroethylene (PTFE) Gore-Tex vascular prostheses

In the last year there have been reports of use of this material for vascular access, some of which give promising results[34-37].

The microstructure of expanded PTFE consists of nodes interconnected by fine fibrils. The open formation allows rapid cellular ingrowth and the grafts become completely incorporated into the tissues. In contrast to bovine grafts the lumen acquires a continuous neointima and this may be a factor contributing to high patency rates when the prostheses are used for reasons other than vascular access[38,39].

We have conducted a pilot study on the use of expanded PTFE (Gore-Tex)* grafts for vascular access (Table 17.2). The aims were: (a) To assess their surgical suitability for anastomosis to the medium and smaller vessels of the limbs. (b) To establish which was the best graft configuration with regard to patency. (c) To assess the effect of dialysis needles on the graft walls.

TABLE 17.2   PTFE Gore-Tex vascular access grafts. Thrombotic loss (follow-up 1 month to $1\frac{1}{2}$ years)

Graft form	No. inserted	No. occlusions	No. lost (weeks)
Forearm straight	2	2	2 (4; 50)
Forearm loop	5	7	1 (17)
Upper arm straight	4	0	0
Thigh loop	2	1	0
Segmental replacement	1	0	0
Totals	14	10	3

Prostheses of 6 mm internal diameter were used in lengths varying between 19 and 58 cm. The period of follow-up was between 1 month and $1\frac{1}{2}$ years. Fourteen grafts were inserted in 13 patients. The majority were in the forearm (Figure 17.13), but latterly we favoured upper arm types. There was one thigh loop from the common femoral artery to the long saphenous vein, and one segmental replacement of a stenotic area in a forearm loop.

The grafts were highly satisfactory from a purely surgical point of view. Fine anastomoses were simple to fashion and there was no tendency for the material to fray (Figure 17.14).

* W. L. Gore and Associates UK Ltd, Pitreavie Industrial Estate, Dunfermline, Fife

Both forearm types had a high incidence of thrombosis with nine occlusive episodes among seven grafts. Thrombectomy by balloon catheter (Figure 17.15) was often successful but three of these grafts were lost. No occlusions occurred earlier than 4 weeks postoperatively. Graft angiograms or direct inspection at operation demonstrated marked stenosis (1–3 cm in length) in the recipient veins of all grafts just central to the end-to-side graft to vein anastomoses (Figures 17.16, 17.17). There were no other complications apart from infection in one occluded graft which was probably introduced by attempted needling, and aneurysm formation in a segment subjected to needling in another (Figure 17.18).

Following this initial experience we placed the venous ends of the grafts into larger proximal limb veins using end-to-end anastomosis to reduce turbulence. The four upper arm straight grafts originated from the brachial artery just proximal to the cubital fossa with venous anastomosis to the transected origin of the axillary vein (Figures 17.19, 17.20). So far all grafts have functioned normally without angiographic evidence of run-off vein stenosis. We now routinely use long-term antiplatelet drugs for these patients and while there is no definite evidence that they are of value in this situation others have demonstrated that they reduce the incidence of thrombosis in Teflon shunts which also develop run-off vein stenosis[40, 41].

Excised grafts were completely infiltrated with fibrous tissue with continuous smooth neointima except at the large defects made by needles which were filled with granulation tissue (Figure 17.21). These defects could be seen on angiography but there were no clinically evident aneurysms. Sections taken through stenotic veins adjacent to graft anastomoses showed platelet deposition and intimal hyperplasia which often reduced the lumen by up to 80%.

Baker et al.[35] reported a series of 84 expanded PTFE grafts (IMPRA)* and among 64 forearm types there were only 15 occlusive episodes. In only one of these was stenosis of the run-off vein cited as a cause of the occlusion. The disparity between these and our own findings is not clear, though the follow-up period in our series is longer. Kaplan et al.[36] reported a smaller series which included 13 forearm grafts (IMPRA) with no occlusions. The period of follow-up however was again shorter than our own.

In spite of our initial problems with expanded PTFE grafts we regard them as potentially the most acceptable alternative to autogenous vein grafts. Their handling properties are superior to those of bovine hetrografts and a more suitable range of diameters is available. When used as straight grafts proximally in the limb the patency may equal that of vein

* International Medical Prosthetic Research Association Inc., 4209 536th Place, Phoenix, Arizona

grafts and their use avoids the inevitable scarring associated with harvesting the saphenous vein.

References

1. Ahearn, D. J. and Maher, J. F. (1972). Heart-failure as a complication of hemodialysis arteriovenous fistula. *Ann. Intern. Med.*, **77**, 201
2. Matold, W., Kastagir, B., Stevens, L. E., Chrysanthakopoulos, S., Weaver, D. H. and Klinkmann, H. (1971). Neurovascular complications of brachial arteriovenous fistula. *Am. J. Surg.*, **121**, 716
2. Storey, B. G., George, C. R. P., Stewart, J. H., Tiller, D. J., May, J. and Shiel, A. G. R. (1969). Embolic and ischemic complications after anastomosis of radial artery to cephalic vein. *Surgery*, **66**, 325
4. Buselmeier, T. J., Najarian, J. S., Simmons, R. L., Rattazzi, L. C., von Hartitzsch, B., Callender, C. O., Goetz, F. C. and Kjellstrand, C. M. (1973). A-V fistulas and the diabetic: Ischemia and gangrene may result in amputation. *Trans. Am. Soc. Artif. Intern. Organs*, **19**, 49
5. Quinton, W. E., Dillard, D. and Scribner, B. H. (1960). Cannulation of blood vessels for prolonged hemodialysis. *Trans. Am. Soc. Artif. Intern. Organs*, **6**, 104
6. Kauffman, Jr, H. M. (1975). Deep inferior epigastric arteriovenous shunt for hemodialysis. *Surgery*, **78**, 675
7. Chavez, M. D. and Bower, J. D. (1969). Femoro-saphenous arteriovenous shunt for hemodialysis. *Sth. Med. J.*, **62**, 345
8. Haimov, M., Burrows, L., Casey, J. D. and Schupak, E. (1973). Vascular access for haemodialysis: Experience with 214 patients special problems and causes for early and late failures. *Proc. E.D.T.A.*, **9**, 173
9. Foran, R. F., Golding, A. L., Treiman, R. L. and De Palma, J. R. (1970). Quinton–Scribner cannulas for hemodialysis; review of four years experience. *Calif. Med.*, **112**, 8
10. Brescia, M. J., Cimino, J. E., Appel, K. and Hurwich, B. J. (1966). Chronic hemodialysis using venipuncture and a surgically created arteriovenous fistula. *N. Engl. J. Med.*, **275**, 1089
11. Haimov, M., Singer, A. and Schupak, E. (1971). Access to blood vessels for hemodialysis: experience with 87 patients on chronic hemodialysis. *Surgery*, **69**, 884
12. Tellis, V. A., Veith, F. J., Soberman, R. J., Freed, S. Z. and Gliedman, M. L. (1971). Internal arteriovenous fistulas for hemodialysis. *Surg. Gynecol. Obstet.*, **132**, 866
13. Someya, S., Bergan, J. J., Kahan, B. D., Yao, S. T. and Ivanovitch, P. (1976). An upper arm arteriovenous fistula for hemodialysis patients with distal access failures. *Trans. Am. Soc. Artif. Intern. Organs*, **21**, 398
14. Beemer, R. K. and Hayes, J. F. (1973). Hemodialysis using a mandril-grown graft. *Trans. Am. Soc. Artif. Intern. Organs*, **19**, 43
15. Morgan, A. and Lazarus, M. (1975). Vascular access for dialysis. Technics and results with newer methods. *Am. J. Surg.*, **129**, 432
16. May, J., Tiller, D., Johnson, J., Stewart, J. and Shiel, A. G. R. (1969). Saphenous vein arteriovenous fistula in regular dialysis treatment. *N. Engl. J. Med.*, **280**, 770

17. Zerbino, V. R. and Tice, D. A. (1973). Successful use of preserved allograft veins for chronic haemodialysis. *Nephron*, **10**, 61

18. Piccone, Jr, V. A., Lee, H., Ramos, S., Ahmed, N., Di Scala, V., Hamanci, M., Piccone III, V. A., Nielsen, E., Le Veen, H. H. and Berger, E. (1975). Preserved allografts of distal saphenous vein for vascular access – an initial experience. *Ann. Surg.*, **182**, 727

19. Bell, P. R. F. and Calman, K. C. (1974). *Surgical Aspects of Haemodialysis.* (Edinburgh and London: Churchill Livingstone)

20. Girardet, R. E., Hackett, R. E., Goodwin, N. J. and Friedman, E. A. (1970). Thirteen months experience with the saphenous vein graft arteriovenous fistula for maintenance hemodialysis. *Trans. Am. Soc. Artif. Intern. Organs*, **16**, 285

21. Santiago-Delphin, E. A., Buselmeier, T. J., Simmons, R. L., Najarian, J. S. and Kjellstrand, C. M. (1972). Modified saphenous vein loop fistula in thigh for chronic hemodialysis. *Surg. Gynecol. Obstet.*, **134**, 835

22. Rosenberg, N., Lord, G. H., Henderson, J., Bothwell, J. W. and Gaughran, E. R. L. (1970). Collagen arterial graft of bovine origin: seven years observations in the dog. *Surgery*, **67**, 951

23. Haimov, M., Burrows, L., Baez, A., Neff, M. and Slifkin, R. (1974). Alternatives for vascular access for hemodialysis: experience with autogenous saphenous vein autografts and bovine heterografts. *Surgery*, **75**, 467

24. Payne, J. E., Chatterjee, S. N., Barbour, B. H. and Berne, T. V. (1974). Vascular access for chronic hemodialysis using modified bovine arterial graft arteriovenous fistula. *Am. J. Surg.*, **128**, 54

25. Vander Werf, B. A. (1973). Bovine graft arteriovenous fistulas for hemodialysis. *Proc. Dial. Transpl. Forum*, **3**, 12

26. Yokoyama, T., Bower, R., Chinitz, J., Schwartz, A. and Schwartz, C. (1974). Experience with 100 arteriografts for maintenance hemodialysis. *Trans. Am. Soc. Artif. Intern. Organs*, **20**, 328

27. Haimov, M. and Jacobson II, J. H. (1974). Experience with the modified bovine arterial heterograft in peripheral vascular reconstruction and vascular access for hemodialysis. *Ann. Surg.*, **180**, 291

28. Merickel, J. H., Anderson, R. C., Knutson, R., Lipschultz, M. L. and Hitchcock, C. R. (1974). Bovine carotid artery shunts in vascular access surgery. *Arch. Surg.*, **109**, 245

29. Rosenberg, N. (1976). The bovine arterial graft and its several applications. *Surg. Gynecol. Obstet.*, **142**, 104

30. De Falco, R. J. (1970). Immunologic studies of untreated and chemically modified bovine carotid arteries. *J. Surg. Res.*, **10**, 95

31. Butt, K. M. H. and Kountz, S. L. (1976). A new vascular access for hemodialysis. The arterial jump graft. *Surgery*, **79**, 476

32. Payne, J. E. and Berne, T. V. (1974). Access to the circulation for haemodialysis. *Med. J. Aust.*, **2**, 667

33. Hermosillo, C. X., Paroa, F., Gordon, H. E. and Wilson, S. E. (1974). Infectability of dacron vs bovine grafts by induced Staphylococcus bacteria. *Surg. Forum*, **25**, 256

34. Jenkins, A. McL. (1976). Gore-Tex: a new prosthesis for vascular access. *Br. Med. J.*, **2**, 280

35. Baker, Jr, L. D., Johnson, J. M. and Goldfarb, D. (1976). Expanded poly-

tetrafluoroethylene (PTFE) subcutaneous arteriovenous conduits: an improved vascular access for chronic hemodialysis. *Trans. Am. Soc. Artif. Intern. Organs*, 22, 382

36. Kaplan, M. S., Mirahmadi, K. S., Winer, R. L., Gorman, J. T., Dabirvaziri, N. and Rosen, S. M. (1976). Comparison of 'PTFE' and bovine grafts for blood access in dialysis patients. *Trans. Am. Soc. Artif. Intern. Organs*, 22, 388

37. Jenkins, A. McL., Picken, C. M. and Halliday, I. M. (1977). Complications following use of expanded polytetrafluoroethylene (Gore-Tex) prostheses for vascular access. *J. R. Coll. Surg. Edin.*, 22, 203

38. Soyer, T., Tempinen, M., Cooper, P., Morton, L. and Eiseman, B. (1972). A new venous prosthesis. *Surgery*, 72, 864

39. Campbell, C. D., Goldfarb, D. and Roe, R. (1975). A small arterial substitute. Expanded microporous polytetralfuoroethylene; patency versus porosity. *Ann. Surg.*, 182, 138

40. Kaegi, A., Pineo, G. F., Shimizu, A., Trivedi, H., Hirsh, J. and Gent, M. (1974). Arteriovenous-shunt thrombosis. *N. Engl. J. Med.*, 290, 304

41. Kaegi, A., Pineo, G. F., Shimizu, A., Trivedi, H., Hirsh, J. and Gent, M. (1975). The role of Sulfinpyrazone in the prevention of arteriovenous shunt thrombosis. *Circulation*, 52, 497

DISCUSSION

J. A. Kanis (Oxford): Antiplatelet drugs were mentioned at the end of the Paper. Mr Jenkins's rate of survival with the Scribner shunt seems to be considerably lower than the experience of many others, where they may survive for many years.

Jenkins: My comment was based on no assessment of figures. I believe it is fairly general experience up to 6 months. There is no formal trial of antiplatelet drugs amongst dialysis patients.

A. Hall (Isle of Man): We have a patient who has had a Scribner shunt for 9 years.

A. M. Martin (Sunderland): Does Mr Jenkins think that there is no longer a need to insert Scribner shunts? It is usually the physicians who do this, and if they lose this skill there may be the not infrequent situation where the patient with acute renal failure requires haemodialysis and ends up with chronic renal failure. If the skill is lost because people such as Mr Jenkins say that the practice is no longer required it will lead to some problems. There will always be a role for a well-inserted Scribner shunt.

Jenkins: I would entirely agree. If the physician is willing to insert the Scribner shunts that is eminently suitable. It depends on the resources of the hospital involved. If someone is willing to be on tap all the time to insert these things then well and good. In Edinburgh the physicians insert a number of Scribners.

Ms Anne T. Lambie (Edinburgh): Perhaps one reason for quoting a 3-month period for the Scribner is that we make no particular attempt to maintain patency for longer periods. They are a transient phenomenon, often abandoned while still working.

Kanis: But for some patients it may be more suitable to have a shunt that can be kept in for many years.

262

J. S. Robson (Edinburgh): Patients make the point that the needle is a major defect – and a defect that could be avoided if we were to get back to the old-fashioned Scribner.

B. H. B. Robinson (Birmingham): Has Mr Jenkins any experience with umbilical vein grafts?

Jenkins: I have not used them. I have tried them experimentally, harvesting our own and putting them into dogs. I know that they are extremely expensive and they do not seem to hold out any great advantage against the other materials that are available.

F. M. Parsons (Leeds): I was a little worried about Mr Jenkins's upper arm Gore-Tex grafts. What rate of flow does he achieve through those grafts? I would suspect that it might produce cardiac embarrassment because the huge lumen of Gor-Tex anastomosed to a very large brachial artery and also to a very large vein. Has he any knowledge of the rate of flow of blood through these?

Jenkins: No. It is very difficult to assess. We have tried out an electromagnetic flowmeter on Gor-Tex but got no recording due to the nature of the conduction of this material.

The graft is only 60 mm internal diameter – no bigger than that. So far we have not seen anyone with cardiac embarrassment indentifiably due to this.

Parsons: I ask because we have put these between femoral artery and femoral vein and have achieved flow rates of between 2 and 2.5 l – which is quite unacceptable to the heart. I would issue a word of caution until flow rates can be given, particularly as a percentage of total cardiac output.

Jenkins: We are cautious about this and we are on the lookout for trouble. They could be banded fairly simply if it should occur.

Parsons: We banded one. It eroded, and that was the end. What material do you use for banding – silk?

Jenkins: I would tend to band with silk. That would be a reasonable thing to do.

Parsons: One of our grafts eroded through the band and that produced an external haemorrhage breaking through the apparently healed incision.

Jenkins: Did the band enter the vascular conduit itself?

Parsons: The whole thing just disrupted.

Miss S. Taber (Cambridge): Can I refer back to the unbilical vein graft. We have one very successful patient in Cambridge. We used 31 cm and it was £250. It is a British-made bovine graft.

Jenkins: We do not use bovine material.

18

The duration of dialysis
A. M. Martin and
J. K. Gibbins

18.1 THE CORRELATION BETWEEN BIOCHEMISTRY AND CLINICAL SYMPTOMS

After periods ranging from 4 months to 2 years on 9–10$\frac{1}{2}$ hours haemo-dialysis weekly, six patients became vaguely unwell over a 2-week period. They developed increasing dyspnoea, anterior chest pain, then pericardial friction. Cardiac tamponade occurred in three cases. The prodromal illness had features not typical of either bronchopneumonia or pulmonary oedema and all had evidence of left ventricular hypertrophy and ischaemia on ECG prior to the illness although only two had previous hypertension. The mean pre-dialysis blood urea at the onset of pericarditis was 39 mmol/l, this being 26% higher than previous levels. These cases represent an incidence of pericarditis of 8% in our dialysis population. Various authors[1] quote an incidence of 10–17% in patients maintained on 'adequate' dialysis.

A 58-year-old mild diabetic was maintained on regular dialysis 10.5 h weekly for 1 year with a mean pre-dialysis blood urea of 33 mmol/l. For a period of 3 months, the first hour of dialysis was replaced by ultrafiltration alone and the pre-dialysis urea levels rose to a mean of 60.1 mmol/l. He was asymptomatic and no pericarditis developed.

These cases are described to illustrate the fact that biochemical status alone does not correlate with clinical symptoms. Perhaps for example in the genesis of pericarditis the state of the left ventricular muscle is of more importance than the blood urea.

We are constantly being confronted with attempts to correlate a great wealth of laboratory data with clinical features in uraemia. The correlations are poor. It is regarded as bad practice to put much emphasis on single case descriptions and instead draw conclusions from large statistically analysed series. This in turn usually provides data inapplicable to the individual patient. Perhaps it is time to pay more attention to the individual patient.

18.2 WORKING GUIDELINES AS TO THE ADEQUACY AND DURATION OF DIALYSIS

Attempts to determine the duration and adequacy of dialysis have been based on inter-related factors. The simplest guide lines are the blood urea, creatinine and potassium concentrations, fluid status and the efficiency of the dialyser. For example, empirically we like the blood urea to be less than 34 mmol/l pre-dialysis. These parameters have been coupled with a consideration of uraemic symptoms, hypertension control and acute dialysis induced symptoms. Tradition and fashion may have had some influence on our use of dialysis and latterly a desire to treat more patients, perhaps with limited facilities, has affected our practice. In our unit, limited facilities stimulated our adoption of a shortened dialysis regime of 3 to $3\frac{1}{2}$ h thrice weekly[2], so that with a staff reduction of 42% and a reduction in renal unit running hours of 40% we were able to increase the number of dialyses by 30%.

18.3 OTHER ELABORATE PARAMETERS

In addition to the simple guidelines I would mention some other elaborate parameters only to discount them as of little practical value in assessing adequacy or duration of dialysis. They include the use of neuro-behavioural probes[3] involving a quantified EEG, photic driving response and continuous performance testing, EMG, motor nerve conduction velocities, the dialysis index[4] which defines middle molecule clearance, kinetic modelling to predict removal rates of urea and creatinine, and finally bone status.

18.4 RANGE OF HAEMODIALYSIS THERAPIES – THE MINIMUM AND OPTIMUM THERAPY

There is no universal optimum duration or type of dialysis. A desire to define this has led to regimens utilizing dialysers with urea clearances ranging from 6 to 180 ml/min at a frequency of one to seven times weekly for dialysis times of 6–168 h per week.

It is probable that the dialysis regime for each patient can be established at two levels. Firstly a type and duration that is the basic minimum which, by controlling dangerous levels of toxins and fluid, keeps the patient alive. Secondly the optimum type and duration which is unique for that patient but variable and results in full rehabilitation. For example, one might say all patients need a minimum of 3–4 h thrice weekly but for optimum therapy this will require variation in duration, ultrafiltration and perhaps even dialysate flow or composition. I think this optimum level can only be arrived at by trial including attending to the patient's own observations. It is possible that an individual adapts in some way to a certain duration and type of dialysis and although they are never normal biochemically, they tolerate regular, similar fluctuations in body chemistry and fluid status.

We have observed one patient who was maintained on an 8h Kiil dialysis thrice weekly and was switched to 3×3 h on a 1.5 m^2 coil. After about 2 weeks he adapted to the therapy in that acute dialysis symptoms were minimal and are now infrequent. He remains well with a blood urea level higher than previously but if we increase the dialysis duration from

3 to 3.5 h the extra half hour induces nausea, vomiting and cramps without any significant ultrafiltration. Initially one was inclined to say this was a psychological reaction to doing an extra half hour. However, I have discounted this and have tried the procedure on several occasions with identical results. We have observed symptoms in one patient on twice weekly 3 h dialysis with a well controlled urea, creatinine and fluid level and little in the way of ultrafiltration required. He regularly developed fatigue and anorexia the day following a dialysis, after a 3 day gap, a phenomenon which did not affect him following the other dialysis of the week. Although urea and creatinine levels were of a similar order it would seem that some change in body chemistry and perhaps metabolism differed between the two dialyses.

On the other hand, two patients were well maintained on 3–3.5 h dialysis thrice weekly for one year. Then without any obvious change in ultrafiltration, dialysate concentration or blood chemistry, they developed regular acute symptoms after about the first hour of every dialysis.

18.5   THE PHYSICAL ADAPTATION TO DIALYSIS

There is no immediate explanation for the occurrences just described and they probably represent two or more different phenomena in the process of physical ADAPTATION to dialysis. I think we are all inclined to explain disturbances on simple grounds and regard most upsets as having similar causes related to excess ultrafiltration, hyponatraemia, exsanguination due to high blood flow rates or hypocalcaemia. However, if we look more carefully at each patient's problems in and around dialysis it is often not possible to relate it to these factors. We may then describe it vaguely as some form of 'disequilibrium' without actually knowing what this means. From the point of view of physical symptoms we can all remember patients who take to dialysis quickly and others who have a prolonged troublesome introduction. It has often been noted that some regular dialysis patients, despite stable biochemistry, require up to 2 years before they are really rehabilitated. There may well be differing rates of metabolic adaptation and once a pattern is set a change may have disturbing effects. It is also possible that intercurrent illness or other disordered function could upset the response to dialysis.

18.6   THE RELATIONSHIP BETWEEN PROTEIN CATABOLISM AND MASS TRANSFER THERAPY

Gotch[6] recently reviewed a series of dialysis–sorbent regimes and analysed the protein catabolic rates in relation to urea removal capacity. He noted that when dialysis was changed from a single pass system to a low volume recirculating system, in addition to a reduction in urea removal there was a reduction in urea production. He suggested that protein catabolic pathways are upset by mass transfer therapy and it is likely that alternative low molecular weight catabolites are formed which are dialysed through standard membranes.

Cambi[7] reviewed the lean body weight of patients treated for up to 9 years by long or short dialysis on free diet. Of his patients 56% commenced treatment above their ideal weight and 44% below. After periods of therapy ranging from 9 months to 9 years on long or short dialysis the body weights were unchanged. It would seem that despite complete symptomatic rehabilitation the patients metabolism may become set at a level consistent with the uraemic and dialysis status but not normal.

It is also probable that the more efficient the dialysis the longer the process of adaptation. Grimsrud[8], using a single pass 100 ml/min dialysate flow, requiring 20–25 l of dialysate for a 3–4 h dialysis thrice weekly with standard dialysers achieved excellent rehabilitation of patients despite high levels of urea and creatinine. Switching from standard high flow to the low flow system resulted in patients having greater ultrafiltration tolerance and a reduction in dialysis related complications.

18.7 CONCLUSION

1. There is probably more uncertainty about the duration and type of dialysis to use now than there was when it was introduced, and there are as many regimens as there are renal units. Perhaps there should be as many regimens as there are patients.

2. Further study of the protein metabolism of the uraemic patient may bring us closer to an understanding of the tolerance and adequacy of dialysis.

3. When Wilhelm Kolff finally perfects the wearable artificial kidney[9] we shall have to think of something other than the duration of dialysis to talk about.

ACKNOWLEDGEMENTS

To Miss J. Davis, Royal Infirmary Sunderland, for constant help and tolerance.

References

1. Hollomby, D., Gonda, A., Morin, J., Long, R. and Dobell, A. R. C., (1975). Uremic pericardial tamponade. *Proc. Dialysis Transplant Forum*, 16–19

2. Martin, A. M., Oduro-Dominah, A., Gibbins, J. K., Devapal, D. and Mitchell, D. C. (1975). Regular short dialysis in end stage renal failure. *Br. Med. J.*, **296**, 758

3. Teschan, P. E., Ginn, H. E., Bourne, J. R., Ward, J. W. and Vaughn, W. K. (1977). Neurobehaviourial probes for adequacy of dialysis. *Trans. Am. Soc. Artif. Intern. Organs.* (In press)

4. Teehan, B., Gracek, E., Heymach, G., Brown, J., Smith, L., Sigler, M., Gilgore, G. and Schleifer, C. (1977). A clinical appraisal of the dialysis index. *Trans. Am. Soc. Artif. Intern. Organs.* (In press)

5. Janssen, H. F., Stanbaugh, G. H. and Holloway, L. S. (1977). Individualised hemodialysis therapy based on Kinetic modelling. *Trans. Am. Soc. Artif. Intern. Organs.* (In press)

6. Gotch, F. (1977). A general review of the progress made in the technical aspects of haemodialysis. Recent Advances in Biochemical Engineering – Technical Aspects of Renal dialysis. University of Newcastle upon Tyne. 4–6 April 1977. (In press)

7. Grimsrud, L., Jørstad, S., Widerøe, T. and Berg, K. J. (1977). Low flow dialysis. *Trans. Am. Soc. Artif. Intern. Organs.* (In press)

8. Cambi, V., Arisl, L., Bignardi, L., Garini, G., Rossi, E., Savazzi, G. and Migone, L. (1975). Short dialysis after 3 years. *Short Dialysis and Uraemic Osteodystrophy.* Opuscula Medico-Technica Lundensia XVI

9. Kolff, W. J. (1977). Honor Lecture. Artificial Organs: Landmarks of the past and prospects of the future. *Trans. Am. Soc. Artifern. Int. Organs.* (In press)

DISCUSSION

Unidentified speaker: What is the attitude of Dr Martin's patients when they find out that other patients spend three to four times as long on the machine at a stretch? Are they pleased or miserable?

Martin: They are quite contented – naturally. We have had patients who have been elsewhere and who have come to us, and they have been exceedingly grateful. It has changed their way of life. There have been spontaneous statements that life is a little more tolerable. I make no exaggerated claims.

A. W. Siemsen (Honolulu): I am curious regarding the patients' reaction when the dialysis regimen is decreased by 30 minutes. This should be done behind a blank wall, with just the tubes coming out through the wall, so that nobody except one person knows how long that patient is on the dialysis.

Martin: That would be essential to really put the finger on whether this was achieving satisfactory dialysis. The problem is that many of our patients control their own dialysis while on the machine. If, for example, they see themselves losing weight they will give themselves saline. I have one particular patient, admittedly he is unique in a group of about 30 patients, who knows when the 3 hours are up even if he cannot see the clock. He knows things are happening and he must stop, and he will look at his weight, and it has not changed.

J. S. Robson (Edinburgh): Surely there are more patients who know when 5 hours are up. I suspect that a number of patients who go to 5 hours then experience cramp, or discomfort, and learn to recognize it.

Martin: Yes. It is quite common. But can one put a finger on why they have cramp?

Robson: No.

J. A. Kanis (Oxford): There are some animal models for the adaptation of protein metabolism that lend credibility to Dr Martin's suggestions. The first is the adaptation of protein metabolism that occurs in the brown bear hibernating in winter.

The other is some fascinating observations presented to the European Society for Clinical Investigation in 1976 whereby uretus transplanted in the peritoneum resulted in a longer survival of uraemic rats than neph-rectomized rats maintained on the same fluid and electrolyte regime[1]. The difference in survival was very marked.

Martin: It would be a very difficult study in the human.

R. Ahmad (Liverpool): Referring to the patient who develops a syndrome after 3 hours, surely he has a positive membrane pressure. Even if there is no dialysate pressure on the machine, he is still ultrafiltrating.

Dr Martin hit the nail on the head. All patients are different and dialysis should be tailor-made for every individual. My patients range from 9 or 10 hours dialysis a week to as much as 24 hours a week. It is connected with the age, sex and muscle mass of the patient, perhaps even the diagnosis, and many other factors.

Martin: Whatever the cause, there would seem to be a variation in how much dialysis is necessary.

Ahmad: I find it increasingly hard to accept $3\frac{1}{2}$ hours of dialysis for every Tom, Dick and Harry. A paper was recently published on someone who started dialysing $3\frac{1}{2}$ hours three times a week and from 16 patients there were four deaths in the first 6 weeks.

Martin: It amounts to how low one can go before one worries.

Ahmad: It has to be determined for the individual patient.

A. C. Kennedy (Glasgow): There are tremendous variations in how much uraemia a patient can stand. We have all seen patients with uraemia who have been remarkably fit, going about a job, and so on, with very high serum creatinines, low haemoglobins, etc. and others who are sick and who present to the doctor as being sick. There is a tremendous difference in acceptability of uraemia.

Robson: Has Dr Martin any advice on how to proceed to find out how much treatment to give to individual patients?

Kennedy: We should go different ways and frequently compare results. It is important for us not to get preset ideas that we must have X or Y. We really do not know. There is need for more flexibility and different approaches.

Robson: But to take one approach and to stick to it for 6 months or 9 months and then change is to go away from individualization because a unit may have a hundred patients.

Kennedy: Even within that.

Ms Anne T. Lambie (Edinburgh): What criteria would Professor Kennedy use in comparing results?

Kennedy: I would have a list of things that I think are very bad to have, such as haemorrhagic pericarditis, uncontrollable hypertension, symptomatic bone disease and so on. I published an article several years ago[2] on a scoring system whereby patients got more adverse points if they developed certain nasty things, or things that I thought were nasty, and the one with the lowest total was doing best. The theme was not taken up. Perhaps there is a need for groups in a country, like the UK, to try to get some agreement and measure a certain number of things subsequently comparing them on a quantitative basis.

Martin: In the North-East (England) we have an ongoing MRC trial comparing acute dialysis symptoms and long-term effects in three groups of patients: home dialysis patients who are entirely on Meltec dialysers, hospital dialysis patients in Newcastle using the polyacrylonitrile dialyser, and our own. My patients have the shortest dialysis time. Information is coming in but the long-term information will be of the utmost value. However, I suspect that we still have not yet found the right things to measure.

Miss Mary E. Selsby (London): What weight gain do Dr Martin's patients have between dialysis?

Martin: From 1 to 1.5 and sometimes 2 kg, with $3-3\frac{1}{2}$ h dialysis thrice a week. We had one patient who was on twice a week, but I have just switched him simply because of the symptom that I described, namely that after a long gap he did not feel good. Now he feels fantastic, yet I have made no difference to his chemistry.

Mrs M. Brown (Manchester): What are the average haemoglobin levels of these patients on short-hour dialysis?

Martin: Overall it is probably 7–8 g/dl.

M. K. Ward (Newcastle-upon-Tyne): There is no real difference between the other two groups in the comparison. The polyacrylonitrile patients are slightly better but this is not yet statistically significant.

Unidentified speaker: We have not heard much about dietary control, or about the heparin control of the patients for the short duration in view of the pericarditis.

Martin: None of our patients are on protein restriction. We are only careful about high potassium intake and fluid. Whether they are on fluid control depends on whether they are making urine. The majority are not. The majority of the patients would be on 750 ml/24 h. The majority of creatinine clearances are zero, although one or two have 2 or 3 ml/minute.

The quantity of heparin used is less than that given for long dialysis and is given as a single bolus injection at the beginning of treatment.

References

1. Schuck, O., Skopkova, J. and Gort, J. (1976). The 'excretory intelligence' of the gut in rats without renal excretion. Abstracts of European Society for Clinical Investigation, no. 194.
2. Kennedy, A. C., Lindsay, R. M., Murphy, A. V., Allison, M. E. M., McLeod, O. (1971). A scoring system for assessing patients on regular dialysis. *Lancet*, i, 701

CONCLUSIONS
A. C. Kennedy

This symposium has been made possible by the generosity and sponsorship of Travenol Laboratories and I am sure that you would wish me to express on your behalf our gratitude to them, and in particular our gratitude to the organizer, Mr Peter Irving. I also know that he would wish me to comment on the help that he received from the committee, Deirdre Jones, John Anderton and Frank Parsons, for the assistance that they gave him. I know that Travenol would be interested in having reactions as to how valuable the Symposium has been, on whether the content of the programme was right, and on the content of the individual papers, bearing in mind the mixed nature of the audience. These comments can either be passed on verbally, when meeting people from Travenol, or they can be sent in in writing.

I shall now use the chairman's privilege to make some remarks that seem to me appropriate.

Speaking as a clinician I think we have had a series of balanced accounts and appraisals of various facets of current practice in the UK. This is always useful. It is a form of painless postgraduate instruction that is very good for clinicians from time to time. It is very useful to realize that the problems I have in my unit are the same problems that everybody else has, and that there is no mysterious magic thing that I should be doing or should have started to do 6 months ago. From the clinician's point of view it was a success.

For the nursing staff, the technical staff, and the other staff relating to dialysis units, I would hope that taken as a whole there was enough in the Symposium to have given them useful guidance on various aspects of practical management. If at times they perhaps felt that the content of the occasional paper had rather too much actual physiology or something that was perhaps not of immediate interest or relevance to them, they should bear with us in this. It is useful for them to understand the complexities that underline these problems and why some of these problems are so difficult to solve.

For those from the Department of Health, the Ministry, in the audience I think that a very clear message came across – a very clear picture of hardworking units, underfinanced. I would hope that the message is taken back, digested and analysed – and even more hopefully, acted on.

Finally, for everyone – doctors, nurses, technical staff, etc., and including the commercial people themselves – there were two clear-cut benefits. First there was the opportunity to meet and make contact with people from other units and related disciplines. This is always enormously valuable. Secondly, we have had the opportunity to hear two very moving but very modest accounts of actually living with renal failure from Mr Baillie and from Dr Henry. Their papers were an inspiration to us all.

Thank you very much.

Index

ELEMENTARY PRINCIPLES OF ECONOMICS

Irving Fisher

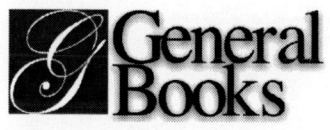

www.General-Books.net

Publication Data:

Title: Elementary Principles of Economics
Author: Irving Fisher
Reprinted: 2010, General Books, Memphis, Tennessee, USA
Publisher: The Macmillan company
Publication date: 1912
Subjects: Economics
Business Economics / Economics / General
Business Economics / Economics / Theory
BISAC subject codes: BUS069000, BUS069030

1

ELEMENTARY PRINCIPLES OF ECONOMICS

: c.

PREFACE

For Teachers

The words " Elementary Principles" in the title of this book indicate the limits of its scope; the book is intended to be elementary, not advanced, and concerns itself with economic principles, not their applications. F v

First, being elementary, it does not attempt to unravel the most difficult tangles of economic theory or to introduce controversial matter. For such studies it should be succeeded by more extensive treatises (e. g., my own: Nature of Capital and Income, Mathematical Investigations in the Theory of Value and Prices, Purchasing Power of Money, and Rate of Interest, which follow out the same general system of thought and exposition as adopted in this book).

Secondly, being devoted to principles, the book is confined to that part or aspect of economics which is now coming to be recognized as capable of scientific treatment in the sense, for instance, in which that term may be applied to physics or biology. The fundamental distinction of a scientific principle is that it is always conditional; its form of statement is: If A is true, then B is true. A principle differs in this respect from a fact which asserts unconditionally that B is true. Science is primarily concerned with the formulation of principles. The aim of this book is to formulate some of the fundamental principles relating to economics.

The method and order of treatment are not altogether traditional. The time-honored order of topics–production, exchange, distribution, consumption–has been found impracticable. Such an order was probably originally intended to parallel the natural course of events from the production of an article to its consumption; but to-day these four topics scarcely retain any traces of such a parallelism. " Distribution," for instance, has, in theoretical discussions, long ceased to be a description of the processes by which food, clothing, and other goods are distributed after being produced and prior to being consumed, and has become simply a study of the determination of rent, interest, and other market magnitudes. It is not, therefore, surprising that many other textbooks on economics have also broken away from this unfortunate order of topics.

Of the many possible methods of writing economic textbooks, there are three which follow well-defined, though widely different, orders of topics. These are the " historical," the " logical," and the " pedagogical." The historical method follows the order provided by economic history; the logical begins with a classification of economics in relation to other studies, explains its methodology, and then proceeds by means of abstract examples from the simplest imaginary case of " Robinson Crusoe economics " to the more complex conditions of real life; the pedagogical begins with the students existing experience, theories, and prejudices as to economic topics, and proceeds to mold them into a correct and self-consistent whole. The order of the first method, therefore, is from ancient to modern; that of the second, from simple to complex; and that of the third, from familiar to unfamiliar. The third order is the one here adopted. That the proper method of studying geography is to begin with the locality where the pupil lives is now well recognized. Without such a beginning the effect on the students mind may be like that betrayed by the schoolgirl, who, after a years study of geography, was surprised to learn that her own playground was a part of the surface of the earth. In like manner we cannot expect to teach economics successfully unless we begin with the material already existing in the students mind. Those textbooks which open with a discussion of the relations of economics to anthropology, sociology, jurisprudence, natural science, and biology, overlook the fact that the beginner in economics is totally unprepared even to understand the meaning of these great subjects, much less their relations to one another. The same sort of error is made by those textbooks which begin with a comparative study of the logical machinery by which truth is ground out in economics and in other sciences. The students logical faculty must be exercised before it can profitably be analyzed.

This book, therefore, aims to take due account of those ideas with which the students mind is already furnished, and to build on and transform these ideas in a manner adapted to the mind containing them. This is especially needful where the ideas are apt to be fallacious. The economic ideas most familiar to those first approaching the study of economics concern money,–personal pocket money and bank accounts, household expenses and income, the fortunes of the rich. Moreover, these ideas are largely fallacious. Therefore, the subject of money is introduced early in the book and recurred to continually as each new branch of the study is unfolded. For the same reason considerable attention is given to cash accounting, and to those fundamental but neglected principles of economics which underlie accounting in general. Every student at first is a natural " mercantilist," and every teacher has to cope eventually with the prejudices and misconceptions which result from this fact. Yet no textbook has apparently attempted to meet these difficulties at the point where they are first encountered, which is at the beginning.

It may be worth while to distinguish the pedagogical procedure here proposed from that recently advocated under the somewhat infelicitous title of the "Inductive Method." I refer to the method by which the student is at first to be taught economic facts without any formulation of principles. This proposal seems to assume that the students mind is quite a blank to start with, and that it is possible on this tabula rasa to inscribe facts without at the same time intimating how they are related. The truth is, however, that the students mind is already familiar with a great mass of economic facts acquired at home, on the street, and from the newspapers. He knows something, not only of money and accounts, but of banks, railways, retail trade, labor unions, trusts, the stock market, speculation, the tariff, poverty, wealth, and innumerable other topics. It is equally true that his head is full of theories as to the relations of these facts,–the working of supply and demand, the nature of money, the operation of a protective tariff, etc. The difficulty is that most of his theories and many of his supposed facts are false; and before we add to his ill-assorted collection of mental furniture we must arrange in orderly fashion that which he already possesses. Moreover, it is almost impossible to impart successfully any considerable mass of disconnected facts. If the teacher does not indicate the true connections, the student will almost inevitably supply false ones; or else the facts without connections will be also without interest.

These objections to the so-called " inductive method" are not, however, intended as militating against the object which its advocates strive to attain, viz., to make the student think for himself, nor against the chief means by which they actually attain this object, viz., the use of original problems. Every teacher can and should illustrate, emphasize, and elaborate every step in the study of principles by propounding problems. Sumners collection of problems, or the more recent collections of Taylor or of the University of Chicago, may profitably be used to sup plement those which every good teacher will readily invent for himself from the suggestions of the text, of current newspapers, or of students questions. These should vary from year to year according to current events and the exigencies of the case as understood by the teacher.

A pamphlet of suggestions as to problems to be used in connection with this book has been prepared for teachers and may be obtained of the publishers. It is submitted that the present treatment of the subject lends itself peculiarly to the use of definite soluble problems in place of the vague "problems" which are usually employed in economics and which call for little more than an expression of opinion. Incidentally, the teacher will find that these definite arithmetical problems are not only much more useful to the student, but are much less trouble for the instructor to correct and grade.

Problems should, I believe, supplement and not supplant a textbook. The effort to substitute problems for textbooks has always failed even in those subjects which, like algebra and geometry, may be said to consist naturally of a series of problems. A preliminary framework of general principles is needed in order to formulate special problems of real value. Problems which are really soluble by the beginner can be little more than applications of general principles to special cases.

What has been said will help explain why greater attention than usual is here paid to certain themes, such as money, bank deposits, accounting, the rate of interest, and the person?! distribution of wealth; as well as why less attention than usual is paid to certain other themes, such as methodology and those obsolete theories like the " wage fund " theory which (unlike some other obsolete theories) has probably never formed any part of the students mental stock in trade.

To some critics the abundant use of curves may seem too advanced for an elementary work. But their use is now so common in the advanced treatises to which the student is, if possible, to be led, that their introduction here is but a necessary part of his preparation. The very fact that there is at present no elementary book in which the nature and use of the graphic method has been made clear for the elementary student is a strong argument for its adoption. Moreover, I am persuaded that the " difficulties " in the elementary use of curves are largely imaginary. Every beginner in economics may be assumed to be familiar with latitude and longitude on a map, and perhaps also with the temperature charts in the daily paper. It is a very easy step from these to curves of supply and demand, provided they be used with sufficient frequency and with sufficient system to take lodgment in the students memory. The student who sees but one diagram in a book will find the initial effort of understanding that diagram scarcely worth while,–not much more worth while than to be taught the use of logarithms without applying them to more than one or two practical examples. As a matter of fact, there are few things which so facilitate the understanding of economic relations at every stage of economic study as the use of diagrams; and it is believed that, with them, the elementary student can proceed both faster and further in economic analysis than without them.

Some friends are inclined to criticize the book as being too cold an analysis. They point out that the students main interest in the subject is a "human interest" and concerned primarily with the practical and immediate solution of great public problems. No one acquainted with my interest in some of these problems can accuse me of lack of appreciation of the "human" element in them all. But the more one studies these problems and the attempts at their solution, the more evident it becomes that most students approach them with an insufficient grounding in fundamental principles. In social as in medical therapeutics a lack of knowledge of anatomy and physiology results in quackery–in remedies worse than the disease which it is proposed to treat. I believe that one of the greatest needs to-day in the teaching of elementary economics is. " to curb this popular tendency to run after remedies before formulating principles. In the present book, therefore, while most of the great practical problems of economics are outlined in connection with the principles which must be employed in their solution, the solutions themselves are not discussed. Full discussion of all these problems is impossible in any textbook, and I earnestly deprecate a general ex cathedra pronouncement of personal opinion by an author on moot questions, especially in a book for immature students. The only proper course, in my opinion, is for the student first to master the fundamental economic. principles on which all or most competent economists can agree, and then, as suggested on the closing page of this book, to take up some one moot question–some burning issue of the day–and, so far as possible, master that also. In the meantime he should, so far as possible, keep an open mind on other problems until, in course of time, they may also be taken up intensively, one by one. A textbook which attempts to supply the student with ready-made opinions on all practical problems "while he waits," may be supplying a real demand, but is not performing a high service.

Possibly the slight emphasis here put on historical, descriptive, and practical economics may decide some teachers against the use of this book and lead them to choose a book in which "the whole subject of economics" is treated. I submit, however, that no such "complete" book exists, since no author exists capable of writing it, and that all which aim to be complete lack at least half of the subject matter here presented and which is taken for granted as if fully known by the student. In many books the terms "assets," "liabilities," "income," "cost," and "rapidity of circulation " are used without discussion or even definition. It would be out of place here to criticize other textbooks, but it has been my hope that the present book may be found a useful introduction to other books, even those which attempt to cover the subject "completely." I would also point out that, by omitting the more "therapeutical" parts of the subject, I have escaped most of its controversies, for the controversies to-day are more as to the solution of 7 practical problems than as to the validity of such elementary,, principles as are contained in this book. Freedom is thus, allowed to each teacher who uses this textbook to follow it up by whichever among others contains the therapeutical treatment which he personally regards as correct. I have been struck by the fact that my critics seldom question the correctness of the propositions here laid down. If this book may afford a common starting point for economic instruction of different schools of thought and different attitudes toward public problems, it will have served one important purpose.

Especial care has been taken in formulating definitions so that the concepts described by these definitions may become firmly fixed in the students minds. These definitions and concepts have been chosen in reference to their usefulness in economic analysis as well as their conformity to practical usage. I am one of those who believe that when the usage of academic economics conflicts with the ordinary usage of business, the latter is generally the better guide. This is not only because business usage has a thousand times the currency of academic usage, but also because in general it comes closer to the needs of economic analysis. Here is not the place to argue why this is true, or even to prove that it is true. I will, however, mention one consideration which appeals increasingly to practical teachers: An academic tradition which is unconvincing to the student is sure later, when he himself becomes a business man and perceives how badly academic traditions are out of tune with modern business usage, to breed a deep distrust, if not contempt, for all academic economics. Thus, expediency, as well as sound theory, should urge teachers to respect the usage of business men.

I have taken so much space to justify those features of this book which will seem new, because several teachers to whom the experimental editions were submitted have condemned it at sight as unteachable. I am glad to report, however, that the teachers who have actually tested the book in classroom have usually become extremely enthusiastic over its "teachableness," although many of them had begun its use with grave misgivings.

The experimental editions, of which there were two, were made possible by special arrangement with the publishers. This gave opportunity for thorough trial for two years in classrooms at Yale, under nearly a dozen different instructors. As a result of this trial and the many valuable suggestions and criticisms which were obtained from teachers, students, and friends, the book has been virtually written three times. The present—the third and final—edition is the first to be offered to the general public.

I am under obligations to President Hadley of Yale for the fundamental idea employed in the discussion of those supply curves which illustrate the willingness to produce "a given amount or more" instead of, as ordinarily assumed, "a given amount or less" ; also for helpful criticism on the presentation of that most difficult subject, the rate of interest. I am also indebted for helpful criticism to my colleagues, Professor Clive Day, Assistant Professors F. R. Fairchild, H. P. Fairchild, W. H. Price, and A. L. Bishop, Dr. H. G. Brown, Dr. E. J. Clapp, now in New York University, and Dr. J. L. Leonard; also to Professor Charles W. Mixter of the University of Vermont, Professor Harvey A. Wooster of De Pauw University, Professor Louis N. Robinson of Swarthmore College, Dean David Kinley of the University of Illinois, Professor E. W. Kemmerer of Cornell University, Professor H. J. Davenport of the University of Missouri, Professors E. R. A. Seligman, H. R. Seager, and H. R. Mussey of Columbia University, R. T. Ely and W. A. Scott of Wisconsin University, and W. M. Adriance of Princeton University, Mr. W. F. Hickernell, now with the Brookmire Economic Chart Company of St. Louis, Mr. Morrell W. Gaines of the Statistical Department of Brown Brothers and Company of New York, Mr. Julius H. Parmelee, statistician of the Bureau of Railway Economics, Washington, D. C., Professor E. B. Wilson of the Massachusetts Institute of Technology, Dr. Leonard Bacon of New Haven, and to Mr. J. M. Shortliffe of the Graduate Department of Yale University.

I endeavored to obtain a clear idea of the undergraduates viewpoint by offering prizes for the best criticisms from students using the book as a textbook, the prizes being awarded by a committee of instructors other than myself. In the college year 1910-1911, the students who won the prizes were R. H. Gabriel, 1913, E. J. Webster, 1913, and G. G. Chandler, 1912, and in the year 1911-1912, Edward Click, 1914, W. Van B. Hart, 1914, and M. W. Brush, 1913. The criticisms of others besides the prize winners were found helpful. To H. Briar Scott, 1913, I am also indebted for suggesting the insertion of Figure 2. My greatest obligations for criticism, especially as to the mode of presentation, are due to my brother, Herbert W. Fisher, who has kindly read and criticized all of the original manuscript and both preliminary editions.

IRVING FISHER. May, 1912.

SUMMARY

Foundation Stones

Introduction

Capital

Income

Capital and Income

CHAPTER I

WEALTH 1. Definition of Economics and of Wealth

Economics may be most simply defined as the Science of Wealth. It is also known under several other titles, of which the most common is " Political Economy." The purpose of economics is to treat the nature of wealth; the human wants served by wealth; the satisfaction of those wants and the efforts required to satisfy them; the forms of the ownership of wealth; the modes of its accumulation and dissipation; the reasons that some people have so much of it and others so little; and the principles that regulate its exchange and the prices which result from exchange. In a word, everything which concerns wealth in its general sense comes within the scope of economics. It is worth emphasizing at the outset, that the chief purpose of economics is to set forth the relations of wealth to human life" and welfare. It is not, however, within the province of economics to study all aspects of human life and welfare, but only such as are connected in some rather direct manner with wealth.

To most persons the chief interest in the subject lies in its practical applications to public problems, such as those connected with the tariff, taxation, currency, trusts, trade-unions, strikes, or socialism. These problems suggest that something is wrong in the present economic order of society and that there is a way to remedy it. But before we can treat of economic diseases, we must first understand the economic principles which these public questions involve. That is, the study of economic principles must precede the application of those principles to problems of public policy. In the end the student will reach more satisfactory conclusions, if at the beginning he will put aside all thought of such applications, and cease to count himself a free trader or a protectionist, an individualist or a socialist, or, indeed, any other kind of partisan.

We must, then, in the first place, distinguish economic principles from their applications to public problems; in the second place, we must distinguish those principles from their applications to private problems. Economics does not concern itself with teaching men how to become rich; nor does a practical skill in the art of becoming rich imply, necessarily, a sound knowledge of economics. Economics, it is true, represents the theory of business; and business, the practice of economics. But, though they are not in the least conflicting–indeed, to some extent they are mutually helpful–economics and business are nevertheless totally different. The primary requisite of a good business man is to master the detailed facts which concern his own individual operations; the primary requisite of a good economist is to master the general principles based on business facts. Some of the wildest economic theories have originated among successful financiers. Men who have been trained in Wall Street are often the most sadly lacking in elementary instruction in economics. This is so because the very matters with which people have longest been familiar are frequently the ones which they have been least disposed to analyze. In business theory, no less than in the theory of public problems, men take too much for granted.

Our first rule, then, in approaching the study of economics is to take nothing for granted. It is quite as important to be careful in defining familiar terms, such as " prices " and " wages," as in explaining unfamiliar ones, such as " index numbers " and " marginal utility."

The chief purpose of this book is to define clearly the fundamental concepts of economics and to state and prove the fundamental principles of the science. These concepts and principles will then serve as a basis for further study. In other books the student will find these concepts and principles applied to problems of public policy, or of business management, or of the economic history of nations. We are not concerned in this book either with practical problems or economic history except as they are used occasionally to illustrate the principles under consideration.

Wealth having been designated as the subject matter of economics, the question at once arises: What is wealth? By wealth in its broader sense is meant material objects owned by human beings. This meaning, however, is broader than the ordinary meaning of the term; for it includes human beings themselves. Every human being is a " material object " and is " owned " either by another human being, as in the case of slavery, or by himself, if he is a freeman. But in ordinary usage men except themselves from the category of " wealth " just as, with equal inconsistency, they except themselves from the category of " animals." Properly speaking man is wealth, just as, properly speaking, man is an animal. But we so seldom need in practice to take account of man as wealth that the ordinary meaning of wealth includes only material objects owned by human beings and external to the owner.1 In this book we shall follow ordinary usage by employing this narrower meaning except occasionally when it will be found convenient to refer to the broader meaning. Any particular article of wealth may be called an" instrument." Thus a locomotive is an article of wealth or an instrument. Other examples are an automobile, a horse, a house, a lot, a chair, a book, a hat, a loaf of bread, a coin.

1 Every writer may define a term as he pleases, except that he should justify his definition in one or both of two ways: (1) by showing that it accords with common practice; and (2) by showing that it leads to useful results. The above def1nition of wealth meets both of these requirements. It agrees substantially with the usual understanding of business men, and it is useful in the development of the science of economics.

Some economists add to the definition that an object, to be wealth, must be useful. But utility is really implied in ownership. Unless a thing is thought to be useful, no one would care to own it. Nothing is owned which is not useful in the sense that its owner hopes to receive benefits from it, and it is only in this sense that utility is to be employed as a technical term in economics. Therefore, as utility is already implied in ownership, it need not be mentioned separately in our definition. Other writers, while including in their definition the idea of utility, omit the idea of ownership and simply define wealth as "useful material objects." But this definition includes too many "objects." Rain, wind, clouds, the Gulf Stream, the heavenly bodies, especially the sun, from which we derive light, heat, and energy, are all useful and material, but are not appropriated, and so are not wealth as commonly understood. Even more objectionable are those definitions of wealth which omit the qualification that it must be material; they do this in order to include stocks, bonds, and other property rights, as well as human and other services. While it is true that property and services are inseparable from wealth, and wealth from them, yet they are not themselves wealth. To include wealth, property, and services all under " wealth," involves a species of triple counting. A railway, a railway share, and a railway trip are not three separate items of wealth; they are respectively wealth, a title to that wealth, and a service of that wealth.

In common parlance " wealth" is often opposed to " poverty," the contrast being between a large amount of wealth and a small amount; precisely as in common parlance " heat" is opposed to " cold," the contrast being between a large degree of heat and a small degree. But just as in physics ice is regarded as having some degree of heat, so in economics a poor man is regarded as having some degree of wealth.

Wealth, then, includes all those parts of the material universe that have been appropriated to the uses of mankind. It includes the food we eat, the clothing we wear, the dwellings we inhabit, the merchandise we buy and sell, the tools, machinery, factories, ships, and railways, by which other wealth is manufactured and transported, the land on which we live and work, and the gold by which we buy and sell other wealth. It does not include the sun, moon, or stars, for no man owns them. It is confined to this little

planet of ours, and only to certain parts of that; namely, the appropriated sections of its surface and the appropriated objects upon that surface.

2. Distinction between Money and Wealth

One of the first warnings needed by the beginner is to avoid the common confusion of wealth with money. Few persons, to be sure, are so naïve as to imagine that a millionaire is one who has a million dollars of actual money stored away; but, because money is that particular kind of wealth in terms of which the value of all other kinds of wealth is measured, it is sometimes forgotten that not all wealth is money.

We are not yet ready for an extended study of money, nor even for a definition of money, but as a warning we shall here enumerate a few of the most common fallacies which beset the subject. The nature of these fallacies the student will understand at a later stage. They are introduced here not with any idea that the student will at once see where the error lies, but chiefly for the purpose of ridding his mind of the ordinary unwarranted assumptions about money.

First among these fallacies, is the assertion that if one man " makes money," some one else must " lose " it, since there is only a fixed stock of money in the world, and it seems clear that " whatever money the money-maker gets must come out of some one elses pocket." The flaw in this reasoning is the assumption that gains in trade are simply gains in actual money, so that in every business transaction only one party can be the gainer. If this were true, we might as well substitute gambling for business and for manufacturing; for in gambling the number of dollars won is equal to the number of dollars lost. As a mattery of fact, however, it is not in order to obtain money that people engage in trade, but in order to obtain what money will buy, and that is precisely what both parties to a normal transaction eventually do obtain.

Again, some persons have tried to prove that the people of the earth can never pay off their debts because these debts amount to more than the existing supply of money. " If we owe money," it is argued, " we cant pay more money than there is." This assertion sounds plausible, but a moments thought will show that the same money can be, and in fact is, paid over and over again in discharge of several different debts; not to mention that some debts are paid without the use of money at all.

A few years ago at a meeting of the American Economic Association a Western banker expressed the opinion that the total amount of money in the world ought to be equivalent to the total wealth of the world; else, he suggested, people would never be able to pay their debts. He explained that in the United States there were twenty dollars of wealth for every dollar of money; and he inferred that therefore there was but one chance in twenty of a debtors paying his debts. " I will give five dollars," he said, " to any one who can disprove that statement." When no one accepted the challenge, a wag suggested that it was because there was but one chance in twenty of getting the promised five dollars I

The attempt to equalize money and wealth by increasing money twenty fold, would, as we shall see later, prove absolutely futile. The moment we increased the amount of money, the money value of all other forms of wealth would rise, and there would, therefore, still be a discrepancy between the amount of money and the amount of wealth.

A very persistent money fallacy is the notion that sometimes there is not enough money to do the worlds business, and that unless at such times the quantity of money is increased, the wheels of business will either stop or slacken their pace. The fact is, however, that any quantity of money, whether large or small, will do the world s business as soon as the level of prices is properly adjusted to that I quantity. In a recent article on this subject, an editor of a popular magazine put this fallacy into the very title: " There is not enough money in the world to do the worlds work." He says, "The money is not coming out of the ground fast enough to meet the new conditions of life." In reality, money is coming out of the ground faster than the " new conditions " require, with the consequent result of raising prices.

A more subtle form of money fallacy is one which admits that money is not identical with wealth, but contends that money is an indispensable means of getting wealth. At a recent meeting of the American Economic Association a very intelligent gentleman asserted that the railways of this country could never have been built in the early fifties had it not been for the lucky discovery of gold in California in 1849, which provided the " means by which we could pay for the construction of the railways." He overlooked the fact that the world does not get its wealth by buying it. J One person may buy from another; but the world as a whole does not buy wealth, for the simple reason that there would be no one to buy it from. The world gets its railways, not by buying them, but by building them. What provides our railways is not the gold mines, but the iron mines. Even though there were not a single cent of money in the world, it would still be possible to have railways. The gold of California enriched those who discovered it, because it en-" abled them to buy wealth of others; but it did not provide the world with railways any more than Robinson Crusoes discovery of money in the ship provided him with food. If money could make the world rich, we should not need to wait for gold discoveries. We could make paper money. This, in fact, has often been tried. The French people once thought they were going to get rich by having the government print unlimited quantities of paper money. Austria, Italy, Argentina, Japan, as well as many other countries, including the American colonies, and the United States, have tried the same experiment with the same results–no real increase in wealth, but simply an increase in the amount of money to be exchanged for wealth.

The idea that money is the essence of wealth was one of the ideas which gave rise to a set of doctrines and practices, called Colbertism or Mercantilism, the earliest so-called " school " of political economy. Colbert was a distinguished minister under Louis XIV of France in the seventeenth century, and a firm believer in the theory that, in order to be wealthy, a nation must have an abundance of money. His theory became known as Mercantilism because it regarded trade between nations in the same light in which merchants look upon their business–each measuring his prosperity by the difference between the amount of money he expends and the amount he takes in. To keep money within the country, Colbert and the Mercantilists advocated the policy now known as " protection."

To-day it is generally understood that, in trade between nations, as in that between individuals, both parties may gain in an exchange transaction; but the mercantilistic fallacy that a nation may get rich by selling more than it purchases, and collecting the " favorable balance of trade " in money, still forms one of the popular bases of protectionism in the United States. The more intelligent protectionists give quite different reasons for a protective tariff, but the old fallacious reason still appeals to the multitude. They continue to think that by putting up a high tariff so that people are prevented from spending money abroad and are compelled to keep it at home, the country will in some way be made richer. One reason for the persistence of this fallacy is the continued use of the misleading phrase " favorable balance of trade " to indicate an excess of exports over imports and " unfavorable balance of trade " to indicate the opposite condition.

Money fallacies of the kinds we have described must be carefully avoided by the student. He should realize that no technical term, such as " money," can be used as a basis

of reasoning without a carefully formulated definition. All catch phrases should be avoided. Especially should the student be on his guard against every proposition concerning money. " Making money," for instance; is a catch phrase used without any definition. Properly speaking, nobody can " make " money except the man in the mint. The rest of us may gain wealth, but, unless we are counterfeiters, we cannot literally " make " money.

We live in a complicated civilization in which we talk in terms of money. Money has come to be a sort of veil which hides the other and more important wealth of the world. Our first task is to take off the veil and see the wealth underneath. We shall then see clearly that wealth can be accumulated only as it is actually produced and saved.

3. Classification of Wealth

Various kinds of wealth may be distinguished. That kind of wealth which consists of portions of the earths surface is called land. Among examples of land are to be included not only farms, city lots and streets, but mines, quarries, oyster beds, fisheries, waterways, etc. All waters which are owned "are in economics called land, being a part of the surface of the earth. Fixed structures upon land are called land improvements. The chief examples of land improvements are houses and other buildings, fences, drains, railways, tramways, macadamized streets, etc. Land and land improvements taken together are called real estate, the word " real " signifying immovable. All wealth which is movable may conveniently be called commodities, although the usage for this term is not altogether certain. Among examples of commodities are wheat, pig iron, food, fuel, furniture, jewelry, clothing, books, chairs, machinery, etc. The term " commodities " also includes slaves, so far as this particular species of wealth exists.

It will be remembered, however, that the definition of wealth which has been adopted excludes free human beings. It was in order to exclude free human beings from the category of wealth that the phrase " external to the owner " was inserted in the definition. Slaves are wealth, for they are external to their owner; but freemen are not wealth in its narrower or ordinary meaning.1

There are, of course, many admissible ways of classifying wealth. That which follows is intended to exhibit the principal groups into which wealth most naturally falls. It is advisable that the student construct other classifications for himself.

f Agricultural land Land Building land 1 Ways of transit
Wealth
Real Estate
Land improve-
ments
Buildings
Improvements
on highways
Miscellaneous
Commodities
Raw materials
Finished products
Mineral
Agricultural
Manufactured

Consumable
Durable 1 In the broader meaning of the term "wealth" all men, even freemen, are, as has been said, wealth. But they are wealth of a peculiar kind because they are not, like ordinary wealth, bought and sold and because the wealth owned and its owner are in this case, identical. It is difficult, however, to draw a strict line of distinction between slaves (human beings owned by other human beings) and freemen (human beings owned by themselves); for in some cases human beings are owned partly by others and partly by themselves; as, for instance, vassals, serfs, indentured servants, long-time apprentices, and men held in peonage. A man bound out to service for thirty years is. almost indistinguishable from a slave, and if his term of service be long enough,. the distinction fades away completely. On the other hand, the shorter the term of service the nearer does his condition approach freedom. As a matter of fact, almost all workers in modern society are bound by contract to some extent and for some period of time, even though it be no more than an hour; and to that extent they are not free. In short, there are many degrees of freedom and many degrees of slavery, with no fixed line of demarcation. This is one reason why the broader meaning of "wealth" is often more useful than the narrower.

It scarcely needs to be stated that these groups are not always absolutely distinct. Like all classes of concrete things, they merge imperceptibly into one another. For this reason the classification is of importance only as it gives a birds-eye view of the subject matter of economics.

4. Measurement of Wealth

Having seen what wealth is and what it is not, and having classified it roughly, we shall next examine separately its two essential attributes, materiality and ownership, devoting the remainder of this chapter to the first of these.

The materiality of wealth provides a basis for a physical measurement of the various articles of wealth. Wealth is of many kinds, and each kind has its own appropriate unit of measurement. Some kinds of wealth are measured by weight. This is true, for instance, of coal, iron, beef, and in fact of most " commodities." Of units of weight, a great diversity has been handed down to us, such as the pound avoirdupois, the kilogram, etc. In England, besides the avoirdupois pound, and the Troy pound, there is the pound sterling, used for measuring gold com. This is much smaller than any other pound, owing partly to the frequent debasements of coinage that have occurred, and partly to changes in the past from silver to gold money. In the United States a dollar of " standard gold " (gold which is Y fine) is a unit of weight employed for measuring gold coin. It is equivalent to 25.8 grains, or to ifffy of a pound avoirdupois, since there are 7000 grains in a pound avoirdupois. We can scarcely put too much emphasis on the fact that the pound sterling and the dollar are units of weight. They should be understood as such before any attempt is made to understand them as units of " value."

For many articles it is not so convenient to measure by units of weight as by units of space, whether of volume, of area, or of length. Thus we have, for volume, milk meas ured by the quart, wheat by the bushel, wood by the cord, and gas by the cubic foot For areas, we have lumber measured by the square foot, and land by the acre. For length, we have rope, wire, ribbons, and cloth measured in feet and yards.

Many articles are already in the form of more or less convenient units. In these cases the measure of their quantity is the number of such units. For instance, eggs or oranges are usually measured by their number, expressed in dozens. Similarly, sheets of writing paper are reckoned by the " quire," pencils and screws by the " gross." In such cases the article is said to be measured " by number." But " number " is by no means peculiar to such cases. All measurement whatever implies an abstract number, as well as a concrete unit. The only peculiarity of so-called measurement " by number " is that the unit, instead of being one which is applied from the outside, as by the yardstick, is one into which the things measured happen to be already conveniently divided.

In measuring the quantity of any particular kind of wealth it is assumed that the wealth measured is homogeneous, or so nearly so as to admit of measurement by a given unit. If different qualities or grades have to be distinguished, the amount of each quality or grade requires separate measurement. A continuous gradation in quality, such as is usually found in real estate, makes it necessary to distinguish a great number of different qualities. A tract of land of 100 acres may consist of a dozen different qualities of land, variously adapted to pasture, crops, or other uses. To describe all this land as simply so many " acres " is misleading. It is necessary to specify separately the number of acres of " pasture-land," " wheat-land," etc.

The unit of measure of any kind of wealth, therefore, when fully expressed, implies a description, not only (1) of size, but also (2) of quality; as, for instance, a " pound of granulated sugar." It is necessary to enumerate the attri

butes of the particular wealth under consideration, or enough of these attributes to distinguish that species of wealth from others with which it might be confused. Thus it is often necessary to specify what " grade " or " brand " is meant, as " grade A," " Eagle brand," etc. Sometimes the special variety is denoted by a " trademark " or " hall-mark."

Some writers have erroneously supposed that the attributes of wealth constitute separate and independent " immaterial " sorts of wealth. But " fertility," for instance, is not wealth, though " fertile land " is wealth. " Sweetness " is not wealth, though " sweet sugar " is wealth; " beauty " is not wealth, although a " beautiful gem " or other object of art is wealth; " strength " and " power " are not wealth, although "powerful horses," automobiles, or waterfalls are wealth.1 5. Price

We have considered articles of wealth as measured separately. Each kind has its own special unit, as the pound, gallon, or yard. But it is convenient also to measure the combined value of aggregations of wealth. The term " value " introduces the subject of exchange. So much mystery has surrounded the term " value " that we cannot be too careful to obtain a correct and clear idea of it at the outset. In the explanation which follows, the concept of value is made to depend on that of price; that of price, in turn, on that of exchange; and finally, that of exchange on that of transfer. In this section we shall treat of price; and, to observe the order of sequence, we must begin with transfer.

1 Some people speak of human qualities–strength, beauty, skill, honesty, intelligence, etc.–as though they were wealth. But these bear the same relation to human beings as similar qualities of articles of wealth bear to those articles; and the only

way we can logically make them even attributes of wealth is, as already stated, to call human beings wealth. Then their attributes become attributes of wealth in the broader meaning of that term.

Wealth is said to be transferred when it changes owners. A transfer is a change of ownership. Such a change does not necessarily imply a change of place. Ordinarily, of course, the transfer of an article is accompanied by a change in its position, the purchase of tea or sugar being accompanied by the physical delivery of these articles across the counter from dealer to customer; but in many cases such a change of position does not occur, and in the case of real estate it is even impossible.

Transfers may be voluntary or involuntary. Examples of involuntary transfers of wealth are: (1) through force and fraud of individuals, as in the case of robbery, burglary, or embezzlement; (2) through force of government, as in the case of taxes, court fines, and " eminent domain." But at present we have to do only with voluntary transfers. These are of two kinds: (1) one-sided transfers, i. e., gifts and bequests; and (2) reciprocal transfers, or exchanges, which are of most importance for economics. An exchange of wealth, then, is a pair of mutual and voluntary transfers of wealth between two owners, each transfer being in consideration of the other.

When a certain quantity of wealth of one kind is exchanged for a certain quantity of wealth of another kind, we may divide either of the two quantities by the other and obtain what is called the price of the latter. That is, the price of wealth of any given kind is the amount of any other kind of wealth supposed to be exchanged for one unit of the given kind of wealth. Thus if 100 bushels of wheat are exchanged for 75 dollars of gold, the price of the wheat in terms of gold is 75-5-100, or three-fourths of a dollar of gold per bushel of wheat. Contrariwise, the price of gold in terms of wheat is 100-5-75, or one and one-third bushels of wheat per dollar of gold. Thus there are always two prices in any exchange. Practically, however, we usually speak only of one, viz., the price in terms of money, obtained by dividing the number of units of money by the number of units of the article exchanged for that money. It follows that, practically, the price in money of any particular sort of wealth is the amount of money for which a unit of that wealth is exchanged. The fact that wealth is exchangeable and in the civilized world is constantly changing ownership is of great importance for our study. Articles of wealth which are seldom exchanged, such as public parks, are not commonly thought of as wealth at all, although logically they must be included in that category.

While it is true that any two kinds of wealth may be exchanged, some kinds of wealth are more acceptable in exchange than others. Money primarily means wealth which is generally acceptable in exchange. Here for the first time we reach a preliminary definition of money. This definition is based on the most important characteristic of money–its exchangeability. An exchange in which money does not figure is called barter. An exchange in which money does figure is called a purchase and sale –a purchase for the man who parts with the money (or its representative, a check), a sale for the man who receives it. Originally, all exchange was barter, but to-day most exchange is, as we all know, purchase and sale.

In order that there may be a price, it is not necessary that the exchange in question shall actually take place. It may be only a contemplated exchange A real estate agent often has an " asking price "; that is, a price at which he tries to sell. This is usually above the price of any actual sale which may occur later. In the same way there is often a " bidding price," which is usually below the price of actual sale. Hence, the price of actual sale usually lies between the price first bid and the price first asked. But it sometimes happens that the bidder refuses to raise his bidding price, and the seller refuses to lower his asking price enough to bring the two together. In such a case no sale takes place, and the only prices are those bid and asked. For many commodities the trade journals report, preferably, prices of actual sales; but, where there have been no sales, they simply report the prices bid or asked, or both.

When there is no sale, especially when there is no price bid or asked, it is not so easy to answer the question: What is the price? Recourse is then had to an " appraisal," which is simply a more or less skillful guess as to what price the article would or should bring. Appraising or guessing at prices is often very difficult. It frequently has to be employed, however, by the government, for the purpose of assessing taxes and customs duties and condemning land; by insurance companies for settling claims and adjusting losses; by merchants for making up inventories and similar statements; and by statisticians for numerous purposes. In fact, some people make a living by appraising wealth on which, for one purpose or another, a price of some sort must be set. The purpose evidently makes a great difference in the appraisal. Sometimes we want to know the price for which an article could be sold in an immediate forced sale; sometimes, the price it might be expected to bring if a reasonable time were allowed; sometimes, the price the owner would probably take; sometimes, the price a purchaser would probably give. These prices may all be different. A family portrait may be worth a big price to the owner, and yet bring next to nothing if sold to strangers. The owner would naturally appraise it at a high figure if he wished to insure it against fire, but if he should try to borrow money on it from a pawnbroker, the appraisal would undoubtedly be low.

Consequently, in applying an appraisal, we encounter many difficulties because the parties involved usually have some interest to serve. When a farmer has land for sale, he will hold it at a high price to prospective purchasers, but will enter it, if the truth must be told, at a low price on the tax list. When a fire loss is adjusted, the two conflict

ing interests, viz., the " insured " and the " company," are usually represented by two experts, who in case of disagreement call in a third.

6. Value

Having succeeded in denning the price of any kind of wealth, we may next proceed to define the value of any given quantity of that wealth. The value of a given quantity of wealth is that quantity multiplied by the price.1 Arithmetically expressed, if the price of wheat is of a dollar per bushel, then a lot consisting of 3000 bushels would have a value of 3000 times of a dollar, or 2000 dollars. Algebraically expressed, if the price of any good is p and its quantity is Q, its value is expressed as pq. In other words, the value of a certain quantity of one kind of wealth at a given price is the quantity of some other kind for which it would be exchanged, if the whole quantity were exchanged at the price set.

The distinctions between quantity, price, and value of wealth may be illustrated by an inventory such as the following:–

QUANTITY PRICE IN TERMS OP WHEAT VALUE IN TERMS OF WHEAT
Shoes lo00 pairs 4 bu. s oer oair -12 0 bu.
Beef 300 Ib. f bu. per pound 60 bu.
Dwelling house. Wheat 1 house 100 bu. 10,000 bu. per house 1 bu. per bushel 10,009 bu. 100 bu.

1 This definition of value departs from the usage of some textbooks, but follows closely that of business men and practical statisticians. Economists have sometimes confined "price" to what is in this book called money price and applied the term "value" to what is here called price. Other economists have used the term "price" in the sense of market price–what an article actually sells for–and "value" in the sense of appraised price or reasonable price–what it ought to sell for. Still others have used the term "price" in the sense employed in this book, but "value" in the sense of the degree of csleem in which an article is held–what in this book will later be called "marginal utility" or "marginal desirability."

1"Bushels" refers to bushels of wheat throughout this table.

The three columns must be carefully distinguished. j

Only in special cases can any two of the three magnitudes, j quantity, price, and value, be identical. The table illus- trates these special cases. Thus in the last line we find 3 quantity and value identical because, in this special case, the value of the good is reckoned in terms of itself,–wheat in wheat. In the line above, price and value are identical because, in this special case, the quantity valued is only one unit. The value of one house is the price per house.

The measurement of various items of wealth in respect of " value," expressed in terms of a single commodity, such as wheat or money, has one great advantage over its measurement in respect of " quantity." This advantage is that it enables us to translate many kinds of wealth into one kind and thus to add them all together. To add up the " quantity " column would be ridiculous, because pairs of shoes, pounds of beef, houses, and bushels of wheat are unlike quantities. But the items in the last column (representing values), being expressed in a single common unit (the bushel), may be added together despite the diversity of the various articles thus valued in bushels of wheat.

Since prices and values are usually expressed in terms of money–the most ex- changeable kind of wealth–money may be said to bring uniformity of measurement out of diversity. In other words, it is not only a medium of exchange, but it can be used also as a measure of value. It serves as a means of comparing values of different things by expressing them both in a common denominator. It would be far more trouble to compare each article directly with every other article, for there would be many more comparisons.

Although this reduction to a common measure is a great practical convenience, we must not imagine that it gives what could in any fair sense be called " the only true measure" of wealth. In fact, to measure the amount of wealth by its value–i. e., its money value–is often misleading. The money value of car wheels exported from the United States in one month was 12,000 and in a later month, 15,000, from which fact we might infer that the quantity of these exports had increased. But the number of car wheels exported in the first of those two months was 2200, and in the second only 2100, showing a decrease. The price had increased faster than the number had decreased. Likewise, the figures for imports of coffee in these periods show a decline in dollars, despite an increase in pounds. Here the price had fallen faster than the number of pounds had risen. It is conceivable that the quantity of every article might decrease, and yet the price simultaneously increase so much that there would be an apparent increase of wealth when there really was nothing of the kind. This is apt to be the case in times of inflation of the currency.

Even when we are confessedly trying to measure the value of wealth and not its quantity, it is difficult or impossible to find a right way. Imports into the United States from Mexico in one year were worth twenty-eight millions of American gold dollars, and ten years later their value was forty millions–an increase in value of forty-two per cent; but these very same imports measured in Mexican silver dollars were forty-one millions in the first year and ninety millions in the second–an increase in value of nearly one hundred and twenty per cent. These two rates of increase, although they represent exactly the same facts, do not agree with each other; yet the American merchant reckons the values one way, and the Mexican merchant, the other. In a sense both are right; that is to say, both are true statements of the value of the articles imported, one of the value in gold and the other of the value in silver. If the value were to be measured in iron, copper, coal, cotton, or any other article, we should have many other different " values," no two of which would necessarily agree. " The

value of wealth," therefore, is an incomplete phrase; to be definite we should say, " the value of wealth in terms of gold," or in terms of some other particular article. Hence we cannot employ such values for comparing different groups of wealth, except under certain conditions, and to a limited degree. To compare the wealth values of distant places or times–as America and China, Ancient Rome and Modern Italy–will inevitably give conflicting and unsatisfactory results.

7. Limit of Accuracy in Economic Measurements

We have learned how the three magnitudes–quantity, price, and value of wealth–are usually measured, and that their measurement is practically a very inaccurate affair. Yet in the minds of most persons, even of business men, the degree of accuracy attainable is exaggerated. Even in the measurement of the mere quantities of wealth there are two sources of error; for every such measurement includes, as we have seen, two elements: a unit and a number or ratio (as the pound, and the number of pounds); and both the unit and the number or ratio may be inaccurate. In modern times the first source of error–that of the unit–is practically eliminated. Our units of weight and measure are standardized by law, and a pound in California is, for all practical purposes, equal to a pound in Connecticut. There is, moreover, at Washington a national bureau and a special building for preserving and testing standards of measurement. Different towns have their sealers of weights and measures, to prevent error through ignorance or fraud. Fraud and error still exist, but are much rarer than in former times. The Egyptians are said to have been unable to test the accuracy of their units of length closer than to 1 part in 350. The Roman weights were true only to 1 part in 50. And when we go back to primitive units, we find that they were very rough indeed. A yard was probably at first the length around the waist, which naturally was apt to vary considerably. So also the distance between the elbow and the end of the finger was taken as a unit and called the ell. Fraud was, therefore, as easy as it was common. At Bergen, in Norway, among other relics of the old Hanseatic League, are the scales used for buying and selling fish, with two sorts of weights used, one considerably heavier than the other. The heavier were used for buying and the lighter for selling! Such tampering with weights and measures is probably much less frequent to-day, although instances of short weights, as in the " sugar trust frauds," are often brought to light.

To-day, therefore, the chief source of error lies not in the unit, but in the ratio of the quantity of wealth to that unit. In retail trade the inaccuracy from this source is very great. If we get our apples or potatoes measured correctly within five per cent, we are fortunate. Wholesale transactions are more accurate. Probably the greatest degree of accuracy ever attained in commercial measurements is on the mint scales employed by the federal government in Philadelphia and San Francisco. These scales weigh accurately to within about one part in two million.

Besides the two sources of error in the measurement of mere quantity, when we proceed from quantity to value, we introduce still a third source of inaccuracy, viz., the price factor by which we multiply the quantity in order to get the value. This is especially true if the price be merely an " appraised " price. The price in an actual sale is an absolute fact and cannot be said to have any inaccuracy; but the price at which we estimate that a thing would sell under certain conditions is always uncertain. In the case of " staple " articles, i. e., articles regularly on the market, a dealer can often appraise correctly within one per cent. Real estate in certain parts of a city where sales are active can sometimes be appraised correctly within five or ten per cent, but in the " dead " or out-of-the-way parts of some towns where sales are infrequent, the appraisement becomes merely a rough guess. Again, in the country districts, while farms in the settled parts of Iowa and Texas can be appraised within ten or fifteen per cent, in the backward parts even an experts valuation is often proved wrong by more than fifty per cent. And where a sale of the article in question is scarcely conceivable, an appraisement is almost out of the question. To estimate the value of Yellowstone Park is impossible, unless we allow ourselves very wide limits of error.1 1 Still wider limits must be allowed when we try to value human beings. We can often give a lower limit, but seldom an upper one. The estimates may vary enormously with the point of view. It is sometimes said, "If I could buy Mr. So-and-so at my valuation and sell him at his, Id get rich."

Freemen are seldom appraised at all. When the slaves in the South became freemen, they ceased to be appraised as wealth. The result has been somewhat confusing to our census statistics. The "Manufacturers Record" of Baltimore recently issued figures showing a sharp drop in the assessed valuations of wealth in the South after the war. The inference was drawn that the value of wealth had immensely decreased; but a large part of this so-called decrease consisted merely in the change of ownership of slaves from their old masters to themselves, and their consequent omission as items of value. Any valuation of freemen, should exceed that of slaves; but even on the basis of slave values the total value of the human beings in any country is always greatly in excess of the total value of all other wealth.

CHAPTER II

PROPERTY 1. The Benefits of Wealth

The definition of wealth which has been given restricts it to concrete material objects owned by man. Accordingly, wealth has two essential attributes: materiality and ownership. Its materiality was the subject of the preceding chapter; its ownership will be the subject of the present chapter.

To own wealth is to have a right to the benefits of wealth, and before proceeding further with the discussion of ownership, we must consider these " benefits " of wealth. To own a loaf of bread means nothing more nor less than to have the right to benefit by it–i. e., to eat it, sell it, or otherwise employ it to satisfy ones desires. To own a suit of clothes is to have the right to wear it. To own a carriage is to have the right to drive in it or otherwise utilize it as long as it lasts. To own a plot of land means to have the right to use it forever. The ultimate objects for which wealth exists are the benefits which it confers. If some one should give you a house on condition that you should never use it, sell it, rent it, or give it away, you might be justified in refusing it as worthless.

Benefits may also be rendered by free human beings (who, according to our broader definition, are included under wealth). Such benefits are then usually called services rendered or work done. When rendered by things rather than persons, benefits are commonly called uses. Some times benefits consist of positive advantages and sometimes of the prevention of disadvantages. Benefits, then, mean desirable events obtained or undesirable events averted by means of wealth or free human beings. For example, when a loom changes yarn into cloth, the transformation is a desirable change due to the loom; it is a benefit conferred or performed by the loom. The benefit from a plow is the turning up of the soil. The benefits or services performed by a bricklayer consist in the laying of bricks. The benefits or uses conferred by a fence around a farm consist in preventing the cattle from roaming away. The dikes in Holland confer the benefit of keeping out the ocean. The benefits conferred by a diamond necklace consist in its pleasing glitter.

Many articles confer benefits on their owners by yielding them money. The benefit to the landlord from the land or building which he lets is the receipt by him of rent. The benefit to the owners of a railway from the railway is the receipt by them of their dividends. But not all benefits, of course, are simply the receipt of money.

To be desirable to the owner, an article must confer benefits on the owner, but not necessarily on the community at large. For instance, the noise of a factory whistle may be a nuisance to the community, but as long as it is serviceable to the owner of the factory, it is for him a benefit. Benefits to the owner and benefits to society may be very different or may be mutually incompatible. The benefits to society are of the greater importance, but, under our present system of ownership, the benefits to the owner control the prices and values of wealth. In order, therefore, to understand prices and values as they are actually determined, we must fix our attention for the present on the benefits to the owner rather than on those to society.

Benefits may be measured just as wealth may be measured, although the units of measurement are, of course, not the same. We measure some benefits by number–as when we

count the strokes of a printing press. We measure other benefits by time–as when we reckon a laborers work by the number of hours or days during which he works. Some benefits we measure by the quantity of wealth which is produced or treated–as when the work of a coal miner is measured by the amount of coal he mines, or when the use of a loom is measured by the number of yards of cloth it weaves, or when the services of a lawn-mowing outfit are measured by the number of acres covered. The measurement of services or benefits is usually rougher than that of wealth, because it is more difficult to establish units of measure. The shelter of a house or the use or " wear" of a suit of clothes is difficult to measure accurately. To save trouble, benefits are usually measured by time, although, as soon as it becomes profitable to do so, the tendency is to establish a more satisfactory measure " by the piece."

When we have measured the benefits of wealth or of free human beings, we may apply to them the same concepts of transfer, exchange, price, and value, which, in the last chapter, we applied to wealth. We have seen that wealth may be exchanged. The same is true of benefits. In fact, every exchange is an exchange of benefits; for to exchange wealth is really to exchange the benefits of wealth, the only object in getting wealth being to get its benefits.

2. The Costs of Wealth

Opposed to the benefits of wealth are its costs. Costs may be called negative benefits. The purpose of wealth is to benefit its owner; that is, to cause to happen what he desires to happen, and to prevent from happening what he desires not to happen. But often wealth can work no benefit without entailing some cost, i. e., preventing what is desirable or occasioning what is undesirable. For instance, one cannot enjoy the benefits of a dwelling without the costs of taking care of it, either through the actual labor of dean

ing, heating, repairing, and keeping it in order, or the pay ment of money to servants for such purposes; one cannot get the benefit of flour without assuming the cost of kneading and baking it into bread; one cannot get the benefit of a farm without the cost of tilling it. Whatever wealth brings about to the pleasure of the owner is a benefit; whatever it brings about to his displeasure is a cost. He assumes the costs only as a means of securing the benefits. Costs are thus the necessary evils which must be if we are to obtain the good which wealth affords.

Like benefits, costs are not only occasioned by wealth, but also by free human beings. An employer can get benefits from a workman only at the cost of paying him wages; an independent workman can get benefits from his own exertions only at the cost of his own labor.

The costs of wealth or of free human beings may, of course, be measured, just as benefits are measured–by number, by time, or by other appropriate units; and costs when thus measured may, by price and value, be translated into terms of money precisely like the opposite items–benefits. We must beware of assuming that cost is always in the form of an expenditure of money. Such money cost has received exaggerated importance in the eyes of business men and has tended to hide the more important and fundamental kind of cost, namely, labor. Even labor appears to the employer in the guise of a money cost–the expenditure of wages. This expenditure, however, is not itself labor. Those who feel a real labor cost are the laborers themselves. It is by their physical and mental exertions that the work of the world is chiefly done.

3. Property, the Right to Benefits

We have said that to own wealth means to have the right to its benefits. We have seen what is meant by " benefits," and shall next examine what is meant by " rights." 1

A property right is the liberty or permit (under the sanction and protection of custom and law) to enjoy benefits of wealth (in its broader sense) while assuming the costs which those benefits entail. The term " property " is merely an abbreviation for " property right " or " property rights." Just as different kinds of wealth are more or less exchangeable, so different kinds of property rights differ greatly in exchangeability. Those forms which are most easily and commonly exchanged are of most importance for our study. Those the exchange of which is infrequent, difficult, or forbidden, are in fact seldom thought of as property rights at all, although logically they must be included in that category. In the modern world the right of a parent over a child or of a husband over a wife is not by ordinary usage called property; for, except in certain remote corners of the earth, their exchange is tabooed.

It will be observed that property rights, unlike wealth or benefits, are not physical objects nor events, but are abstract social relations. A property right is not a thing. It is that relation of man to things, called ownership. It is in this human relationship to wealth that we are most interested, and not in the physical objects as such.

The benefits flowing from wealth require time for their occurrence and are therefore either past or future. The past and the future are separated by the present, which is a mere point of time. The only benefits from wealth which can be owned at this present point of time are future benefits. Past benefits have vanished. When a man owns any form of property, he owns a right to future benefits. The idea of " futurity " is, therefore, implied in our definition of property, which may, therefore, be more explicitly expressed as follows: Property is the right to future benefits of wealth (in its broader sense). It is also to be observed that the future is always uncertain; no man can ever tell in advance exactly how much future benefit he can obtain; he can only take the chances and risks involved. Consequently, the idea of uncertainty is also implied in our definition of property, which may, therefore, be still more explicitly expressed as follows: Property is the right to the more or less probable future benefits of wealth (in its broader sense).

1 As we have seen that "benefits" may be occasioned not only by wealth in its narrow sense, but by free human beings, we shall consider "rights" to benefits from both of these sources.

If a man has the right to all the benefits which may come in the future from a particular article of wealth, he is said to have its complete ownership, or its ownership without encumbrance. If he has a right to only some of the benefits from a particular article of wealth, he is said to own that wealth partially, or to " have an interest " in it. When two brothers own a farm equally in partnership, each is a part owner; each has a half interest in the farm; that is, each has a right to half of the benefits to be had from the farm. What is divided between the two brothers is not the farm, but the benefits of the farm. To emphasize this fact, the law describes each brothers share as an " undivided half interest." Partnership rights are usually employed only when the number of coowners is small. When the number is large, the ownership is usually subdivided into shares of stock; but the principle is the same–each individual owns a right to a certain fraction of the benefits which come to the owners.

After the quantities of property of different kinds are measured, we may apply the same concepts of transfer, exchange, price, and value which have already been applied to wealth and benefits, each particular kind being measured in its own particular unit. Consider, for example, the property called stock in the Pennsylvania Railway Company. This is measured by the " number of shares," the share here being the unit of measurement.

It is important that the student should become accus tomed to see the real basis underlying property rights. This basis is either wealth or free persons, or both. Practically it is usually wealth. A mortgage is based on land, and great care is taken not to have the mortgage too large for the basis on which it rests. Railroad stocks and bonds are based on the real railway. Personal notes are based partly on the person issuing them and partly on his wealth. A street railway franchise is a property right, the physical basis of which consists in the streets. Sometimes the property rights are removed several steps from the real basis. If a number of factories are combined into a " trust," the original stockholders surrender their stock certificates to trustees and receive in their place trust certificates. Their rights are then a claim against the trustees who hold the stock which represents the factories. The ultimate basis for their rights is still the factories, but their ownership is indirect.

The future benefits flowing from wealth may be compared to a pennant attached to a flagstaff–a long streamer stretching out into the future. Two of the possible ways in which the present ownership of these benefits may be subdivided are indicated in Fig. 1. Here are two " streamers " representing the streams of benefits which may come from a dwelling house. These begin at the present and stretch out indefinitely into the future. If two brothers own the house in partnership, each has a right to half the shelter of the house, i. e., to half of its benefits; the benefits are therefore divided, so to speak, longitudinally in time.

But if the house is rented, the division of benefits between the tenant and the landlord is transverse, as shown in the lower " streamer " of the diagram. The tenant has ah the shelter of the house until the time when his lease is to expire, while the right to all shelter beyond the time of the lease rests in the landlord, either to use himself or to sell to others by new leases.

These are not, of course, the only ways in which future benefits may be parceled out among their several owners,

Bo SHARE OF FUTURE BENEFITS

As Share. Of Future Benefits.

but they are the principal and usual modes of subdivision.

In common speech, the minor rights to wealth are not ordinarily dignified as rights of ownership. Thus a tenants right in the dwelling he occupies is sharply distinguished from the right of the owner. Yet, strictly speaking, every right to the benefits of wealth or to the services of free human beings, however insignificant that right may be, is a part ownership. When an

Tenants Landlords 1
SHARE SHARE V
Fig. 1.

Present INSTANT owner of land wishes to give an unencumbered title, he finds it necessary to extinguish all outstanding leases, or claims for future benefits, often at considerable cost. It is the total ownership which he is selling, and the total ownership always includes the ownership which the tenant enjoys. Thus the tenant of a dwelling is, to a very slight extent, a part owner of that dwelling. In the same way the employer is, to a very slight extent, a part owner of the employee.

4. The Relation between Wealth and Property

We have thus far considered three very important and fundamental concepts: wealth, benefits, and property. A convenient collective term for all of them is " goods."

Wealth and property are only present representatives of future benefits and future costs. Wealth (in its broader sense) is the present means by which we secure future benefits; while property is the present right to these benefits, and so to the wealth (in its broader sense) which yields them. It follows that wealth (in its broader sense) on the one hand, and property rights on the other, may be said to correspond to one another. The wealth (including free human beings) consists in real tangible things, while the property rights represent intangible, abstract relations which persons, as owners, hold toward them (the wealth, including free human beings). Wealth and persons are the important things; property is the human right of ownership of the wealth or of the services of free human beings. In specific cases we can readily see the correspondence between the wealth and its ownership. In fact, in cases where wealth is owned unencumbered or completely, the correspondence is altogether too obvious; so obvious that in ordinary parlance the two terms, " wealth" and " property," become confused, as when speaking of a piece of wealth, in the form, say, of land, we call it a " piece of property."

On the other hand, where the ownership is minutely subdivided, the wealth and the property rights to that wealth become so dissociated in our minds that we are apt to fall into the opposite error, and entirely lose sight of their connection. For instance, when railway shares are sold in Wall Street, the investor rarely thinks of those shares as connected with any actual wealth. All that he sees are the engraved certificates of his property rights; he has no visual picture of the railway. Sometimes the rights are so far separated from the thing to which the rights relate, that people are unaware that there is anything behind the rights at all, and delude themselves with the notion that there need not be anything behind them. A government bond, for instance, is often regarded as a kind of property behind which there is no wealth. But if we examine the case, we shall find that the wealth of the entire community is behind this property right; for it is by means of the taxing power that the bonds are to be paid, and this taxing power can only be effective by means of wealth (including freemen) as sources of income. For cities, in fact, this is definitely recognized; there is usually a legal debt limit expressed in terms of the value of taxable wealth, to insure the creditors that there shall always be sufficient real wealth behind the city bonds to make their ultimate payment secure.

Not only should the student clearly distinguish in his mind between the three important concepts, wealth (including man), benefits and property, but he should avoid confusing any of these with a fourth relatively unimportant concept, namely, certificates of ownership. To avoid misunderstanding, it is often necessary that property rights should be evidenced by written documents. Examples of such written evidence or certification of property rights are deeds for real estate, receipted bills for goods bought and paid for, engraved stock certificates, railway tickets, signed promissory notes, written contracts with laborers to "work out" a sum of money advanced, etc. It is clear, however, that such written evidence of property rights is very different from the property rights themselves; and in many cases such rights exist without any written evidence. Thus, the farmer who rears his own cattle, or horses, or sheep, usually has no written evidence of property rights in them. Or, two brothers might own and operate a farm in partnership, without any written evidence as to their partnership rights, i. e., their respective rights in the products of the farm. Or, again, one person might, without written evidence, lease (say) a cottage for a season from a friend. In all these cases, there are no documentary evidences of property rights. Yet in all three cases property rights exist. In the first case the right is complete; in the other two cases partial, the benefits being subdivided,–in one case longitudinally, in the other, transversely.

5. Table of Typical Property Rights

The following table indicates the most important types of property, and shows in each case the wealth on which the property right is based and the benefits accruing from that wealth. The most important forms are: unencumbered, stocks, bonds, notes, leases, and partnership rights.

TYPICAL CASES ILLUSTRATING THE EXISTENCE OF WEALTH BEHIND PROPERTY RIGHTS

Name Of Case	Wealth On Which The Property Right Is Based	Benefits Of That Wealth	Description Of Property Right	Certificate Of Ownership, If Any
Unencumbered	Farm	Yielding crops	Right to all use of farm forever	Deed
Partnership	Dry goods	Yielding profits from sale	One partner's "undivided " fractional interest	Articles of agreement
Joint Stock stock	Railway	Yielding profits	The shares of stock	Stock certificate
Street Franchise	Street	Use of same for passage, etc.	Right to run cars through it	Charter
Lease or Hire	Dwelling	Use of same for shelter, etc.	Right of tenant till fixed date	Lease
Railway Ticket	Railway	Transportation	Right to speci-	Ticket

fied trip

Railway Bond Railway Payment of " in-Right to same Bond certifi-
terest " and and contin-cate
"principal " gent right to
foreclose

Personal Note All the posses-Payments Right to same Note
sions of the and in de-
signer fault thereof,
right to collat-
eral security

Work due from Workmen Work Right of employ-Written con-
Contract Labor er to perform-tract
ance of same

6. Practical Problems of Property

We have seen that wealth (including man), on the one hand, and property rights, on the other, correspond to each other. When we treat of the welfare of a community, we think rather of wealth (in its broader sense) than of property. When we treat of the welfare of an individual, we think rather of property than of wealth. This fact of correspondence between property rights, on the one hand, and wealth (including man), on the other, should be emphasized, because it will save us from confusions which are all too common, and it will save us also from many practical blunders growing out of these confusions. If our State legislators understood this, there would be less of the iniquitous double taxation that is the bane of the present systems of State and local taxation. Such unjust taxation is illustrated by the case of the Massachusetts factory owner who decided to transfer his property to a stock company of which he himself should hold all the stock. Previously he paid taxes only on the factory itself; but when the " company" was formed (under a Maine charter), the tax collector came along and informed him that henceforth not only must the " company " pay taxes on the factory, but that he personally must pay taxes on the stock also, since stock in a Maine company is taxable "personal property." Thus the owner was taxed both on the stock which represented the factory and on the factory itself. Instances of double taxation are quite common in the United States, though they are not all so self-evident as this. It is not within the scope of this book to discuss taxation or other practical problems of economics. The object of this section is merely to point out what practical problems are related to " property."

Many of the ir ost important problems of economic policy are problems of the form of ownership of wealth. The great question of slavery, for instance, turned upon the question whether one man should be owned by another.

A more modern problem of property is that of perpetual franchises. Is it, for instance, good public policy to grant to a street railway company in perpetuity the right to use a citys streets? Or ought we to fix a time limit, say fifty years, after which the right shall revert to the city? A kindred question has been raised as to private property in land. Is it wise public policy that the present form of land ownership in fee simple should continue? Ought a man to have the right to a piece of land forever, perhaps abusing that right, obstructing others, and neglecting the opportunities which it affords; or should the government own the land and lease it to individuals for limited periods? This question is now being discussed with reference to our mineral lands, and particularly our coal lands in Alaska. Questions of land ownership "have in all ages vexed mens minds and been the source of social unrest. Rome had her agrarian troubles, not unlike those of modern England and Ireland.

The right to bequeath property is also a prime source of trouble. This right to dispose of property by will has not always been recognized. It was developed by the Romans, from whose system of law we borrowed it. Even now it is a limited right, and its exercise differs with law and custom. These differences are responsible for peasant proprietorship in France and for primogeniture in England. The right has, indeed, been limited so as to prevent the perpetual tying-up of an estate by a testator. Its further limitation will probably be one of the problems of the future.

An even broader question of the same sort is the question of socialism. Shall we discontinue what is called private property, except in the things that we wear and eat, and possibly the houses in which we live? That is, shall we allow our railways and our factories to be owned by private individuals? Or shall they be owned by the community at large so that we may all have shares in them, as we already have in the post office and the government printing office? These are some of the greatest problems in economics; and they are problems concerning the ownership of wealth. The answers to these questions do not come within the purpose of this book, which is concerned merely with principles. The problems are mentioned, however, as illustrating the application of principles here discussed.

CHAPTER III

CAPITAL 1. Capital and Income In the foregoing chapters we have set forth several fundamental concepts of economics–wealth, property, benefits, price, and value. We have seen that wealth in its broader sense includes human beings, and that property in its broader sense includes all rights whatsoever; that benefits are the desirable occurrences which happen through wealth (in its broader sense); that prices are the ratios of exchange between quantities of goods of various kinds (wealth, property, or benefits); and that value is price multiplied by quantity. These concepts are the chief tools needed in economic study.

Little has yet been said about the relation of these various magnitudes to time. When we speak of a certain quantity of wealth, benefits, or property, we may refer either (1) to a quantity existing at a particular instant of time, or (2) to a quantity produced, exchanged, transported, or consumed during a particular period of time. The first is a stock of " goods "; the second is a flow of " goods." Examples of stocks are the stock in trade of a merchant on a certain date, the cargo of wheat on board a ship, the amount of food in a pantry at a particular instant, the number of shares of stock owned by a particular individual in a particular corporation at a particular date. Examples of flows are the sales of merchandise made in the course of a given month by a given merchant, the amount of wheat imported into a given country during a given year, the quantity of food consumed by a family in a given week, the sales of a given kind of stock on the New York Stock Exchange during a given number of days, the transportation accomplished by a railway in the course of a certain year, the work done by a given man in a given time.

The most important purpose of the distinction between a stock and a flowis to differentiate between capital and income. Capital is a stock, and income a flow. This, however, is not the only difference between capital and income. There is another, equally important; namely, that capital consists of wealth, while income consists of benefits. We have, therefore, the following definitions: A stock of wealth existing at a given instant of time is called capital; a flow of benefits from wealth through a period of time is called income. Many authors restrict the name capital to a particular kind or species of wealth, or to wealth used for a particular purpose, such as the production of new wealth; in short, to some specific part of wealth instead of any or all of it. Such a limitation, however, is not only difficult to make, but cripples the usefulness of the concept in economic analysis.1

A dwelling house is capital; the shelter or the rent it affords, during any given period of time, is income. The railways of the country are capital; their benefits (in the form of transportation or its equivalent in dividends) are the income they yield.

The term capital is also applied to a stock or fund of property existing at an instant of time. But such " capital property " is not, of course, in addition to "cap 1 Just as wealth may be considered in a broader sense as including freemen, so capital may also be considered in this broader sense. Thus an individual, because of his ability to work, may be considered as capital, while the benefits resulting from his labor (services rendered employer or self) should be considered as income. However, in the following discussion of " capital," we shall, except where the contrary is expressly stated, use the term in its narrower sense.

ital wealth," but merely instead of it; for we have seen that wealth and property are coextensive. The only true capital of society as a whole is its capital-wealth,–its lands, railways, factories, dwellings, and in its broader sense its human inhabitants also; but since the ownership of many of these things is subdivided, the capital of an individual can often be stated only in terms of property–his stocks, bonds, mortgages, personal notes, etc.

2. Capital-goods, Capital-value, Capital-balance

We have defined capital as a stock of wealth existing at a given point of time. An instantaneous photograph of wealth would reveal, not only a stock of durable wealth, but also a stock of wealth more rapid in consumption. It would disclose, not the annual procession of such wealth, but the members of that procession that had not yet passed off the stage of existence, however swiftly they might be moving across it. It would show trainloads of meat, eggs, and milk in transit, as well as the contents of private storerooms, ice chests, and wine cellars. Even the supplies on the table of a man bolting his dinner would find a place. So the clothes in ones wardrobe, or on ones back, the tobacco in a smokers pouch or pipe, the oil in the can or lamp, would all be elements in this flashlight picture.

We have seen in the last two chapters that wealth and property may be measured either by quantities (such as so many bushels or pounds or so many shares or bonds of a particular description) or by value (such as so many dollars worth). When a given collection of capital is measured in terms of the quantities of the various goods of which it is 1 composed, it is called capital-wealth or capital-property or, j to include pitv1pr r. npiin l. nndi-when it is measured in/ terms of its value, it is sometimes called ftltaja u r J

One of the best methods of understanding the nature of capital is to understand the method of keeping capital ac counts. We shall, therefore, in the remainder of this chapter indicate some of the principles of capital accounting. Such a study is useful not only because it enables us to keep our own capital accounts and to understand the accounts of banks, railways, and other institutions as published, but, what is more important for our present purpose, because it shows how in the present complicated world of divided ownership of capital, with its interrelated arrangement of stocks, bonds, debts, and credits, the capitals of individuals dovetail into one another, forming together the capital of the community.

A capital account or balance sheet is a statement of the quantity and value of the wealth of a specific owner at any instant of time. It consists of two columns–the assets and the liabilities–the positive and negative items of his capital. The liabilities of an owner are his debts and obligations to others; that is, they are the property rights of others for which this owner is responsible. The assets or resources of the owner include all his capital, irrespective of his liabilities. These assets include both the capital which makes good the liabilities, and that, if any, in excess of the liabilities.

The owner may be either a physical human being or an abstract entity called a " fictitious person " made up of a collection of human beings and keeping a balance sheet distinct from those of the individuals composing it. Examples of fictitious persons are an association, a partnership, a joint stock company, a government. With respect to a debt or liability, the person who owes it is the debtor, and the person owed is the creditor. The difference in value between the total assets and the total liabilities in any capital account is called the net capital, or capital-balance of the person or company whose account it is.

A fictitious person is to be regarded as owning all the capital nominally intrusted to it and as owing its individual members for their respective shares; consequently, there is no net capital-balance belonging to the fictitious person, although in most cases there is a liability item called capital which represents what is owed to those most responsible for the management of the business. The most important example of a fictitious person is a joint stock company. This may be roughly described as an aggregation of individuals uniting for the purpose of holding property jointly, and so organized that the individual shares of ownership and management are represented by "stock certificates." Associated with the stockholders are usually also bondholders without voting power, but with the right to receive fixed payments stipulated in the bonds which they hold. The " capital" item in the capital account of a joint stock company is a liability due to the stockholders. It represents what is left after the value of all other liabilities is deducted from the value of the assets.

The items in a capital account are constantly changing, as also their values; so that, after one statement of assets and liabilities is drawn up, and another is constructed at a later time, the balancing item, or net capital, may have changed considerably. However, bookkeepers are accustomed to keep this recorded "capital" or "capital-balance" item unchanged from the beginning of their account, and to characterize any increase of it as " surplus " or " undivided profits " rather than as capital. There are several reasons for this bookkeeping policy. In the first place, the less often the bookkeepers entries are altered, the simpler the bookkeeping. Again, by stating separately the original capital and its later increase, the books show at a glance what the history of the individual or company has been as to the accumulations of net capital. Finally, in the case of joint stock companies, the stockholders capital is represented by stock certificates, the engraved " face value " of which cannot conveniently be altered to keep pace with changes in real value. Consequently, it is customary for bookkeepers to maintain the book value of the recorded " capital," or " capital-balance," equal to the face value of the certificates. But this bookkeeping policy does not alter the fact that at a given instant the stockholders capital consists of the entire excess of assets over liabilities, including in that excess the accumulated surplus and undivided profits. If the excess of assets over liabilities be added to the liabilities, the two sides of the account will exactly balance. A capital account so made out is therefore called a " balance sheet."

The following two balance sheets illustrate the accumulation in a year of that part of capital which bookkeepers separate from the " capital " item and call " surplus."

JANUARY 1, 1910

Assets Liabilities

Plant 200,000 Debts 100,000

Capital (owed to the stockholders). 100,000 200,000 200,000

JANUARY 1, 1911

Assets Liabilities

Plant, etc 246,324 Debts 100,000

Capital 100,000

Surplus 46,324 246,324 246,324

Not only is the book item, " capital," maintained intact as long as possible, but often the surplus also is put in round numbers and kept at the same figure for several successive reports. This leads bookkeepers to distinguish a third part of the capital, namely, the odd sum usually existing in addition to the surplus. This third item is called " undivided profits," and is subject to constant fluctuation from one date to another. The distinction between surplus and undivided profits is thus merely one of degree. The three items–capital, surplus, and undivided profits–together make up the total capital-balance due the stockholders. Of this, " capital " represents the original capital, "surplus " the earlier and larger accumulations, and " undivided profits " the later and minor accumulations. The undivided profits are more likely soon to disappear in dividends, i. e., to become divided profits, although this may also happen to the surplus, or even in certain cases to the " capital " itself.

We see, then, that the capital of a company, firm, or person, is to be understood in two senses: first, as the item entered in the balance sheet under that head–the original capital; and secondly, this sum plus surplus and undivided profits–the true net capital at the instant under consideration.

In the case of a joint stock company, since the stock certificates were issued at the time of the formation of the company, and cannot be perpetually changed, they ordinarily correspond to the original capital instead of the present capital. Recapital-ization may be effected, however, by recalling the stock certificates and issuing new ones. In this way the nominal or book value may be either decreased or increased. It is sometimes scaled down because of shrinking assets, and sometimes increased because of new subscriptions or expanding assets. If, for instance, the original capital was 100,000, and the present capital (including the surplus and undivided profits) is 300,000, it would be possible, in order that the total certificates outstanding might become 300,000, and the surplus and undivided profits be enrolled as capital, to issue additional stock certificates to the amount of 200,000 free to the holders of the original stock. Such an issue of stock is called a stock dividend. Ordinarily, however, the stock certificates remain as originally, and merely increase in value. Thus, if the present capital is 300,000, whereas the original capital or the outstanding certificates amounted to only 100,000, the " market value " of the shares will be triple the " face

value "; for the stockholders own a total of 300,000, represented by certificates the face value of which is 100,000.

3. Book and Market Values If, however, we attempt to verify such a relation by reference to the companys books, we shall find some discrepancies in the results. For instance, a certain bank of New York recently reported a total capital, surplus, and undivided profits of 1,295,952.59, of which the original capital was only 300,000. We should expect, therefore, that the stock certificates, the total face value of which was 300,000, would be worth 1,295,952.59; or, in other words, that each stock certificate with a face value of 100 would be worth 432. The actual selling price, however, was about 700. The discrepancy between 432 and 700 is due to the fact that there are two estimates of the value of capital—one that of the bookkeeper, which is seldom revised and usually conservative, and the other that of the market, which is revised almost daily. The stockholders of this bank were credited by the bookkeeper with owning 1,295,952.59, whereas in reality, the total value of their property was more nearly 2,100,000. The bookkeeper systematically undervalued the assets of the bank, and even omitted some valuable assets altogether, such as " good will." The object of a conservative business man in keeping his books is not to obtain mathematical accuracy, but to make so conservative a valuation as to be well within the requirements of the law and expediency. The law discountenances the valuation of assets above their original cost; and sometimes there is an additional motive to undervalue,—the wish to conceal a large surplus, from fear either of competition or of taxation.

Of the two valuations of the capital of a company, the bookkeepers and the markets, the latter, being more frequently revised, is apt to be the truer of the two, although it must be remembered that each of them is merely

an appraisement. The ordinary bookkeepers figures, which have so imposing an appearance of accuracy, are, in reality, and often of necessity, very wide of the mark. For instance, a certain bank recently reported its capital, surplus, and undivided profits at 444,814.40, but at the same time the president of the bank boasted that the banking house was entered among the assets at 20,000, while its real value was probably 50,000. Thus the figure giving the capital, surplus, or undivided profits, instead of being correct to the last cent or even the last dollar, was not correct even to the last ten thousand dollars.

4. Case of Decreasing Capital-balance

We have seen that the effect upon the balance sheet of an increase in the value of the assets is to swell the surplus or the undivided profits. Conversely, a shrinkage of value tends to diminish thdse items. For instance, if the plant of a company having a capital of 100,000 and a surplus of 50,000 depreciates to the extent of 40,000, the effect on the account will be as follows:–

ORIGINAL BALANCE SHEET

Assets Liabilities

Plant. 200,000.00 Debts. 150,000.00

Miscellaneous. 101,256.42 Capital. 100,000.00

Surplus. 50,000.00

Undivided profits. 1,256.42 301,256.42 301,256.42

PRESENT BALANCE SHEET

Assets Liabilities

Plant 160,000.00 Debts. 150,000.00

Miscellaneous. 101,256.42 Capital. 100,000.00

Surplus. 10,000.00

Undivided profits 1,256.42 261,256.42 261,256.42

Here the shrinkage in the value of the plant, as recorded on the assets side, " comes out of the surplus," as recorded on the liabilities side.

In case the surplus and undivided profits have both been wiped out, the capital itself becomes impaired. In this case the bookkeeper may indicate the result by scaling down the capitalization. This sometimes occurs in banks and trust companies, but not often in ordinary business. It is often avoided by making up the deficiencies through assessment of stockholders or postponement of dividends. Such measures are sometimes required by law, as in the case of insurance companies.

Dishonest concerns, however, often conceal their true condition by the reverse process of exaggerating the value of the assets. Sometimes this is done systematically, as in the case of stock-jobbing concerns. The sums intrusted to unscrupulous promoters by confiding stockholders are often invested in unwise or fraudulent ways. For instance, take an Oil Well Company in California, of the illegitimate type called " stock-producing wells." Suppose it borrows 50,000 and collects 50,000 more from the sale of stock (at par), and with this 100,000 purchases land at a fancy price from friends who collusively agree that a part of the proceeds shall be secretly returned to the promoter. In such a case the books of the bubble concern will show the following figures:–

Assets Liabilities

Land 100,000 Debts 50,000

Capital 50,000 100,000 100,000

But if the land is worth, say, only 60,000, these accounts should have been quite different, viz.:–

Assets Liabilities

Land 60,000 Debts 50,000

Capital 10,000 60,000 60,000

In other words, the investor has only 10,000 worth of property, instead of the 50,000 which he put in, or 20 cents for every dollar invested. The rest has been diverted into the pockets of the promoter and of those in collusion with him.

This is stock jobbing. It is one example of what, in commercial slang, is called " stock watering," being an issue of stock whose nominal or face value is greater than the actual capital. Another and more usual use of the term " stock watering" makes it meamnj. an issue of stock beyond the original cost value of the capital as shown by the actual money paid in, whether or not this be beyond the real commercial capital-value. Thus a " trust" may buy up a number of factories and then capitalize them far beyond that cost, because the combination of the factories gives them a monopoly value beyond the sum of their values when separate. By this kind of stock watering, concealment is made of the fact that the trust is earning an enormous rate of dividends in proportion to the original investment; for the dividends make a much smaller rate on the inflated, or watered, capitalization than on the cost value. Stock watering is usually employed to prevent a knowledge of the original value of the capital, for instance, to avoid public displeasure, taxation, or legal regulation of the rates charged. It is sometimes said that there is no wrong in such stock watering, so long as it is fully known. This is much like saying that to lie is not wrong, provided everybody knows you are lying. Stock watering of the kind described is the exaggeration of the " capital " item entered on the liabilities side of the balance sheet; and, since the two sides must balance, it involves the exaggeration of the assets also. It usually represents an intention to deceive, and through this deceit injury may be done both to buyers of stock and buyers of bonds. The buyers of stock are injured if they buy without knowledge of the proposed stack watering, and the bond buyer

is injured if the watering of the stock, having given him a false idea of the actual capital, induces him to lend more money than the capital can satisfactorily secure.

5. Insolvency

The original capital of a concern may be either increased or decreased. It may even disappear altogether if the assets shrink so much as no longer to exceed the liabilities (other than the capital liability itself). Insolvency is the condition in which the assets fall short of the liabilities other than capital. The capital-balance is intended to prevent this very calamity; it is for the express purpose of guaranteeing the value of the oiher liabilities–those to bondholders and other creditors.

These other liabilities, for the most part, are fixed blocks of property, carved, as it were, out of assets, the value of which property the merchant or company has agreed to keep intact at all hazards. The fortunes of business will naturally cause the whole volume of assets to vary in value, but all the " slack " ought properly to be taken up or given out by the capital, the surplus, and the undivided profits. A mans capital thus acts as a safety fund or buffer to keep the liabilities from overtaking the assets. It is the " margin " he puts up as a guarantee to others who intrust their capital to him.

The amount of capital-balance necessary to make a business reasonably safe will differ with circumstances. A capital-balance equal to five per cent of the liabilities may, in one kind of business, such as the business of a mortgage company, be perfectly adequate, whereas fifty per cent may be required in another kind. Much depends on how likely the assets are to shrink, and to what extent; and much, likewise, depends on the character of the liabilities.

The risk of insolvency is the chance that the assets may shrink below the liabilities–to others than stockholders. This risk is the greater, the more shrinkable the assets, and the less the margin of capital-value between assets and liabilities.

Insolvency must be distinguished from insufficiency of cash. The assets may comfortably exceed the liabilities, and yet the cash assets at a particular moment may be less than the cash liabilities due at that moment. This condition is not true insolvency, but only insufficiency of cash. In such a case, a little forbearance on the part of creditors may be all that is necessary to prevent financial shipwreck.

A wise merchant, however, will not only avoid insolvency, but also insufficiency of cash. He will not only keep his assets in excess of his liabilities by a safe margin, but he will also see that his assets are invested in such a manner that he shall be able, by exchanging them for cash, to cancel each claim at the time and in the manner agreed upon.

From this point of view there are three chief forms of assets; namely, cash assets, quick assets, and slow assets. A cash asset is in actual money, or what is acceptable in place of money. A quick asset is one which may be exchanged for cash in a relatively short time, as, for instance, gold or silver bullion, wheat, short-time loans, and other marketable securities. A slow asset is one which may require a relatively long time to be exchanged for cash. Such are real estate, office fixtures, and manufacturers equipment.

If all property were as acceptable as money, there would be no need of classifying assets into these three groups. But since the creditor will not accept railway stock or bonds, when he has contracted for payment in money, the debtor must maneuver so as to keep on hand a sufficient quantity of cash assets to enable him to meet his immediate obligations and enough quick assets to enable him to exchange them for cash in time to meet obligations soon to fall due. A large part of the skill of a business man consists in marshaling his assets so that he always has enough cash and enough quick assets to provide for impending debts, while maintaining at the same time enough slow assets to insure a satisfactory income from his business.

Originally, before business was separated from private life, all of a debtors assets, even including his own person, were regarded as pledged to the payment of a debt. An insolvent debtor could be imprisoned. To-day, however, laws exist in most countries by which a bankrupt may, under certain conditions, be discharged; free from further liability.

Since the liabilities of one man are also the assets of another, when one man fails and is able to pay only fifty cents on the dollar, the unlucky man who is his creditor–who has the first mans notes as assets–suffers a shrinkage in his own assets which may in turn mean embarrassment or even bankruptcy to him. It is usually true in a panic that the failures start with the collapse of some big firm, involving a shrinkage in the assets of others. This indicates why assets ought usually to be undervalued. A man who is in debt has no right to exaggerate his means of payment. A conservative and honest business man will always undervalue rather than overvalue his assets, in order to be fair to his creditors.

6. Real and Fictitious Persons It is well to note here the distinction between the accounting of real persons and of fictitious persons. For a real person, the assets may be, and usually are, in excess of the liabilities, and the difference is the capital-balance of that person. This capital is not, in the case of real persons, to be regarded as a liability, but as a balance or difference between the liabilities and the assets. For a fictitious person (i. e., a corporation, partnership, association, etc., regarded as independent of the real persons comprising it), on the other hand, the liabilities are always exactly equal to the assets; for the balancing item called capital

is as truly an obligation (from the fictitious person to the real stockholders) as any of the other liabilities. For instance, the items entered as " capital," " surplus," and " undivided profits" in the accounts of a joint stock company do not belong to the company, as such, but to the stockholders. So far as the " company " is concerned, they are its liabilities; they represent what it owes to the stockholders, just as truly as the other items of liabilities represent what it owes to the bondholders, etc. A fictitious person, in fact, is a mere imaginary being, holding certain assets and owing all of them out again to real persons, including the stockholders. A joint stock company may, it is true, be regarded as consisting of real persons (stockholders, etc.). But if we prefer, it may be regarded as a separate entity. In this case, of course, the " company " becomes a mere bookkeeping dummy having no capital-balance of its own and apart from what it owes the stockholders.

7. Two Methods of Combining Capital Accounts

We have seen how the capital account of each person in a community is formed. Our next task is to express the total net capital of any community. This is the sum of the net capitals of its members, i. e., all the innumerable assets of all the persons less all the liabilities of those persons. This net sum will be the same, of course, in whatever order the items are added and subtracted. We might write each item on a slip of paper, marking each asset item as positive and each liability item as negative, and, shuffling them into any random order, add and subtract them one by one according as they are positive or negative. But there are two ways in particular which need to be emphasized.

The simplest is, first, to obtain the net capital-balance of each person by subtracting the value of his liabilities from that of his assets, and then to add together these net capitals of different persons to get the capital of society. This method of obtaining societys net capital may be called the method of balances;, for we balance the books of each individual. The other method is to cancel each liability against an equal and opposite asset, which equal and opposite asset, as we shall see, must exist somewhere in another individuals account, and then add the remaining assets. This method may be called the method of couples; for we couple items in two different accounts. The method of couples is based on the fact that every liability item in a balance sheet implies the existence of an equal asset in some other balance sheet. This is true because every debit implies a credit. A debt may be owed to somebody, a creditor, as well as from somebody, a debtor, and the debt of the debtor is the credit of the creditor. It follows that every negative term in one balance sheet may be canceled against a corresponding positive term in some other. Each of these two methods–of balances and of couples–is important in its own way.

Let us illustrate each by the balance sheets of three real persons, say X, Y, and Z.

PERSON X

Assets Liabilities

Zs note. 30,000 A Mortgage held by Y. 50,000 b

Residence. 70,000

Railroad shares. 20.000 120,000 50,000

Capital-balance. 70,000

PERSON Y

Assets Liabilities

Xs mortgage. 50,000 B Debt to Z. 40,000 c

Personal effects. 20,000

Railroad shares. 10,000 80,000 40,000

Capital-balance. 40,000

PERSON Z

Assets Liabilities

Ys debt. 40,000 C Debt to X. 30,000 a

Farm. 50,000

Railroad bonds. 20,000 1 10,000 30,000

Capital-balance. 80,000

As the persons are real, not fictitious, the " capital" is in this case not a true liability, but is the excess of the total assets over the total liabilities. The sum of these capital-balances is the total net capital of X, Y, and Z, and is thus obtained by the method of balances. To show the method of couples in the table, each couple of corresponding items–i. e., each item which appears twice, once as a liability of one man and again as an asset of another–is indicated in both places by the same letter. Thus, " A " in Xs assets is matched by the equal and opposite item " a " in Zs liabilities. The method of couples thus consists in canceling, and, therefore, omitting from societys balance sheet, these pairs of items, and entering and adding only those which remain uncanceled. These, in the present case, are all assets. Adding these, we again obtain a sum representing the total net capital of X, Y, and Z, this time by the method of couples.

The results of summing up the capital accounts by the two methods are shown in the following tables:–

Method Of Balances Method Of Couples

Xs capital. 70,000 Residence 70,000

Ys capital. 40,000 Personal effects. 20,000

Zs capital. 80,000 Farm 50,000

Railroad shares. 30,000

Railroad bonds. 20,000 190,000 190,000

The totals are the same by both methods, but the method of balances exhibits the share of this total capital which is

owned by each individual, while the method of couples exhibits the portion ascribable to each different capital-good.

8. Ultimate Result of Method of Couples

Let us now introduce into our addition the capital accounts of the railroad whose stocks and bonds were included among the assets of persons X, Y, and Z. For simplicity, we shall suppose that these three persons are the only persons interested in the road. The balance sheet of the railroad company will accordingly appear as follows:–

RAILROAD COMPANY

Assets Liabilities

Railway 50,000 Bonds (held by Z). 20,000

Capital stock (held by X) 20,000 (held by Y) 10,000 30,000 50,000 50,000

Capital-balance of the R. R. Co. itself 00,000 If now, by the method of balances, we combine this balance sheet with those of X, Y, and Z, we shall see that its inclusion does not affect the results which were obtained by the same method before the railroad was introduced into the discussion. The totals will stand as follows:–

Xs capital-balance 70,000

Ys capital-balance 40,000

Zs capital-balance 80,000

Railroad Co. s capital-balance. 00,000 190,000

When we apply the method of couples, we find, however, that the inclusion in our consideration of the railway companys capital account will affect the items, though not the final sum. The stocks and bonds, as assets of X, Y, and Z, will then pair off or couple with the corresponding liabilities of the railroad company, and their place will be taken by the concrete railroad itself, as follows:–

Method Of Couples

Residence, 70,000

Personal effects 20,000

Farm 50,000

Railway 50,000 190,000

The appearance of the capital inventory is thus changed. Formerly, the items of property rights in it included such /ar/-rights as stocks and bonds; now they consist only of complete property rights. But the complete right to any article of wealth is best expressed in terms of the article of wealth itself. Consequently, instead of the long phrase, the " right to a residence," we may merely use the term " residence." The property no longer veils the wealth beneath it; and the inventory, which before was an inventory of both capital wealth and capital property becomes an inventory of only capital wealth.

Such a result is sure to follow when we combine capital accounts, provided we combine enough of them to supply, for every liability item, its counterpart asset, and for every asset which has one, its counterpart liability. Those assets which have no counterparts are what we have called the complete rights to wealth; while those assets which do have canceling counterparts are the partial rights to wealth. The reason is that partial rights to wealth necessarily have canceling counterparts in that whenever any partial ownership of a given article of wealth is held by a particular person, its whole ownership must be supposed to be held by some fictitious person even if specially created for the purpose. Thus, if a farmer named Smith owns an undivided half interest in a farm jointly owned by himself and brother, we conceive of the whole farm as owned by the fictitious person, the partnership, known as the " Smith brothers." The owner of the half interest, "John Smith," thus holds a claim against the partnership "Smith brothers." This claim is an asset to Smith but a liability to the partnership. It is clear that an individual cannot own a part interest in any given wealth without its being true that the fictitious owner of it all is liable to him to that extent. Therefore every partial right to wealth, while an asset to the owner of that right, is a liability to the fictitious person owning the whole. Every article of concrete wealth has to be regarded as owned by some one, even if we have to set up a fictitious person or dummy for that very purpose.

To follow out totals of capital thus requires the inclusion of many fictitious persons, for it is often only the fictitious persons who hold the complete rights. Locomotives and railway stations, for instance, are owned by corporations, not individuals. In fact, these fictitious persons–partnerships, corporations, trusts, municipalities, associations, and the like–are devices for the express purpose of holding large aggregations of concrete wealth and parceling out its ownership among a number of real persons.

If, then, we suppose balance sheets so constructed as to include all the real and fictitious persons in the world, with entries in them for every asset and liability,–even public parks and streets, household furniture, and other possessions not formally accounted for in ordinary practice,–it is evident that we shall obtain, by the method of balances, a complete account of the distributionof capital-value among real persons; and, by the method of couples, a complete list of the articles of actual wealth thus owned. In this list there will be no stocks, bonds, mortgages, notes, or other part-rights, but only land, buildings, and other land improvements, and commodities. All debit and credit items being two faced–positive and negative–cancel out in the total. This self-effacement, however, does not mean that the total would be just the same if there were no stocks, bonds, mortgages, notes, or other two-faced items. On the contrary, the existence of such property rights indirectly adds a great deal to the effectiveness of wealth. They make

possible the cooperative ownership of great aggregations of capital which without such ownership could scarcely exist, and thus result in increasing greatly the total benefits we enjoy from capital.

9. Confusions to be Avoided

Among the forms of part-rights in real wealth is "credit." Credit is simply a debt looked at from the standpoint of the creditor. There has been much discussion as to the nature of credit. It has been sometimes regarded as an item of wealth; and an increase or inflation of credit has been looked on as a real addition to the wealth of the community. But, of course, since every credit is also a debit, it cannot be regarded as a simple addition to the wealth of the community as a whole. The phenomenon of credit means nothing more nor less than a specific form of divided ownership of wealth. Credit merely enables one man temporarily to control more wealth or property than he owns –., some part of the wealth or property of others.

It is, therefore, a cardinal error to regard credit as increasing the capital of the debtor. Indirectly, of course, credit may result in an increase of societys capital, by stimulating trade and production, as well as by getting the management of capital into the right hands and its ownership into the most effective form. In these ways the earth is made to yield up more wealth, or greater benefits from the same wealth–in either case entailing an increase of capital; but the amount of any such increase of capital thus indirectly produced bears no necessary relation to the amount of the credit which facilitated its production. Even when capital is increased through credit, the credit does not constitute the increase.

A great deal of confusion in legislation and discussion could be avoided if the two methods of combining capital accounts were distinguished and their interrelations recognized. In taxation, the two methods are often confused. An impor tant problem of efficient taxation of property is how to avoid unintentional double taxation and at the same time not to allow some property unintentionally to escape any taxation. There are two solutions. One is to tax the amount owned by each real person as obtained by the method of balances; this method seeks out the real owners or part-owners of wealth. The other is to tax the actual concrete wealth as obtained by the method of couples; this method seeks out the real wealth owned. In short, one method follows the person, the other the thing. At present the two methods are much confused. Legislators too often fail to perceive that under the first, or owner-method, corporations should not be taxed, for they are not true owners; and that under the second, or wealth-method, bonds, stocks, and other part-rights to wealth should not be taxed, for these are already taxed when the actual railways and other items of physical wealth underlying such part-rights are taxed. It is not claimed, of course, that a complete system of taxation can be worked out merely by choosing one of the two methods just indicated. But the distinction between the two should be borne in mind, whenever any scheme of taxation is considered; for where one system is applied, the other cannot also be applied without double taxation.

The study of capital accounting, therefore, enables us to avoid many common confusions. More important still, it gives us a clear picture of the relations between the capital of a community and the capital of the individuals of which the community is composed, i. e., between the stocks of actual wealth in a community and the stocks of property representing the ownership of this wealth among different individuals. In short, it enables us to see both individually and as a whole the items which make up private and collective property, as stocks, bonds, mortgages, debts, etc., on the one hand, and land, ships, dwellings, and other concrete wealth, on the other.

In the light of the foregoing principles we are in a position to take a birds-eye view of the capital in any country. In America, for instance, we find a stock of wealth of various kinds with an estimated value of over 100,000,000,000. More than half of this consists of real estate; about ten per cent consists of railways and their equipment; manufactured products make up about 8,000,000,000; furniture, carriages, and kindred articles about 6,000,000,000; live stock on farms about 4,000,000,000; tools, implements, and machinery in factories about 3,000,000,000; clothing and personal adornments about 2,500,000,000; street railways about 2,000,000,000; agricultural products about 2,000,000,000; gold and silver coin and bullion about 2,000,000,000; and there are numerous other smaller items. The ownership of this real wealth is divided up in various ways. To a very large extent, especially in the case of farms, the real estate is owned completely by the occupier. In other cases it is mortgaged, the occupier then owning merely the excess of value over the mortgage. Of the national capital apart from real estate, on the other hand, probably by far the greater part is owned by corporations, which means, of course, simply that its ownership is parceled out among the stockholders and bondholders of these corporations. From what has been said the student will not make the mistake of adding the value of stocks and bonds to the value of the tangible wealth which these represent. Stocks, bonds, mortgages, and other items which are assets to some persons are liabilities to others., and thus cancel themselves out for the country as a whole. The student will also notice how insignificant is the stock of gold and silver as compared with the total capital, although the value of all is measured in terms of gold.

CHAPTER IV INCOME 1. Concepts of Income and Outgo

The income from any particular article of wealth has been denned as the flow of benefits from that article. These benefits may sometimes consist of money payments; but it is important to avoid the mistaken notion that they always consist of money payments. Income is the flow of whatever benefits accrue from any article, whether these benefits happen to be in the form of money payments or not. A self-supporting farmer, for instance, may not receive or expend a single dollar from one years end to the other. He has, nevertheless, an income. He gets a " living "–the very essence of income–from the farm. A windmill pumps water; the pumping is the benefit or income resulting from the windmill. A derrick hoists coal from a mine; the hoisting is the income from the derrick. A wife does housework; her work is an item of the familys income, for, as was stated in the last chapter, the services of a human being are income. The warmth and shelter that a house provides for its occupants constitute the income furnished by the house. All the operations of industry and all the transactions of commerce are items of income. When axes fell trees and sawmills turn them into lumber, these changes constitute items in the income flowing from the agencies which produce them. When a manufacturing plant converts raw materials into food or into fabrics or into imple ments, these changes constitute income produced by the plant. What we call agriculture, mining, commerce, and domestic operations constitute large and important classes of income.

Practically, of course, most of the examples given of benefits or services are not income to the owner of the instruments rendering those services; for, practically, those services are not enjoyed by the owner, but are sold to some one else, the owner receiving a money payment instead. Thus, although a farmer may get his living directly from the farm, it is more usual for him to sell some of the farm products and to receive money payments instead. Likewise it may be that the owner of the windmill pumps water for others and receives money payments in return; and that the owner of a house sells its use for a money rental. Similarly the owners of the derrick, axes, sawmill, manufacturing plant, etc., do not get the direct benefit of the hoisting, cutting, sawing, manufacturing, etc., but exchange these for money payments. In such cases the owners get their income in the form of money payments by selling to others the direct benefits of their capital. Thus their capital yields them an indirect money income through the sale of the direct income produced by the capital. So usual is it for the owner of capital to sell his direct or natural income for a money income that ordinarily we think of income as consisting only of such money return. One of the early economists seriously maintained that the owner of a house could receive no income from it except by renting it, forgetting that to let a house is merely to sell the shelter income for money income. A man who lives in his own house gets the shelter income directly. A man who lets his house to another secures a money income as the equivalent of the shelter income which he sells to the tenant.

Income, being a flow of benefits, implies a stock or fund which produces the flow. This stock or fund may consist partly of instruments of external wealth, which we have designated as capital (in the narrow sense), and partly of the population itself, which is also capital (in the broader sense).

It has already been noted that income differs from capital in two respects. In the first place, income is a flow relating to a given period, whereas capital is a stock or fund relating to a given instant. In the second place, income consists of (intangible) benefits, whereas capital consists of (tangible) instruments; not farms, therefore, nor houses, nor food, nor railroads, nor artesian wells, nor instruments of any sort can, strictly speaking, ever constitute income. Income consists rather in the yielding of crops by the farms; the warming and sheltering of people by the houses; the nourishing of people by the food; the transporting of passengers and freight by the railroads; the raising of water by the wells; and benefits of any sort rendered by instruments of wealth.

Although income consists partly of other benefits than money receipts, all income, like all capital, may be translated into terms of money. For, as was pointed out in chapter II, 1, to all items of income, i. e., benefits, may be applied the concepts of price and value.

Income, as well as capital, is subject to accounting. Thus far we have considered only such items as would belong to the positive side of income accounts. But just as in our capital account we found a negative side–comprising the liabilities–so we shall find a negative side to income. The negative of income is called outgo, and the items which constitute outgo are called costs. A cost occasioned by an article has already been defined as the opposite of a benefit. It is an undesirable event occasioned by that article. Labor, trouble, expense, and sacrifices of all sorts are entailed by wealth and are counted among its costs. An instrument seldom confers benefits without also involving costs. A dwelling, while it gives shelter, compels its owner to assume important costs in keeping it in repair, painting it, cleaning it, caring for it, insuring it, and paying taxes upon it. A saddle horse yields income to the owner when it gives him a pleasure ride, but it requires feeding, stabling, and shoeing–the negative side of the account, constituting the outgo or flow of costs occasioned by the horse. A farm produces benefits in yielding crops; but it requires fertilizing, tilling, and seeding, all of which are costs occasioned by the farm. A railroad produces benefits called " transportation"–hauling passengers and commodities; but it involves an expenditure of money, it burns coal, it requires labor; and these are the outgo, or the negative side of its account.

Costs, too, may be measured in money just as income may be measured in money; and some costs, whether of dwellings, farms, railways, or other articles, consist in the actual expenditure of money, just as some benefits consist in the receipt of money. Strictly speaking, neither consists of actual money. We must, therefore, distinguish carefully three money items: (1) money on hand at an instant of time, which is an example of capital; (2) the receipt of money during a period of time, which is an example of income (from whatever instrument occasions the receipt of the money); and (3) the expenditure of money during a period of time, which is an example of outgo (on the part of whatever instrument occasions the expense).

In general, the costs of a given item of capital are outweighed by its benefits. For if it should occasion more costs than benefits, it would be thrown away, thereupon ceasing to be wealth according to our definition. Or if it should still remain in any ones possession, it might be called negative wealth, of which ashes, rubbish, garbage, etc., are familiar examples.

Costs, then, are never voluntarily assumed except in the hope of benefits which will make them worth while. The total value of all the benefits flowing from a given instrument in a given time is called gross income-value or simply gross income, during that time. Similarly, the total value of its costs is called outgo-value or simply outgo. The total gross income during a given time minus the total outgo (i. e., the value of its costs), constitutes net income. Thus, just as net capital is found by subtracting the liabilities from the assets in a capital account, so net income in an income account is found by subtracting the value of the costs from the value of the benefits. Both benefits and costs, moreover, are attributable to a definite capital source. In income-accounting the benefits or income-items are credited to capital, and the outgo or cost-items are debited to capital. In keeping income accounts, therefore, it is important to know to what category of capital any item of income should be credited, or any item of outgo debited.

2. Income Accounts

We are now in a position to apply the foregoing definitions to income accounts. Perhaps no other subject in economics has been so fraught with confusion, misunderstanding, and double counting, as income. It will help the student to understand these accounts if he will bear in mind that they show the income and outgo which any given capital (or free human being) yields. We are apt to think of income and outgo too much with reference to the owner of the income instead of the source of the income. It will be easy later to make up the owners income-account; but first we must construct the income account for an isolated article of capital.

We may begin by imagining a certain " house-and-lot " as one composite instrument or article of wealth, and may first consider its income and outgo during the calendar year 1910. The instrument is capital, and the income which this capital brings to its owner may be either a money rental or the direct shelter and similar benefits of the house enjoyed by himself and his family. In either case the income may be measured in money, although in the case of occupancy by the owner this measurement requires a special appraise ment. The house, let us suppose, was built many years ago, and is now nearly worn out. It yields an income worth 1000 a year. Against its income there are offsets in the form of repairs, taxes, etc.–costs which it occasions. We have, then, the following " income account ":– INCOME ACCOUNT FOR HOUSE AND LOT DURING THE
YEAR 1910
Income Outgo
  Use of house and lot. 1000 Repairs 200
  Taxes 180 Insurance 20 1000 400 Net income. 600

Next year the house is found to have rotten timbers, is condemned, and must be abandoned or torn down. Its benefits are ended, but the land is still good, and the owner can build a new house. The period consumed by this operation is the first six months of the year 1911, so that during such period there is no income attributable to the house and lot, but only outgo. During the second half of the year the house is occupied, and its use is valued at 600. In the first six months not only did the " house-and-lot " fail to yield any income, but it occasioned a cost. This cost was the cost of production of the new house.

We have, then, the following account:– INCOME ACCOUNT FOR HOUSE AND LOT DURING THE

YEAR 1911 Income Outgo

Use of house and lot (six Expense of building months) 600 house 10,000

Taxes and insurance. too 600 10,100

Net outgo 9,500

During this year, then, the house causes a net outgo of 9500. As we know, all costs are " necessary evils "; they lead to good, though not good themselves; and this cost of constructing the house was incurred only for the sake of expected future benefits. The adverse balance it creates is only temporary, and should be more than made up in the years which follow.

For the year 1912, for instance, we may have the following:– INCOME ACCOUNT FOR HOUSE AND LOT DURING THE

YEAR 1912

Income Outgo

Use 1300 Repairs 50

Taxes and insurance. 250

Net income.

1300

1000 300

These figures remain about the same for forty-nine years and give 49,000 net income during that time, offsetting the INCOME

Kit 1813 1814 1815 1916 1817 Kit

Fig. i.

OUTGO

excess in cost for 1911 (9500) and leaving a large margin besides. Then the house is worn out a second time and has to be rebuilt. The same cycle is repeated, one year of excess of cost being offset by forty-nine years of excess of income. Figure 2 shows a part of this cycle, picturing graphically the figures in the above income-and-outgo accounts.

It will be observed that the cost of reconstructing the house was entered in the accounts in exactly the same way as the cost of repairing it or as any other costs. This may be puzzling at first, because most of the other costs are fairly regular year by year, whereas the cost of reconstruction occurs only once, or at any rate only once in a long while. It may also seem puzzling because the cost of reconstruction is so large in comparison with other costs. But the irregularity or size of costs is, of itself, no reason for omitting them from our accounts. The only way in which we can escape recording such a cost–for instance, the cost of constructing the house–is by substituting in its place an equivalent series of smaller and more regular costs. What is called a depreciation fund is sometimes created for this very purpose. This fund is accumulated during the existence of the house by setting aside annually small portions of the Income yielded by the house, sufficient in the aggregate to replace the house when it is worn out. The depreciation fund, combined with the " house-and-lot " renders the flow of costs uniform or regular. But even when a depreciation fund is used, we can only say that the combination of the two things (the fund and the house) has a regular cost. We cannot say that this is true of the house by itself; and when no such device as a depreciation fund at all is used, there can be no escape from charging the cost of reconstruction in precisely the same way as we charge any other cost. If this still seems puzzling, it is because we are in the habit of seeing the cost of reconstruction entered as the value of the house and, hearing it called, for that reason, a " capital cost." It is true that the value of the new house must be entered on the capital-balance sheet; but the cost of producing it belongs properly to the income account. The value relates to an instant of time (which may be any instant from the time the house is begun till the time when it ceases to exist); the cost relates to a period of time (which may be all or any part of the time during which the labor and other sacrifices occasioned by the house occur). The value of the house is quite distinct from the series of costs by which it was built, although the confusion between the two is natural in view of the bookkeeping practice of entering capital at its " cost value." The house on which 10,000 was expended for construction may be worth either more or less than 10,000. In either case the income account should contain 10,000 on the outgo side, and the capital account a larger or smaller figure, as the case may require.

3. Devices for Making Net Income Regular

We have seen that the irregularities in the net annual income or outgo flowing from the " house-and-lot" may be combined with the opposite irregularities of the net annual outgo or income from a " depreciation fund," so that the net result from the two combined is a steady net income. The same result may be secured in other ways. For instance, if the owner of the house-and-lot happens to own a large number of other houses-and-lots in different degrees of repair, the irregularities in income from them individually may tend to offset each other. Thus, if a man owns fifty houses, each lasting fifty years, and every year one wears out and has to be rebuilt, it is then evident that he will have an expense of 10,000 every year for the rebuilding of a house, which will be a regular item; and he will have a regular income balance as a consequence, because he will get the benefit of forty-nine houses, which will far outweigh the cost of building only one. The difference will be his net income, which will be a fairly regular amount year after year.

This example ought to set at rest any lingering doubts as to the correctness of our including the cost of reconstructing a house as an item of outgo, to be entered as such in a true and complete income account. The only reason this may, at first, seem wrong is that the cost of reconstruction is not usually a regular item. In the case of the fifty houses it becomes a more or less regular item. But if it is correct to call it outgo when there are fifty houses, it must be correct to call it outgo when there are ten houses or when there is only one. Irregularity of income is an inconvenience and we usually seek to avoid it b depreciation funds, by having a large number of articles at different stages of repair, or otherwise. But so long as irregularity of income exists it must be entered as such. The effect of reducing irregularities by combining a large assortment of articles is present wherever a sufficiently large assortment exists. Professor Clark of Columbia University suggests a helpful simile when he compares a stock or fund of capital to a waterfall: the drops of water,-or component parts of the waterfall or fund, are constantly changing; but the waterfall or fund remains substantially the same.

4. How to Credit and Debit

Before leaving the subject of income accounts, we shall speak of one particular kind of capital, namely, a stock of cash. This will furnish an opportunity to illustrate anew some of the principles of accounting which we have just discussed. What puzzles the novice in accounting is the manner of debiting and crediting a stock of cash, or what is called the " cash drawer." At first sight the usage seems to be the opposite of what it should be. To understand the practice of accountants in this particular is to go a long way toward understanding the main principles of accounting. It will help us to understand it if we liken a cash drawer to a gold mine. We credit a gold mine with all the gold extracted, and we debit it with all the costs put into it. In the case of the gold mine, what it costs to run it is outgo; all of the yield of gold is gross income; and the difference is the net income. Similarly, the gross income from the cash drawer consists of what the cash drawer yields, or whatever comes out of it. It benefits us whenever it pays our bills; it costs us whenever we pay its bills, i. e., whenever we pay some thing into it. All the payments which we have to make to the drawer are a cost of that drawer to us, whereas all the payments that we make by the drawer are the benefits which it produces for us. As long as we pay money into the drawer, we realize no income, but merely accumulate capital for future use. If we should only pay money into the drawer and never throughout our life take any out, the "drawer " would benefit us nothing. Its benefits would go to our descendants whenever they should take the money out. Ordinarily, however, the money is taken out soon after it is put in. What net benefit, then, does the cash drawer yield in the long run? Seldom anything at all. We pay out just as much as we put in; and if we subtract one amount from the other, the net annual income from the cash drawer will be about zero, unless during a certain year we store up more than we take out, or take out more than we put in.

The reason that these credits and debits of " cash " seem at first the reverse of what they should be is that we are accustomed to think of money receipts and expenditures, not in their relation to the stock of cash into or out of which they are paid, but in their relation to some other item of wealth on account of which the payments are made. If a lodging-house keeper receives 10 from a lodger and puts it into her cash drawer, she finds it hard to debit 10 to " cash." She thinks of the 10 as income; and it is income with respect to her lodging-house, for the latter has yielded it to her. Her stock of cash, however, has not yielded the 10 to her. On the contrary, it has taken that amount from her. Later on it will yield back that amount or some portion of it, and at that time may properly be credited with the sum it yields up.

We are now ready to understand how to derive a mans total income. It is simply the combined income from all the capital he owns. We could obtain a full account of it by keeping a separate income account for each item of capital he owns, crediting and debiting each such item with its re spective benefits and costs. The difference of all the benefits and costs of all his capital is his net income. In these accounts we should include, therefore, all positive and negative items of income pertaining to all positive and negative items of capital. The negative items of capital are the liabilities. Liabilities yield a net outgo instead of a net income. In order, then, to find out the net income of any person during a certain day or month or year, the proper method is to make a complete statement of all his assets and all his liabilities; and for each asset as well as each liability, credit all the benefits and debit all the costs. The net result will be the net income of the person.

A real person will have a net income, but a fictitious person will not. We have seen, in the case of fictitious persons, that there is no net capital because the liabilities always equal the assets; for what is often called the capital of a " company " really means the capital of its stockholders. As there is no net capital of the company, as such, the " company " owing it all to the stockholders, so there is no net income of the company, as such, the " company " paying it all to the stockholders or others.

The following is an imaginary income account of a railroad company:– INCOME ACCOUNT OF A RAILROAD CORPORATION Income

By passenger and freight service 1,246,147

Outgo

To operating expenses 800,000

To interest to bond-

holders. 100,000 1,246,147

To dividends to stock-

holders. 200,000

To surplus applied to (1) purchase of land 140,000 (2) cash paid into treasury. 6,147 1,246,147

The passenger and freight service has yielded 1,246,147. That is the gross income of the road. All the benefits flowing from that road are worth this amount of money. On the other side of the railroad account we find the costs of the road to the company; they exactly equal the benefits, for the company is an abstraction–a mere holding concern–not a real individual. The outgo consists principally of operating expenses, 800,000; interest to bondholders, 100,000; dividends to stockholders, 200,000. The words by and to are usual in income accounts. The receipts are benefits; they come by virtue of the services designated. The costs represent something which has to be given to these several items in order to make the benefits possible. These items leave a surplus, part of which is expended for land (140,000); this is a cost just as much as anything else. Then there is cash left in the treasury to the amount of 6147. It must not be concluded that this cash is a net income. The cash drawer swallows it up. The company loses 6147, so to speak, in feeding its cash drawer. Therefore the two sides of the account balance, and there is no net income at all to the "company."

5. Omissions and Errors in Practice

Practically, however, it is not convenient to enter in an income or a capital account everything which theoretically ought to be entered there. Moreover, capital and income accounts are not always treated consistently in practice. For instance, in a capital account a man would not ordinarily enter his own person, as a free human being is not ordinarily counted as wealth; and yet in his income account he will enter the money he earns or the work that he does. That is, work and wages are entered in the income accounts, but the corresponding items representing the agencies which do this work or earn these wages are not entered in the capital accounts. The correspondence be tween the two accounts is, therefore, obscured. On the other hand, a man never, in practice, enters in his income account the shelter of his own house as a benefit, and yet he may include the house among his assets in his capital account. In ideal accounting we should insist upon recording every benefit of any kind, every cost, and every source of benefit or cost. As we have already indicated, an early economist fell into error when he said that a dwelling occupied by the owner yields no income. He claimed that, on the contrary, it is a source of expense. Evidently he had in mind only those costs and benefits which come in the form of money payments. One certainly gets no money benefits by living in his own house, while he does suffer a money cost to run it. So far as money receipts and expenditures are concerned, therefore, the house costs more than it brings in. But no man would keep his house if it did not afford him benefits greater than its costs. We should, therefore, appraise the shelter of the house and enter this as its gross income. If we do not, we reach the absurd conclusion that if I live in my own house and you live in your own house, neither of us receives any income; but if you rent your house to me and I rent mine to you, then we shall each be receiving income! Obviously the income is really there, all the time, in the form of shelter; and when one man rents another mans house, he gets the shelter-income and gives the other man a money-income in its place.

An account of money received and expended by a given person can sometimes furnish a fairly complete picture of his income; but only when two conditions exist; namely, that all the income from his property is in the form of money, and all the outgo is in the form of money spent for personal satisfactions (i. e., goes directly to pay for clothes, food, shelter, amusements, and the like, and is not expended in investments, repairs, and the expenses of running a business). Under these conditions the cash drawer and the cash account constitute a kind of money meter of income. These conditions are approximately fulfilled when people live in a city and rent the houses or furniture of others instead of owning them themselves. Such people get practically all of their income in the form of money receipts, as salaries, dividends, and interest. This money is spent for benefits, as food, clothing, theater going, etc. The cash drawer (or bank account) then intervenes between the money-income on the one hand, and the final income which this money-income buys, on the other hand; much as a cogwheel intervenes to transmit motion from one part of a machine to another. A man who receives 5000 a year in money or checks and spends it all on food, clothing, shelter, amusements, and other final or enjoyable benefits, and gets no such benefits from any other source, evidently receives a real income of 5000 a year. His money income correctly measures his real income. But if he " saves " part of the 5000, i. e., expends it for stocks, bonds, or a savings bank account or any other capital, the benefits from which are greatly deferred, his real income may be less than 5000; while if he derives shelter from his own house, or food from his own garden, his real income may be greater than his money income. Thus money income is an unsafe indication of real income. The only method, then, of constructing income and outgo accounts which will be correct and which can serve as a basis for economic analysis is the method already indicated–the method by which are recorded, for each article of capital (including human beings), the values of all its benefits and all its costs. These benefits and costs are of many kinds. Sometimes they consist of money payments–not in themselves enjoyable to anybody; sometimes they consist of merely intermediate or productive operations; and sometimes, of truly final or enjoyable elements. All these items should be entered in the accounts on the same footing; but we shall see that all except the " enjoyable " elements will cancel among themselves.

CHAPTER V

COMBINING INCOME ACCOUNTS 1. Methods of "Balances" and "Couples" "Interactions "

We have now learned how to reckon the income of either a real or a fictitious person. Of reckoning the income of all society, on the other hand, there are many ways, including, in particular, two that correspond to the two ways which we discussed in Chapter III of reckoning societys capital. These are the method of balances and the method of couples. The method of balances is very easy to apply. All that is necessary is to make up an income account for any given period for each instrument or article of wealth so as to include all possible income or outgo in society and, deriving from each such account the net balance, add these net balances together. The result is the total income of society. Its constituent parts are the net incomes from the several articles of societys wealth.

The " method of couples " is somewhat more difficult to follow. But it is also more important. Just as it often happens that the same item in capital accounts is both asset and liability, according to the point of view, and is therefore self-canceling, so it often happens that the same item in income accounts is both benefit and cost, and is, therefore, likewise self-canceling. In fact, the reader may have felt that, in many of the examples cited, what we called costs were really benefits. He may have asked himself: Why should we call repairing a house a cost? When a carpenter and his tools repair it, do we not credit him and them with a service performed? Is not any production a benefit? Have we not, then, placed repairs on the wrong side of the ledger? It all depends upon which of two accounts we are considering. When a carpenter with his plane, hammer, and saw helps to rebuild a house, we have to consider two groups of capital.1 One group, the carpenter and tools, is acting on the other group, the house. The carpenter and tools certainly perform a service or benefit, but the house does not. Considered as occasioned by the house, the repairs are costs. The house absorbs or soaks up these costs, promising to compensate for them by benefits to be yielded later on. The renailing of loose shingles is certainly not what the house is for; with respect to the house, it is a necessary evil; with respect to the hammer, however, it is a service rendered. Therefore the repairing of the house is at once a benefit and a cost.

Such double-faced events are so important as to require a special name. We shall call them interactions. Each interaction takes place between two instruments or groups of instruments.

An interaction, then, is a double-faced event, at once a benefit or service of the acting instrument, and a cost or disservice of the instrument acted on. There can never arise the slightest doubt as to when it is to be regarded as positive and when negative. The definitions of benefit and cost settle this question in each case. If it is desired by the owner of a given instrument that this instrument should occasion a given event, then the event is "desirable" or a benefit. If it is desired that an instrument should not occasion a given event, then the event is "undesirable" or a cost. Thus, since the house owner desires that the house should not occasion repairs, these repairs are costs of the house; and since he desires that the tools should produce repairs, such repairs are the benefits from those tools.

1 In this instance and throughout the following discussion we shall consider capital in its broader sense as including free human beings.

The example given is typical of the general relations between interacting instruments. The mental picture we should construct is that of two distinct groups of capital. Group A acts on, and, so to speak, benefits Group B. Whatever the nature of this interaction, A, the giver of the benefit, is credited with it and B, the recipient, is debited with it as a cost. These two items of credit and debit are equal and simultaneous because they are the selfsame event looked at from opposite sides.

Interactions constitute the great majority of the elements which enter into income and outgo accounts. The only benefits which do not form merely the positive side of such canceling interactions, and so do not cancel out, are satisfactions –desirable conscious experiences–often called " consumption " (these are credited to the things enjoyed–for instance, a house); and the only costs which do not form merely the negative side of such canceling interactions, and so do not cancel out, are " labor and trouble " (these are debited to human beings). But these two final elements–" satisfactions," on the one hand, and "labor and trouble," on the other–are only the outer edges of the series of interactions. Between them lies a connective chain of productive processes and commercial transactions, every link of which has two sides, a positive side of benefits or services and a negative side of costs, always mutually canceling.

2. Production: Interactions which Change the Form of
Wealth

The interactions between two articles or groups of articles are of three chief kinds: changes in the form of wealth, changes in the position of wealth, and changes in the ownership of wealth; in other words, transformation, transporta tion, and transfer or exchange. All three may be called "production," although this term is sometimes confined to the first two and sometimes even to the first alone. These we shall take up in order, and show how each is a two-faced event or an interaction.

First, what is here called " transformation " of wealth is practically identical with what is usually understood by " production " or " productive processes." By this transformation or change in the form of wealth is meant the change of relative position of its parts. Weaving, for instance, is the transformation of yarn into cloth by a rearrangement in the relative positions of the warp and woof. Spinning, likewise, consists in moving, stretching, and twisting fibers into yarn; sewing, in changing the position of thread so that it may hold cloth together; and so it is with carding, wool sorting, shearing, and all the other operations which constitute the manufacture of fabrics. All these operations–which include all manufacture and all agriculture

–consist simply of a series of transformations of wealth, each transformation being a two-faced operation. With respect to the transformed instrument or instruments, the transformation is a cost; with respect to the transforming instrument or instruments it is a benefit. So it is when a loom produces cloth out of yarn, or when land renders a service in producing wheat. So it is, not only when a carpenter and his tools build or repair a house, but also when the painter decorates it or the janitor cleans it; or when a cobbler transforms leather into shoes, or when a bootblack transforms dirty shoes into clean and polished ones.

The principle is not altered when the interaction consists, not in producing a change, but in preventing one. A warehouse renders its service as a means of storing bales of cotton, i. e., protecting them from the elements; and this storage is, on the part of the stock of cotton, an element of outgo, or expense, as on the part of the warehouse it is an item of income.

Nor is the principle altered when there are, as indeed is usually the case, more articles than one in either or both of the two interacting capitals. Plowing, or the transformation of land into a furrowed form, is performed by a plow, a horse, and a man. The plowing is a cost debited to the land, on the one hand, and at the same time a service credited to the group consisting of the plow, horse, and man, on the other.

Nor is the principle altered if one or more of the transforming agents perish in the transformation and another comes for the first time into existence. Bread making is a transformation debited to the bread and credited to the cook, the range, the flour, and the fuel, of which the last two are consumed as soon as they perform their services. Agents which disappear in the transformation, but reappear in whole or in part in the product (as here the flour), are called " raw materials." The production of cloth from yarn is a transformation effected by means not only of the loom, but also of a number of other agents, among them the yarn itself, which thus vanishes as yarn and reappears as cloth. The cost of weaving includes the consumption of raw material–yarn; and this consumption of yarn is, on the part of the yarn itself, not cost, but service. It is the use for which the yarn existed. When cloth is turned into clothes, this transformation is a service to be credited to the cloth, and a cost to be debited to the clothes. All raw materials yield benefits as they are converted into finished products. Their conversion is, however, on the part of these products, always outgo and not income.

In general, production consists of a succession of stages, and at each stage there is an interaction. The finished product of one stage passes over as the raw material of the next, and its passage from the earlier to the later stage is an interaction between the capitals of the two. Each operation is credited to the group of instruments earlier in the series and debited to the group next later in the series.

3. Transportation: Interactions which Change the Position of Wealth

The second class of interactions we have called " transportation." It is a very slight distinction which separates this class from the preceding class. Transforming or producing wealth consists in changing the position of its parts as related to one another; transporting wealth consists mechanically in changing the position of that wealth as a whole. But " part " and "whole " are themselves loose and relative terms. Bookbinding is a transformation or production of wealth; it assembles the paper, leather, thread, and paste into a whole book. Delivering the finished book to a library is transportation. Yet the library is, in a sense, a whole; and to assemble books into a classified and organized library is to make a whole out of parts and may be regarded as a transformation or production of wealth. The distinction between transformation and transportation is thus merely one of convenience. Many writers prefer to include them both under " production." We prefer to include them under the less ambiguous and more inclusive head of " interactions," and our object here is not to emphasize their difference but their similarity. The principles already discussed of coupling and canceling equal and opposite items apply also to transportation. The following are examples. When merchandise is transmitted from one warehouse to another, the stock in the first warehouse is credited with the change and that in the second, debited. The stock which has rendered up the merchandise has done a service; that which has received it is charged with a cost. A banker who takes money from his vault and puts it into his till will, if he keeps separate accounts for the two, credit the vault and debit the till. When wheat is carried from wheatfield to barn the wheatfield is credited and the barn debited. When wheat is imported from Canada, Canada is credited, and the United States debited.

4. Exchange: Interactions which Change the Ownership of Wealth

The third class of interactions is the change of ownership of wealth or of property. This has been called " transfer." Every transfer is a species of interaction. If two dollars are transferred from Smiths cash drawer to Joness, Smiths cash drawer is credited with the two dollars yielded up, and Joness is debited with receipt of the same. Transfers usually occur in pairs, and involve two objects transferred in opposite directions between two owners. One transfer pertains to each object. Such a double transfer we have called an exchange. Since an exchange consists of two transfers, and since a transfer is a species of interaction and as such is self-canceling, every exchange is self-canceling, and hence cannot be counted as a part of the total income of society unless it be counted out again (although it may lead to later items which are not self-canceling). Whatever is credited on one side is debited on the other. This is shown in the following scheme which gives the credits and debits involved when goods worth 2 are sold. The dealer credits his stock of goods and debits his " cash," while the buyer does the

	Stocks or Goods	Stocks Of Cash
Sellers	Cr. 2	Dr. 3
Buyers	Dr. 2	Cr. 2

opposite. We see, then, that an exchange, whether of goods against goods or of goods against money, occasions an element of income to the seller equal to the corresponding element of outgo to the purchaser, and an element of outgo to the seller equal to the corresponding element of income to the purchaser, and therefore no immediate income at all to society.

The effect of canceling these items–the credit item of the seller and the debit item of the purchaser–is to free the income account for any article from all entanglements with exchange, to wipe out all money-income, and to leave exposed to view the direct or natural income from that article. Thus books yield their natural income, not when the book dealer sells them, but later when the reader peruses them. The sale is a mere preparatory service, a credit item to the book dealer, and a debit item to the buyer.

Only the book remains in the hands of the purchaser. Again, a forest of trees yields no natural income until the trees are felled and pass into the next stage of logs. The owner of the forest may, to be sure, " realize " on the forest long before it is ready to be cut, by simply selling it to another. To the seller the forest has then yielded income; but, as the purchaser has suffered an equal outgo, the net result of this interaction, as of every other, is zero. Only the forest remains ready for future use. Similarly, the money " rent " of a rented house is, for society, not income at all. It is income to the landlord, but outgo to the tenant–outgo which he is willing to suffer solely because of the shelter he receives. As we may cancel the landlords money-income against the tenants money-outgo, it is clear that the shelter alone remains as the income from the house. The shelter-income is the essential and abiding item, and without it there could be no rent-income to the landlord. Thus we see clearly the fallacy of the old view that a dwelling yields income only when it is rented. In like manner, a railway yields as its natural income solely the transporting of goods and passengers. Its owners sell this transportation service for money, and regard the railway simply as a money-maker; but to the shippers and passengers this same money is an expense, and exactly offsets the railways money earnings. Of the three items–money-income of the road, money-outgo of its patrons, and transportation–the first two mutually cancel and leave only the third, transportation, as the real contribution of the railway to the sum total of income.

We do not mean, of course, that interactions are useless, but simply that in the accounting of society they are self-canceling. They are a necessary step toward achieving the final income which remains uncanceled, but they themselves disappear under the method of couples. We see that capital is not a money-making machine, but that its income to society is simply its services of production, transportation, and gratification. The income from the farm is the yielding of its crops; from the mine, the giving up of its ore; from the factory, its transformation of raw into finished products; from commercial capital, the passage of goods between producer and consumer; from articles in consumers hands, their enjoyment or so-called " consumption." Although these items are all measured in terms of money, they do not consist of money receipts. Those items which do consist of money receipts are money receipts for individuals, never for the world as a whole; since each dollar received by one person implies that some other person–the one from whom it was received–expended it.

Similar principles apply to outgo, no part of which, for society, occurs in money form. The great bulk of what merchants call " cost of production," expense, or outgo, consists of money costs which, as concerns society, carry with them their own cancellation, and so are not ultimate costs at all. For manufacturers, merchants, and other business men, almost every outgo is an expense, i. e., consists of a money payment. But such money payments are for wages, raw materials, rent, and interest charges, all of which are incomes for other people. The wages are the earnings of labor; the payment for raw material is received by some other manufacturer, farmer, or miner; the rent is received by the landlord; the interest charges, by the creditor. Labor itself–human effort, not the payment for it–remains, however, uncanceled.

5. Accounts Illustrative of Interactions in Production

Not only do money transactions completely cancel themselves out in reckoning the total income of society, but the great majority even of the natural benefits of capital do the same. Even these natural benefits of capital consist for the most part of " interactions "; they are transformations or transportations of wealth. They are intermediate stages, merely preparatory to the final enjoyable benefits of wealth, and, after the interactions have been canceled out, do not enter as items either on the income or the outgo side of the social balance sheet. In order to show the effect of canceling out the equal and opposite items entering into every interaction throughout all productive processes, let us observe the various stages of production which begin with the forest above referred to. The gross income produced by the forest is the series of events called the turning out of logs. This log production is a mere preparatory service, a credit item to the forest and a debit item to the stock of logs of the sawmill, to which the logs next pass. Next the sawmill turns its logs into lumber, and is therefore credited with its share in this transformation while the lumber yard is debited with the production of lumber. Intermediate categories may, of course, be created, and we may follow, in like manner, the further transformation, transportation, and exchange to the end of the stages of production–or rather, to the ends; for these stages split up and form several streams flowing in different directions. To follow one only of these streams, let us suppose that the lumber which goes out from the yard is used in repairing a certain warehouse. The warehouse is used for storing cloth; the cloth goes from the warehouse to the tailor; the tailor converts the cloth into suits for his customers; and his customers receive and wear those suits. In this series of productive services, all the intermediate services cancel out in " couples " and leave as the only uncanceled ele ment, or fringe of final services, the use of clothes in the consumers possession.

Should we stop our accounts, however, at earlier points in the series, the uncanceled fringe at which we should find ourselves would be some other item. The uncanceled income item in a production series is always the positive side of some intermediate service or interaction whose negative side does not appear, as it belongs to a later stage in the series. This will be clear if we put the matter in figures, stage by stage. The following are the items for the logging camp above mentioned, in the accounts of its owner.

INCOME ACCOUNT FOR LOGGING CAMP Income

Outgo

Yielding of logs to sawmill. 50,000

The income from the logging camp is here seen to consist in the production of 50,000 worth of logs. Of course there are usually large outgoes; but as these do not concern our present point, for simplicity we leave them out of account. If we now combine the account of the logging camp with that of the sawmill, we shall have accounts like the following, in which, to avoid irrelevant complications, no mention is made of any outgoes which do not happen to be interactions between the groups of capital considered:– INCOME ACCOUNT FOR LOGGING CAMP AND SAWMILL

Capital Source Income Outgo

Logging camp. Sawmill Yielding logs to saw-mill. 50,000 Yielding lumber to lumber yard 60,000

Receiving logs from camp. 50,000

0 O O
8 8 8
a 8 o 0 0 Q
o0 0 o
p . Si .
c. E 3 M . 2
S i U 2 . j
to i
8 ff rt P . 0
S o S S 1
a O t-. s o
0 1 E
c V Q +3
XI XI a (/
S 3 p S o 3
o 5 a en
. f I 60 to no
. V o.-
8 1 o 1 O 4;
o 6 W3 s M
o 1 0 oooo6 8 1
vo S 10 and
t 1 .
3 C
b 0
Income to sawmill ler to lumb(ier t0 ware! O TJ J to custome
o 3
4-1 pb "o 2 a
a E S en 1
i a i
u
to bo bfi 3 tc eo to
C . s o c . S . S
J3 2 1 3 2 2
4) w V o "a "o
x
. , . . w . a
u
i B , B O B g
H . S Q 2
I a i
and . s o o
tfi
Capital Logging camp Sawmill. Lumber yard Warehouse. 0 T3 0 St0ck 0f cl0the
3

0 –

O

1 en 1

C/3 In this case, canceling the two log items of 50,000 each, we have left only the lumber item; that is, the net income from the combined logging camp and sawmill consists only of the production of lumber, their final product. The transfer of logs from one department to the other no longer appears. This transfer is like the taking of money from one pocket and putting it into another–a fact which would be particularly evident in case the logging camp and sawmill were combined under the same management.

Extending the same principles to the entire series, we have the accounts as given in the table on the preceding page.

In this table we may successively cancel each pair of items constituting an inter-action. An item on the left is the positive side of an interaction of which the item on the right in the line next below is the negative side. Thus, as previously, the 50,000 in the first line on the left cancels the 50,000 in the second line on the right. Similarly, the two items of 60,000 cancel in the two lines next below, to the right and left, respectively. If we stop after the first two cancellations, thus restricting the account to the first three horizontal lines of the table, we shall find that the net income from logging camp, sawmill, and lumber yard consists only of the production of retail lumber, worth 70,000; it includes neither the transfer of logs from the camp to the mill nor the transfer of lumber from the mill to the yard. In like manner, if we proceed one stage further, i. e., if we stop our cancellations at the end of the first three interactions, the production of retail lumber no longer appears as an element of income; and so on, step by step to the end, when the only surviving item will be the " wear " of the suits.

It is, of course, true that in any actual accounts there will be other items besides those which have been exhibited in this simple, chainlike fashion. Were it worth while, we might insert these additional entries of income and outgo elements. Most of them would likewise consist of the positive or the negative side of interactions; and if we were to

introduce their respective mates, the opposite aspects of the same interactions, it would be necessary to include the accounts of still other instruments. If we should follow up all such leads, we should soon have, instead of the simple chain represented in the table, an intricate network of related accounts; but the same principle of the interaction as a self-effacing element would continue to apply.

6. Preliminary Results of Combining these Income

Accounts

The table given will throw light on the question: Of what does income consist? or, to be more definite: Of what does the income from a particular group of capital-goods consist? Whether the yielding of logs by the logging camp to the sawmill is income or not depends upon what capital we are including. It is income with respect to the first link of capital in our series (the logging camp); it is not income with respect to the first two links (the logging camp and the sawmill taken together), but merely a self-canceling interaction between the two. Likewise the use of the warehouse is income with respect to the first four links of capital, but is not income with respect to the first five links.

We see, therefore, that in reckoning up the income from any group of capital we may as well omit all interactions taking place within it, and confine ourselves to the outer fringe of services performed by the group as a whole. As the group is enlarged, this particular outer fringe disappears by being joined to the next part of the economic fabric, and another fringe still more remote appears. To answer the question whether any particular item is or is not income–as, for instance, the question, "Is sawing lumber income?"–we must first ask, "Income from what?" Income is always relative to its source.

Contrasting the method of couples with the method of balances, we may say that the method of couples is useful in showing of what elements income consists in any given case. The method of balances, on the other hand, is useful in exhibiting the amount of income contributed from each capital source. The two methods, as applied to the example just given, are as follows:– (Summarized from Table on p. 86)

METHOD OF BALANCES

Capital ncome Outgo Net Income
Logging camp i;0.000 "; o,000
Sawmill 60,000 50.000 10,000
Lumber yard 70,000 60,000 10,000
Warehouse 80,000 70,000 10,000
Stock of cloth in warehouse Stock of cloth of tailor. Stock of clothes of customers
90,000 500,000 600,000 80,000 90,000 500,000 10,000 410,000 100,000
600,000

METHOD OF COUPLES Income

Outgo

The two methods–balances and couples–show the same final result (600,000), but from different points of view. By means of the method of balances we are enabled to see that, of this 600,000, the part contributed by the logging camp is 50,000, that contributed by the sawmill, 10,000, and so on. By means of the method of couples, we are enabled to see that, canceling by the oblique lines, we have left but one item, 600,000, representing the

"wear" of the suits. Thus the entire 600,000 consists of the use or "wear" of the suits, although five-sixths of it is contributed by other kinds of capital than the stock of clothes of customers. Combining the results of both methods, we may state that the total net income from the specified group of instruments consists of 600,000 worth of

"wear " of suits, and that this is due partly to the stock of clothes and partly to other capital. Of course our table does not give all the capital to which the wear of the suits is indebted. We have, as already noted, omitted, for the sake of simplicity, all items of cost which do not belong to our chosen series. But the inclusion of other items, while it complicates the accounts, does not change the principle of cancellation. It merely introduces other chains of interactions.

7. Analogies with Capital Accounting

The two methods correspond in a general way to the two methods for canceling liabilities and assets in capital accounts. Applied to capital, the method of balances gave, it will be remembered, the amount of capital belonging to each individual; the method of couples showed of what elements the total capital consists. Similarly, applied to income, the method of balances shows what share of the resulting income is contributed by any articles or groups of articles of capital; while the method of couples shows wherein that resulting income consists.

Let us consider for a moment the method of couples as applied to the two sorts of accounts. In capital accounts the self-effacing items were debts; in income accounts the self-effacing items were interactions. These concepts– debts and interactions– supply the key for the mutual cancellations between accounts. A debt is both positive and negative and so is self-canceling. An interaction is likewise both positive and negative and so self-canceling. A realization of the two-faced nature of debts helps us to avoid the confusions of double counting in capital accounts and double taxation; a realization of the two-faced nature of interactions saves the confusions of double counting in income accounts.

It is important here to observe of income, as was previously observed of capital (Chapter III, 8), that the self-effacement of the self-effacing elements (interactions in the case of income) does not mean that the total income would be just the same if there were no interactions. On the contrary, the existence of interactions–the operations of industry and commerce–are essential steps toward the final goal of uncanceled income to which they lead. Without them the final uncanceled income would be very much less and often nonexistent. Debts mean subdivided ownership of capital and interactions mean subdivided steps in income. They make capital and income respectively more abundant and effective.

We may illustrate what has been said by two simple examples. If a man owns a piece of real estate worth 10,000 and mortgages it for 6000, this debt must be entered in his accounts as a liability of 6000 and in the accounts of the mortgagee as an asset of 6000. Consequently, as between the two men the item cancels out. But this does not mean that the mortgage is of no account. It does not mean that the two men would be just as well off if there were no mortgage. If we should force them against their will to cancel the debt, it would be an inconvenience to both. The owner would find it difficult to make the payment and the mortgagee would have the inconvenience of finding another investment for the 6000 returned to him. The inconvenience to the owner might be so great that he would be forced to sell his land perhaps at a sacrifice below the 10,000 which is its real worth, while if the mortgage is allowed to stand, he might not be willing to sell even for a sum considerably above the 10,000. The inconvenience to the mortgagee might be less.

We find the same thing true of interactions. A bookseller who sells 2000 worth of books in the course of a year credits his business with this sum while his customers debit their libraries with 2000 worth of books. These entries are evidently correct accounting, and the receipts of the bookseller and the expenditures of his customers exactly offset each other. But this does not mean that the transactions are of no account. Without them the bookseller would find a great accumulation of books which would be entirely useless to him while his customers would be deprived of the satisfaction of reading these books. If we could force the reversal of the normal process and make the customers resell their books to the dealer, there would be an obvious loss to both parties. The dealer would refuse to take them except at a price far below the 2000, while their possessors would not be willing to sell them unless for more than 2000.

8. Double Entry in Accounts of Fictitious Persons

We have now followed the cancellations to which interactions lead, whether they be interactions of exchange or of production. The case of exchange, however, needs further consideration. Since every exchange consists of two transfers, and every transfer of two items, a credit and a debit, the exchange evidently consists of four items in all, two of which are credits and two of which are debits. These four may be paired off in two ways, only one of which has thus far been mentioned. They stand, as it were, at the four corners of a square, as in the scheme given in 4.

The two transfers into which any exchange may be resolved are represented by the second and third columns of that scheme. The second column indicates that a 2 article has been transferred from the stock of the seller to that of the buyer, being, therefore, credited to the one and debited to the other; the third column indicates that 2 of money has been transferred from the stock of cash of the buyer to that of the seller and credited and debited accordingly. But this same exchange may also be resolved into two pairs of items represented by the two horizontal lines of the scheme. The upper line indicates that the seller has exchanged goods for cash crediting his goods with the sale and debiting his cash; the lower line indicates the reverse conditions for the buyer.

Every exchange, then, consists of four items, and may be resolved either into two transfers (one for each good exchanged) or into two transactions (one for each person exchanging those goods).

These latter items, namely, transactions represented by the horizontal lines, we must now consider more fully. Each of the previous income accounts is an account of income flowing from a specified good owned, not of the entire income received by a given person as owner. But it is easy now to form the income accounts of any given person, i. e., the income and outgo of all his assets and liabilities, simply by combining in each case, by the method of balances, the accounts of all his items of property (whether assets or liabilities). We must distinguish, however, the accounts of real and of fictitious persons. We begin with the income account of a fictitious person.

The following account represents the entries during a given year for a dry goods company. In this account we observe that every item on the income side is balanced by an equal and opposite item on the outgo side. All items thus paid are represented by the same letters, the capitals being used for positive items and the small letters for negative.

INCOME AND OUTGO OF A DRY GOODS COMPANY FOR 1910

Capital Source Income Outgo

Stock of goods By goods sold 10,000 A To goods bought 5,000 b
Cash. By cash taken out for purchases 5,000 B for profits 2,000 C To cash received from sales. 10,000 a
Capital Stock. (a liability) To dividends 2,000 c

The rule we have learned in Chapter IV for making complete income accounts is to start with the capital account, taking each item of assets and each item of liabilities, and to enter for each item of either kind all the items of income to which they give rise, plus or minus, as the case may be. For simplicity, it is here assumed that, instead of fifty or one hundred different items of capital, there are only three items; namely, the stock of goods, the stock of cash, and the " capital stock," which is " negative capital." The stock of goods yields 10,000 worth of sales. But, on the other hand, it costs 5000 to replenish this stock of goods. Therefore it is credited with a plus item of 10,000, and debited with a minus item of 5000. The student will notice, moreover, that each of these items is entered twice, once on each side. The doubly entered items may be mutually canceled. A cancels with a; that is, though the stock of goods is credited with bringing in 10,000 (A) in cash, the cash drawer must be debited with the 10,000 (a) which it swallows up. Likewise the stock of goods costs 5000 (b), which must therefore be debited to it; but the cash drawer has to supply this 5000, and is therefore credited with 5000 (B), so that items B and b cancel. Finally, when the profits are paid, they also come out of the cash drawer, and the cash drawer is

credited with exactly that amount, 2000 (C); while the " capital stock " is debited with that amount as a cost (c). So we see that all six items cancel one another in pairs. The two sides of the account of such a fictitious person necessarily balance. Even if the company accumulates its profit instead of paying it in dividends to the shareholders, the two sides of its account still balance; for, as has been seen, all money received is not only credited to the capital source which brought it in, but is also debited to the cash account. Here, for instance, the 2000 item (doubly entered as C and c) would merely be omitted. There would be no 2000 dividends, but the cash drawer would be 2000 fuller.

9. Double Entry in Accounts of Real Persons In the case of real persons, however, the two sides do not balance, for the accounts do not then consist solely of double entries. To show this, let us consider the accounts of a real person as given in the next table. In these accounts, as in the previous ones, both of which are much simplified, we have indicated the like items on opposite sides by like letters, the positive items being represented by capitals and the negative by small letters. We observe that, as in the accounts of the previous company, many of the items will " pair." But, unlike the companys accounts, the present accounts contain a residue of items which will not pair. The letters representing these unpaired items are designated on the next page by being inclosed in square brackets. They show that B and C–the shelter of the house, and the use of food–constitute a kind of income which does not appear elsewhere as outgo.

When studying the accounts of goods owned, we found in considering the chain of productive services of a lumber camp, etc., that there always remains some outer fringe of uncanceled income. We have now reached this same kind INCOME AND OUTGO OF A REAL PERSON FOR THE YEAR 1910

Capital Source Income Outgo
Stocks and bonds By receipt of money from stocks and bonds 2000. 1 To money expended for stocks and bonds. 500./
Lease right. By shelter. 100 B To money rent paid. Si oo e
Food. By use of food. f15o C To money cost of food. 150 /
"Cash". By cash taken out for stocks and bonds 500 I) To receipt of money from stocks and bonds. 2000 a To receipt of money for work done. 2000 g
By payment for rent 100 E By payment for food 150 F

Self. By receipt of money for work done. 2000 G
Uncanceled items: Shelter B. 100
   Use of food C. 150
   Total uncanceled income. 250 of outer fringe in studying the accounts of owners, provided they are real persons. This outer fringe consists of the final benefits of their goods. All other items are merely interactions preparatory to such final benefits, and pass from one category of capital to another. Thus the income from investments, being paid into the cash drawer, is outgo with respect to the drawer; the drawer yields income by paying for stocks and bonds, food, etc., but in each case the same item enters as outgo with respect to these or other categories of capital. In all these cases the individual receives no income which is not at the same time outgo. It is only as he receives shelter from the house, consumes food, wears clothes, or uses furniture, or some other article, that he receives income. And these final benefits are, of course, the end and goal of all the preceding economic processes and activities.

We have thus reached what may be called the stage of final or enjoyable income. This is the stage at which wealth at last acts upon the person of the recipient. This final income is that of which the economist is in search, and is that which the ordinary statistics of workingmens expenditures represent. It has been made clear that, in the final net income which we derive from wealth, all interactions between different articles of wealth drop out–all the transformations of production, such as the operations of mining, agriculture, and industry, all the operations of transportation, and all transfers and exchanges in business. For in all such cases the debits and credits inevitably occur in pairs of equal and opposite items. Each pair consists of the opposite facets of the same interaction. The only items which survive are the final personal uses of wealth. The chief classes of such uses or benefits are those of nourishment, shelter, and clothing.

Having reached the action of wealth on the human body, we may, as students of economics, be content to stop. But, theoretically, there is one step more before the process of tracing a series of interactions has reached its final goal. Indeed, no benefits outside ourselves are of significance to us except as they lead to feelings within our minds. And if we regard the human body in the same light in which we have regarded articles of wealth, we could extend our accounts by conceiving wealth as interacting with the human body. We would then debit the human body with the nourishment, shelter, protection from cold, etc., which it receives from food, dwellings, clothing, etc., and credit it with the satisfactions experienced through the brain, i. e., the feelings of enjoyment of food or avoidance of pain, etc. As, however, we have in general, in this textbook, limited the concept of wealth to its narrower definition, excluding free human beings, we shall not attempt to follow these transformations of income after they reach the person of the owner. Usually the mental satisfactions follow so closely after the physical effects of wealth on the human body that practically we scarcely need to distinguish between those physical effects and the resulting satisfactions. Hereafter we shall speak of satisfactions of food, shelter, clothing, etc., as if they flowed directly from these external objects.

   10. Ultimate Costs and Income

We have now reached a convenient place at which to emphasize a point of great importance, but one which is seldom understood; namely, that most of what is called " cost of production " is, in the last analysis, not cost at all. We have found, in using the method of couples, that every item of money cost is also an item of income, and that in the final total no such items survive cancellation. It costs the baker flour to produce bread; but the cost of flour to the baker is a benefit to the miller. To society as a whole, on the other hand, it is neither cost nor benefit, but a mere interaction.

As has been said, in the last analysis, payments of wages, interest, rent, or any other payments from one member of society to another, are not costs to society as a whole. This fact should now be clear; yet it is commonly overlooked. When people talk of the cost of producing coal or wheat, they usually think of money payments. The items called costs of production are mostly payments from person to person, or interactions, at various stages of production. We have seen that each such item is two-faced and, in the final total, wipes itself off the slate. The only ultimate item of cost is labor cost or efforts; that is, all the experiences of an undesirable nature which are undergone in order that experiences of a desirable nature may be secured. We may conclude, therefore, that in the last analysis income consists of satisfactions and outgo of efforts to secure satisfactions. Between efforts and satisfactions may intervene innumerable interactions, but they all must cancel out in the end. They are merely the machinery connecting the efforts and satisfactions. At bottom, economics treats simply of efforts and satisfactions. This is evident in the case of an isolated individual like Robinson Crusoe, who handles no money; but it is equally true of the most highly organized society, though obscured by the fact that each member of such a society talks and thinks in terms of money.

In the light of the foregoing principles we are now in a position to take a birds-eye view of the income of any country. Unfortunately, there are no available statistics for income in the United States. We can only guess as to what the amount of it may be. Possibly 20,000,000,000 worth of final income is annually enjoyed in the United States, of which about one third is in the form of nourishment or food uses, about one sixth in the form of shelter, and about one eighth in the form of clothing. These and the other items of the direct uses of wealth constitute the real income of society. In other words, our real income is what is often called our " living." Money-income, as we have seen, is not real income, but is converted or spent for real income in what we call our " bread and butter," which, more exactly expressed, means the use of our " bread and butter " and of the other goods contributing direct benefits to human beings. These uses include the necessaries, comforts, luxuries, and amusements of life. These are what make up our " living." The more money wages it costs to acquire a given amount of real wages, the higher the "cost of living" of which we hear so much to-day. The money which the workman is paid in wages is not his real wages, but only his nominal wages. The real wages are the workmans living for which that money is spent. Money payments, as we have seen, cancel themselves out when we take a view of the whole, for they are not only receipts, but also payments. They therefore disappear, just as in our view of capital the bonds and stocks disappear, being not only assets, but also liabilities. And in exactly the same way the operations of production and transportation cancel themselves out in the total production of the farms. The ten billions of dollars worth of farm products, for instance, which we are producing are not a part of the income of the country to be added to our consumption of food, etc., any more than they are a part of the costs of the country. To the farmer they represent income, but to those who buy of the farmer they represent outgo, while to the country as a whole they represent neither income nor outgo. By the method of couples they vanish, and in their stead we have the consumption of bread and the other finished products which originated with the farm; and should we, as is sometimes erroneously done, try to add together the value of these finished products and the value of the farm products, we should be guilty of double counting, as would be the case in capital accounting if we should add the value of mortgages to the value of real estate.

The method of couples thus provides us with a view of real income, making clear what it consists of and what it does not consist of. If, however, we wish to know the extent to which various agencies have produced this income, we must look at the matter from the standpoint of the method of balances. From this standpoint, perhaps three quarters of the total income enjoyed in the country is nroduced by human beings, the workers of sor1 ider being produced by capital in its nar this capi tal that which produces the greater part of our income is land, but some of our income must also be credited to railways, ships, factories, shops, dwellings, etc. It does not matter whether the capital is or is not itself the product of other capital, of human beings, or of nature. There will usually be a net income to be credited opposite each, kind of capital, as shown in the table of the Method of Balances in 6.

CHAPTER VI

CAPITALIZING INCOME 1. The Link between Capital and Income

We have now learned what capital and income are, and how each is measured. We have seen that the term " capital " is not to be confined to any particular part or kind of wealth, but that it applies to any or all wealth existing at a given instant of time, or to property rights in that wealth, or to the values of that wealth or of those property rights. We have seen that income is not restricted to money-income, but that it consists of all kinds of benefits of wealth. We have seen that, like capital, income may be measured either by the mere quantity of the various benefits or by the value of those benefits. We have seen that in the addition both of capital-value and of income-value there are two methods available for canceling positive and negative items, called respectively the " method of balances " and the " method of couples." By the method of balances the negative items in any individual account are deducted from the positive items in the same account, and the difference or " balance " gives the net capital (or income, as the case may be) with which that account deals, whether this net capital (or income) pertains to a particular instrument or instruments, or to all the property of a particular owner. The method of couples, on the other hand, cancels items in pairs and is founded on the fact that, as to capital, every liability relation has a credit as well as a debit side– namely, as related to creditor and debtor respectively; and that, as to income, every interaction is at once a benefit and a cost–a benefit occasioned by that good (or person) by which the event originates; a cost occasioned by that good (or person) for which it originates.

We observed that it is the method of couples alone which, if fully carried out, reveals wherein capital and income ultimately consist. This method, applied to capital, gradually obliterates all partial rights, such as stocks and bonds, and exposes to view the concrete capital-wealth of a community. The same method applied to income obliterates the "interactions" such as money payments between persons, and exposes to view an uncanceled outer fringe of benefits and costs. It leaves simply the final benefIts of the wealth, poured, so to speak, into the human organism—the satisfactions and the efforts of human life.

We have seen that capital and income are in many re-pects correlative; that all capital yields income and that all income flows from capital including human beings.

In spite of this close association between them, capital and income have thus far been considered separately. The question now arises: How can we calculate the value of capital from that of income or vice versa? The bridge or link between them is the rate of interest. The rate of interest is the ratio between income and capital, both the income and the capital being expressed in money value. Business men, therefore, sometimes call the rate of interest the "price of capital " or the " price of ready money." Suppose, for instance, that a merchant wants a capital worth 10,000 and is willing to pay a bank 400 per year for it perpetually; then the price the merchant pays for the capital (or the ratio between the annual payment to the bank and the capital received from it) is 400-=-10,000 = T, or four per cent, and the rate of interest is, therefore, said to be four per cent.

We may also define the rate of interest as the premium on goods in hand at one date in terms of goods of the same kind to be in hand one year later. Present and future goods seldom exchange at par. One hundred dollars, if in hand to-day, is worth more than if due one year hence. To-days ready money will always buy the right to more than its full value of next years money. If, then, 100 to-day will exchange for 104 to be received one year hence, the premium —or rate of interest—is four per cent. That is, the price of to-days money in terms of next years money is four per cent above par; for 104-r-100 exceeds 100-5-100 by tfa, which is four per cent.

We have, then, two definitions of the rate of interest, viz., " the price of capital in terms of income " and " the premium which present goods command over similar goods due one year hence."

But the two definitions are quite consistent, and either definition may be converted into the other. The rates of interest in the two senses are, in fact, normally equal. For instance, if a man borrows 100 to-day and agrees to pay it back in one year with interest at four per cent, we may conceive of him as selling for 100 a perpetual income of 4 a year—and at the same time agreeing to buy it back for 100 at the end of one year. But these two stipulations—to sell and to buy back—amount simply to an exchange of 100 to-day for 104 next year–i. e., an exchange of present for future money at four per cent. Thus the rate of interest in the price sense becomes equivalent to the same rate in the premium sense. Or, beginning at the other end, conversely if we suppose 100 to-day to be exchanged for 104 due one year hence, so that the rate of interest in the premium sense is four per cent, we may suppose that when the time comes to receive the 104, only 4 of it is really kept, the 100 being again exchanged for 104 due the year following. If this process is repeated indefinitely, the man will continue to receive simply 4 a year; and thus the rate of interest in the premium sense becomes equivalent to the same rate in the price sense.

By means of the rate of interest we can evidently translate, as it were, present money-value into its equivalent future money-value, or future money-value into its equivalent present money-value. To translate any present value into next years value, when interest is four per cent, we multiply this years value by the factor 1.04; to translate any next years value into this years value, we divide next years value by the factor 1.04. Thus if the rate of interest is four per cent, 25 to-day is the equivalent of 25 X 1.04 due one year hence, i. e., 26. Or, vice versa, 26 due one year hence is worth in the present 26-1-1.04, or 25. Again, 1 due one year hence is worth in the present 1-5-1.04, or 0.962. In general we may obtain the present worth of any sum due one year hence by dividing that sum by one plus the rate of interest. This latter operation is what we learned in our school arithmetics as " discounting," by which is meant finding the "present worth " of a given future sum. The rate of interest is thus a link between values at any two points of time–a link by means of which we may compare values at any different dates.

The rate of interest, however defined, may be regarded as a species of price; but it is a very different species from any prices mentioned in previous chapters. We have seen that the price of wheat enables us to translate any given number of bushels of wheat into so many dollars worth of wheat; and the prices of other goods in like manner, to translate their respective quantities into their money equivalents. Any price thus serves as a bridge or link between the quantity of any good and its value in some other good, as money. By means of prices we can convert a miscellaneous assortment of goods at any time into their money-value for that same time, or convert a miscellaneous assortment of benefits occurring through a period of time into their money-value for that same period. By such prices we may only convert quantities into simultaneous money-values. We cannot, by them, pass from one time to another. By means, however, of that unique price called the rate of interest, we may convert the money-values found for one time into their equivalent at another time. The rate of interest is thus the hitherto missing link necessary to make our reckoning of money equivalents universal.

We are not yet ready to explain how the rate of interest comes about. In fact, we are not yet ready to explain how any prices come about. We must, for the present, take the rate of interest ready-made, as it were, just as we have taken other prices ready-made. In the preceding chapters we have seen how to form capital accounts and income accounts by assuming the prices necessary in each case to turn quantities into money-values. We are now ready, by assuming a rate of interest, to show the relations between these two sets of accounts–i. e., to turn income into capital. It is worth while, however, at the outset to rid our minds of the idea that money is the one and only source of interest, just as we have already rid our minds of the idea that money is the only kind of wealth. We may, as we have seen, express a great many things in terms of money-value which are not themselves money. This habit leads us unconsciously into the fallacy of thinking of these things as though they were actual money. If we question a man who says, "I have 10,000 of money invested, and from it I get 500 of money each year as interest," implying a rate of interest of five per cent, he will be forced to admit that he has not really got 10,000 of money at all, and, perhaps, even that the 500 of money interest which he says he gets each year is not at first in money form. The true form of statement is simply that he has a farm (or other capital-wealth) which yields crops (or other products), and that both of these may be measured in terms of money, the farm being worth 10,000 and the crops 500. Money need not enter at all except as a matter of evaluating in bookkeeping. Hence, if we are careful, we shall avoid thinking and speaking of a fund of 10,000 producing an interest of 500, but will instead think and speak of actual capital, such as farms, factories, railways, or ships, worth 10,000 and producing actual benefits (such as yielding crops, manufacturing cloth, or transporting goods) which are worth 500.

There is another confusion to be carefully avoided, viz., the confusion between interest and the rate of interest. If the interest from 10,000 worth of capital is 500 worth of benefits, the rate of interest is five per cent. Interest and the rate of interest are as distinct as value and price and in the same way.

The rate of interest, then, is a sort of universal time price representing the terms on which men consider this years values exchangeable in next years or future years values. By assuming this rate, we are enabled to convert future values into present, and present values into future.

2. Capital as Discounted Income

But although the rate of interest may be used either for computing from present to future values, or from future to present values, the latter process is far the more important of the two. Accountants, of course, are constantly computing in both directions, for they have both sets of problems to deal with; but the problem of time valuation which nature sets us is that of translating the future into the present; that is, the problem of ascertaining the value of capital. The value of capital must be computed from the value of its expected future income. We cannot proceed in the opposite direction and derive the value of future income from the value of present capital.

This statement may at first puzzle the student, for he may have thought of income as derived from capital, and, in a sense, this is true. Income is derived from capital-goods. But the value of the income is not derived from the value of those capital-goods. On the contrary, the value of the capital is derived from the value of the income. These re

lations are shown in the following scheme in which the arrows represent the order of sequence–from capital-wealth to its future benefits, from its benefits to their value; and from their value back to capital-value:–

Capital-wealth. Flow of benefits (income)

Capital-value—Income-value

Not until we know how much income an item of capital will bring us can we set any valuation on that capital at all. It is true that the wheat crop depends on the land which yields it. But the value of the crop does not depend on the value of the land. On the contrary, the value of the land depends on the value of its crop.

The present worth of anything is what men are willing to give for it. In order that each man may decide what he is willing to give, he must have: (1) some idea of the value of the future benefits his purchase will bring him, and (2) some idea of the rate of interest by which these future values may be translated into present values by discounting.

With these data he may derive the value of any capital from the value of its income by means of the connecting link between them called the rate of interest. This derivation of capital-value from income-value is called " capitalizing" income or " discounting " income.

3. The Discount Curve

Let us assume that, for any given article of wealth or property, the expected income is foreknown with certainty, and that the rate of interest is also known. With these provisos, it is very easy, by the use of the rate of interest, to compute the capital-value of said wealth or property; and this, whether the income accrues continuously or discon-tinuously; whether it is uniform or fluctuating; whether the installments of it are few or infinite in number.

We begin by considering the simplest case; namely, that in which the future income consists of a single item becoming due at some particular time. If, for instance, one holds a property right by virtue of which he will receive at the end of one year a benefit worth 1.04, the present value of this right, if the rate of interest is four per cent, will be 1. Or if the future benefit one year hence is worth 1, its present value (interest being at four per cent) is found, as we have seen in 1, by dividing the 1 by the factor 1.04. The result is 1-5-1.04, or 0.962. If the value to which the right entitles the owner is any other amount than 1, its present value is simply that given amount divided by 1.04. Thus the present value of 432 due in one year is 432-=-1.04, which is 415.38.

Let us now take a period of two years instead of one. We know by " compound interest " (at 4 per cent) that not only will 1 amount to 1.04 next year, but that this 1.04 next year will amount to 1.04 X 1.04 or 1.082 the year after,–in short, that 1 to-day amounts in two years to 1 X (1. c 4)2 or 1.082. Conversely, of course, the sum of 1.082 due two years hence is worth in present value 1.082-5-(1.04)2, or 1. Similarly, the present value of, let us say, 1000 due two years hence is 1000 -t-(1. o4)2 or 924.21. We see then that, if interest is 4 per cent, we can. by multiplying by (1. O4)2, translate any present sum into its equivalent two years hence, and we can, by dividing by (1. o4)2, translate any sum due two years hence into its equivalent present value.

By the same reasoning it is easy to show that we must multiply any sum in hand to-day by (1.04) to obtain the equivalent sum due three years hence, and must divide any sum due three years hence by (1.04) to obtain its present value. If the period is four years, we must multiply or divide by (1. O4)4; for five, by (1. o4)6, etc. For our present purposes we shall need to apply the process of division by (1.04) or (1. o4)2 or (1. o4)3, etc.; for our chief object is to translate future sums into present, not the reverse.

We may illustrate this process by a diagram, much in the same way as geography is illustrated by a map. Curves sometimes puzzle beginners, but they are very important in economics, and render the subjects which they illustrate so clear and simple that the student should not fail to make himself master of their use at the outset.

In Figure 3 the vertical distances measure the money and the horizontal distances measure the lapse of time. The sum of 100 (represented as bb) is supposed to be due at the beginning of the year 1001. The problem is to find its value at the point of time represented by a; that is, at the beginning of the year 1900, which we shall consider the "present instant " or simply the "present." This discounted value is a A. If we draw the line BA, its slope downward from right to left pictures the fact that a future sum becomes smaller and smaller in present value the longer the period of time involved. This line BA is called the discount curve. It is not a straight line, but a line such that its height at any point represents the discounted value of bb for the particular instant corresponding to that point. If the 100 due in 1001 be discounted in 1900 at four per cent, its value in the latter date will be 96.15, the difference in value between the two points of time being 3.85, as indicated in the diagram, where ac is equal to bb, and AC is the difference between ac or bb, the amount due in 1901, and a A, the discounted value of that amount in 1900.

We shall understand the nature of this curve better if, instead of taking merely the interval of one year, we consider a longer interval such as ten years. This is represented

3.85 c B

zr —.—-

b

00 60

70 60

50

40

30

1900 1901

Flo. 3.

in Figure 4. In this figure, as in the preceding figure, the vertical distances (or "latitudes") above the base line represent sums of money and the horizontal distances (or " longitudes") represent periods of time. The curve, ABC DM is the discount curve. The latitudes of these points (or their vertical distances above the base line, abcdm) represent the values of the same capital-good at different instants of time; and the longitudes or horizontal distances between them represent the intervals of time between those 1.50 I9OO 01

O7 OS O9 lo

Fig. 4.

instants. Thus, let the point a represent the present instant, say the beginning of the year 1900, and let the longitude interval, ab, represent a year, say from the beginning of 1900 to the beginning of 1901. Using equal intervals for successive years, we have aa representing any capital-value at the beginning of the year 1900, say 1, bb representing its equivalent next year, say 1.04, cc, the equivalent two years hence, and so on. We see that bb is what we have called the " amount," 1.04, of a A put out at interest for one year, and cc is the " amount " of the same compounded for two years. Conversely aa represents the present value in 1900, or discounted value, of any one latitude on the curve, such as bb, as well as of any other, such as cc or dd. The latitude of any point on the curve may thus be regarded as the " amount " of the sum represented by any preceding latitude or as the "present value" of the sum represented by any succeeding latitude. Thus, if the total breadth of the diagram am represents ten years, we may either say that mm is the amount, at the end of the ten years, of the present sum aa, or that a A is the "present value " of the future sum, mm, discounted for ten years. The line AM not only ascends, but at an accelerating rate–i. e., it does not ascend in a straight line, but gradually bends upward, being continually steeper toward the right. The slope of the curve is due to the rate of interest, and the greater the interest in any given period of time, the more steeply will the curve slope. This curve, if prolonged to the left to show what the " present value " was prior to the time a, will, of course, never reach the bottom line. It keeps becoming flatter and flatter, so that its distance above the line can never become zero.

If there were no rate of interest or if the rate of interest were zero, the curve would not slope at all, but would be a horizontal line.

4. Application to Valuing Instruments and Property

The principles which have been explained for obtaining the present value of a single future sum apply to many commercial transactions, such as to the valuation of bank assets, which exist largely in the form of " discount paper," or short-time loans of other kinds. The value of such a note is always the discounted value of the future payment to which it entitles the holder. Similarly, the value of any article of wealth, reckoned when that wealth is in course of construction, is the present value of what it will bring when com pleted (less the present value of the cost of completion). For instance, the maker of an automobile will, at any of its stages in the course of construction, appraise it as worth the discounted value of the price expected for it when finished and sold, less the discounted value of the costs of construction and selling which still remain. Thus, if an automobile is to be sold for 5000 and requires a year before this sum will be realized, while it will cost to complete a sale 2000, which sum for simplicity, we also assume is payable at the end of the year, the present value of the automobile will be the present value of 5000 minus 2000, which, at four per cent, will be (50x30–2000)-r-1.04, or 2884.62. The element of risk should not, of course, be overlooked; but its consideration does not belong here.

Another application of these principles of capitalization is to goods in transit. A cargo leaving Sydney for Liverpool is worth the discounted value of what it will bring in Liverpool, less the discounted value of the cost of carrying it there. Another good example is a young forest, which is worth the discounted value of the lumber it will ultimately form.

Ordinarily, however, we have to deal, not with one future sum, but with a series of future sums. A man who buys a bond or a share of stock is really buying the right to a series of future items of income. But we can treat a series of items of income by discount curves in exactly the same way that we can treat one such item.

For instance, let us consider a 100 " flve per cent" ten year bond. Such a bond is simply a promise to pay 5 each year for ten years and at the end of these ten years to pay in addition the "principal" sum of 100. The problem is to discover the present value of the bond. This is evidently the discounted value of the eleven sums which the owner will receive from the bond; in other words, the discounted value of the " principal," due ten years hence, together with the discounted values of the ten separate in terest payments due respectively one year, two years, three years, etc., up to and including ten years from date. As we have just seen how to get the discounted value of any one of these sums, it is simply a question of arithmetic to calculate them all and then add them together. Before we can perform the calculations, however, we must know what rate of interest to use. The mere fact that the bond is called a " five per cent" bond does not mean that those who buy the bond will calculate its present value to them by discounting its benefits at five per cent. The five per cent named in the bond is called the nominal rate of interest. It may or may not be the same as the rate of interest used by investors in ascertaining the present value of the bond. This latter rate is called the rate " realized."

If the rate realized happens to be the same as the nominal rate of interest, i. e., that named in bond, the present value of the bond will be par, or 100. This can be shown in various ways, as by calculating separately all the eleven different sums to which the bond entitles the owner; namely, the ten interest payments of 5 each and the final principal of 100. Such a calculation shows that the present value of the first interest payment of 5 (namely, that due one year hence) is 5 -s-1.05, or 4.76; that the present value of the second interest payment of 5 is 5–(1.05)2, or 4.55; that the present value of the third interest payment is 5-s-(1.05)3, or 4.32; that the present value of the fourth interest payment is 5-=-(1.05), or 4.11; and so on up to the tenth, the present value of which would be 5.5-(1.05)10 or 3.07. To this series must be added the present value of the principal, which, being discounted for ten years, is 100-=-(1.05)10, or 61.39. The sum of all these will be 4.76 + 4.55 + 4.32 + 4.1 1 + 3.92 + 3.73 + 3.55 + 3.38 + 3.22 + 3.07 + 61.39 = 100, which is the present value of the bond.-x

Another method of getting the same result is, beginning our calculation at the time when the bond falls due in the future, to proceed backwards, discounting year by year. It is evident that just before the payment of the bond it will be worth 105; for at that time there is immediately due 5 of interest and 100 of principal. Any time earlier in the ninth year, the value of the bond will evidently be the discounted value of this 100 and this 5, the discount being for whatever portion of the year may be involved. Just after the ninth interest payment, and just one year before the date when the 105 are due, the value of the bond will evidently be found by discounting 105 for one year at five per cent. This gives 105–1.05, or 100. In other words, the value of the bond at the end of nine years, just after the ninth interest payment, will be par, or 100. The instant preceding, namely, just before the ninth interest payment, the value of the bond will be more by the amount of interest payment, 5. That is, the value of the bond will be 105 just before the ninth interest payment and 100 just after. This sudden drop of 5 is due to the abstraction of the 5 of interest. For this reason, care is always taken by brokers at or near the time of interest payments to specify whether the bond is to be sold with the interest payment or without it, the higher price being paid if the bond is bought before the interest has been abstracted.

Thus, the instant before the ninth payment of interest the bond is worth 105, just as was the case the instant before the tenth and last payment. By the same reasoning, therefore, its value one year earlier, just after the eighth interest payment, will be 100 and just before, 105. In this manner we may proceed year by year back to the present, finding that the value of the bond will be 100 just after any interest payment and 105 just before. Its value will therefore be 100 just after the first interest payment, which occurs one year hence, and 105 just before that payment. The value of this 105 at the present instant will therefore be 100.

Reviewing these figures in the reverse order, we see that the value of the bond begins at 100, ascends to 105 one year from date, then drops suddenly to 100, ascends during the next year to 105, and then drops, and so on, ascending and dropping, as it were, by a series of teeth until the whole ten years have elapsed, when the value reaches its last height of 105 and then disappears altogether. In these oscillations, the gradual rise of 5 each year is evidently the interest accrued, while the sudden fall of 5 at the end of each year is the income taken out.

It is appropriate, here, to remind the student, that the entire height from the base line to any point in this tooth- 5 5 s 5 -, r: S c

too . r- 5

90 80 TO N B

60 50

40 SO 20 IO – g t

5 5 5 S 5 5 S 5 5

C 1 1 234-S678AA

Fig. 5.

like curve–whether at highest or lowest or anywhere between–represents the value of the capital at the corresponding instant of time. This should be constantly borne in mind.

The life history of such a bond can best be seen by the aid of Figure 5. The ten small, dark lines marked "5" standing on the base line MA (or the equivalents of these above the par line) and the long, dark line A B represent the eleven sums to which the bondholder is entitled; in other words, the small, dark lines representing the interest payments in the ten successive years, and AB, the principal, 100, due at the end of the ten years. The problem is: Given these eleven sums to which the bondholder is entitled, to show in the diagram the value of the bond at different dates. Assuming as before that the rate of interest used in computing is 5 per cent, we obtain the results seen in Figure 5. We observe that the value of the bond, just before it becomes due, is the sum of Aa (or BC, 5 of interest), and AB (the 100 of principal). This sum is represented by the vertical line AC. One year earlier, just after the ninth interest payment A a (or BC), the value of the bond is.4. B, or 100, being the discounted value of AC obtained by drawing the discount curve CB1. The value just before the ninth interest payment will be AC, or 105. Continuing in this manner backward, we obtain the series of " teeth," as indicated in the diagram.

If the various discount curves in Figure 5 are all continued to the left (as in Fig. 6), they will divide the line MN, representing the present value (100) of the bond, into the eleven parts of which it is composed, each part representing the present value of one of the eleven payments to which the bond entitles the owner. Thus the present value of the principal is seen to be 61.39, this being the height above M at which the lowest discount curve meets MN; the present value of the last or tenth interest payment is 3.07, this being the difference in height between the two lowest discount curves; the present value of the ninth interest payment is 3.22, as indicated in the next space above. Similarly, the present value of each of the other future payments is indicated in the diagram. The parts into which MN is divided thus form a picture of the eleven present values calculated earlier in this section.

As we pass from left to right in the diagram, we see that the value of the bond at the beginning of each year is 100, made up of the discounted values of all the remaining future receipts; and that the value increases each year along a discount curve to 105 at the end of the year, im- 1 v

t, 1 x"

x x" x S X X X X V, X

5, 5 and" 5 5 S

100 v g

,

90 , z . - e;

80 ,- 92. b. S- .

H -r

u i-. , "" " ,- "

;-. –"

EJ

. I.3S n q

5 5 5 S S 5 5 5 5 5

s e

Fig. 6.

A A mediately before the annual payment is made. The value then drops again to 100, when this annual income is received. It thus continues to oscillate (just as in Figure 5) between 100 and 105 each year to the end, when the final income of 105 is received.

But often the bond is not sold at par because the rate of interest used by the purchaser in calculating what he is willing to pay for it may be more or less than the five per cent named in the bond; in other words, the rate realized by the purchaser may be more or less than the nominal rate. When a bond is sold above par, this fact shows that the rate of interest realized by the investor is less than five per cent. In this case the bond is only nominally a " five per cent bond." If the rate used in calculating the value of the bond is four per cent, that value 108.17– n ? 5 x-and X 5-! and 3 2 . x-t 5. X 5, g 1

Par 1 Value 100 y 5

90 6

60 TO

60

80

40 40 2O IO ——

s 5 5 s – 5 s 5 S d s a 5

M i 3 A-S

F1G. 7.

will be found to be 108.17; so that if the bond is sold at 108.17, the purchaser is said to " realize" four per cent. It will be seen that the rate realized is that market rate which is actually used for discounting eleven items, namely the ten annual items of 5 each and the final item of 100. The value of the bond, 108.17, is found in the way already explained and is illustrated by the discount curves in Figure 7. Expressed arithmetically the calculation consists in adding together the following: the present value of the first payment of 5 (namely that due one year hence) which is 5-t-1.04, or

4.81, then that of the second which is 5.+. (r.04)2 and so on up to and including the present value of the principal which is 100–(1.04)0. The sum is 108.17.

Here the five per cent bond is said to be sold on a four per cent basis. Its capital-value (108.17), at the beginning of the period represented (i. e., the value of a five per cent bond, valued on a four per cent basis), is obtained just as before, except that we now reckon by discounting at four per cent instead of at five per cent. Thus, in Figure 7, we see that the value of the bond, just before it becomes due, is 105, or AC; that its value one year earlier, just after the ninth interest payment, is AB, or 105-5-1.04, or 100.96, and, just before the interest payment, is AC, or 100.96 + 5, or 105.96; and so on back to its value at the beginning, MN, which is thus found to be 1o8.17.1 This is greater by 8.17 than the value of the bond as reckoned on the five per cent basis. The fact that four per cent has been used in our calculations instead of five per cent has made all of the discount curves less steep.

We see, therefore, that nominally the rate of interest of the bond is not necessarily the actual rate of interest used in buying or selling that bond, and if the value of the bond is calculated on the basis of a rate of interest below the nominal rate of interest in the bond, the resulting value of the bond will be above par. Nominally the rate of interest is that named in the bond and, as previously noted, this is the actual rate of interest if the bond is worth par, but not otherwise. The actual rate is always that rate by which the actual value of the bond is calculated from the payments to which it entitles the holder. Tracing the history of the capital-value of the ten-year-five-per-cent bond reckoned at four per cent from the present toward the future, we may say that the rise in value during each 1 Of course, the same result could be obtained by discounting separately at four per cent each of the eleven items to which the bondholder is entitled and adding the results together. The elements of which MN is composed may then be easily indicated just as, for the previous example, in Figure 6.

X s 34s

Fro. 8.

year is the interest accrued during the year on the capital-value at the beginning of the year. Thus, the rise in value during the first year is four per cent of 108.17, or 4.32, and in the last year is four per cent of 100.96, or 4.038. It is also clear that the fall in the capital-value at the end of each year (except the last), when the payment of the nominal interest is made, is exactly 5. That is, the income taken out each year is greater than the interest accruing during the year; hence the general decline in the capital-value of the bond. In the last year the income taken out is 105; although if the investor is wise, he will put back at least 100 into some other bond or equivalent property.

The reverse is true if the present value of the bond is calculated on a six per cent basis, or on any other higher than the five per cent named in the bond. Figure 8 represents the case of a five per cent bond valued on a six per cent basis. In this case the discount curves are steeper than in Figure 5, and the value of the bond at present, ten years before it becomes due, is 92.61. In Figure 8, as in the preceding diagrams, we know that the rise of capital-value during any year is always the accruing interest on the capital-value at the beginning of that year. Thus, the rise in the first year will be six per cent of 92.61, that is, 5.55, and the rise during the last year will be six per cent of 99.05, namely, 5.95. It is also clear that the drop in capital-value at the end of each year is, as before, equal to the income taken out, or 5; that is, the income taken out each year is less than the interest accrued during the year; hence the general increase in the capital-value of the bond.

It will be seen (as shown in the three figures, 5,7, and 8) that the final value of the bond just before it becomes due will be 105 in all three cases, but that the present value is different in each case; namely, 100, 108.17, and 92.61. In each case the value zigzags year by year, but approaches in a general way 105 as its final value. If the " five per cent" bond is sold on an actual five per cent basis, the value of the bond is maintained year by year, as seen in Figure 5, where the curve indicating capital-value runs in general horizontally; if it is sold on a four per cent basis, its value in general decreases, as shown by the descending trend of the curve in Figure 7; while, if it is sold on a six per cent basis, it tends to increase in value, as shown by the general upward trend in Figure 8.

Elaborate tables have been constructed, called " bond-value books," calculated on the foregoing principles. They are used by brokers for indicating the true value of bonds on different bases; that is, the prices a man ought to pay for bonds, at different rates of interest and having different times in which to mature, in order to realize on them the market rate of interest. These tables are also used for solving the converse problem, viz., for finding the true rate of interest " realized " when a bond is bought at a given price. This rate realized will be the market rate, if the man has paid the right price, but sometimes he pays a wrong price. Given the market rate, we can deduce the right price to pay. Given the actual price paid, we can deduce the actual rate realized. The following table is an abridgment of these brokers tables, for a five per cent bond. The prices of such a bond are in all cases the prices immediately after an installment of interest has been received. In all cases the gradual increase in capital-value during any time is equal to the interest accruing during that time, while the sudden decrease at any time is equal to the value

RATES OF INTEREST

Five Per Cent Bond

Year . To Maturity

i s IO

102 3.0 4.6 4.8

101 4.0 4.8 4.9

100 S.0 S.0 S.0

99 6.1 5.2 5.1

98 7.1 5.5 5.3

of the income taken out at that time. The only exceptions to these statements are when capital-value varies up or down because of changed opinion as to the chances of future income; but we are here assuming that there are no uncertainties to be reckoned with.

From this table we see that if the so-called five per cent bond is sold at 102, and has one year to run, it will " yield " the investor three per cent; that is, if three per cent is used in calculating its value, th;s value will be 102. Again, if the bond has five years to run and is sold at 102, it will yield the investor 4.6 per cent; and if ten years, 4.8 per cent. If the bond is sold at 98 and has one year to run, it will yield the investor 7.1 per cent; if ten years, 5.3 per cent. If it is sold at par, it will yield five per cent, whatever may be the number of years it has to run.

The same principles as have just been applied to valuing bonds apply also to valuing any other article of property or wealth. The student will find it a useful exercise to draw diagrams for other cases. He may construct a series of diagrams, the vertical lines representing the successive items of income expected, and beginning at the last item proceed backward year by year, by a series of teeth, to obtain the present value of the capital. The value of the capital must always be first traced backward, but, after it has been obtained, we may retrace our steps.

The zigzag curves which have been indicated for bonds and which could be constructed for exhibiting the valuation of any other property right entitling the owner to definite sums of money or benefits of definite value at definite times are visual representations of the fact that the present value of any future benefit or collection of benefits gradually rises as the time grows near for their realization and suddenly falls as the realization occurs. The rate at which the value thus grows with time (between benefits-realized) is the rate of interest employed in these market valuations.

5. Effect of Changing the Rate of Interest

From what has been said, it is evident that the value of any article of capital depends very greatly on the rate of interest. If there were no rate of interest, or if, in other words, the rate of interest were zero, the value of the capital would be simply the sum of the values of the anticipated benefits. In the case of the five per cent bond, for instance, running for ten years, if reckoned on a zero per cent basis, its value would be simply the sum of the 100 and the ten interest payments, amounting to 50, or a total of 150. Since the rate of interest is always higher than zero, the value of the bond will always be lower than 150. To change the rate of interest will always change the value of capital in the opposite direction. For several generations the rate of interest has been falling, and consequently the value of bonds and of capital in general has tended to rise. Of course, the change in value of capital will be due also to many other circumstances than the change in the rate of interest, and, moreover, the effect of the change in rate of interest will not be the same on all articles of capital. For instance, the capital, the income from which is most remotely future, will be most affected. The following table shows : the effect of lowering the rate of interest from 5 per cent to 25 per cent on five typical articles, whose incomes have different degrees of remoteness.

Capital Rate Of Nkt Income Peb Year Total Incomb Capital-valce Capital-valu (INT. AT 5) (INT. AT 2J)
Land House 1000 per yr. forever 1000 per yr. for 50 yrs. 100 per yr. for 6 yrs. 20 1st yr.; 10 zd yr Infinite 20,000.00 40,000.00
Horse Suit of clothes Loaf of bread 30,000.00 600.00 18,3OO. OO SOS. OO 28,4OO. OO 551-00
36.50 per yr., for 1 dav. 30.00.10 28.00.10 29. OO. IO
1 The figures in this table are worked out by the principle of discounting previously explained.

If the value of the benefits derivable from these various articles continues in each case uniform, but the rate of interest is suddenly cut down from 5 per cent to 2 per cent, there will result a general increase in the capital-values, but a very different increase for different articles. The more enduring ones will be affected the most. These effects are seen in the last two columns of the table. When the rate of interest is halved, the value of the land will be doubled, rising from 20,000 to 40,000, but the value of the house will rise by only about sixty per cent, namely, from 18,300 to 28,400; the value of the horse will rise only ten per cent, namely, from 508 to 551; the value of the suit will rise only from 28 to 29; and, finally, the value of the loaf of bread will not rise at all, but will remain at 10 cents. We see from the changes in the values of these five types of articles that the sensitiveness of capital-value to a change in the rate of interest is the greater, the more remote the income. A high rate of interest requires a high premium on income near at hand as compared with income remotely future; or, expressed the other way about, a high rate of interest diminishes the attractiveness of remotely future income as compared with income close at hand.

CHAPTER VII

VARIATIONS OF INCOME IN RELATION TO CAPITAL 1. Interest Accrued and Income Taken Out

We have seen how the value of capital is derived from that of income. We have also seen that the value of capital rises in anticipation of income and falls after its realization. The alternate rise and fall may or may not be equal. From the principles explained it is evident that the rise of the capital-value as it ascends on the discount curve is equal to the interest accrued on that capital during that time, while the fail in that capital value due to the taking out of income is equal to the income taken out. If the income taken out is just equal to the interest, the capital is thereby restored to its original value. // more than this amount of income be taken out, the capital-value will be impaired, that is, made less than it was at the beginning of the period under consideration; if less, the capital-value will increase.

When a man is said to own a capital fund of 1000, this means simply that he owns capital-goods worth that much; and these capital goods are worth that much simply because, in terms of money, the discounted value of the expected income from them is that much. The income which he expects may be a perpetual income flowing uniformly or in recurring cycles; or it may be an income like that from the bond, flowing recurrently for a limited time, at the end of which a large lump sum, ordinarily called the "principal," is returned in addition; or it may be any one of innumerable other forms. Thus if we assume that five per cent is the rate of interest used in calculating the capital-value, then any one of the following investments will have a present value of 1000: a perpetual annuity of 50 per year; or an annuity of 50 a year for ten years, together with 1000 at the end of that period; or 100 a year for fourteen years, after which nothing at all; or 25 a year for ten years, followed by 167.50 a year for ten years, after which nothing at all; or any one of innumerable other forms. The student can easily prove that any one of these series of incomes, when discounted at five per cent, will make up a present value of 1000.

In the first case the income taken out (50 a year) is exactly equal to the annual accrued interest, for 50 is the interest for one year at five per cent on 1000. The same is true of the second instance mentioned, that of the five per cent bond, except in the last year when the income taken out (1050) exceeds the interest for the year by 1000, thereby reducing the value of the bond to zero.

In the third case the income taken out the first year is S100, while the interest accrued in that year is only 50. Thus the income taken out exceeds the accrued interest by 50. This excess of 50 involves a reduction of 50 in the capital-value of the property, which therefore becomes 950 instead of 1000. Thus, at the end of the first year and after the 100 of income has been taken out, 950 is the discounted value of the remaining thirteen items of 100 a year for each year. In the second year the interest (on 950) is 47.50; whereas the income taken out is 100, the difference being 52.50. Hence, at the end of the second year, the capital-value of the remaining payments has been reduced by 52.50, becoming 897.50. Similarly, the capital-value of the property decreases each year by the excess of the income over the accrued interest until the last income item of 100 is received; after which, no more income being anticipated, the capital-value is zero.

In the fourth case, the interest accruing during the first year is 50, whereas only 25 income is taken out at the end of the year, the difference being 25. Hence, at the beginning of the second year the capital-value of the bond goes up to 1025. During the second year, the interest (on 1025) is 51.25. After the receipt of the second income item of 25, therefore, the capital-value of the bond is increased by the difference (26.25) and becomes 1051.25. Similarly, the value of the bond increases until after the payment of the tenth income item of 25, when it becomes 1314.43. The interest on this amount in the eleventh year is 65.72; whereas the income taken out that year, and each of the remaining nine years, is 167.50. Hence, from the beginning of the eleventh year to the end of the twentieth, the capital-value of the bond decreases, finally reaching zero at the end of the period.

The principle here shown may be summarized as follows: (1) When a property yields a specified foreknown income, and is valued by discounting that income at a specified rate of interest, if the income taken out is equal to the interest accrued, the value of the capital will be restored each year to the level of the year before. (2) If the income taken out exceeds the interest accrued, the value of the capital will fall below that of the year before, the amount of the fall being equal to the amount of the excess. (3) If the amount of income taken out is less than the interest accrued, the value of the capital will rise above that of the year before, the amount of the rise being equal to the amount of the deficiency.

Briefly, the general principle connecting income taken out and interest accrued is that they differ by the net appreciation or depreciation of capital. It is thus possible to describe interest accrued as income taken out less depreciation of capital, or as income taken out plus appreciation of capital.

2. Illustrations In order that these important relations may be as clear and vivid as possible, we shall illustrate them by concrete examples, and by business accounting. The following table gives the income supposed to be taken out for five selected kinds of capital-wealth; the capital-value found by discounting that income at five per cent; the accrued interest for the first year; the resulting change or net appreciation or depreciation of capital-value; and the ratio of the first years income to the original capital-value.

The student will readily understand how the figures in the successive columns are calculated although the actual calculation of the third column (capital-value) from the second (income) is a tedious process involving in most cases the discounting of a large number of separate items.

Increase Ratio Of

Capital- Wealth Income Taken Out Per Year Capital- Value Interest (+) Or De- Crease (-) Of Capital- Value IN First Year First Years Income To Original Capital- Value ACCRUED

Forest land 1000 a yr. for (1ST. AT S) K r First Year

14 yrs. and

then 3000 a

yr. forever. 40,000.00 2OOO. OO + 1000.00 2-5

Farm land 1000 per yr.

forever. 2O, OOO. OO IOOO. OO o.00 5-o

House 1000 per yr.

for 50 yrs. 18,300.00 915.00 -85.00 5-4

Horse 100 per yr. for

6 yrs. 508.00 25-40 -74.60 19.6

Suit of 201styr.; 1o

clothes 2d yr. 28.00 1.40 -18.60 71-4

1. The forest land yields 1000 worth of income the first year on a capital-value of 40,000, from which, on the five per cent basis assumed, the interest accrued would be five per cent of 40,000, or 2000. Consequently, the income taken out (1000) is less than the interest accrued (2000) by 1000. Therefore the forest will appreciate in the year by the excess, 2000–1000, or 1000, and will be worth 41,000 at the end of the year. Similarly, it will continue to appreciate for fourteen years, when it will be worth 60,000; after which the income that is annually taken out (3000) will be equal to the annual accrued interest on 60,000.

2. The farm land yielding 1000 a year in perpetuity is, on the five per cent basis, worth 20,000, and continues to be worth that amount each succeeding year. The income taken out (1000) is always equal to the interest accrued from 20,000.

3. The house yields an income of 1000 on a capital-value the first year of only 18,300. The interest accrued on 18,300 would be five per cent of 18,300, or only 915. The consequence is an excess of income taken out over interest accrued of 1000-915, or 85, and a corresponding fall of 85 in the value of the capital. That is, the house depreciates by 85 in the year, or from 18,300 to 18,215. It will continue to depreciate each year until its value vanishes entirely at the end of fifty years.

4. The horse also depreciates, and very fast. Its owner realizes from the horse an income of 100 on a capital-value of 508, from which the interest accrued would be only 25.40. The difference between the income taken out and the interest accrued is 100-25.40, or 74.60, and the horse will lose that much in value during the year, and will continue to depreciate in value for all of the six years during which it yields income.

5. The suit of clothes yields an income the first year of 20 on a capital of 28, from which the interest accrued would be only 1.40. It therefore depreciates by the difference, 20-1.40, or 18.60.

In all cases the interest accrued is 5 per cent of the capital-value, while the income taken out is in some cases a higher, and in some cases a lower, percentage. Expressed in percentages, the actual rate of value-return (i. e., ratio of income taken out to capital) on the forest land is 2.5 per cent; on the farm land, 5 per cent; on the house, 5.4 per cent;

on the horse, 19.6 per cent; and on the suit of clothes, 71.4 per cent. The more rapidly the income is taken out, the greater the rate of value-return realized; but (if that rate exceeds the rate of interest) the more rapidly will the capital be exhausted. The house yields a rate but slightly higher than the rate of interest, and lasts 50 years; the horse yields a rate nearly 4 times the rate of interest, but it lasts only 6 years; and the clothes yield a rate over 14 times the rate of interest, but last only 2 years. The farm land, which yields a rate exactly equal to the rate of interest, lasts forever, while the forest land, which yields a rate only half the rate of interest, not only lasts forever, but also increases in value for the first 14 years.

The various cases supposed may also be illustrated by the dividends declared by a joint stock company. If a company declares dividends of five per cent, when it earns five per cent, these dividends will be the interest accrued on the capital and will leave it intact. If the dividends are less than five per cent, capital will be accumulated; that is, a " surplus " will be added to the original capital. If the dividends are greater than five per cent, the capital or surplus previously accumulated will be decreased. In the last-named case the company is said to pay its dividends partly " out of capital." Such a practice is unusual, and when it occurs is generally condemned because of an assumed intention to deceive as to the ability to pay dividends.

A case at the opposite extreme occurs when the dividends are made unusually small in order that the capital may be increased. There is in New York City a company which has never declared any dividends, but has been rolling up a large surplus for years, and whose stock is for this reason much above par.

3. Confusions to be Avoided

With all the preceding explanations and illustrations the distinction between income taken out and interest accrued should be clear. Interest accrued is the income which, if it were taken out, would maintain capital intact, neither impaired nor increased, at the value it had at the beginning of the period under consideration.

Of the two concepts, income taken out and interest accrued, the former is by far the more fundamental. Everything else depends upon income expected to be taken out. We cannot, as would at first seem possible, begin with capital-value and derive the actual income from it; nor can we begin with interest accrued, for interest accrued presupposes some capital-value. That is, interest accrued depends on capital-value, and capital-value depends on income to be taken out. The order of dependence, then, is income taken out, capital-value, interest accrued. It is not uncommon to confuse these three concepts. The illustrative table (2) of this chapter will help to keep us from confusing them. For instance, from this table we see clearly one reason why certain articles have been erroneously identified with income. Clothes have nearly the same capital-value as income-value, so that, if a person were not accustomed to fine distinctions, he might think it unnecessary to discriminate between the 30, which is the total value of the use of the clothes for two years, which is, therefore, income, and the 28, which is the value of the clothes themselves, and which is, therefore, capital. There is almost as much danger of such confusion in the case of the horse; for there is no very great difference between the 600, the value of the use of the horse, and the 508, which is the value of the horse. As we pass to the more enduring articles, there emerges so wide a difference between the value of the use of an article and the value of the article itself, that there is no difficulty in distinguishing between them. But if the distinction is valid in one case, and all acknowledge that it is, it is valid in the others. We find no difficulty in distinguishing between the shelter of a house, which is income, and the house itself, which is capital; nor between their values. Thus the shelter is worth 1000 a year for 50 years (or 50,000 in all), whereas the house itself is the discounted value of all this 50,000, or only 18,300. We ought to find no greater difficulty in distinguishing between the horse and the use of the horse, nor between the clothes and the use of the clothes.

The more rapidly any capital yields up its benefits, that is, the greater the rate at which its income is taken out, the more the danger of confusing the capital with the income it yields.

We have shown the tendency to confuse three concepts—interest accrued, income taken out, and capital-value. We have also dealt with a fourth concept, which must not be confused with the other three, viz., appreciation or depreciation. Appreciation is also sometimes called savings, for savings in its broadest sense includes more than simply saved money. It includes all the net increase in capital-value after all income has been detached. It is the net appreciation, or the difference between the interest accrued and the income taken out. Savings are therefore still a part of capital. They are the part of capital saved from being taken out for income. They are not a part of income taken out. The individual is always struggling between saving more capital and taking out more income. He cannot do both—have his cake and eat it too. A savings bank depositor is sometimes thought to draw income from his deposit when the interest merely " accumulates " in the bank. This is an error. The bank renders income to the depositor when, and only when, money is drawn out of it. It occasions him outgo when, and only when, money is put into it. If the depositor merely lets his deposit accumulate, he derives no income and suffers no outgo. There is no effect on income. The only effect is upon capital, which is made to increase. If we accept the fiction that the man who allows his savings to accumulate virtually receives the interest, we must, to be consistent, also accept the fiction that he re-deposits it and so cancels the receipt. If the teller hands over the interest across the counter, the depositors account or claim against the bank certainly yields up income " to him, but if the depositor hands it back, the account occasions " outgo," and the net result is simply a cancellation. To allow a deposit to accumulate is evidently equivalent to this double operation. We see, then, that net appreciation is not. income, but is an addition to capital. Likewise, net de-T preciation is not outgo, but is a subtraction jrorncarjital. jl Almost every article except land ultimately deprec1ates in value, owing to the fact that the services which it still remains capable of rendering gradually diminish in number and value. The approaching cessation of services may be due to physical wear and tear, but not always. Sometimes the expression " wear and tear " is a misnomer. There are articles which suffer no physical change, but of which the services, nevertheless, last only a limited period. On the Atlantic coast the fishermen sometimes construct temporary platforms which are pretty sure to disappear in the September gales. It is evident that without any physical deterioration during the summer the value of such property must, nevertheless, decrease rapidly as the end of the fishing season approaches. The " Worlds Fair " buildings. at St. Louis depreciated, during the brief period of the fair, from 15,000,000, which was first paid for their construction, to 386,000, for wluch they were sold after they had served their main purpose during the few months of the Fair. The buildings equipping a mine become worthless when the mine is exhausted. " Wear and tear," therefore, is a phrase which we should use only in a metaphorical sense. Even when there is actual physical deterioration, this deterioration affects the value only in so far as it decreases or terminates the flow of income, and not directly because of a physical change in the capital which bears the income.

There are, then, four concepts which we must keep distinct. Stated in the order of dependence on income taken out, these concepts are:– (1) Income (value) taken out.

(2) Capital-value (the discounted value of expected income to be taken out).

(3) Interest accrued (the interest on capital-value).

(4) Appreciation (the excess of interest accrued over income taken out), and its opposite, depreciation (the excess of income taken out over interest accrued).

This order of dependence together with the dependence of the first element (income taken out) on antecedent elements previously explained may be conveniently expressed in a scheme as follows:–

Capital wealth–Benefits (income)

C tal al Income (value) taken out If Appreciation or. l a v.lu interest accrued j 1 depreciation 4. Standardizing Income

Various devices have been used to make income taken out agree with interest accrued. The method of the depreciation fund has already been mentioned under income accounts, and before the relation of income to capital was explained. By means of a depreciation fund, an irregular net income is converted into a regular net income; and we know that the capital-value of a perpetually regular income will remain constant. For instance, the possessor of 18,300 purchases a house and obtains at first an income worth 1000 a year. He knows, however, that by the end of 50 years the house will need to be rebuilt, and therefore sets aside a depreciation fund into which he pays annually a sum equal to the depreciation of his house. This, in the first year, is 85, as we have seen. The depreciation fund costs him this sum as outgo the first year. At the end of 50 years his depreciation fund, accumulated at interest, is large enough to rebuild the house. Although the house by itself does not yield him a uniform income of 915 for ever, but instead 1000 a year for 50 years, yet the house and the depreciation fund taken together yield him the 915 in perpetuity, or as long as he keeps up the system.

In this way, any article of capital may be made to yield a uniform perpetual income, not by itself, but conjointly with a depreciation fund. The latter is often forgotten. Only by actually paying into this fund can income taken out be made to agree with interest accrued. Merely to reckon what the depreciation is will not make the income taken out agree with the interest accrued. Reckoning depreciation is as poor a substitute for providing a fund to meet depreciation as Beau Brummels keeping a dinner hour was a substitute for a dinner. Of course, depreciation payments only rectify or change the distribution in time of one mans income at the expense of some other mans income. That is, every addition and subtraction caused in the one mans income implies equal and opposite changes in some other mans. A banker must be found who is willing to take the 85 and succeeding payments into the depreciation fund and to pay back 18,300 at the end of 50 years.

Another and simpler method of keeping income steady is to take care that ones capital shall consist of a large number of instruments at different stages of production or consumption. If a weaving mill is equipped with twenty looms of the same degree of wear, the value of this plant will evidently diminish, and a depreciation fund may be necessary. But if the twenty looms are evenly distributed throughout the different stages of wear, and if we assume that one loom wears out each year and is replaced at a regular cost, no depreciation fund will be necessary. The replacement of one loom annually is equivalent to such a depreciation fund, and the capital is thereby maintained at a uniform level. This method, which consists in properly assorting and combining a large number of instruments, is the chief reliance for steadying the income of society as a whole, for to society as a whole purely shifting devices,

such as borrowing, are inapplicable, since society can find no outside party on whom to shift the fluctuations.

In a new country just being opened up, such as the early American colonies, little income can at first be obtained because almost all the stock of wealth, especially the land, is, with respect to ability to yield income, in an embryonic stage, so to speak. The first settlers must, therefore, wait several years before they can get a comfortable living. An older country, on the other hand, such as the United States to-day, will have its capital better assorted. Only part of its capital will be in the embryonic stage–young forests, new mines, railways in process of construction. Other capital will be in full operation, yielding a large stream of benefits–older forests, mines, railways, factories, farms, dwellings, etc.

5. The Risk Element

There is one important feature in the relation between capital-value and income-value which has not yet been mentioned. This is the fact that at any point of time when we take account of capital-value, the future income from which it is obtained is only imperfectly foreknown. The capital-value is the discounted value of the future expected income, with all the chances of loss or gain included in present expectations.

Hitherto we have assumed that the entire future history of the capital in question is definitely known in advance; in other words, we have ignored chance. The articles of capital which were taken for illustration were supposed to yield definite future income which could be counted upon, precisely as the interest payments on a bond may be counted on by the bondholder. But as every enterprise offers chances of both gain and loss, we cannot close our discussion of the relation of income to capital without some account of how these chances affect the matter.

It has been explained that capital-value increases with the approach of an anticipated installment of income, and diminishes when that installment is taken out or received. These changes in capital-value take place when the future income is regarded as certain. The introduction of the element of chance will bring other and even more important changes in capital-value. If we take the history of the prices of stocks and bonds, we shall find it to consist chiefly of a record of changing estimates due to what is called chance, rather than of a record of the foreknown approach and detachment of income. Few, if any, future events are entirely free from uncertainty. In fact, property, by its very definition, is simply the right to more or less probable future benefits. The owner of a mine takes his chances as to what the mine will yield; the owner of an orange plantation in Florida takes his risk of winter frosts; the owner of a farm assumes risks as to the effect of sun and rain and other meteorological conditions, as well as the risks of the ravages of fire, insects, and pests generally. In buying an overcoat a man takes some risk as to its effectiveness in excluding cold, and as to the length of time it will continue to be serviceable. Even what are called " gilt-edged " securities are not entirely free from risk. Strictly speaking, therefore, every owner of property is a risk bearer.

We may now take a birds-eye view of the capital and income of any country, such as the United States. We have seen that the capital of the United States consists of over a hundred billion dollars worth of articles of various kinds, mostly real estate, and that the income consists of several billion dollars worth of nourishment, clothing, shelter, and other satisfactions. We now see how the capital is related to the income. All income comes from capital (in its broader sense) whether, as is frequently the case, the capital is a human being, or some other form of wealth. The income produced by capital gives value to that capital; for instance, the fruit borne by a tree gives value to the tree. Business men seldom assign value to human beings by capitalizing their earning power, although statisticians occasionally do this. But other forms of capital are commonly valued by capitalizing the income which they yield, that is, the one hundred and odd billions of dollars which our national capital is worth represent merely the discounted value of the nations net future satisfaction which, it is expected, that capital will ultimately produce. The value of our capital is merely the present value of the future " living " of ourselves and our descendants. Most of the capital does not directly produce that " living "–does not turn out bread and butter ready-made; but contributes to it only indirectly–by growing the wheat which will be made into bread or pasturing the cows from whose milk the butter will be churned. But all of the capital has as the goal toward which its services aim the production of bread and butter and the other necessities, comforts, and amusements of life the enjoyment of which constitutes our " living " or real income; and each individual article of this capital derives its value from the value of the services it is expected to render in helping toward this goal. These expectations may never be realized, and often are not realized, or the expectations may be surpassed by realization. But in either case it is expectation and not realization which gives the value to capital; and any change in expectations, whether occasioned by a shock to business confidence, a rumor of war, or any other cause, will tend to change the value of our national capital.

6. Review

The preceding chapters are intended to give a definite picture of the mass of capital and its benefits to man. In such a picture we see man standing in the midst of a physical universe; the events of this universe affect his life favorably or unfavorably. Over many of these events he can exercise no control or selection; they constitute his natural environment. Over others he exercises selection and control by assuming dominion over part of the physical universe and fashioning it to suit his own needs. The parts of the material world which he thus appropriates constitute wealth, whether they remain in their natural state or are "worked up" by him into products to render them more suitable to his needs. This mass of instruments will consist, first, of the appropriated parts of the surface of the earth, the buildings and structures attached to the soil, and the movable objects or "commodities" which man possesses and stores up; and, secondly (if we take wealth in its broader sense), of human beings.

This mass of instruments serves mans purpose in so far as its possession enables him to modify the stream of occurrences. By means of land and the modifications to which he subjects it he is enabled to increase and improve the growth of the vegetable and animal kingdoms in such a way as to supply him with food and the materials for constructing other instruments. By means of dwellings and other buildings he is enabled to avert or minimize the unfavorable effects of the elements upon his body and upon the articles of wealth which he stores in those buildings. By means of machinery, tools, and other instruments of production, he is enabled to fashion new instruments, to add to his store of goods or to supply the place of those destroyed or worn out. By means of the final finished products which minister to his more immediate enjoyments–such, for instance, as food, clothing, books, ornaments–he is enabled to consummate the purposes for which the entire mass of wealth is produced and kept in existence; namely, the satisfaction of his desires, whether these be for the necessities, the comforts, the luxuries, or the amusements of life. In these and other ways the stock of wealth will modify the course of natural events in a manner more or less agreeable to the owner. These desirable changes in the stream of events which occur by means of wealth constitute the benefits of wealth.

But these benefits are obtained by dint of certain costs. In the last analysis, costs are simply human efforts, and benefits are simply human satisfactions; but the interval between efforts and satisfactions is divided into so many stages, and at each of these stages there are so many processes of production or exchange, that these intermediate occurrences, or interactions, are much more in evidence than either the efforts which precede them or the satisfactions which follow. Each interaction is accounted as a benefit with respect to the producing article or agent, and a cost with respect to that on account of which it occurs.

The whole economic structure therefore–all that is represented in capital and income accounts–rests on two ultimate elements, namely, efforts and satisfactions. These enter our accounts, transformed simply by means of factors called prices, including that important price called the rate of interest. By means of such price factors, we reach from these elements, first, the interactions which depend on them, then the complete income and outgo accounts (containing the values not only of interactions, but of efforts and satisfactions as well), and then the capital accounts (containing the discounted values of the items in the income accounts).

To recapitulate in a few words the nature of capital and income, we may now say that those parts of the material universe which at any time are under the dominion of man, constitute his capital-wealth; its ownership, his capital-property; its value, his capital-value. Capital-value implies anticipated income, which consists of a stream of benefits or its value. When values are considered, the causal relation is not from capital to income, but from income to capital; not from present to future, but from future to present. In other words, the value of capital is the discounted value of the expected income. The fluctuations of this capital-value will, barring chance, be equal and opposite to the divergencies of " income taken out" from "interest accrued." When the influence of chance is included, there will be in addition to these fluctuations still others which mirror the successive changes in the outlook for future income.

CHAPTER VIII

PRINCIPLES GOVERNING THE PURCHASING POWER OP MONEY 1. Introductory

We have now finished the first great division of our subject–a study of the foundation stones of Economics and how they fit together. These foundation stones are wealth, property, benefits, costs, capital, and income. Our study has so far consisted in pointing out the nature and relations between these various concepts, and particularly between capital and income.

All of these relations find expression by means of prices. By prices, as we have seen, a miscellaneous collection of goods may be translated into a homogeneous mass of money-values. Only by such reduction to a common money basis are capital and income accounts possible. Capital accounts and income accounts are groups of heterogeneous elements reduced to common terms by means of prices. But in all the capital and income accounts to which reference has thus far been made, and in all our previous discussions, we have taken prices for granted. We have, in other words, started out in our investigations upon the assumption that prices were fixed and known. But inasmuch as prices themselves are the outcome of economic forces, they must in turn be made the subject of analysis, and we must consequently now take up the second part of our task, which consists in discovering the principles that determine prices.

If one were to ask how the price of wheat is determined, the immediate answer would probably be: By supply and demand. This answer, though correct so far as it goes, is superficial. It is well to be on ones guard against glib phrases which are so often substituted for real analyses. " Supply and demand " is such a phrase. A long time ago, when economics consisted rather of glib phrases than of real analyses, a critic of the study said, "If you want to make a first-class economist, catch a parrot and teach him to say supply and demand in response to every question you ask him. What determines wages? Supply and demand. What determines the distribution of wealth? Supply and demand." In every instance the answer is right, but it explains nothing. We must discover the forces which determine supply and demand. In so doing we shall learn that to determine the price even of one simple commodity, like wheat, involves practically all the principles of economic science.

We are now ready to undertake–not the full study of the supply and demand of any article–but one of the important forces underlying the supply and demand of all articles. That force is the purchasing power of money, a force as subtle as it is omnipresent. As every price is expressed in money, it is evident that the willingness to take or give a certain amount of any article at a given price in money depends on the willingness to give or take a certain amount of money in exchange. This willingness to give or take money depends on the purchasing power of money over other things. Will a man pay ten cents for a pound of sugar? That depends on whether or not he wants the sugar more than something else purchasable with the ten cents. The man, in other words, balances in his mind the sugar and the money–the latter standing in his mind for any goods he could spend it for. If the purchasing power of money is high, he will conceive so high a regard for money as to be reluctant to part with a given amount of it for a given quantity of sugar, i. e., he will be willing to pay only a low price for sugar. The seller, on the other hand, is more eager to take a unit of money when it has a high purchasing power, i. e., he is more willing to take a low price for sugar. Hence, if in a given year money has a high purchasing power, the price of sugar will be low. We see then that the price of any particular article will tend to be low if money has a high purchasing power; that is, if the prices of articles in general are low. It is therefore clear that the money price of every particular commodity depends partly on the prices of oiher commodities, i. e., on the general level of prices; just as the actual height reached by a particular wave of the sea depends partly on the general level of the tides, or as the actual height of a spire depends on the elevation of the ground on which it stands.

The phrases " the purchasing power of money " and " the general level of prices " are reciprocal. To say that the purchasing power of money is high or low is the same thing as to say that the general level of prices is low or high, respectively. If the price level is doubled, the purchasing power of money will be halved, and vice versa.

It is possible to study the general level of prices independently of particular prices, just as it is possible to study the general tides of the ocean independently of its particular waves. Moreover, it is not only more logical to study the general price level first, but this order of study has also the advantage of acquainting us as early as possible with the nature of money. Therefore, before we attempt to explain even the price of wheat in particular, we shall first take up the study of prices in general.

In practice, money is a most convenient device, but in theory it is always a stumbling-block to the student of economics, who is exceedingly prone to misunderstand its functions. At the beginning of this book we pointed out some of the imagined functions of money that do not belong to it. We are now in a position to ask: What are the real functions of money?

2. The Nature of Money

We define money as goods generally acceptable in exchange for other goods. The facility with which it may thus be exchanged, or its general acceptability, is the chief characteristic of money. The general acceptability may be reenforced by law, the money thus becoming "legal tender" (i. e., money which may be legally tendered or offered by a debtor to his creditor as a means of discharging his obligations expressed in terms of money units and which the creditor must accept). But such reenforcement is not essential. All that is necessary in order that any good may be money is that general acceptability shall attach to it. On the frontier, without any legal sanction, money is sometimes gold dust or gold nuggets. In the colony of Virginia it was tobacco. Among the Indians in New England it was wampum.

How does it happen that any particular commodity comes into use as money? Not originally because a government so decreed, but because the commodity was very salable for other uses than money and could be readily resold. Thus gold was readily sold and resold. Many wanted it for jewelry, and many others could easily be induced to accept it in exchange, even if they had no personal use for it themselves, for they knew they could resell it at any time to some one who had such a use for it. Gradually it became customary to accept it with no thought of any other use than to resell it or pass it on indefinitely. Gold has finally survived as the most important form of money. It is easily transportable and is durable.

There are various degrees of exchangeability which must be transcended before we arrive at real money. Of all kinds of goods, one of the least exchangeable is real estate. It is often difficult to find a person who wants to buy a particular piece of real estate. A mortgage on real estate is one degree more exchangeable. Yet even a mortgage is less exchangeable than a well-known and safe corporation security, or a government bond. One degree more exchangeable than a government bond is a time bill of exchange; one degree more exchangeable than a time bill of exchange is a sight draft; while a check is almost as exchangeable as money itself. Yet no one of these is really money, for none of them is " generally acceptable."

If we confine our attention to present and normal conditions, and to those means of exchange which either are money or most nearly approximate it, we shall find that money itself belongs to a general class of goods which we may call " currency " or " circulating media." Currency may be any kind of goods which, whether generally acceptable or not, do actually, for their chief purpose and use, serve as a means of exchange.

Currency consists of two chief classes: (1) money; (2) bank deposits, which will be treated fully in the next chapter. By means of checks, bank deposits serve as a means of payment in exchange for other goods. A check is the evidence of the transfer of bank deposits. It is acceptable to the payee only by his consent. It would not be generally accepted by strangers. Yet by checks, bank deposits, even more than money, do actually serve as a medium of exchange. In this country bank deposits subject to check, or, as they are sometimes called, " deposit currency," are by far the most important kind of currency or circulating media.

But although a bank deposit transferable by check is included in circulating media, it is not money. A bank note, on the other hand, is both circulating medium and money. Between these two lies the final line of distinction separating what is money and what is not. The line is delicately drawn, especially in the case of such checks as cashiers checks or certified checks. For the latter are extremely similar, in respect to acceptability, to bank notes. Each is a demand liability on a bank, and each confers on the holder the right to draw money. Yet while a bank note is generally acceptable in exchange, a check is acceptable only by special consent of the payee. Real money is what a payee accepts without question, because he is induced to do so by " legal tender " laws or by a well-established custom.

Of real money there are two kinds: primary and fiduciary. Money is called primary if it is a commodity any given unit of which has just as much value in some use other than money as it has in monetary use; that is, primary money is a commodity which has its full value even if it is not used as money or even if it is changed to a form in which it will not circulate as money. For instance, gold coins in the United States are primary money, since their value will be undiminished even if they are melted into gold bullion. In the same way, the tobacco money of Virginia in old days was primary, having as much value as tobacco as it had as money. Fiduciary money, on the other hand, is money the value of which depends partly or wholly on the owners confidence that he can exchange it for primary money, or at any rate for other goods, e. g., for primary money at a bank or government office or for discharge of debts or purchase of goods of merchants. For instance, a silver dollar in the United States is fiduciary money, since it is worth a dollar only because of the public confidence that the government will take it in taxes and the people in discharge of debts and for other purposes on equal terms with a dollar of gold. If a silver dollar be melted into bullion, it will, unlike the gold dollar, lose a large part of its value. That is, the bullion in a silver dollar is not worth a dollar; it is only worth about forty cents. Our other silver coins are worth as bullion even less in proportion to their value as money, and our nickel and bronze coins are worth still less in proportion. Bank notes, government notes, and other forms of paper money are still more striking examples of fiduciary money, being practically worthless as paper, but having a high value as money, owing to the con fidence that they can be exchanged for gold at the banks or the government treasury. The larger part of the money in use in the United States is fiduciary money, the chief examples being silver dollars, fractional silver, minor coins, silver certificates, gold certificates, government notes (nicknamed "greenbacks"), and bank notes. The exact nature of these various kinds of money constitutes a subject outside the purpose of this book. The student can, however, learn much as to their nature for himself, by reading the inscriptions on the various forms of money, which, from time to time, pass through his hands.1

The qualities of primary money which make for exchangeability are numerous. The most important are portability, durability, and divisibility. The chief quality of fiduciary money, which makes it exchangeable, is its redeemability in primary money, or else its imposed character of " legal tender."

Figure 9 indicates the classification of all circu-lating media in the United States. It shows that the total amount of circulating media is about eight and one half billions, of which about seven billions are bank deposits subject to check, and one and one half billions, money; and that of this one and one half billions of money one billion is

BANK
DEPOSITS.
SEVEN
BILL1ONS.

1 Some economists have proposed that what is here called " fiduciary " money should not be called money at all; that is, that the term " money " should be restricted to primary money. It seems preferable, however, here as elsewhere, to follow ordinary usage. There are instances where countries have for a time had no primary money, but only fiduciary money.

FidUCIARY
MONEY
PRIMARY
MONEY.

ONE-HM. F
Bh. uon.
ONE 3ILUON
Fig. Q.
fiduciary money and only about half a billion primary money.

In the present chapter we shall exclude the consideration of bank deposit or check circulation and confine our attention to the circulation of money, primary and fiduciary. In the United States, the only primary money is gold coin. The fiduciary money includes token coins and paper money.

Checks aside, we may classify exchanges into three groups: the exchange of goods against goods, or barter; the exchange of money against money, or " changing " money; and the exchange of money against goods, or purchase and sale. Only the last-named species of exchange involves what we call the circulation of money. The circulation of money signifies, therefore, the aggregate amount of its transfers against goods. All money held for circulation, i. e., for use in payment for goods purchased is called money in circulation. This includes the money in the pockets and purses of the people or the tills and safes of merchants. In the United States this includes all money except what is in the vaults of the banks and of the United States government.

3. The Equation of Exchange Arithmetically Expressed

Having learned something of the nature of money, we are ready to study the causes which determine the purchasing power of money; in other words, the causes which determine the general level of prices.

If we overlook for the present the influence of checks, we may say that the price level depends on only three sets of causes: (1) the quantity of money in circulation; (2) its " efficiency " or velocity of circulation (or the average number of times a year a dollar is exchanged for goods); and (3) the volume of trade (or amount of goods per year bought by money). The so-called " quantity theory " (i. e., the theory that prices vary proportionally to money) has often been incorrectly formulated, but it is correct in the sense that the level of prices varies directly with the quantity of money in circulation, provided the velocity of circulation of that money and the volume of trade effected by means of it are not changed. This theory will be made clearer by the equation of exchange, which is now to be explained.

The equation of exchange is a statement, in mathematical form, of the total transactions effected in a certain period in a given community. It is obtained simply by adding together the equations of exchange for all individual transactions. Suppose, for instance, that a person buys 10 pounds of sugar at 7 cents per pound. This is an exchange transaction, in which 10 pounds of sugar have been regarded as equivalent to 70 cents, and this fact may be expressed thus: 70 cents = 10 pounds of sugar multiplied by 7 cents a pound. Every other sale and purchase may be expressed similarly, and by adding them all together we get the equation of exchange for a certain period in a given community; that is, the left side represents all the money spent and the right represents the value of all goods bought within the given period. During this period, however, the same money may serve, and usually does serve, for several transactions. For that reason the left or money side of the equation is, of course, greater than the total amount of money in circulation.

The equation has a goods side and a money side. The money side is the total money exchanged, and may be considered as the product of the quantity of money multiplied by the rapidity of its circulation, i. e., the number of times it is exchanged for goods. This important magnitude, called the velocity of circulation or rapidity of turnover, means simply the quotient obtained by dividing the total money payments for goods in the course of a year by the average amount in circulation by which these payments are effected. This velocity of circulation in an entire community is a sort of average of the rates of turnover of different persons. Each person has his own rate of turnover which he can readily calculate by dividing the amount of money he expends per year by the average amount he carries. The goods side of the equation is made up of the quantities of goods multiplied by their respective prices.

Let us begin with the money side. If the number of dollars in a country is 5,000,000, and the velocity of circulation of these dollars is twenty times per year, then the total amount of money expended (for goods) during any year is 5,000,000 times twenty, or 100,000,000. This is the money side of the equation of exchange.

Since the money side of the equation is 100,000,000, the goods side must be the same. For if 100,000,000 has been spent for goods in the course of the year, then 100,000,000 worth of goods must have been sold in that year. In order to avoid the necessity of writing out the quantities and prices of the innumerable varieties of goods which are actually exchanged, let us assume for the present that there are only three kinds of goods–bread, coal, and doth; and that the sales are:– 200,000,000 loaves of bread at.10 a loaf, 10,000,000 tons of coal at 5.00 a ton, and 30,000,000 yards of cloth at 1.00 a yard.

The value of these transactions is evidently 100,000,000,–i. e., 20,000,000 worth of bread plus 50,000,000 worth of coal plus 30,000,000 worth of cloth. The equation of exchange, therefore, is as follows:– 5,000,000X20= 200,000,000 loaves X.10 a loaf
+ 10,000,000 tons X 5.00 a ton
+ 30,000,000 yards X 1.00ayard.

This equation contains on the money side two magnitudes, viz., (1) the quantity of money, and (2) the number of times it circulates or is " turned over " in a year; and on the goods side two groups of magnitudes in two columns, viz., (1) the quantities of goods exchanged in a year (loaves, tons, yards), and (2) the prices of these goods (.10 per loaf, 5.00 per ton, and 1.00 per yard). The equation shows that these four sets of magnitudes are mutually related. Because this equation must be fulfilled, the prices must bear a relation to the three other sets of magnitudes–quantity of money, rapidity of circulation, and quantities of goods exchanged. Consequently, these prices must, as a whole, vary proportionally with the quantity of money and with its velocity of circulation, and inversely with the quantities of goods exchanged.

Suppose, for instance, that the quantity of money were doubled, while its velocity of circulation and the quantity of goods exchanged remained the same. Then, since the equation of exchange must continue to hold true, it would be quite impossible for prices to remain unchanged. The money side would now be 10,000,000 X 20 times a year, or 200,000,000; whereas, if prices should not change, the goods would remain 100,000,000 and the equation would be violated. Since exchanges, individually and collectively, always involve an equivalent quid pro quo, the two sides must be equal.

Not only must purchases and sales be equal in amount–since every article bought by one person is necessarily sold by another–but the total value of goods sold must equal the total amount of money exchanged. Therefore, under the given conditions, prices must change in such a way as to raise the goods side from 100,000,000 to 200,000,000. This doubling may be accomplished by an even or an uneven rise of prices, but some sort of a rise of prices there must be. If the prices rise evenly, they will evidently all be exactly doubled, so that the equation will read:– 10,000,000 X 20 = 200,000,000 loaves X.20 per loaf + 10,000,000 tons X 10.00 per ton + 30,000,000 yards X 2.00 per yard. If the prices rise unevenly, the doubling must evidently be brought about by compensatioe; if some prices rise by less than double, others must rise by enough more than double to exactly compensate.

But whether all prices increase uniformly, each being exactly doubled, or some prices increase more and some less (so as still to double the total money-value of the goods purchased), the prices are doubled on the average. This proposition is usually expressed by saying that the " general level of prices " is raised twofold. From the mere fact, therefore, that the money spent for goods must equal the quantities of those goods multiplied by their prices, it follows that the level of prices must rise or fall according to changes in the quantity of money, unless there are changes in its velocity of circulation or in the quantities of goods exchanged.

If changes in the quantity of money affect prices, so will changes in the other factors–quantities of goods and velocity of circulation–affect prices. In the case of a change in the velocity of circulation, the change is very similar to that seen in the case of a change in the quantity of money. Thus a doubling in the velocity of circulation of money will double the level of prices, provided the quantity of money in circulation and the quantities of goods exchanged for money remain as before. The equation will change (from its original form) to the following:– 5,000,000 X 40 = 200,000,000 loaves X.20 a loaf + 10,000,000 tons X 10.00 a ton + 30,000,000 yards X 2.00 a yard; or else the equation will assume a form in which some of the prices will more than double, and others less than double by enough to preserve the same total value of the sales.

Again, a doubling in the quantities of goods exchanged will cut in two the height of the price level, provided the quantity of money and its velocity of circulation remain the same. Under these circumstances the equation will change (from its original form) to:– 5,000,000 X 20 = 400,000,000 loaves X.05 a loaf
+ 20,000,000 tons X 2.50 a ton
+ 60,000,000 yards X.50 a yard; or else it will assume a form in which some of the prices are more than halved, and others less than halved, so as to preserve the equation.

Finally, if there is a simultaneous change in two or all of the three influences, i. e., quantity of money, velocity of circulation, and quantities of goods exchanged, the price level will be a compound or resultant of these various influences. If, for example, the quantity of money is doubled, and its velocity of circulation is halved, while the quantity of goods exchanged remains constant, the price level will be undisturbed. Likewise it will be undisturbed if the quantity of money is doubled and the quantity of goods is doubled, while the velocity of circulation remains the same. To double the quantity of money, therefore, does not always double prices. We must distinctly recognize that the quantity of money is only one of three factors, all equally important in determining the price level.

4. The Equation of Exchange Mechanically Expressed

The equation of exchange has now been expressed by an arithmetical illustration. It may be represented visually by a mechanical illustration. This is embodied in Figure 10 which represents a mechanical balance in equilibrium, the two sides of which symbolize respectively the money side and the goods side of the equation of exchange. The weight at the left, symbolized by a purse, represents the money in circulation; the leverage or distance from the fulcrum at which the purse is hung represents the efficiency of this money, or its velocity of circulation. The product

Fig. 10.

of the weight by its leverage is exactly balanced by or equal to corresponding products on the opposite side. On the right side are three weights, representing bread, coal, and cloth, and symbolized respectively by a loaf, a coal scuttle, and a roll of cloth. The leverage, or distance of each from the fulcrum, represents its price. In order that the leverages at the right may not be inordinately long, we have found it convenient to reduce the unit of measure of coal from tons to hundredweights, and that of cloth from yards to feet, and consequently to enlarge correspondingly the number of units (the measure of coal changing from 10,000,000 tons to 200,000,000 hundredweights, and that of the cloth from 30,000,000 yards to 90,000,000 feet). In these new units the price of coal becomes 25 cents per hundredweight and that of cloth becomes 333 cents per foot. If the purse at the left becomes heavier, it is evident that, in order to maintain the balance, some of the weights at the right must be heavier also or must be moved toward the right, or else the purse itself must be moved toward the right. If, now, we assume that the last and first of these three changes do not occur, the middle one must occur. In other words, if the position of the purse remains unaltered (i. e., if the velocity of circulation of money does not change) and if the weights at the right remain unaltered (i. e., if the volume of trade does not change), then some or all of these weights must move to the right (i. e., the prices of goods must increase). If these prices increase uniformly, they will increase in the same ratio as the increase in money; if they do not increase uniformly, some will increase more and some less than this ratio, maintaining an average. Likewise it is evident that if the velocity of circulation of money increases, i. e., if the leverage at the left lengthens, and if the money in circulation (the purse) and the trade (the various weights at the right) remain the same, there must be an increase in prices (lengthening of the leverages at the right). Again, if there is an increase in the volume of trade (represented by an increase in weights at the right), and if the velocity of circulation of money (left leverage) and the quantity of money (left weight) remain the same, there must be a decrease in prices (right leverages).

In general, any change in one of these four sets of magnitudes must be accompanied by such a change or changes in one or more of the other three as shall maintain equilibrium.

As we are interested in the average change in prices rather than in the prices individually, we may simplify this mechanical representation by hanging all the right-hand weights at one average point, so that the leverage shall represent the average of prices. This average, of 10 cents per loaf, 25 cents per hundredweight, and 33 cents per foot, is found by dividing the total value (10 cents times 200 million loaves, plus 25 cents times 200 million hundredweight, plus 33! cents times 90 million feet,–or 100,000,000)

Fig. 1t.

by the total number of units (200 million plus 200 million plus 90 million–or 490 million), which is 100,000,000-5-

490,000,000, or 20.4 cents per unit. This leverage is a so-called " weighted average " of the three original leverages, the " weights " being literally the weights hanging at the right. This averaging of prices is represented in Figure 1 1 which visualizes the fact that the average price of goods (right leverage) varies directly with the quantity of money (left weight), directly with its velocity of circulation (left leverage), and inversely with the volume of trade (right weight).

5. The Equation of Exchange Algebraically Expressed

To put these relations in general terms, let

M stand for money in circulation,

V, its velocity of circulation,

P, p, p", etc., the prices of various goods,

Q, Q, Q", etc., the quantities of those goods sold.

Then we may write the formula as follows:–

$MV = pq$
$+ PQ + P"Q"$
$+$ etc.

M V evidently represents the amount of money expended for goods during the year. On the other side of the equation, pq, p Q, and so on, represent the values of the various goods bought. If in this equation M is doubled (and V and the Qs remain unchanged), then the ps will, on the average, be doubled; if V is doubled (and M and the Qs are unchanged), the ps will be doubled also; while if the Qs are doubled (and M and V are unchanged), the ps will be halved.

The right side of this equation is the sum of terms of the form pq –a price multiplied by a quantity bought. It is customary in mathematics to abbreviate a sum of terms (all of which are of the same form) by using " S " as a prefix to pq. The Greek letter sigma is the equivalent of the English letter " S," the initial letter of sum and is employed as a symbol of summation. This symbol does not signify a magnitude as do the symbols M, V, p, Q, etc. It signifies merely the operation of addition, and should be read " the sum of terms of the following type." The equation of exchange may therefore be written:–

MV-

We may, if we wish, further simplify the right side by writing it in the form PT, where P is a weighted average of all the ps, and T is the sum of all the Qs. P then represents in one magnitude the level of prices, and T represents in one magnitude the volume of trade of the community within or without its borders. The equation thus simplified $(MV = PT)$ is the algebraic interpretation of the mechanical illustration given in Figure 11, where all the goods, instead of being hung separately, as in Figure 10, were combined and hung at an average point representing their average price.

6. The "Quantity Theory of Money"

To recapitulate, we find then that, under the conditions assumed, the price level varies: (1) directly as the quantity of money in circulation (M), (2) directly as the velocity of its circulation (V), (3) inversely as the volume of trade done by it (T. The first of these three relations needs special emphasis. It constitutes the "quantity theory of money."

So important is this principle, and so bitterly contested has it been, that we shall illustrate it further. By " the quantity of money " is meant the number of dollars (or other given monetary units) in circulation. This number may be changed in several ways, of which the four named below are most important. A statement of these four will serve to picture to our mind the meaning of the conclusions we have reached and to reveal the fundamental peculiarity of money on which they rest.

I. As a first illustration, let us suppose the government to double the denominations of all money; that is, let us suppose that what has been hitherto a half dollar is henceforth called a dollar, and that what has been hitherto a dollar is henceforth called two dollars. Evidently the number of " dollars " in circulation will then be doubled; and the price level, measured in terms of the new " dollars," will be double what it would otherwise be. Every one will pay out the same coins as if no such law were passed. But he will, in each case, be paying twice as many " dollars." For example, if 3 formerly had to be paid for a pair of shoes, the price of this same pair of shoes will now become 6. The proof that prices must in general be doubled rests on the equation of exchange. Money in circulation (M) having doubled (its velocity of circulation (V) and the volume of trade (T) remaining the same), the average of the prices (P) must be doubled. The same reasoning applies to the three illustrations which follow.

II. For a second illustration suppose the government cuts each dollar in two, coining the halves into new " dollars "; and, recalling all paper notes, replaces them with double the original number–two new notes for each old one of the same denomination. In short, suppose money not only to be renamed, as in the first illustration, but also reissued. Prices in the debased coinage will again be doubled just as in the first illustration. The subdivision and re-coinage is an immaterial circumstance, unless it be carried so far as to make counting difficult, and thus to interfere with the convenience of money. Wherever a dollar had been paid before debasement, two dollars–i. e., two of the old halves coined into two of the new dollars–will now be paid instead.

In the first illustration, the increase in quantity was simply nominal, being brought about by renaming coins. In the second illustration, besides renaming, the further fact of recoining is introduced. In the first case, the number of actual pieces of money of each kind was unchanged, but their denominations were doubled. In the second case, the number of pieces is also doubled by splitting each coin and reminting it into two coins, each of the same nominal denomination as the original whole of which it is the half, and by similarly doubling the paper money.

III. For a third illustration, suppose that, instead of doubling the number of dollars by splitting them in two and recoining the halves, the government duplicates each piece of money in existence and presents the duplicate to the possessor of the original. (We must in this case suppose, further, that there is some effectual bar to prevent the melting or exporting of money. Otherwise the quantity of money in circulation will not be doubled; much of the increase will escape.) If the quantity of money is thus doubled, prices will also be doubled just as truly as in the second illustration, in which there were exactly the same number of coins as now under consideration as well as the same denominations. The only difference between the second and the third illustrations will be in the size and weight of the coins. The weights of the individual coins, instead of being reduced, will remain unchanged; but their number will be doubled. This doubling of coins must have the same effect as the fifty per cent. debasement; that is, it must have the effect of doubling prices.

IV. The force of the third illustration becomes even more evident if, in accordance with the presentation of the great economist Ricardo, we pass back by means of a seigniorage from the third illustration to the second. That is, after duplicating all money, let the government subtract half of each coin, thereby reducing the weight to that of the debased coinage in the second illustration, and removing the only point of distinction between the two. This " seigniorage" or charge for coinage made by the sovereign will not affect the money value of the coins, so long as their number remains unchanged. Prices will remain at exactly the same level as before the abstraction of seigniorage.

Thus to double the quantity of money will double prices in whatever way the doubling may be brought about,–unless there should occur at the same time some change in the velocity of circulation of money or in the volume of trade.

The student may ask whether some change in the velocity of circulation of money or in the volume of trade will not necessarily occur as a direct consequence of the increased quantity of money. The answer to this question is in the negative, but this answer will be better understood after we have seen on what causes velocity of circulation and volume of trade depend. In the present chapter we are concerned merely to show that an increase in money will necessitate a rise in prices provided the velocity of circulation and volume of trade do remain the same.

There are many historical instances of raising the prices by inflating the currency. At present, Argentina has an inflated paper currency, and prices in paper pesos are a little more than double the prices in the original gold pesos.

The quantity theory, then, asserts that (provided ve-locity of circulation and volume of trade are unchanged) if we increase the number of dollars, whether by renaming coins, by cutting them in two, by duplicating them, or by any other means, prices will be increased in the same proportion. It is the number, and not the weight, that is essential. This fact needs great emphasis. It is a fact which differentiates money from all other goods and explains the peculiar manner in which its purchasing power is related to other goods. The desirability of sugar depends upon its sweetening power, which is a specific quality in the sense that a given weight of sugar, such as a pound, always possesses the same sweetening power. The desirability of money, on the other hand, depends merely on its purchasing power; but purchasing power is not a specific quality of gold or of other money, for we cannot say that a given quantity of gold, such as an ounce, always possesses the same purchasing power. If the quantity of sugar is changed from 1,000,000 pounds to 1,000,000 hundredweight, it does not follow that a hundredweight will have the value previously possessed by a pound, for the sweetening power of a hundredweight cannot be the same as that of a pound. But if the money in circulation is changed from 1,000,000 units of one weight to 1,000,000 units of a lighter weight, the value of the new and lighter coins will be just as great as was the value of the old and heavy ones, for we have seen from the equation of exchange that their purchasing power will be unchanged.

The quantity theory of money thus rests, ultimately, upon the fundamental peculiarity which money alone of all goods possesses–the fact that it has no definite relation to the satisfaction of human wants, but only the power to purchase things which do have such satisfying power.

CHAPTER DC INFLUENCE OF DEPOSIT CURRENCY 1. The Mystery of Circulating Credit

We are now ready to explain the nature of bank-deposit currency, or circulating credit. Credit, in the sense here employed, is the promise of one party (called the debtor) to pay money to another party (called the creditor). Bank deposits subject to check are the claims against the bank of a special class of creditors known as depositors, by virtue of which they may, on demand, draw by check specified sums of money from the bank. Since no other kind of bank deposits will be considered by us, we shall usually refer to " bank deposits subject to check " simply as " bank deposits." They are also called " circulating credit."

It is to be observed that bank checks are merely presumptive evidences of rights to draw money on the basis of bank deposits or to transfer such rights. The checks themselves are not the ultimate currency. It is the bank-deposits themselves, or credit balances on the books of the banks, that constitute the ultimate currency. As has been noted, these deposits subject to check are not money, since they are not generally acceptable; they always require the special consent of the payee. But they are currency, because their chief purpose and use is to act as a medium of exchange. Closely analogous to checks are post office orders and money orders issued by express companies. They are distinguishable only by two facts: that they are not issued by ordinary banks, and that they originate in special deposits of money (or checks). For this reason, and because they are not of great importance, we prefer to place them in the same category with bank checks rather than to place them in a separate class, which otherwise they might occupy.

It is in connection with the transfer of bank deposits that there arises that so-called " mystery of banking" called circulating credit. Many persons, including some economists, have supposed that credit is a special form of wealth which may be created out of whole cloth, as it were, by a bank. Others have maintained that credit has no foundation in actual wealth at all, but is a kind of unreal and inflated bubble with a precarious if not wholly illegitimate existence. As a matter of fact, bank deposits are as easy to understand as bank notes, and what is said in this chapter of bank deposits may in substance be taken as true also of bank notes. The chief difference is a formal one, the notes circulating freely from hand to hand, while the deposit currency circulates only by means of specially indorsed orders called " checks."

To understand the real nature of bank deposits, let us imagine a hypothetical institution–a kind of primitive bank existing mainly for the sake of deposits and the safekeeping of actual money. The original bank of Amsterdam was somewhat like the bank we are now imagining. In such a bank a number of people deposit 100,000 in gold, each accepting a receipt for the amount of his deposit. If this bank should issue a " capital account " or statement, it would show 100,000 in its vaults and 100,000 owed to depositors, as follows:–

Assets Liabilities

G0ld 100,000 Due depositors. 100,000

The right-hand side of the statement is, of course, made up of smaller amounts owed to individual depositors. Assuming that there is owed to A 10,000, to B 10,000, and to all others 80,000, we may write the bank statement as follows:–

Assets Liabilities

Gold 100,000 Due depositor A. 10,000

Due depositor B. 10,000

Due other depositors. 80,000 100,000 100,000

Now assume that A wishes to pay B 1000. A could go to the bank with B, present certificates or checks for 1000, obtain the gold, and hand it over to B, who might then redeposit it in the same bank, merely handing it back through the cashiers window and taking a new certificate in his own name. Instead, however, of both A and B visiting the bank and handling the money, A might simply give B a check for 1000. B would then send the check to the bank and the bank would simply reduce As credit on its books by 1000 and increase Bs by the same amount. The transfer in either case would mean that As holding in the bank was reduced from 10,000 to 9000, and that Bs was increased from 10,000 to 11,000. The statement would then read:–

Assets Liabilities

Gold 100,000 Due depositor A. 9,000

Due depositor B. 11,000

Due other depositors. 80,000 100,000 100,000

Thus the certificates, or checks, would circulate in place of money among the various depositors in the bank. What really changes ownership, or "circulates," in such cases is the right to draw money. The check is merely a presumptive evidence of this right and of the transfer of this right from one person to another. The man who receives the check uses it as evidence of a right to draw at the bank against the account of the man who drew the check.

In the case under consideration, the bank would be conducted at a loss. It would be giving the time and labor of its clerical force for the accommodation of its depositors, without getting anything in return. But such a hypothetical bank would soon find– much as did the bank of Amsterdam–that it could make profits by lending at interest some of the gold on deposit. This could not offend the depositors; for they do not expect or desire to get back the identical gold they deposited. What they want is simply to be able at any time to obtain the same amount of gold. Since, then, their arrangement with the bank calls for the payment not of any particular gold, but merely of a definite amount, and that but occasionally, the bank finds itself free to lend out part of the gold that otherwise would lie idle in its vaults. To keep it idle would be a great and needless waste of opportunity.

Let us suppose, then, that the bank decides to loan out half the money which it has in its vaults. In this country this is usually done in exchange for promissory notes of the borrowers. Now a loan is really an exchange of money (or credit–which is immediately convertible into money) for a promissory note which the lender–in this case the bank–receives in place of the gold. Let us suppose that so-called borrowers actually draw out 50,000 of gold. The bank thereby exchanges this money for promises, and its books will then read:–

Assets Liabilities

Gold 50,000 Due depositor A. 9,000

Promissory notes. 50,000 Due depositor B. 11,000

Due other depositors. 80,000 100,000 100,000 It will be noted that now the gold in bank is only 50,000, while the total deposits are still 100,000. In other words, the depositors now have more " money on deposit" than the bank has in its vaults! But, as will be shown, this form of expression involves a popular fallacy, in the word " money." Something of equivalent value is behind each loan, but not necessarily money.

Next, suppose the borrowers become, in a sense, lenders also, by redepositing the 50,000 of money which they borrowed, in return for the right to draw out the same sum on demand, preferring to use the same in making payments by check rather than by money. In other words, suppose that after borrowing 50,000 from the bank, they lend it back to the bank. The banks assets will thus be enlarged by 50,000, and its obligations (or credit extended) will be equally enlarged; and the balance sheet will become:–

Assets Liabilities

Gold 100,000 Due depositor A. 9,000

Promissory notes. 50,000 Due depositor B. 11,000

Due other depositors. 80,000

Due new depositors, ., the borrowers. 50,000 150,000 150,000

What happened in this case was the following: Gold was borrowed in exchange for a promissory note and then handed back in exchange for a right to draw. Thus the gold really did not budge; but the bank received a promissory note and the depositor, a right to draw. Evidently, therefore, the same result would have followed if each borrower had merely handed in his promissory note and received, in exchange, a right to draw. As this operation most frequently puzzles the beginner in the study of banking, we repeat the tables representing the conditions before and after these " loans," i. e., these exchanges of promissory notes for present rights to draw.

BEFORE THE LOANS

Assets Liabilities

Gold 100,000 Due depositors. 100,000

AFTER THE LOANS

Gold 100,000 Due depositors. 1 50,000

Promissory notes. 30.000

Clearly, therefore, the intermediation of the money in this case is a needless complication, though it may help to a theoretical understanding of the resultant shifting of rights and liabilities. Thus the bank may receive deposits of gold or deposits of promises to pay. In exchange for these promises it may give, or lend, either a right to draw, or gold–the same that was deposited by another customer. Even when the borrower has " deposited " only a promise to pay money, by fiction he is still held to have deposited money; and, like the original depositor of actual money, he is given the right to make out checks to draw out money. The total value of rights to draw, in whichever way arising, is termed "deposits." Banks more often lend rights to draw (or deposit-rights) than actual money, partly because of the greater convenience to borrowers, and partly because the banks wish to keep their actual money on hand, or " cash reserves" large, in order to meet large and. unexpected demands. It is true that if a bank loans money, part of the money so loaned will be redeposited by the persons to whom the borrowers pay it in the course of business; but it will not necessarily be redeposited in the same bank. Hence the average banker prefers that the borrower should not withdraw actual money.

Besides lending deposit rights, banks may also lend their own notes, called " bank notes." And the principle governing bank notes is the same as the principle governing deposit rights. The holder simply gets a pocketful of bank notes instead of a credit on his bank account. The bank

must always be ready to pay, on demand, either the note holders–i. e., to " redeem its notes "–or the depositors, and in either case the bank exchanges a promise for a promise. In the case of the note, the bank has exchanged its bank note for a customers promissory note. The bank note carries no interest, but is payable on demand. The customers note bears interest, but is payable only at a definite date.

Assuming that the bank issues 50,000 of bank notes, the balance sheet will now become:–

Assets Liabilities

Gold 100,000 Due depositors. 150,000

Loans (promissory notes) 100,000 Due bank note holders 50,000 200,000 200,000

2. The Basis of Circulating Credit

We repeat that by means of credit the deposits and notes of a bank may exceed its cash. There would be nothing mysterious or obscure about this fact, if people could be induced not to think of banking operations as money operations. To so represent them is metaphorical and misleading. They are no more money operations than they are real estate transactions. A bank depositor, A, has not ordinarily " deposited money "; and whether he has or not, he certainly cannot properly say that he " has money in the bank." What he does have is the banks promise to pay money on demand. The bank owes him money. When a private person owes money, the creditor never thinks of saying that he has it on deposit in the debtors pocket.

The same principles of property which apply to bank deposits also apply to bank notes. There is wealth somewhere behind the mutual promises, though in different degrees of accessibility. The note holders promise (his promissory note) is secured by his assets; and the banks promise (the bank note) is secured by the banks assets. The note holder has " swapped" less-known credit for better-known credit.

If this fact is borne in mind, the reader will be able to conquer the doubt which may already have arisen in his mind–the doubt as to the legitimacy of the banks procedure in " lending some of its depositors money." It cannot be too strongly emphasized that, in any balance sheet, the value of the liabilities rests on that of the assets. The deposits of a bank are no exception. We must not be misled by the fact that the cash assets may be less than the deposits. When the uninitiated first learn that the number of dollars which note holders and depositors have the right to draw out of a bank exceeds the number of dollars in the bank, they are apt to jump to the conclusion that there is nothing behind the notes or deposit liabilities. Yet behind all these obligations there is always, in the case of a solvent bank, full value; if not actual dollars, at any rate, dollars worth of property. By no jugglery can the liabilities exceed the assets except in insolvency, and even in that case only nominally, for it still holds that the true value of the liabilities will be only what can be paid on them–perhaps only 25 cents on the dollar. This true value of the liabilities will rest upon and be equal to the true value of the assets behind them by means of which they will be paid, so far as may be. Debts which cannot or will not be paid in full are often called " bad debts "; and the value of " bad debts " is not their face value, but their actual value to the creditor.

These assets, as already indicated, are, and ought to be, largely the notes of merchants, although, so far as the principles here discussed are concerned, they might be any property whatever. If they consisted in the ownership of real estate or other wealth unencumbered so that the tangible wealth which property always represents were clearly evident, all mystery would disappear. But the effect would not be different. Instead of taking grain, machines, or steel ingots on deposit, in exchange for the sums lent, banks prefer to take interest-bearing notes of corporations and individuals who own, directly or indirectly, grain, machines, and steel ingots; and by the banking laws the banks are even compelled to take the notes instead of the ingots. The bank finds itself with liabilities which exceed its cash assets; but this excess of liabilities is balanced by the possession of other assets than cash. These other assets of the bank are the liabilities of business men. These liabilities are in turn supported by the assets of the business men. If we continue to follow up the chain of liabilities and assets, we shall find the ultimate basis of the banks liabilities in the concrete tangible wealth of the world.

This ultimate basis of the entire credit structure is kept out of sight, but the basis exists. Indeed, we may say that banking, in a sense, causes this concrete, tangible wealth to circulate. If the acres of a landowner or the iron stoves of a stove dealer cannot circulate in literally the same way that gold dollars circulate, yet the landowner or stove dealer may give to the bank a note on which the banker may base bank notes or deposits; and these bank notes and deposits will circulate like gold dollars. Through banking, he who possesses wealth difficult to exchange can create a circulating medium based upon that wealth. He has only to give his note, for which, of course, his property is liable, get in return the right to draw, and lo! his comparatively unexchangeable wealth becomes liquid currency. To put it crudely, deposit banking is a device for coining into dollars land, stoves, and other wealth not otherwise generally exchangeable.

We began by regarding a bank as substantially a cooperative enterprise, operated for the convenience and at the expense of its depositors. But, as soon as the bank reaches the point of lending money to X, Y, and Z on time, while itself owing money on demand, it assumes toward X, Y, and Z risks which the depositors would be unwilling to assume. To meet this situation, the responsibility and expense of running the bank are taken by a third class of people–stockholders–who are willing to assume the risk for the sake of the chance of profit. Stockholders, in order to guarantee the depositors against loss, put in some cash of their own. The object is to make good any loss to depositors, while reserving the right to keep the profits earned by loaning at interest.

Let us suppose that the stockholders put in 50,000, viz., 40,000 in gold and 10,000 in the purchase of a bank building. The accounts now stand:–

Assets Liabilities
Gold 140,000 Due depositors.
Loans 100,000 Due note holders.
Building 10,000 Due stockholders.
250,000

The accounts as they now stand include the chief features of an ordinary modern bank–a so-called " bank of deposit, issue, and discount."

3. Banking Limitations

We have seen that there are assets to meet the liabilities. We now should note that the form of the assets must be such as will insure meeting the liabilities promptly. Since the business of a bank is to furnish easily exchangeable property (cash or credit) in place of the " slower " property of its depositors, it fails of its purpose when it is caught with insufficient cash, by which is meant money. Yet it makes profits partly by tying up its quick property, i. e., lending it out in quarters where it is less accessible. Its problem in policy is to tie up enough to increase its earnings, but not to tie up so much as to get tied up itself. So far as anything has yet been said to the contrary, a bank might increase indefinitely its loans in relation to its cash or in relation to its capital. If this were so, deposit currency could be indefinitely inflated.

There are, however, limits to such expansion of loans imposed by prudence and sound economic policy. Insolvency and insufficiency of cash must both be avoided. As has been noted in Chapter III, 5, insolvency is that condition which threatens when liabilities are extended with insufficient capital. Insufficiency of cash is that condition which threatens when liabilities are extended unduly relatively to cash. Insolvency is reached when the assets no longer cover the liabilities (to others than stockholders), so that the bank is unable to pay its debts. Insufficiency of cash is reached when, although the banks total assets may be fully equal to its liabilities, the actual cash on hand is insufficient to meet the needs of the instant, and the bank is unable to pay its debts on demand.

The risk of insolvency is the greater the less the ratio of the stockholders interests to all liabilities to others. The risk of insufficiency of cash is the greater, the less the ratio of the cash to the demand liabilities. In other words, the leading safeguard against insolvency lies in a large capital and surplus, but the leading safeguard against insufficiency of cash lies in a large cash reserve. Insolvency proper may befall any business enterprise. Insufficiency of cash relates especially to banks in their function of redeeming notes and deposits.

Let us illustrate insufficiency of cash. In our banks accounts as we left them there appeared cash to the extent of 140,00x3, and 200,000 of demand liabilities (deposits and notes). The managers of the bank may think this fund of 140,000 unnecessarily large, or the loans unnecessarily small. They may then increase their loans (extended to customers partly in the form of cash and partly in the form of deposit accounts) until the cash held by the bank is reduced, say to 40,000, and the liabilities due depositors and note holders increased to 300,000. If, under these circumstances, some depositor or note holder demands 50,000 cash, immediate payment will be impossible. It is true that the assets still equal the liabilities. There is full value behind the 50,000 demanded; but the understanding was that depositors and note holders should be paid in money on demand. Were this not a stipulation of the deposit contract, the bank might pay the claims thus made upon it by transferring to its creditors the promissory notes due it from its debtors; or it might ask the customers to wait until it could turn these securities into cash.

Since a bank cannot follow either of these plans, it tries, where insufficiency of cash impends, to forestall this condition by " calling in " some of its loans, or if none can be called in, by selling some of its securities or other property for cash. But it happens unfortunately that there is a limit to the amount of cash which a bank can suddenly realize. No bank could escape failure if a large percentage of its note holders and depositors should simultaneously demand cash payment. The paradox of a run on a bank is well expressed by the case of the man who inquired of his bank whether it had cash available for paying the amount of his deposit, saying, "If you can pay me, I dont want it; but if you cant, I do." Such was the situation in 1907 in Wall Street. All the depositors at one time wanted to be sure their money " was there." Yet it never is there all at one time.

Since, then, insufficiency of cash is so troublesome a condition–so difficult to escape when it has arrived, and so difficult to forestall when it begins to approach–a bank must so regulate its loans and note issues as to keep on hand a sufficient cash resene, and thus prevent insufficiency of cash from even threatening. It can regulate the reserve in various ways. For instance, it can increase its reserve relatively to its liabilities by " discounting " less freely–by raising the rate of discount and thus discouraging would-be borrowers, by outright refusal to lend or even to renew old loans, or by " calling in " loans subject to call. Reversely, it can decrease its reserve relatively to its liabilities by discounting more freely–by lowering the rate of discount and thus attracting borrowers. The more the loans in proportion to the cash on hand, the greater the profits, but the greater the danger also. In the long run a bank maintains its necessary reserve by means of adjusting the interest rate charged for loans. If it has few loans, and a reserve large enough to support loans of much greater volume, it will endeavor to extend its loans by lowering the rate of interest. If its loans are large, and it fears too great demands on the reserve, it will restrict the loans by a high interest charge. Thus by alternately raising and lowering the rate of interest, a bank keeps its loans within the sum which the reserve can support, but endeavors to keep them (for the sake of profit) as high as the reserve will support.

If the sums owed to individual depositors are large, relatively to the total liabilities, the reserve should be proportionately large, since the action of a small number of depositors can deplete it rapidly. The reserve in a large city of great banking activity needs to be greater in proportion to its demand liabilities than in a small town with infrequent banking transactions. No absolute numerical rule can be given. Arbitrary rules are often imposed by law. Banks in the United States, for instance, are required to keep a ratio of reserve to deposits, varying from twelve and a half per cent to twenty-five percent, according as they are state or national banks, and according to their location. For the whole country the reserves in banks are about one fifth of the deposits. These reserves are all in defense of deposits. In defense of bank notes, which are issued only by national banks, the method of protection is different. True, the same economic principles apply to both bank notes and deposits, but the law treats them differently. The gov

ernment itself chooses to undertake to redeem the national bank notes on demand, imposing on the banks certain obligations to deposit with itself a redemption fund and government bonds.

As previously stated the cash reserves of banks, though money, are not, properly speaking, money in circulation. The reason is that they are not held for the purchase of goods, but for the redemption of another kind of currency–deposits. Thus the money in any society is divided into two chief parts; money in circulation and money in banks. In the United States these two are approximately equal, both being about one and a half billion dollars.1 4. The Total Currency and its Circulation

The study of banking operations, then, discloses two species of bank currency: one, bank notes, belonging to the category of money; and the other, deposits, belonging outside of that category but constituting an excellent substitute. Referring these to the larger category of goods, we have a threefold classification of goods: first, money; second, deposit currency, or simply deposits; and third, all other goods. Among these, then, there are six possible types of exchange:– (1) Money against money, (2) Deposits against deposits, (3) Goods against goods, (4) Money against deposits, (5) Money against goods, (6) Deposits against goods.

For our purpose, only the last two types of exchange are important, for these constitute the circulation of currency. As regards the other four, the first and third have been previously explained as " money changing " and " barter," respectively. The second and fourth are banking transactions: the second being such operations as the selling of drafts for checks or the mutual cancellation of bank clearings; and the fourth being such operations as the depositing or withdrawing of money, by depositing cash or cashing checks.

1 In the United States there is a third though smaller stock of money, the hoard in the United States Treasury, amounting at present to about a third of a billion of dollars. In other countries the government money is usually almost all deposited in banks.

The analysis of the balance sheets of banks has prepared us for the inclusion of bank deposits or circulating credit in the equation of exchange. We shall still use M to express the quantity of actual money, and V to express the velocity of its circulation. Similarly, we shall now use M to express the total deposits subject to transfer by check; and V to express the average velocity of their circulation. The total value of purchases in a year is therefore no longer to be measured by MV, but by M V + MV. The equation of exchange, therefore, becomes

PT.

Let us again represent the equation of exchange by means of a mechanical picture. In Figure 12, trade, as before, is represented on the right by the weight of a miscellaneous

Flo.

assortment of goods; and their average price by the distance to the right from the fulcrum, or the leverage at which this weight hangs. Again at the left, money (M) is represented by a weight in the form of a purse, and its velocity of circulation (V) by its leverage; but now we have a new weight at the left, in the form of a bank book, to represent the bank deposits (M"). The velocity of circulation (V) of these bank deposits is represented by its distance from the fulcrum or the leverage at which the book hangs.

This mechanism makes clear the fact that the average price (right leverage) increases with the increase of money or bank deposits and with the velocities of their circulation, and decreases with the increase in the volume of trade.

Recurring to the left side of the equation of exchange, or M V + M V, we see that in a community without bank deposits the left side of the equation reduces simply to M V, the formula of Chapter VIII; for in such a community the term M V vanishes. The introduction of M tends to raise prices; that is, the hanging of the bank book on the left requires a lengthening of the leverage at the right.

5. Deposit Currency Normally Proportional to Money

With the extension of the equation of moneuly circulation to include deposit circulation, the influence Ixerted by the quantity of money on general prices becomes less direct; and the process of tracing this influence becomes more difficult and complicated. It has even been argued that this interposition of circulating credit breaks whatever connection there may be between prices and the quantity of money. This would be true if circulating credit were independent of money. But the fact is that the quantity of circulating credit, M, tends to hold a definite relation to M, the quantity of money in circulation; that is, deposits are normally a more or less definite multiple of money.

Two facts normally give deposits a more or less definite ratio to money. The first has been already explained, viz., that bank reserves are kept in a more or less definite ratio to bank deposits. The second is that individuals, firms, and corporations preserve more or less definite ratios between their cash transactions and their check transactions, and also between their money and deposit balances. These ratios are determined by motives of individual convenience and habit. In general, business firms use money for wage payments, and for small miscellaneous transactions included under the term " petty cash "; while for settlements with each other they usually prefer checks. These preferences are so strong that we could not imagine them overridden except temporarily, and to a small degree. A business firm would hardly pay car fares with checks and liquidate its large liabilities with cash. Each person strikes an equilibrium between his use of the two methods of payment, and does not greatly disturb it except for short periods of time. He keeps his stock of money or his bank balance in constant adjustment to the payments he makes in money or by check. Whenever his stock of money becomes relatively small and his bank balance relatively large, he cashes a check. In the opposite event, he deposits cash. In this way he is constantly converting one of the two media of exchange into the other. A private individual usually feeds his purse from his bank account; a retail commercial firm usually feeds its bank account from its till. The bank acts as intermediary for both.

Another reason why money and checks each have separate spheres, tending at any given time to maintain a fairly definite relation to each other, is that they are used in definitely different ways by different classes. Thus wage earners for the most part use only money, while the professional and propertied classes and the fictitious persons (corporations, partnerships, etc.) use mostly checks. At present probably over half of the families in the United States use no checks.

For any one individual the adjustment of cash-in-pocket to deposits-in-bank will be extremely rough; for sometimes the one or the other will be much too large or too small. But, for the community as a whole, the adjustment of the cash to deposits used will be very delicate; for the temporary aberrations of many thousands of individuals will ordinarily almost completely neutralize each other.

In a given community the quantitative relation of deposit currency to money is determined by several considerations of convenience. In the first place, the more highly developed the business of a community, the more prevalent the use of checks. Where business is conducted on a large scale, merchants habitually transact their larger operations with each other by means of checks, and their smaller ones by means of cash. Again, the more concentrated the population, the more prevalent the use of checks. In cities it is more convenient both for the payer and the payee to make large payments by check; whereas, in the country, trips to a bank are too expensive in time and effort to be convenient, and therefore more money is used in proportion to the amount of business done. Again, the wealthier the members of the community, the more largely will they use checks. Laborers seldom use them; but capitalists, professional and salaried men, use them habitually, for personal as well as business transactions.

There is, then, a relation of convenience and Custom between check and cash circulation, and a more or less stable ratio between the deposit balance of the average man or corporation and the stock of money kept in pocket or till. This fact, as applied to the country as a whole, means that by convenience a fairly definite ratio is fixed between M and M. If that ratio is disturbed temporarily, there will come into play a tendency to restore it. Individuals will deposit surplus cash, or they will cash surplus deposits.

Hence, both money in circulation (as shown above) and money in reserve (as shown previously) tend to keep in a fixed ratio to deposits. It follows that the two must be in a more or less definite, though elastic, ratio to each other.

6. Summary

The contents of this chapter may be formulated in a few simple propositions:– (1) Banks supply two kinds of currency, viz., bank notes –which are money; and bank deposits (or rights to draw) –which are not money.

(2) A bank check is merely presumptive evidence of a right to draw.

(3) Behind the claims of depositors and note holders stand, not simply the cash reserve, but all the assets of the bank.

(4) Deposit banking is a device by which wealth, incapable of direct circulation, may be made the basis of the circulation of rights to draw.

(5) The basis of such circulating rights to draw or deposits must consist in part of actual money, and it should consist in part also of quick assets readily exchangeable for money.

(6) Six sorts of exchange exist among the three classes of goods, money, deposits, and other goods. Of these six sorts of exchange, the most important for our present purposes are the exchanges of money and deposits against other goods.

(7) The equation of money circulation, extended so as to make it include bank deposits, reads thus: MV + MV = I. pq = FT.

(8) Bank deposits (M) tend to keep a normal ratio to bank reserves and to the quantity of money (M); because, in the first place, cash reserves are necessary to support bank deposits, and these reserves must bear some more or less constant ratio to the amount of such deposits; and because, in the second place, business convenience dictates that the circulating medium or currency shall be apportioned between deposits and money in a certain more or less definite, even though elastic, ratio.

CHAPTER X

CAUSES AND EFFECTS OF PURCHASING POWER DURING TRANSITION PERIODS

1. Transition Periods In the preceding chapter it was shown that the quantity of bank deposits normally maintains a more or less definite ratio to the quantity of money in circulation and to the amount of bank reserves. As long as this normal relation holds, the existence of bank deposits merely magnifies the effect on the level of prices produced by the quantity of money in circulation and does not in the least distort that effect. Moreover, changes in velocity or trade will have the same kind of effect on prices, whether bank deposits are included or not.

But during periods of transition this relation between money (M) and deposits (Af) is by no means rigid. By a period of transition is meant the interval of time during which a disturbance in any of the six magnitudes in the equation of exchange (for instance, an increase in the quantity of money in circulation) works out its effects. It takes time for any such disturbance to completely work out its results, just as it takes time after a locomotive engineer has put on more steam for the full effects to be felt by the train which is drawn. There is always a transition period which must elapse before any new cause completes its influence, and, during this transition period, the effects are somewhat different from the final result after the transition period is over. Thus, though the final result of suddenly putting on the increased steam will be to increase the speed of the train from thirty miles per hour to forty miles per hour, this effect will not be felt immediately. There will be a transition period of several minutes before this speed is attained. During this transition period the speed will gradually increase, the couplings will expand and then contract, the passengers will feel jolted, and so forth. After the transition period is over, the train will run smoothly again.

We are now ready to study periods of transition for the equation of exchange. Our concern is with rising or falling prices. Rising prices mark the transition between a lower and a higher level of prices, just as a hill marks the transition between flat lowlands and flat highlands.

The study of these acclivities and declivities is bound up with the study of business loans. Now when prices are rising borrowers are benefited and lenders injured, while when prices are falling the opposite is true. It must be borne in mind that although business loans are made in the form of money, yet whenever a man borrows money he does not do this in order to hoard the money, but to purchase goods with it. Suppose A borrows 100 from B. What has really been borrowed is purchasing power. If at the end of a year A returns 100 to B, but prices have meanwhile advanced, then B has lost a fraction of the purchasing power originally loaned to A. Even though A should happen to return to B the identical coins in which the loan was made, these coins represent somewhat less than the original quantity of purchasable commodities. Bearing this in mind, let us suppose that prices are rising. Then every lender will lose by the rise in prices unless he can safeguard himself against this loss by making sufficiently hard terms with the borrower. Usually, however, when prices are about to rise, neither the lender nor the borrower fully realizes that prices are going to rise as much as they actually do.

2. How a Rise of Prices Generates a Further Rise

We are now ready to study temporary or transitional changes in the factors of our equation of exchange. Let us begin by assuming a slight initial disturbance, such as would be produced, for instance, by an increase in the quantity of gold. This, through the equation of exchange, will cause a rise in prices. As prices rise, profits of business men measured in money will rise also, even if the costs of business were to rise in the same proportion. Thus, if a man who sold goods for 10,000 which cost 6000, clearing 4000, could get double prices at double cost, his profit would double also, being 20,000–12,000, which is 8000. Of course, such a rise of profits would be purely nominal, as it would merely keep pace with the rise in price level. The business man would gain no advantage, for his larger money profits would buy no more than his former smaller money profits bought before. But, as a matter of fact, the business mans profits will usually rise more than this, because many of his expenses will tend to remain the same. In particular his payments to creditors for past loans and his payments to employees for work will for a time remain unaffected or little affected by the general rise in prices. Consequently, he will find himself making greater profits than usual, and be encouraged to expand his business by increasing his borrowings. These borrowings are mostly in the form of short-time loans from banks; and, as we have seen (Chapter IX, 1), short-time loans engender deposits. Therefore, deposit currency (Af) will increase. But this extension of deposit currency tends further to raise the general level of prices, just as the increase of gold raised it in the first place. This further rise of prices enables borrowers who are now receiving greater profits to receive still greater profits. Borrowing, already stimulated, is stimulated still further. More loans are demanded, and, with the resulting expansion of bank loans, deposit currency (M), already expanded, expands still more. Hence prices rise still further.

This sequence of events may be briefly stated as follows:– (1) Prices rise (whatever the first cause may be; we have chosen for illustration an increase in the amount of money in circulation).

(2) "Enterprisers," i. e., persons who undertake business enterprises of various kinds, get much higher prices than before, without having much greater expenses, and therefore make much greater profits.

(3) Enterpriser-borrowers, encouraged by large profits, expand their loans.

(4) Deposit currency (M) expands relatively to money (M). " f (5) Because of this expansion of deposit currency (M) prices continue to rise; that is, phenomenon No. 1 is repeated. Then No. 2 is repeated, and so on.

In other words, a slight initial rise of prices sets in motion a train of events which tends to repeat itself. Rise of prices generates rise of prices, and continues to do so as long as the enterprisers profits continue abnormally high.

3. How a Rise of Prices Culminates in a Crisis

The expansion in deposit currency indicated in this cumulative movement abnormally increases the ratio of M to M. This, however, is not the only disturbance caused by the increase in M. There are disturbances to some extent in the Qs, in V, and in V". In particular, trade (the Qs) will be stimulated by the stimulation of loans. New constructions of buildings, etc., are entered upon. These effects are always observed during rising prices, and people note approvingly that " business is good " and " times are booming." Such statements represent the point of view of the ordinary business man who is an " enterpriser borrower." They do not represent the sentiments of the creditor, the salaried man, or the laborer, most of whom are silent but long-suffering, paying higher prices, but not getting proportionally higher incomes.

But the expansion cannot proceed forever. It must ultimately spend itself. A check upon its continued operation lies in making loans harder to get. As soon as this occurs, the whole situation is changed. The banks are forced in self-defense to refuse loans (or at any rate to discourage loans by making harder terms for them.) because they cannot stand so abnormal an expansion of loans relatively to reserves. Then borrowers can no longer hope to make great profits, and loans cease to expand.

There are other forces placing a limitation on further expansion of deposit currency and introducing a tendency to contraction, but those above mentioned are the most important.

Now an enterprise, as it is started by borrowing, is expected to be continued by renewed borrowing. But with loans hard to get, those persons who have counted on renewing their loans on the former terms and for the former amounts are unable to do so. It follows that those of them who cannot contract new debts and, without contracting such new debts, cannot pay old ones are destined to become insolvent and fail. The failure (or prospect of failure) of firms that have borrowed heavily from banks induces fear on the part of many depositors that the banks will not be able to realize on these loans. Hence the banks themselves fall under suspicion, and for this reason depositors demand cash. Then occur " runs on the banks," which deplete the bank reserves at the very moment they are most needed to pay the demands of the depositors. Being short of reserves, the banks have to curtail their loans. Renewed borrowing becomes difficult or impossible, and even the original loans may be " called " by the banks. Those enterprisers who are caught must have currency to liquidate their obligations or else become insolvent. Some of them are destined to become bankrupt, and, with their failure, the demand for loans is correspondingly reduced. This culmination of an upward price movement is what is called a crisis, a condition characterized by failures which are due to a lack of cash when it is most needed. Bankruptcies, as shown in Chapter III, 5, tend to spread from debtor to creditor.

4. Completion of the Credit Cycle

After the crest of the wave is reached, a reaction sets in. Bank loans tend to be small, and consequently deposits (M) are reduced. The contraction of deposit currency makes prices fall still more. Those who have borrowed for the purpose of buying stocks of goods, now find they cannot sell them for enough even to pay back what they have borrowed. The sequence of events is now the opposite of what it was before:– (1) Prices fall.

(2) Enterprisers get much lower prices than before without having much lower expenses, and therefore make much lower profits.

(3) Enterpriser-borrowers, discouraged by small profits, contract their borrowings.

(4) Deposit currency (M) contracts relatively to money (M).

(5) Because of this contraction of deposit currency (M) prices continue to fall; that is, phenomenon No. 1 is repeated. Then No. 2 is repeated, and so on.

Thus a fall of prices generates a further fall of prices. The cycle evidently repeats itself as long as the enterprisers profits remain abnormally low. The man who loses most is the business man in debt. He is the typical business man, and he now complains that " business is bad." There is a " depression of trade."

The contraction becomes self-limiting as soon as loans are easier to get. Banks are led to make loans easy in order to get rid of their accumulated reserves. After a time, normal conditions begin to return. The weakest producers have been forced out, or have at least been prevented from expanding their business by increased loans. The strongest firms are left to build up a new credit structure. Borrowers again become willing to take ventures; failures decrease in number; bank loans cease to decrease; prices cease to fall; borrowing and carrying on business becomes profitable; loans are again demanded; prices again begin to rise, and there occurs a repetition of the upward movement already described.

The upward and downward movements taken together constitute a complete credit cycle, which resembles the forward and backward movements of a pendulum.

Many historical examples could be cited. The discovery of gold in California in the middle of the last century was followed by an inflation of the worlds currency, first through the new gold and later through expansion of deposit currency as well. Prices rose rapidly; business men made high profits; times were good until 1857, when a crisis occurred both in the United States and Europe. This was followed by a sharp fall in prices, a depression in trade, a recovery and another period of inflation culminating in a second crisis in 1866. Again the pendulum swung back, only to return again in the crisis of 1873. A more recent example is found in the gold inflation beginning in 1896 in consequence of the enormous gold production in the Transvaal, in Cripple Creek, and in the Klondike. The money in circulation in the United States doubled in eleven years (1896-1907), bank deposits subject to check nearly trebled, prices rose 50 per cent. "Prosperity" (that is, profitable business from the point of view of the enterpriser) seemed boundless. In 1907 the wave broke in the crisis of that year, followed by a contraction of deposits and a fall of prices in the next year with a gradual recovery in the years immediately following.

We have considered the rise, culmination, fall, and recovery of prices. In most cases the time occupied by the swing of the commercial pendulum to and fro is about ten years. While the pendulum is continually seeking a stable position, practically there is almost always some occurrence to prevent perfect equilibrium. Oscillation s are set up which, though tending to be self-corrective, are continually perpetuated by fresh disturbances.

The factors in the equation of exchange are continually seeking normal adjustment. A ship in a calm sea will " pitch " only a few times before coming to rest. But in a high sea the pitching never ceases. While continually seeking equilibrium, the ship continually encounters causes which accentuate the oscillation.

The foregoing sketch of prices gives, of course, only the elementary features of price cycles. In any actual case numerous special factors enter. The factors which we have studied are those in the equation of exchange.

CHAPTER XI

REMOTE INFLUENCES ON PRICES 1. Influences which Conditions of Production and Consumption Exert on Trade and therefore on Prices

Thus far we have considered the level of prices as affected by the volume of trade, by the velocity of circulation of money and of deposits, and by the quantity of money and of deposits. These are the only influences which can directly affect the level of prices. Any other influences on prices must act through these five. There are myriads of such influences (outside of the equation of exchange) that affect prices through the medium of these five. It is our purpose in this chapter to note the chief among them, excepting those that affect the volume of money (M); the latter will be examined in the next chapter.

We shall first consider the outside influences that affect the volume of trade and, through it, the price level. The conditions which determine the extent of trade in the world or within any particular area are numerous and technical. The most important may be classified as follows:– 1. Conditions affecting producers.

(a) Geographical differences in natural resources.

(b) The division of labor.

(c) Knowledge of the technique of production.

(d) The accumulation of capital.

2. Conditions affecting consumers.

(a) The extent and variety of human wants. 3. Conditions connecting producers and consumers.

(a) Facilities for transportation.

(b) Relative freedom of trade.

(c) Character of monetary and banking systems.

(d) Business confidence.

1. (a) Geographical differences. If all localities were exactly alike in their natural resources, no trade would be set up between them. Cattle raising in Texas, the production of coal in Pennsylvania, of oranges in Florida, of apples in Oregon, etc., promote trade among these communities.

1. (b) Division of labor. By division of labor is meant the system by which different individuals in society perform different kinds of work. It is based in part on differences in comparative costs or efforts of different men producing different goods–corresponding to geographic differences as between countries. Because of such differences, natural and acquired, some men devote themselves to farming, others to weaving, others to carpentry, others to mason work, plumbing, typesetting, moving pianos, or driving aeroplanes, and exchange their products.

1. (c) Knowledge of technique. Besides local and personal differentiation, the state of knowledge of the means and methods of production will stimulate trade. For

instance, mines of Africa and Australia were left unworked for centuries by ignorant natives, but were opened by white men possessing a knowledge of metallurgy.

1. (d) Accumulation of capital. But knowledge, to be of use, must be applied; and its application usually requires the aid of capital. The greater and the more productive the stock of capital in any community, the more goods it can put into the currents of trade. A mill will make a town a center of trade. Docks, elevators, warehouses, and railway terminals help to transform a harbor into a port of commerce.

Since increase in trade tends to decrease the general level of prices, it is obvious that anything which tends to increase trade likewise tends to decrease the general level of prices. We conclude, therefore, that among the various causes which tend to decrease prices are greater geographical or personal specialization, improved productive technique, and the accumulation of capital.

2. (a) Extent and variety of human wants. Wants are, as it were, the mainsprings of economic activity which in the last analysis keep the economic world in motion. The desire to have clothes as fine as the clothes of others, or finer, or different, leads to the multiplicity of silks, satins, laces, etc.; and the same principle applies to furniture, amusements, books, works of art, and every other means of gratification.

The increase of wants, in so far as it leads to an increase in trade, tends to lower the price level.

2. Influences which Conditions Connecting Producers and Consumers Exert on Trade and therefore on Prices 3. (a) Facilities for transportation. As Macaulay said, with the exception of the alphabet and the printing press, no set of inventions has tended to alter civilization so much as those which abridge distance–such as the railway, the steamship, the telephone, the telegraph, and that conveyer of information and advertisements, the newspaper. These all tend, therefore, to decrease prices.

3. (i) Relative freedom of trade. Trade barriers are not only physical, but legal. A tariff between countries has the same influence in decreasing trade as a chain of mountains. The freer the trade, the more of it there will be. In France, many communities have a local tariff (octroi) which tends to interfere with local trade. In the United States, trade is free within the country itself, but between the United States and other countries there is a high protective tariff. The very fact of increasing facilities for transportation, lowering or removing physical barriers, has stimulated nations and communities to erect legal barriers in their place. Tariffs not only tend to decrease the frequency of exchanges, but to the extent that they prevent international or interlocal division of labor and make countries more alike as well as less productive, they also tend to decrease the amounts of goods which can be exchanged. The ultimate effect is thus to raise prices. This is the effect on the general level of prices. Besides this general effect are the particular effects on those articles on which duties are laid, but with these particular effects we have here nothing to do.

Another sort of restriction on trade is the " restraint of trade " of monopolies or combinations. These, of course, like any other reduction in the amounts of goods sold, tend to raise the general level of prices.

3. (c) Monetary and banking systems. The development of efficient monetary and banking systems tends, among other effects, to increase trade. There have been times in the history of the world when the money was in so uncertain a state that people

hesitated to make many trade contracts because of the lack of knowledge of what would be required of them when the contract should be fulfilled. In the same way, when people cannot depend on the good faith or stability of banks, they will hesitate to use deposits and checks.

3. (d) Business confidence. Confidence, not only in banks in particular, but in business dealings in general, is truly said to be " the soul of trade." In South America there are many places waiting to be developed simply because capitalists do not feel any security in contracts there. They are fearful that by hook or by crook the fruit of any investments they may make will be taken from them.

We see, then, that prices will tend to fall through an increase in trade, which may in turn be brought about by improved transportation, by increased freedom of trade, by improved monetary and banking systems, and by business confidence.

3. Influence of Individual Habits on Velocities of Circulation, and therefore on Prices

Having examined those causes outside the equation which affect the volume of trade, our next task is to consider those outside causes which affect the velocities of circulation of money and of deposits. For the most part, the causes affecting one of these velocities affect the other also. These causes may be classified as follows:– 1. Habits of the individual (a) As to hoarding, (b) As to book credit and loans, (c) As to the use of checks.

2. Systems of payments in the community (a) As to frequency of receipts and of disbursements, (b) As to regularity of receipts and of disbursements, (c) As to correspondence between receipts and disbursements.

3. General causes.

(a) Density of population,

(6) Rapidity of transportation.

1. (a) Hoarding. Taking these up in order, we may first consider what influence hoarding has on the velocity of circulation. Velocity of circulation of money is the same thing as its rate of turnover. It is found (Chapter VIII, 3) by dividing the total payments effected by money in a year by the average amount of money in circulation in that year. It is an average of the rates of turnover of the individuals which compose the society. This velocity of circulation or rapidity of turnover of money is the greater for each individual, the more he expends with a given average amount of cash on hand, or the less average cash he keeps for a given yearly expenditure. One man keeps an average of 10 in his pocket and expends 500 a year; he, therefore, turns over the contents of his pocket fifty times a year. Another, while expending the same sum (500), keeps the more prudent average of 20; he, therefore, turns over his stock of cash only twenty-five times a year.

Some people are by habit always impecunious or short of ready money and tend to have a high rate of turnover; others carry a full purse and have a slow rate of turnover. When, as used to be the custom in France, people put money away in stockings and kept it there for months, the velocity of circulation must have been extremely slow. The same principle applies to deposits.

Hoarded money is sometimes said to be withdrawn from circulation, but this is only another way of saying that hoarding tends to decrease the velocity of circulation. The only real distinction between " hoarding" money in a stocking or safe and " carrying " money in a purse is one of degree. The money remains in the stocking or safe longer than in the purse. In either case it may be said to be in circulation, but when " hoarded" it circulates much more slowly. In the case of individual hoards, as of misers, it is convenient to consider them as in circulation. Only in the case of the larger government hoards is it worth while to consider them as excluded from " money in circulation."

1. (6) Book credit and loans. The habit of " charging," i. e., using book credit, tends to increase the velocity of circulation of money, because the man who gets things "charged" does not need to keep on hand as much money as he would if he made all payments in cash. A man who daily pays cash needs to keep cash for daily contingencies. The system of cash payments, unlike the system of book credit, requires that money shall be kept on hand in advance of purchases. Evidently, if money must be provided in advance, it must be provided in larger quantities than when merely required to liquidate past debts. In the system of cash payments a man must keep money idle in advance, lest he be caught in the embarrassing position of lacking it when he most needs it. With book credit he knows that even if he should be caught without a cent in his pocket, he can still get supplies on credit. These he can pay for when money comes to hand. As soon as this money is received there is a use awaiting it to pay debts accumulated. For instance, a laborer receiving and spending 7 a week, if he cannot " charge," must make his weeks wages last through the week. If he spends 1 a day, his weekly cycle must show on hand on successive days at least 7, 6, 5, 4, 3, 2, and 1, at which time another 7 comes in. This makes the average balance 4. The rate of turnover (ratio of expenditure to cash carried) is 7-5-4 or about twice a week. But if he can charge everything, and then wait until pay day to meet the resulting obligations, he need keep nothing through the week, paying out his 7 when it comes in. His weekly cycle need show no higher balances than 7, o, o, o, o, o, o, averaging only 1, and the turnover is 7-5-1 or seven times a week.

Analogous to book credit is the use of loans of any kind. In a highly organized center of trade, like the New York stock or produce exchanges, credit is extended to an extreme degree in order to facilitate the transactions of a large volume of business without the necessity of keeping on hand a large cash balance of money or deposits subject to check. Credit is extended by loans, by allowing purchases on small payments called " margins," and in other ways. All these extensions of loan credits tend to increase the velocity of circulation of money and deposits.

Through book credit and loans, therefore, 1e average amount of money or bank deposits which each g rson must keep on hand to meet a given expenditure is made less. This means that the rate of turnover is increased; for if people spend the same amounts as before, but keep smaller amounts on hand, the quotient of the amount spent divided by the amount on hand must increase.

1. (c) Use of checks. The habit of using checks rather than money will also affect the velocity of circulation of money, because a depositors surplus money will immediately be put in the bank in return for a right to draw by check.

Banks thus offer an outlet for any surplus pocket money or surplus till money, and tend to prevent the existence of idle hoards. In like manner, surplus deposits may be converted into cash–that is, exchanged for cash–as desired. In short, those who make use both of cash and deposits have the opportunity, by adjusting the two, to prevent either from being idle.

We see, then, that these three habits–the habit of being impecunious, the habit of charging, and the habit of using checks–all tend to raise the level of prices through their effects on the velocity of circulation of money, or of deposits.

4. Influence of Systems of Payments on Velocities of Circulation and therefore on Prices 2. (a) Frequency of receipts and of disbursements. The more frequently money or checks are received and disbursed, the shorter is the average interval between the receipt and the expenditure of money or checks, and the more rapid is the velocity of circulation.

This may best be seen from an example. A change from monthly to weekly wage payments tends to increase the velocity of circulation of money. If a laborer is paid weekly 7, and reduces this evenly each day, ending each week empty-handed, his average cash, as we have seen, would be a little over half of 7, or about 4. This makes his turnover nearly twice a week. Under monthly payments, the laborer who receives and spends an average of S1 a day will have to spread the 30, more or less evenly, over the following thirty days. If, at the next pay day, he comes out empty-handed, his average money during the month has been about 15. This makes his turnover about twice a month. Thus the rate of turnover is more rapid under weekly than under monthly payments provided, of course, the introduction of weekly payments does not disturb some other factor influencing velocity. If it leads to cash payments in place of book credit, the rate of turnover may really decrease instead of increasing.

2. (b) Regularity of receipts and of disbursements. When the workingman can be fairly certain of both his receipts and expenditures, he can, by close calculation, adjust them so precisely as safely to end each payment cycle with an empty pocket. This habit is extremely common among certain classes of city laborers. On the other hand, if the receipts and expenditures are irregular, either in amount or in time, prudence requires the worker to keep a larger sum on hand to insure against mishaps. Even when foreknown with certainty, irregular receipts require a larger average sum to be kept on hand. We may, therefore, conclude that regularity, both of receipts and of payments, tends to increase velocity of circulation.

2. (c) Correspondence between receipts and disbursements. We next consider the synchronizing of receipts and disbursements, i. e., making the payments come at nearly the same times as the times when receipts are obtained. It is manifestly a great convenience to the spender of money, or of deposits, if dealers to whom he is in debt will allow him to postpone payment until he has received his money or his check. This arrangement obviates the necessity of keeping much money or deposits on hand, and therefore increases their velocity of circulation. Where payments, such as rent, interest, insurance, and taxes, occur at periods irrespective of the times of receipts of money, it is often necessary to accumulate money or deposits in advance, thus increasing the average on hand, withdrawing money from use for a time, and decreasing the velocity of circulation.

We conclude, then, that synchronizing and regularity of payment, no less than frequency of payment, tend to increase prices by increasing velocity of circulation.

5. Influence of General Causes on Velocities of Circulation and therefore on Prices

3. (a) Density of population. The more densely populated a locality, the more rapid will be the velocity of circulation, because there will be readier access to people from whom money is received or to whom it is paid. In the country, although there are no statistics on this subject, the velocity of circulation must be much slower than in the city. A lady who has a city house and a country house states that in the country she keeps money in her purse for weeks, whereas in the city she keeps it but a few days. Pierre des Essars has worked out the velocity of circulation at banks in many European cities. Examination of his figures reveals the fact that, in almost all cases, the larger the town in which the bank is situated, the more active the deposits. The bank of Greece has a turnover whose rate of rapidity is only four times a year, while that of the bank of France is over one hundred times a year.

3. (b) Rapidity of transportation. Again, the more extensive and the speedier the transportation in general, the more rapid the circulation of money. Anything which makes it easier to pass money from one person to another will tend to increase the velocity of circulation. Railways have this effect. The telegraph has increased the velocity of circulation of deposits, since these can now be trans ferred thousands of miles in a few minutes. Mail and express, by facilitating the transmission of bank deposits and money, have likewise tended to increase their velocity of circulation.

We conclude, then, that density of population and rapidity of communication tend to increase prices by increasing velocities of circulation.

6. Influences on the Volume of Deposit Currency and therefore on Prices

We have to consider lastly the specific outside influences on the volume of deposits subject to check. These are chiefly:– (1) The system of banking and the habits of the people in utilizing that system.

(2) The habit of charging.

(1) Systems and habits of banking. It goes without saying that a banking system must be devised and developed before deposits can affect prices or even exist. The invention of banking has undoubtedly led to a great increase in deposits and a con-sequent rise of prices. This has been true, in spite of the fact that, as pointed out in 1, the development of efficient monetary and banking systems tends to increase trade and to that extent to lower the price level. Here, as in many other instances, the effects of improving monetary and banking facilities are complex, affecting more than one factor in the equation of exchange. The price-raising effect is far more important than the price-depressing effect. In the future one of the chief causes tending to raise prices will doubtless be the expansion of deposits subject to check.

(2) Habit of charging. We have already seen that " charging " increases the velocity of circulation of money. It is also a means of increasing the volume of deposits sub ject to check; that is, "charging" is often a preliminary to payment by check rather than by cash. If a customer did not have his obligations " charged," he would pay by money and not by check. The ultimate effect of the practice of charging, therefore, is to increase the ratio of check payments to cash payments and the ratio of deposits to money carried (M to M) and therefore to increase the amount of credit currency which a given quantity of money can sustain.

This effect, the substitution of checks for cash payments, is probably by far the most important effect of " charging," and exerts a powerful influence toward raising prices.

Anything which tends to increase bank deposits tends, to that extent, to raise prices. Thus the creation of " trusts " has resulted in the issue of a great mass of stocks and bonds which are more readily accepted by bankers as " collateral" for loans than the stocks and bonds of the smaller and less known companies from which the " trusts " are formed. The consequence is: more bank loans, greater deposits, and a higher level of prices. Besides these and the other effects of " trusts," which have been mentioned elsewhere, on the general level of prices there are the more obvious and direct effects on the particular prices of the goods dealt in by the " trusts." But we have here nothing to do with particular prices. We may observe, however, that when trusts raise particular prices it does not follow that they raise the general level of prices. Unless they disturb the five factors, M, M, V, V, or T, they cannot affect the general level of prices; for, in that case, the general level of prices, as the equation of exchange shows, could not be disturbed either, and the raising of prices of particular trust-made articles would have to result indirectly in lowering the prices of some other goods enough to compensate in the general level.

CHAPTER XII

REMOTE INFLUENCES (Continued) 1. Influence of " The Balance of Trade " on the

Quantity of Money and therefore on Prices

We have now considered those influences outside the equation of exchange which affect the volume of trade (the Qs), the velocities of circulation of money and deposits (7 and V), and the amount of deposits (M1). We have reserved for separate treatment in this chapter the outside influences which affect the quantity of money (M).

The chief of these may be classified as follows:– (1) Influences operating through the exportation and importation of money.

(2) Influences operating through the melting or minting of money.

(3) Influences operating through the production and consumption of money metals.

(4) Influences of monetary and banking systems.

The first to be considered is the influence of foreign trade on the quantity of money in a country and therefore on its price level. Hitherto we have confined our studies of price levels to an isolated community, having no trade relations with other communities. In the modern world, however, no such community exists, and it is important to observe that international trade gives present-day problems of money and of the price level an international character. If all countries had their own irredeemable paper money and no money that was acceptable elsewhere, price levels in different countries would have no intimate connection. Indeed, the connection is actually slight as between countries which have different metallic standards, for example, between a gold-basis and a silver-basis country. But where two or more nations trading with each other use the same standard, there is a tendency for the price levels of each to influence profoundly the price levels of the other.

The price level in a small country like Switzerland depends largely upon the price level in other countries; for if the price level in these other countries is higher or lower than in Switzerland, the difference will set up trade currents which will increase or decrease the quantity of money in Switzerland and therefore raise or lower its level of prices to correspond to the levels outside. Gold, which is the primary or full-weight money in most civilized nations, is in this way constantly sent from one country or community to another. When a single small country is under consideration, while it is quite correct to say that the quantity of money in that country determines the price level, we must not fail to note that the quantity of money within its borders is in turn dependent upon the level of prices outside. An individual country bears the same relation to the world that a lagoon bears to the ocean. The level of the lagoon depends, of course, upon the quantity of water in it. But the quantity of water in it depends in turn upon the level of the ocean. As the tide in the outside ocean rises and falls, the quantity of water in the lagoon will adjust itself accordingly.

To simplify the problem of the distribution of money among different communities, we shall, for the time being, ignore the fact that money consists ordinarily of material capable of nonmonetary uses. We shall therefore omit consideration of the disappearance of money through melting; likewise, for the present, we shall omit consideration of the production of money through minting.

Let us, then, consider the causes that determine the quantity of money in a state like Connecticut. If the level of prices in Connecticut temporarily falls below that of the surrounding states, Rhode Island, Massachusetts, and New York, the effect is to cause an export of money from these states to Connecticut, because people will buy goods wherever they are cheapest and sell them wherever they are dearest. With its low prices, Connecticut becomes a good place to buy from, and a poor place to sell in. But if outsiders buy of Connecticut, they will have to bring money to buy with. There will, therefore, be a tendency for money to flow to Connecticut until the level of prices there rises to a level which will arrest the influx. If, on the other hand, prices in Connecticut are higher than in surrounding states, it becomes a good place to sell in and a poor one to buy from. But if outsiders sell in Connecticut, they will receive money in exchange. There is then a tendency for money to flow out of Connecticut until the level of prices in Connecticut is lower. In general, money flows away from places where the level of prices is high, and towards places where it is low. Men sell goods where they can get most money, and buy goods where they will have to give least money. We say " money," for in the long run we do not need to consider the interflow of bank deposits; as we have seen, in the long run deposit currency in each country will maintain a definite ratio to money. In the long run an increase or decrease of money in a country will increase or decrease its deposits.

But it must not be inferred that the prices of various articles or even the general level of prices will become precisely the same in different countries. Distance, ignorance as to where the best markets are to be found, tariffs, and costs of transportation, help to maintain price differences. The native products of each region tend to be cheaper in that region. They are exported as long as the excess of prices abroad is enough to more than cover the cost of transportation. Ordinarily a commodity will not be exported at a price which will not at least be equal to the price in the country of origin, plus the freight. Many commodities are shipped only one way. Thus, wheat is shipped from the United States to England, but not from England to the United States. It tends to be cheaper in the United States. Large exportations raise its price in America toward the price in England, but the American price will usually remain below the English price by the cost of transportation. A few commodities may be sent in either direction, according to market conditions.

But, although international or interlocal trade will never bring about exact uniformity of price levels, it will, to the extent that it exists, produce an adjustment of these levels toward uniformity by regulating, in the manner already described, the distribution of money. If one commodity enters to any considerable extent into international trade, it alone will suffice, though slowly, to act as a regulator of money distribution; for, in return for that commodity, money may flow, and, as the price level rises or falls, the quantity of that commodity sold is correspondingly adjusted. In ordinary intercourse between nations, even when a deliberate attempt is made to interfere with it by protective tariffs, there will always be a large number of commodities thus acting as outlets and inlets. And since the quantity of money itself affects prices for all sorts of commodities, the regulative effect of international trade applies, not simply to the commodities which enter into that trade, but to all others as well. It follows that nowadays international or interlocal trade is constantly regulating price levels throughout the world.

We must not leave this subject without emphasizing the effects of a tariff on the purchasing power of money. When a country adopts a duty on imports, the tendency is for the level of prices in that country to rise. A tariff obviously raises the prices of the " protected " goods. Thus the high duties on wool and woolen goods have kept American prices of wool and woolens higher than European prices. But the tariff does more than that—it tends also to raise the prices of wwprotected goods. Thus, the tariff first causes a decrease in imports. This sudden decrease in imports will lead to a corresponding but gradual decrease in exports. This gradual check on exports will come about indirectly. The foreigner will, for a time, continue to buy from the protected country almost as much as before. This unchecked buying of goods means unchecked export of goods while the imports have suddenly been checked. There will result, therefore, a temporary excess of the protected countrys exports over its imports, or a so-called " favorable " balance of trade, that is, a net inflow of money. This inflow will eventually raise the prices, not alone of protected goods, but of unprotected goods as well. The rise will continue till it reaches a point high enough to put a stop to the " favorable " balance of trade,–that is, until foreigners cease to send in their money.

Although the " favorable balance " of trade created by a tariff is temporary, it leaves behind a permanent increase of money and of prices. This is, perhaps, the chief reason why a protective tariff seems to many a cause of prosperity. It furnishes a temporary stimulus not only to protected industries, but to trade in general, which is in reality simply the stimulus of money inflation. The permanent effect is to keep prices in general, including wages, at a higher level in the protected country than in free trade countries. This is doubtless one reason why American wages and prices are higher than English.

We have shown how the international or interlocal equilibrium of prices may be disturbed by changes in the distribution of money alone. But it may also be disturbed by changes in the volume of bank deposits, or in the velocity of circulation of money, or in the velocity of circulation of bank deposits, or in the volume of trade. But whatever

may be the source of the difference in price levels, equilibrium will eventually be restored through an international or interlocal redistribution of money and goods brought about by international or interlocal trade. Elements in the equation of exchange other than money and commodities cannot be transported from one place to another.

2. Influence of Melting and Minting on the Quantity of Money and therefore on Prices

We have seen how M in the equation of exchange is affected by the importation or exportation of money. Considered with reference to the M in any one of the countries concerned, the Ms in all the others are " outside influences."

Proceeding now one step farther, we must consider those influences on M that are not only outside of the equation of exchange for any particular country, but also outside that for the whole world. Besides the monetary inflow and outflow through importation and exportation, there is an inflow and outflow through minting and melting. In other words, not only do the stocks of money in the world connect with each other like interconnecting bodies of water, but they connect in the same way with the outside slock of bullion. In the modern world one of the precious metals, such as gold, usually plays the part of primary money, and this metal has two uses–a monetary use and a commodity use. That is to say, gold is not only a money material, but a commodity as well. In their character of commodities, the precious metals are raw materials for jewelry, works of art, and other products into which they may be wrought. It is in this unmanufactured or raw state that they are called bullion.

Gold money may be changed into gold bullion, and vice versa. In fact, both changes are going on constantly, for if the value of gold as compared with other commodities is greater in the one use than in the other, gold will immediately flow toward whichever use is more profitable, and the market price of gold bullion in terms of gold money will determine the direction of the flow. Since 100 ounces of gold, i9o fine, can be transformed into 1860 gold dollars, the market value of so much gold bullion,-and fine, must tend to be 1860. If it costs nothing to have bullion coined into money, and nothing to melt money into bullion, there will be an automatic flux and reflux from money to bullion and from bullion to money that will prevent the price of bullion from varying greatly. On the one hand, if the price of gold bullion is greater than the money which could be minted from it, for instance, if 100 ounces of gold sell for 1861, the users of gold who require bullion–notably jewelers–will save the 1 difference by melting 1860 of gold coin into 100 ounces of bullion. Contrariwise, if the price of bullion is less than the value of gold coin, say 1859, the owners of bullion will save the 1 difference by taking 100 ounces of bullion to the nunt and having it coined into 1860 gold dollars. The effect of melting coin, on the one hand, is to decrease the amount of gold money and increase the amount of gold bullion, thereby lowering the value of gold as bullion and raising the value of gold as money; and thereby also lowering the price level and restoring the equality between bullion and money. The effect of minting bullion into coin is, by the opposite process, to bring the value of gold as coin and the value of gold as bullion into equilibrium.

When a charge called " seigniorage " is made for changing bullion into coin, or where the process involves expense or delay, the flow of bullion into currency will be to that extent impeded. But under a modern system of free coinage and with modern methods of reducing coin to bullion, both melting and minting may be performed so inexpensively and so quickly that there is practically no cost or delay involved. In fact, there are few instances of more exact price adjustment than the adjustment between gold bullion and gold coin. It follows that the quantity of money, and therefore its purchasing power, is directly dependent on that of gold bullion.

This stability of the price of gold bullion expressed in gold com causes confusion in the minds of people, giving them the erroneous impression that there is no change in the value of money. Indeed, this stability has often been cited to show that gold is a stable standard of value. Dealers in objects made of gold seem to misunderstand the significance of the fact that an ounce of gold (fine) always costs 18.60 in the United States or (fine) 3, 175., io d. in England. This means nothing more than the fact that gold in one form and measured in one way will always bear a constant ratio to gold in another form and measured in another way. An ounce of gold bullion is worth a fixed number of gold dollars, for the same reason that a pound sterling of gold is worth a fixed number of gold dollars, or that a ton of large steel ingots is worth a fixed number of pounds of small steel ingots.

Except, then, for extremely slight and temporary fluctuations, gold bullion and gold money must always have the same value. Therefore, in the following discussion respecting the more considerable fluctuations affecting both, we shall speak of these values interchangeably as " the value of gold."

3. Influence of the Production and Consumption of Money Metals on the Quantity of Money and therefore on Prices

The stock of bullion is not the ultimate outside influence on the quantity of money. As the stock of bullion and the stock of money influence each other, so the total stock of both is itself influenced by production and consumption. The production of gold consists in the output of the mines, which constantly tends to add to the existing stocks both of bullion and coin. The consumption of gold consists in the use of bullion in the arts by being wrought into jewelry, gilding, etc., and in losses of coin by abrasion, shipwreck, etc. If we consider the amount of gold coin and bullion as a sort of reservoir, production would be the inflow from the mines, and consumption the outflow to the arts and by destruction and loss. To the inflow from the mines should be added the re-inflow from forms of art into which gold had previously been wrought, but which have since become obsolete. This is illustrated by the business of producing gold bullion by burning gold picture frames.

We shall consider, first, the inflow or production, and afterward the outflow or consumption. The regulator of the inflow (which practically means the production of gold from the mines) is its estimated cost of production. Wherever the estimated cost of producing a dollar of gold is less than the existing value of a dollar in gold, the gold will (normally) be produced. Wherever the cost of production exceeds the existing value of a dollar, the gold will (normally) not be produced. In the former case the production of gold is profitable; in the latter it is unprofitable.

This holds true, in whatever way cost of production is measured, whether in terms of gold itself, or in terms of some other commodity such as wheat, or of commodities in general. In gold-standard countries the gold miner does actually reckon the cost of producing gold in terms of gold. From his standpoint it is a needless complication to translate the cost of production and the value of the product into some other standard than gold. He is interested in the relation between the two, and this relation will be the same whichever standard is employed. To illustrate how the producer of gold measures everything in terms of gold, suppose that the price level rises. He will then have to pay more dollars for wages, machinery, fuel, etc., while the prices obtained for his product (expressed in those same dollars) will, as always, remain unchanged. Conversely, a fall in the price level will lower his cost of production (measured in dollars), while the price of his product will still, as always, remain the same. Thus we have a variable number expressing the cost of production and a constant number expressing the price of gold product.

If we express the same phenomena, not in terms of gold, but in terms of wheat, or rather, let us say, in terms of goods in general, we shall have the opposite conditions. Then a fall in the price level cannot be said to affect his cost of production (measured in goods), while the " price, " or purchasing power, of his product over goods will rise. A constant number expresses the cost of gold and a variable number, its price (purchasing power).

Thus the comparison between price and cost of production is the same, whether we use gold or other commodities as our criterion. In the one view–i. e., when prices of labor and commodities are measured in gold–a rise of these prices appears as a rise in the gold miners cost of production–the money cost to him of labor and materials–while the price of his product, gold, appears constant; in the other view–i. e., when labor and commodities are measured in other goods–the same phenomenon is expressed as a fall in the purchasing power of his product, gold, while the cost of labor and materials in terms of themselves is the constant quantity. In the one view his costs rise relatively to his product; in the other his product falls relatively to his costs. In either view he will be discouraged. He will look at his troubles in the former light, i. e., as a rise in the cost of production; but we shall find it more useful to look at them in the latter, i. e., as a fall in the purchasing power of the product. In either case the comparison is between the cost of the production of gold and the purchasing power of gold. If this purchasing power is above the cost of production hi any particular mine, it will pay to work that mine. If the purchasing power of gold is lower than the cost of production in any particular mine, it will not pay to work that mine.

So much for the inflow of gold and the conditions regulating it. We turn next to outflow or consumption of gold. This has two forms, viz., consumption in the arts and consumption for monetary purposes.

First we consider its consumption in the arts. If objects made of gold are cheap–that is, if the prices of other objects are relatively high–then the relative cheapness of the gold objects will lead to an increase in their use and consumption. Expressing the matter in terms of money prices, when prices of everything else are higher and peoples incomes are likewise higher, while gold leaf and gold ornaments remain at their old prices, people will use and consume more gold leaf and ornaments.

These are instances of the consumption of gold in the form of commodities. The consumption and loss of gold as coin is a matter of " abrasion " (gradual waste by wearing or rubbing against other coins or the hands, pocket, or purse), of loss by shipwreck and other accidents. They change with the changes in the amount of gold in use and in its rapidity of exchange.

A fall, therefore, in the purchasing power or value of gold, affects both consumption and production. It stimulates consumption (that is, the turning of bullion into articles of commerce); and it discourages production. An increase of purchasing power, of course, acts in the opposite way. Conversely, consumption and production affect purchasing power. Consumption, or the withdrawal of bullion into commerce, raises the purchasing power of what is left, while production from the mines lowers the purchasing power.

The purchasing power of money, being thus played upon by the opposing forces of production and consumption, is driven up or down as the case may be.

4. Mechanical Illustration of these Influences In any complete picture of the forces determining the purchasing power of money we need to keep prominently in view three groups of factors: (1) the production or the " inflow" of gold (i. e., from the mines); (2) the consumption or " outflow " (into the arts and through destruction and loss); and (3) the " stock " or reservoir of gold (whether

Fig. 13.

coin or bullion) which receives the inflow and suffers the outflow. The relations among these three sets of magnitudes can be set forth by means of a mechanical illustration, as shown in Figure 13. This represents two connected reservoirs of liquid, Gt and Gm. The contents of the first reservoir represent the stock of gold bullion, and the contents of the second the stock of gold money. Since purchasing power increases with scarcity, the distance from the top of the cisterns, OO, to the surface of the liquid (which evidently increases as the liquid grows more scarce) is taken to represent the purchasing power of gold over other goods. A lowering of the level of the liquid indicates the corresponding increase in the purchasing power of money, since we measure this purchasing power downward from the line OO to the surface of the liquid. We shall not attempt to represent other forms of currency explicitly in the diagram. We have seen that normally the quantities of other currency are proportional to the quantity of primary money, which we are supposing to be gold. Therefore the variation in the purchasing power of this primary money may be taken as representative of the variation of all the currency. The cistern Gm must be of such a form as will make the distance of the liquid surface below OO decrease with an increase of the liquid, in exactly the same way as the purchasing power of gold decreases with an increase in its quantity. That is, as the quantity of liquid in Gm doubles, the distance of the surface from the line OO should decrease by one half. In a similar manner the form of the gold bullion cistern must be such as will make it represent faithfully the facts for which it stands; that is, it must be such that the distance of the liquid surface below OO will decrease with an increase of the liquid exactly as the value of the gold bullion decreases with an increase in the stock of gold bullion. The shapes of the two cisterns need not, and ordinarily will not, be the same, for we can scarcely suppose that doubling the amount of bullion in existence will always exactly halve its purchasing power.

Both reservoirs have inlets and outlets. Let us consider those belonging to the bullion reservoir (G6). Here each inlet represents a particular mine, supplying bullion, and each outlet represents a particular use in the arts, consuming gold bullion. Each mine and each use has its own distance from OO. There are, therefore, three sets of distances from OO: the inlet-distances, the outfet-distances, and the liquid-surface-distances. Each inlet-distance represents the cost of production, measured in goods, for some particular mine; each outlet-distance represents the value which gold has or would have in the particular use represented, likewise measured in goods. The surface distance, as we have already explained, represents the value of bullion, likewise measured in goods–in other words, its purchasing power.

It is evident that among these three sets of levels there will be discrepancies. These discrepancies serve to interpret the relative state of things as bullion flows in and out. If an inlet at a given moment be above the surface-level, i. e., at a less distance from OO than is the surface, the interpretation is that the cost of production is less than the purchasing power of the bullion. Hence the mine owner will turn on his spigot and keep it on until, perchance, the surface-level rises to the level of his mine–i. e., until the surface-distance from OO is as small as the inlet-distance–in other words, until the purchasing power of bullion is as small as the cost of production. At this point there is no longer any profit in mining. So much for inlets; now let us consider the outlets. If an outlet at a given moment be below the surface-level, i. e., at a greater distance from OO, the interpretation is that the value of gold in that particular use is greater than the purchasing power of bullion. Hence gold bullion will flow into those uses where its value may happen for the moment to be greater than its value as bullion. That is, it will flow out of all outlets below the surface in the reservoir.

It is evident, therefore, that at any given moment, only the inlets above the surface-level, and only the outlets below it, will be called into operation. As the surface rises, therefore, more outlets will be brought into use, but fewer inlets. That is to say, the less the purchasing power of gold as bullion, the more it will be used in the arts, but the less profitable it will be for the mines to produce it, and the smaller will be the output of the mines. As the surface falls, more inlets will come into use and fewer outlets.

We turn now to the money reservoir (Gm). The fact that gold has the same value either as bullion or as coin, because of the interflow between them is represented in the diagram by connecting the bullion and coin reservoirs, in consequence of which the stock in both will (like water) find a common level; the surface of the liquid in both reservoirs will be the same distance below the line OO, and this distance represents the value of gold (or its purchasing power). Should the inflow at any time exceed the outflow, the result will necessarily be an increase in the stock of gold in existence. This will tend to decrease the purchasing power or value of gold. But as soon as the surface rises, fewer inlets and more outlets will operate. That is, the excessive inflow on the one hand will decrease, and the deficient outflow or consumption on the other hand will increase, checking the inequality between the outflow and inflow. If, on the other hand, the outflow should temporarily be greater than the inflow, the reservoir will tend to become less full. The purchasing power will increase; thus the excessive outflow will be checked, and the deficient inflow stimulated–restoring equilibrium. The exact point of equilibrium may seldom or never be realized, but as in the case of a pendulum swinging back and forth about a position of equilibrium, there will always be a tendency to seek it.

It need scarcely be said that our mechanical diagram is intended merely to give a picture of some of the chief variables involved in the problem under discussion. It does not of itself constitute an argument, or add any new element; nor should one pretend that it includes explicitly all the factors which need to be considered. But it does enable us to grasp the chief factors involved in determining the purchasing power of money. It enables us to observe and trace the following important variations and their effects:–

First, if there be an increased production of gold–due, let us suppose, to the discovery of new mines or improved methods of working old ones–this may be represented by an increase in the number or size of the inlets into the bullion reservoir; the result will evidently be an increase of " inflow " into that reservoir, and from that into the currency reservoir, a consequent gradual filling up of both, and therefore a decrease in the purchasing power of money. This process will be checked finally by an increase in consumption and by discouraging production. When production and consumption become equal, an equilibrium will be established. An exhaustion of gold mines obviously operates in exactly the reverse manner.

Secondly, if there be an increase in the consumption of gold–as through some change of fashion–it may be represented by an increase in the number or size of the outlets of Gb. The result will be a draining out of the bullion reservoir, and consequently a decreased amount in the currency reservoir; hence an increase in the purchasing power of gold, which increase will be checked finally by an increase in the output of the mines as well as by a decrease in consumption. When the increased production and the decreased consumption become equal, equilibrium will again be reached.

If the mints are closed, that is, if the connection between the bullion reservoir and the currency reservoir is closed by a valve so that gold cannot flow from the former to the latter (although it can flow in the reverse direction), then the purchasing power of the gold as money may become greater than its value as bullion. Any increase in the production of gold will then tend only to fill the bullion reservoir and decrease the distance of the surface from the line OO, i. e., lower the value of gold bullion. The surface of the liquid in the money reservoir will not be brought nearer OO. It may even by gradual loss be lowered farther away. In other words, the purchasing power of money will by such a circumstance be made entirely independent of the value of the bullion out of which it was first made.

We have now discussed all but one of the outside influences upon the equation of exchange. That one is the character of the monetary and banking system which affects the quantity of money and deposits. This we reserve for special discussion in the following chapter.

Meanwhile, it is noteworthy that almost all of the influences which at the present time actually affect either the quantity or the velocities of circulation have been and are predominantly in the direction of higher prices. Almost the only opposing influence is the increased volume of trade. We may also point out that some of those influences discussed in this and the preceding chapter operate in more than one way. Consider, for instance, technical knowledge and invention, which affect the equation of exchange by increasing trade. So far as these increase trade, the tendency is to decrease prices; but so far as they develop metallurgy and the other arts which increase the production and transportation of the precious metals, they tend to increase prices. So far as they make the transportation and circulation of money and deposits quicker, they also tend to increase prices. So far as they lead to the development of the art of banking, they likewise tend to increase prices both by increasing deposit currency (Af) and by increasing the velocity of circulation both of money and deposits. So far as they lead to the concentration of population in cities, they tend to increase prices by accelerating circulation.

CHAPTER XIII
OPERATION OF MONETARY SYSTEMS

I. Greshams Law

Thus far we have considered the influences that determine the purchasing power of money when the money in circulation is all of one kind. The illustration given in the previous chapter shows how the money mechanism operates when a single metal is used. We have now to consider the monetary systems in which two or more kinds of money are used.

One of the first difficulties in the early history of money was that of keeping two or more metals in circulation at the same time. The monetary unit in one of the two would become cheaper than in the other, and the cheaper would drive out the dearer.

To this tendency has been given the name of " Greshams Law" in honor (rather undeservedly) of Sir Thomas Gresham, a financial adviser of Queen Elizabeth of England. He called attention to the tendency in the middle of the sixteenth century, although it is now known that many others had anticipated him. In fact, the law seems to have been recognized among the ancient Greeks. It is mentioned in the " Frogs " of Aristophanes:–

"For your old and standard pieces, valued and approved and tried,
Here among the Grecian nations and in all the world beside
Recognized in every realm for trusty stamp and pure assay,
Are rejected and abandoned for the trash of yesterday;
For a vile, adulterate issue, drossy, counterfeit and base
Which the traffic of the City passes current in their place I "

Greshams Law is ordinarily stated in the form, "Bad money drives out good money," for it was usually observed that the badly worn, defaced, light-weight, " clipped," " sweated," and otherwise deteriorated money tended to drive out the full-weight, freshly minted coins. This formulation, however, is not accurate. " Bad " coins, e. g., worn, bent, defaced, or even clipped coins, will drive out other money only so far as they are less valuable. Sometimes bright, freshly minted coins drive out old, dull defaced coins, as, for instance, when new gold drove out silver from the United States shortly after 1837, the new gold dollars being cheaper than the old silver dollars. Accurately stated, the Law is simply this: The cheaper dollar (or whatever the monetary unit) lends to drive out the dearer. The reason why the cheaper of two moneys always prevails is that the choice of the use of money rests chiefly with the man who gives it in exchange, not with the man who receives it. When any one has the choice of paying his debts in either of two moneys, motives of economy will evidently prompt him to use the cheaper. If the initiative and choice lay principally with the person who receives instead of the person who pays the money, the opposite would hold true. The dearer or " good " money would then drive out the cheaper or " bad" money. It is because the payer of money exercises the choice that the cheaper money tends to be passed on and the dearer money to be withdrawn. Any individual into whose hands the two moneys may chance to fall may exercise this choice and withdraw the newly minted coins. But there are two classes especially interested and most instrumental in withdrawing the " good " money from circulation; namely, those who wish it either for export or for melting,–the bankers and the goldsmiths.

What then becomes of the dearer money? It may be hoarded, or go into the melting pot, or go abroad–hoarded and melted from motives of economy, and sent abroad be cause, where foreign trade is involved, it is the foreigner receiving the money, rather than ourselves giving it, who dictates what kind of money shall be accepted. He will take only the best, because our legal-tender laws do not bind him.

Until " milling " the edges of coins (making the edges finely corrugated so that they cannot be filed or otherwise rubbed off without detecting) was invented, and a " limit of tolerance " of the mint (the deviation from the standard weight beyond which the coin is rendered unacceptable in law as legal tender) was adopted, much embarrassment was felt in commerce from the fact that the clipping and debasing of coin was a common practice. Nowadays, however, any coin which has been so " sweated" or clipped as to reduce its weight appreciably ceases to be legal tender, and, being commonly rejected by those to whom it is offered, ceases to be money. Within the customary or legal limits of tolerance, however,–that is, as long as the cheaper money continues to be money,–it will tend to drive out the dearer.

Greshams Law applies not only to two rival moneys of the same metal; it applies to all moneys that circulate concurrently.

2. Bimetallism

The obvious effect of Greshams Law is to decrease the purchasing power of money at every opportunity. The history of the worlds currencies is largely a record of money debasements, often at the behest of the sovereign. Our chief purpose now, in considering Greshams Law, is to formulate more fully the causes determining the purchasing power of money under monetary systems subject to the operation of Greshams Law. The first application is to " bimetallism." Under bimetallism, governments open their mints to the free coinage of two metals (usually gold and silver) at a fixed coinage ratio, and make both sorts of coin unlimited legal tender at that ratio.1 Under this system, the debtor has the option, unless otherwise bound by contract, of making payment either in gold or in silver money. These, in fact, are the two requisites of complete bimetallism, viz.: (1) the free and unlimited coinage of both metals at a fixed ratio, and (2) the unlimited legal tender of each metal at that ratio.

The object of bimetallism is to render the purchasing power of money more stable; but in order to understand fully the influence of any monetary system on the purchasing power of money, we must first understand its mechanism and mode of operation. It has been denied that bimetallism ever did or can work successfully so that gold and silver dollars circulate side by side at equal values. This denial is based on Greshams Law by which the cheaper metal will drive out the dearer. Our first task is to show, quite irrespective of its desirability, that bimetallism can and does " work " under certain circumstances, but not under others. To make clear when it will work and when it will not, we shall state the effects of a bimetallic law first in words and then, for the sake of greater clearness and exactness, in terms of a mechanical illustration.

Suppose that, at first, gold alone is freely coined (and is unlimited legal tender) and that then (as proposed in the United States by the " free silver" party in 1896 and 1900) silver is put on exactly the same basis, the mints being opened to its free coinage also.

The results of thus opening the mints to silver at a ratio of 16 to 1 with gold will be different, according to the relative market value of gold and silver before the mints are opened. If 412 grains of silver were dearer than 25.8 grains of gold, there would be no silver coined at all, for no one will take 412 grains of silver to be coined and used as a dollar of money when he can get more than a gold dollar for it by selling it as silver bullion.

1 By the " coinage ratio " is meant the ratio of the weight of the silver dollar to that of the gold dollar. This is at present 16 to 1; for a silver dollar weighs 412 J grains, which is almost exactly sixteen times the weight of a gold dollar, 25.8 grains.

But if (as happens to be the case to-day) 412 grains of silver are cheaper than 25.8 grains of gold, every owner of silver bullion will make a profit by taking it to the mint. In this way he can get a silver dollar for every 412! grains of silver bullion, while in the silver bullion market he can get only, let us say, fifty cents. The result will be a wild scramble among all owners of silver bullion to get it coined, in order to transform each 412. grains of it into a full-fledged dollar instead of the fifty cents which previously was all they could get for it. It is true that the new silver dollar may not be worth as much in purchasing power as a gold dollar; but, being legal tender, it will have just as great debt-paying power.

There can be no doubt, then, that silver, being cheaper than gold, will be taken to the mint as soon as the bimetallic law takes effect. The question now is: What will be the result? To this question the answer is briefly as follows:– I. The first effect (as has been emphasized by " mono-metallists ") will be the operation of Greshams Law, by which the cheap silver dollars will tend to expel the dear gold dollars from circulation.

II. But (as emphasized by " bimetallists ") this very operation of Greshams Law tends to reduce the disparity between the values of the gold and silver dollars. Owing to the eagerness of debtors to use silver instead of gold in paying their debts, the value of silver is increased and that of gold decreased. This mutual approach of the values of gold and silver dollars may result in making them equal.

III. But (as pointed out by the " monometallists ") the next result will be a great stimulus to the mining of silver and a great discouragement to the mining of gold. Con sequently, silver will gradually become more plentiful, and therefore cheaper again, and gold scarcer, and therefore dearer again. Consequently, silver will again tend to expel gold.

IV. But (as insisted by " bimetallists ") this increase of the stock of silver (coin and bullion) and decrease of the stock of gold are self-limiting; for the increased production of silver will be checked by increased cost of production, and consumption will tend to overtake production, while the opposite adjustments apply to gold.

We shall consider these results in their order.

3. When Bimetallism Fails I. In accordance with Greshams Law, the cheap silver money will drive the dearer gold money out of circulation–either abroad or into the melting pot, or both. If there is a sufficient amount of silver bullion available, it will drive gold completely out of circulation, and the country which enacted the law will find itself converted from a gold standard country into a silver standard country. There are many historical examples of such a breakdown of bimetallism, both in the United States and elsewhere.

But even when bimetallism thus fails of its object (keeping both metals in circulation, with silver and gold dollars of equal value), it will, nevertheless, have had the effect of making them more nearly equal. A tendency toward equalization will have come about from two causes, one the fact that from the worlds stock of silver bullion there has been taken away a great mass of silver (i. e., the silver turned into coin), thus making the remaining silver bullion scarcer and dearer; and the other the fact that to the worlds stock of gold bullion there is suddenly added a great mass of gold (i. e., the gold melted from coin), thus making the gold bullion more abundant and cheaper in its purchasing power over other things. The result is that, though the law has failed to raise 412 grains of silver from the equivalent of half a dollar of gold to the equivalent of a whole dollar of gold, it may at any rate raise it a little.

These effects can be more exactly shown by means of. the mechanical illustration of the last chapter carried a little further. In this the amount of gold bullion is represented by the contents of reservoir Gb (Figs. 14, 15). Here, as before, we represent the purchasing power or value of gold by the distance of the liquid level below the zero level, OO. In the last chapter, our figure represented only one metal, gold, and represented that metal in two reservoirs–the bullion reservoir and the coin reservoir. We shall now, one step at a time, elaborate that figure. First we add a reservoir for silver bullion (56). This reservoir may be used to show the relation between the value or purchasing power of silver and its quantity considered as bullion.

Here, then, are three reservoirs. At first (Fig. 140) the silver reservoir is entirely isolated. For the present, let us suppose that the middle one, which contains money, is filled with gold money only (Figs. 140, 150), no silver being yet used as money. In other words, the monetary system is the same as that discussed in the last chapter. The only change here introduced is to add to the picture another reservoir (56), entirely detached, showing the quantity and value of silver bullion.

We next suppose a pipe opened at the right, connecting Sb with the money reservoir; that is, we introduce bimetallism. These new conditions are represented in Figure 146, where a pipe gives silver an entrance into the money or central reservoir. Thus the a part of the figure represents conditions before the mints are opened to silver. The b part represents conditions after they have been opened.

The liquids representing gold and silver money are separated by a movable film/. In Figure 140 this film is at the extreme right; in Figure 146, at the extreme left.

We may disregard for the present all inlets and outlets except the connections between the bullion reservoirs and the coin reservoir; because what we are about to represent is merely the relations between bullion (two kinds) and coins.

Now in these reservoirs the surface-distances below OO. represent, as has been said, the purchasing powers of gold and silver. A unit of liquid represents that quantity of gold or of silver which constitutes a unit of money. Of ( )

Fig. 14.

course a silver dollar is physically larger than a gold dollar, but they are both represented in our diagram by the same unit, or drop, of liquid; that is, each drop of liquid on the right side of the film / represents a dollar of silver (412 J grains), while each drop of liquid on the left of this film represents a dollar of gold (25.8 grains).

In the figure the situation represented is such that the level of the silver bullion in the right reservoir is above the level of the other two reservoirs, which are filled with gold; that is, the silver bullion is so abundant and cheap as to be ready to flow into the money reservoir as soon as the mint or connecting pipe is opened. Were this not the case (that is, if the silver level in the right reservoir were below the gold level in the other two reservoirs), it is evident that the (6)

Fig. 1s.

statute introducing bimetallism would be inoperative; the silver bullion would not, as it were, flow uphill into the money reservoir. But if, as is represented in Figure 140, the silver level is the higher, then, as soon as the mints are opened to silver (that is, as soon as the connecting pipe is inserted),

silver will flow into circulation (into the money reservoir), and in accordance with Greshams Law, will displace gold. It will continue to displace gold as long as it is cheaper than gold (that is, as long as the level of the inflowing silver liquid is above that of the gold liquid which it displaces). The gold money will be melted and turned into bullion (that is, pushed out through the left tube into the bullion market).

It is evident that this operation of Greshams Law may proceed so far that the money reservoir will be wholly cleared of gold and filled instead with silver, the film/ having been swept completely to the left. This result is pictured in Figure 146, which illustrates the failure of bimetallism.

4. When Bimetallism Succeeds II. But such a result would not in all cases occur. It will occur only when, as is represented in Figure 14, there exists, to start with, a sufficiently great disparity between the silver and gold levels and a sufficiently large amount of silver bullion.

These conditions need not always hold true. Let us suppose, for instance, that prior to the introduction of bimetallism 412 grains of silver bullion, instead of being worth only fifty cents in terms of gold, should be worth ninety-five cents. Under these conditions the introduction of the free coinage of silver would mean introducing a new dollar worth, at the outset, at least ninety-five cents, or nearly par. It would still be true that the owner of silver bullion would be impelled to take it to the mint by the prospect of a profit of five cents on each 412 grains, but it would not require much such coinage to raise the price of silver to par. The eagerness to get the new silver dollars would tend to raise their value, while the discarding of the old gold dollars would tend to lower their value. Just as soon as enough silver dollars had been coined out of silver bullion to bring them up to par in terms of gold, Greshams Law would, of course, cease to operate, and we should have both silver and gold dollars circulating on equal terms, side by side.

This result is pictured in Figure 15. The upper part (Fig. 150) shows the situation before the introduction of free coinage of silver, and the lower part (Fig. 156) shows what will be the result if silver has been allowed to flow into circulation. In this case the film/ has been pushed only part way to the left,–to such a point as to bring the silver and gold levels into coincidence. As the film has been swept to the left, and more room has thus been made for silver, the silver level has fallen, while as the film has crowded out gold, the gold level has risen and the two levels have come into coincidence on the line mm. In other words, the premium on gold bullion has disappeared, and bimetallism has, for the time being at least, succeeded.

While such an equality in the value of gold and silver dollars continues, neither completely expels the other, although both are freely coined. If the levels of the two metals on opposite sides of the film / should, for a moment, differ slightly, the difference would be automatically corrected, for the cheaper metal having the higher level would simply crowd against the dearer metal having the lower level and the separating film / would need to shift only a little before the two levels would again coincide. For these reasons, no matter which of the metals tends from time to time to become more plentiful and cheaper, and, therefore, to expel the other, the only result would be a slight shifting of the film. This will move from right to left or left to right, as the case maybe, but as long as it does not move completely to the right or the left limit, bimetallism will continue to be successful. The film being movable (that is, gold and silver being mutually replaceable as money), the three reservoirs act as one and keep a common level for all three.

We see, then, that those are wrong who maintain that Greshams Law always results in complete expulsion from circulation of one metal by the other. The expulsion can continue only so long as there is a difference in value between the two metals, but as the expelling proceeds (that is, as the film / shifts) the very difference of level which shifts it tends to disappear. Sometimes (as in Fig. 146) the film will be pushed to its extreme limit before the difference of level between the two liquids disappears, but sometimes on the other hand (as in Fig. 156) the difference of level between the two liquids will disappear before the film reaches its limit. Which of these two results will happen, depends on circumstances. To distinguish the two cases we may suppose the line mm to be drawn in all of the four cases (Figs. 140, 146, 150, 156). This line is the mean level of the liquids in the reservoirs (that is, the common level which the liquids contained in the three reservoirs would find if intercommunication among them were entirely free).

The case represented in Figure 14 is the case where the amount of silver bullion x above the mean line mm equals or exceeds the total capacity of the money reservoir below that line. In such a case, as soon as x is allowed to flow into the money reservoir it is sufficiently great to wholly displace all the gold in that reservoir.

The case represented in Figure 15 is the case where the amount of silver bullion x above the line mm is less than the total contents of the money reservoir below the line mm. In this case when x is given access to the money reservoir it is inadequate to wholly sweep gold out of circulation.

The first case undoubtedly represents what would have happened in the United States if we had attempted free coinage of silver, at 16 to 1, as proposed by one political party in 1896 and 1000. It also represents what actually did occur in the United States after the adoption of the Bimetallic Law (at a ratio of 15 to 1) in 1792. In that case it was gold which expelled silver.

5. Changes in Production and Consumption III. Thus far in our discussion we have taken no account of the production and consumption of the precious metals. We have taken account only of the distribution of the existing stocks of these metals as between money in circulation and gold and silver bullion. As has already been hinted, as soon as the first effects of free coinage have been felt and the existing available stock of silver has been coined, there will be at once a great stimulus to silver mining and discouragement to gold mining. If, for instance, as above supposed, before the introduction of bimetallism, the value of 412 grains of silver had been ninety-five cents in gold, but, as a consequence of the free coinage of silver, its value has improved to a dollar, it is evident that producers of silver will, in consequence of this rise in price of their product, be encouraged to mine a larger product than before the introduction of bimetallism. Through its new monetary use their market for silver has been greatly increased. At the same time the market for gold will have been decreased and its production discouraged. While the value of silver in terms of gold has increased, the value of gold in terms of silver has decreased, or, what is more to the point, while the value of silver in terms of goods in general has increased, the value of gold in terms of goods in general has decreased. We have already seen (in Chapter XII, 4) that this decrease in the value of gold will discourage its production just as the increase in the value of silver will encourage its production.

Since, then, the output of silver increases and that of gold decreases, there will be a still further expulsion of gold by silver. In the mechanical illustration some of the silver inlets at the right, formerly unused (below the liquid surface) will have been uncovered and will pour their streams into the reservoir Sj, while some gold inlets at the left formerly open will be submerged and cease their flow. Consequently, the film will be shifted toward the left.

IV. But this movement of the film, or displacement of gold by silver, will not necessarily proceed far. The increased production of silver will tend to be self-limiting, for with increased production comes increased cost. The consumption of silver on the other hand may increase and overtake production; for the greater the stock of silver in circulation, the larger the amount which will be used up by abrasion, losses, etc. Therefore it may soon come about that the production and consumption of silver will again be equal. When this occurs the stock of silver will again be stationary. The same may happen to gold by the opposite process. Its lessened production is self-limiting, for the mines where gold is most cheaply produced will continue to operate at a profit; moreover, the lessening in production will be followed by a lessening of stock, and the lessening of stock may lead to a lessening of consumption which may fall to equality with production. When this occurs the stock of gold will again be stationary.

As a matter of fact, however, such ideal equilibrium, in which the stocks of both metals remain stationary, never occurs. Changes in production and consumption of the precious metals are constantly adding to and subtracting from the stocks of these metals in the form of money and bullion. Any such disturbance of the stocks of the precious metals will, as we have seen, tend to make one metal displace the other, but whether the displacement will be complete or not depends, as we have seen, upon circumstances.

Consequently, the film will be driven to the right or the left as gold or silver flows in from one side or the other. In this way, by moving the film back and forth, bimetallism may remain in successful operation for a long time, as, in fact, it did in France for three fourths of a century ending in 1873. In this period gold and silver money circulated at par in France, sometimes silver partially displacing gold and sometimes gold partially displacing silver. Never until the end of the period did either completely displace the other. For a long time the film shifted back and forth without reaching its limit on either side. But such a fate is in the end almost inevitable. This is what happened in France in 1873.

6. The " Limping " Standard

Bimetallism is to-day a subject of historical interest only. It is no longer practiced; but its former prevalence has left behind it in many countries, including France and the United States, a monetary system which is sometimes called the " limping " standard. Such a system comes about when, in a system of bimetallism, before either metal can wholly expel the other, the mint is closed to the cheaper of them, but the coinage that has been accomplished up to date is not recalled. Suppose silver to be the metal thus excluded–as in France and the United States. Any money of that metal already coined and in circulation is

Flo. 16.

kept in circulation at par with gold. This parity may continue even if limited additional amounts of silver be coined from time to time. There will then result a difference in value between silver bullion and silver coin, the silver coin being overvalued. This situation is represented in Figure 16. Here the pipe connection between the money reservoir and the silver bullion reservoir has been, as it were, cut off, or, let us say, stopped by a valve which refuses passage of silver from the bullion reservoir to the money reservoir, but not the reverse (for no law ever can prevent the melting down of silver coins into bullion). Newly mined silver cannot now become money, and thus lower the purchasing power of money.

On the other hand, new supplies of gold continue to affect the value of currency as before–the value, not only of the gold, but also of the concurrently circulating overvalued silver. If more gold should flow into the money reservoir, it would raise the currency level. Should this level ever become higher than the level of the silver bullion reservoir, silver would flow from the money reservoir into the bullion reservoir; for the passage in that direction (i. e., melting) is still free. So long, however, as the money level is below the silver level, i. e., so long as the coined silver is worth more than the uncoined, there will be no flow of silver in either direction. The legal prohibition prevents the inflow of silver, and the loss which would be sustained by melting prevents its outflow.

In the case just discussed, the value of the coined silver will be equal to the value of gold at the legal ratio. Precisely the same principle applies in the case of any money the coined value of which is greater than the value of its constituent material. Take the case, for instance, of paper money. So long as it has the distinctive characteristic of money–general acceptability at its legal value–and is limited in quantity, its value will ordinarily be equal to that of its legal equivalent in gold. If its quantity increases indefinitely, it will gradually push out all the gold and entirely fill the money reservoir, just as silver would do under bimetallism if produced in sufficiently large amounts. Likewise credit money and credit in the form of bank deposits would have this effect. To the extent that they are used, they lessen the need for gold, decrease its value as money, and cause more of it to go into the arts or to other countries.

So long as the quantity of silver or other token money, e. g., paper money, is too small to displace gold completely, gold will continue in circulation. The value of other money in this case cannot fall below that of gold. For if it should, it would by Greshams Law displace gold, which we have supposed it is not of sufficient quantity to do. The parity between silver coin and gold coin, under this " limping " standard is, therefore, not necessarily dependent on any redeemability in gold, but may result merely from limitation in the amount of silver coin. Such limitation is usually sufficient to maintain parity, despite irredeemability. This is not always true, however; for if for any reason (such as its novelty and strangeness or rumors of further inflation) the people should not have confidence in some form of irredeemable paper or token money, even though it were not overissued, it would depreciate and be nearly as cheap in money form as it is in the raw state. It might even be so completely rejected that it would cease to circulate and cease to be money. A man is willing to accept money at its face value so long as he has confidence that every one else is ready to do the same. But it is possible, for instance, for a mere fear of overissue to destroy this confidence. The payee, who under ordinary circumstances submits patiently to whatever money is a customary or legal tender, may then take a hand and insist on " contracting out " of the offending standard. That is, he may insist on making all his future contracts in terms of the better metal–gold, for instance–and thus contribute to the further downfall in value of the depreciated paper.

Irredeemable paper money, then, like our irredeemable silver dollars, may circulate at par with other money if limited in quantity and not too unpopular. If it is gradually increased in amount, such irredeemable money may expel all metallic money and be left in undisputed posses sion of the field. But though such a result–a condition of irredeemable paper money as the sole currency–is possible, it has never proved desirable. On the contrary, irre-deemability is a constant temptation toward abuse, and this fact alone causes business distrust and discourages long-time contracts and enterprises. Irredeemable paper money has almost invariably proved a curse to the country employing it. While, therefore, redeemability is not absolutely essential to produce parity of value with the primary money, it is practically a wise precaution.

The lack of redeemability of silver dollars in the United States is one of the chief defects in our unsatisfactory monetary system. Our paper silver certificates are redeemable in silver dollars, but these silver dollars are not redeemable in gold. The absurdity of the situation consists in the fiction that somehow the redemption of the silver certificates in silver dollars keeps them both at par with gold. The truth is that the paper would keep its parity with gold just as well if there were no redemption in silver. A silver dollar as silver is worth less than a gold dollar just as truly as a paper dollar, as paper, is worth less than a gold dollar. The fact that the silver is worth half a dollar, while the paper is worth only a fraction of a cent, will not avail in the least to make either the silver or the paper worth a whole dollar. A pillar which reaches halfway to the ceiling cannot hold the ceiling up any more than a pillar an inch high. The silver certificates and silver dollars keep at par with gold merely because they are not sufficient in quantity to displace gold. If their quantity should ever be made great enough, they would displace gold and depreciate; and the redeemability of one of them in the other will not avail to prevent such depreciation.

The system of the limping standard, now obtaining in the United States and some other countries, logically forms a connecting link between complete bimetallism and those " composite " systems by which any number of different kinds of money may be simultaneously kept in circulation. Most modern civilized states have solved the problem of concurrent circulation by using gold as a standard and silver, nickel, and copper chiefly as a subsidiary money, limited in quantity, with, in most cases, limited amounts of paper money, the latter being usually redeemable. The possible variations of this composite system are unlimited. In the United States at present we have a system which is very complicated, consisting of gold dollars freely coined, silver dollars, fractional silver, minor coins of nickel and of copper, United States notes, national bank notes, gold certificates and silver certificates. The system is not only complicated, but objectionable in many of its features, especially in its lack of elasticity, which characteristic is due to the fact that national bank notes are based upon the inelastic national debt rather than upon the elastic general assets of the bank.

CHAPTER XIV

CONCLUSIONS ON MONEY 1. Can "Other Things Remain Equal"?

The chief purpose of the preceding six chapters is to set forth the causes determining the purchasing power of money. This purchasing power has been studied as the effect of three, and only three, groups of causes. The three groups center on currency, on its velocity, and on the volume of trade. These and their effects, namely, prices, we saw to be connected by an equation called the equation of exchange, $MV + MV = Zpq$. The three causes, in turn, we found to be themselves effects of antecedent causes lying entirely outside of the equation of exchange, as follows: the volume of trade will be increased, and therefore the price level correspondingly decreased by the differentiation of human wants; by diversification of industry; and by facilitation of communication. The velocities of circulation will be increased, and therefore the price level increased by improvident habits; by the use of book credit; and by rapid transportation. The quantity of money will be increased, and therefore the price level increased, by the import and minting of money, and, antecedently, by the mining of the money metal; by the introduction of another and initially cheaper money metal through bimetallism; and by the issue of bank notes and other paper money. The quantity of deposits will be increased, and therefore the price level increased, by extension of the banking system and by the use of book credit. The reverse causes produce, of course, reverse effects.

Thus, behind the three sets of causes which alone affect the purchasing power of money, we find over a dozen antecedent causes. If we chose to pursue the inquiry to still remoter stages, the number of causes would be found to increase at each stage in much the same way as the number of ones ancestors increases with each generation into the past. In the last analysis myriads of factors play upon the purchasing power of money; but it would be neither feasible nor profitable to catalogue them. The value of our analysis consists rather in simplifying the problem by setting forth clearly the three proximate causes through which all others whatsoever must operate. At the close of our study, as at the beginning, stands forth the equation of exchange as the great determinant of the purchasing power of money. With its aid we see that normally the quantity of deposit currency varies directly with the quantity of money, and that therefore the introduction of deposits does not disturb the relations we found to hold true before. That is, it is still true that (1) prices vary directly as the quantity of money, provided the volume of trade and the velocities of circulation remain unchanged; (2) that prices vary directly as the velocities of circulation (if these velocities vary together), provided the quantity of money–and therefore deposits–and the volume of trade remain unchanged; and (3) that prices vary inversely as the volume of trade, provided the quantity of money and therefore deposits and the velocities of circulation remain unchanged.

But the question now arises, Can the factors supposed to " remain unchanged " in these three cases actually remain unchanged? To this question the answer is, "Yes, with one exception." A change in the volume of trade per capita seems to affect, besides prices, the velocities of circulation, so that these velocities cannot " remain unchanged." At a given price level, the greater the per capita trade, the more rapid is the individual turnover. Statistics seem to show this.

Thus an increase in trade, unlike an increase in currency or in velocities, may have other effects than simply on prices; for, in fact, it may increase the magnitudes on the opposite side of the equation. But with this exception and apart from transition periods, the three groups of magnitudes which determine the price level–(1) money and deposits, (2) their velocities, (3) volume of trade–are independent of each other. That is to say, a change in the quantity of money,–and therefore of deposits,–though it may temporarily affect velocities and trade, will not do so in the long run. Instead it will expend all its effects on prices, which will therefore change in the same proportions. Similarly, a change in velocities, though it may temporarily affect money and deposits as well as trade, will not do so in the long run, but will also expend all its effects on prices.

The proof of these conclusions consists simply in the fact that investigation fails to show any other relations among the factors in the equation of exchange than those which have been mentioned.

2. An Increase of Money does not Decrease its Velocity It cannot be shown, for instance, that (except during transition periods) there is any tendency for an increase in the quantity of money to decrease its velocity of circulation. Some persons who have never investigated the subject imagine that if money were suddenly doubled in quantity,

prices need not rise at all, as the effect might be simply to cut the velocity of circulation in two. This would be true if the public should, for some unaccountable reason, decide to carry double the former quantity of money while expending precisely the same amounts, but we have found that the velocity of circulation of money is determined by the habits of the people. They find for themselves what is the most convenient amount to carry in order that it shall be best adapted to meet their particular expenditures. If, then, money and expenditure are mutually adjusted to suit the convenience of the people, this implies that any increase in the amounts carried would (for a given price level) be inconveniently large.

To make the picture definite, let us suppose that the average per capita amount of money in actual circulation in the United States, outside of the United States Treasury and the banks, is about 15, and that some mysterious Santa Claus suddenly doubles the amount in the possession of each individual. This means that the average individual will have 30 where before he had 15. Now, statistics show that the average per capita amount in circulation changes only slightly from month to month. While the amount of money carried by an individual will necessarily fluctuate because of his expenditures and receipts, in a large group of people the average amount carried by the several individuals composing the group will fluctuate but little. If, then, so large an addition to the total circulation is suddenly made as to put fifteen extra dollars per capita in the hands of the public, the first thought of most people will be how to get rid of this inconvenient addition to the money which they are carrying. If they should be inclined to hoard it in stockings or safes or to bury it in the earth or to drop it into the sea, it would have no tendency to raise prices. Instead, however, they will seek to make some use of it either by expending it for goods or by depositing it in banks. Thus a few days after the supposed visit of Santa Claus, the surprised recipients of the extra money will, in most cases, have disposed of it in one of these two ways. To the extent that they dispose of it in the first way–in the purchase of goods–it is evident that there will be a tendency to raise prices, for the sudden expenditure of 15 per capita, even by a small fraction of the people of the United States, will mean a phenomenal rush upon the shops.

The average individual does not expend in actual money more than 15 in two weeks. This is about a dollar a day, or about 100,000,000 a day for the entire country. If within, let us say, five days from his windfall of 15 the average man should try to spend this extra sum, the result would be 3 per day per capita, or 300,000,000 a day for the nation. This, in addition to the usual 100,000,000 a day, would make 400,000,000 a day, or four times the ordinary rate of expenditure. Such a sudden briskness in trade would astonish the shopkeepers and lead them promptly to raise their prices; otherwise, in many cases their stocks would be entirely depleted.

At first sight, it might seem that it would only require a few days for each one to get rid of his extra money so that the flurry in prices would, therefore, be only temporary; but such reasoning would be fallacious; for we must not forget that the only way in which the individual can get rid of his money is by handing it over to somebody else. Society is not rid of it. If the shopkeepers, who under our Santa Claus hypothesis have already had their till money doubled mysteriously, receive in addition the surplus cash of their customers, they will now be the ones embarrassed with a surplus of cash and will, in their turn, endeavor to get rid of it, by purchasing goods for their business or by depositing it in banks. Since, then, the effort to get rid of money by transferring it merely results in somebody else having a surplus, the surplus in the community remains unchanged. Therefore, the effort to get rid of it and the consequent effect on prices will continue until prices have reached a sufficiently high level.

This conclusion cannot be avoided by supposing that most of the money is not spent in trade, but deposited in banks. The bankers whose deposits are thus suddenly swollen will now be the ones who will strive to get rid of the surplus cash. No banker wishes to have idle reserves, and each will make the increase in reserves the basis for an in crease of business, including an increase of deposits. We have seen that this tendency results ultimately in preserving the relative amounts of the three magnitudes: money in circulation, money in bank reserves, and deposits based on these reserves. In the end, then, the doubling of societys money will mean a doubling (1) of the money in circulation, (2) of the money in banks, and (3) of the deposits based on this money. In a short time it will also mean a doubling of prices, for as long as prices fail to be double what they were, there will be the same phenomenon of inconvenient surpluses. Individuals, tradesmen, bankers, etc., will be trying to get rid of these surpluses, and their efforts to get rid of them must tend to raise prices. When, however, prices have reached double their original level, there will be no longer any effort to get rid of surplus cash; for there will be no surplus cash. The 30 per capita which has thus been created will no longer seem excessive, in view of the fact that prices are double what they formerly were and that the persons carrying this money will, on the average, find their wages or incomes doubled likewise. Thus, if formerly the average individual was accustomed to spend 300 and to carry an average balance of 15, he will now spend 600 and cany an average balance of 30. The adjustment of the 30 to 600 is exactly the same as the former adjustment of the 15 to 300. In either case the relation is one to twenty, which means that the individual turns his money over, on the average, twenty times a year. Thus, in the end, a doubling of the quantity of money does not expend its effect in disturbing the velocity of circulation, but in raising the general level of prices.

It is worth noting that the imaginary example we have given represents, except in its details, exactly what actually happens when new gold is discovered. Gold miners convert their product into money, sometimes using it as such in the form of nuggets or gold dust and sometimes taking it to the mint and converting it into coin. They find themselves in possession of bags full of money far beyond what they need as the most convenient amount of pocket money. If, for instance, one of these men has just received from the mint a thousand dollars in gold, he is almost sure to get rid of at least 950 of it as speedily as possible, either by spending it or by depositing it in the bank. In either case, he and the hundreds of others who are doing the same thing tend to raise prices in the community where they are spending their money or where they and others spend checks on the banks in which they deposit their money.

It was thus that prices rose in the mining camps of California a half dozen decades ago and one or two decades ago in Colorado and the Klondike. This local rise of prices then communicated itself to other places; for, as we have seen, the price level cannot in one locality greatly exceed that in a neighboring locality without causing an export of money to the cheaper locality. Thus, new money gradually finds its way into circulation throughout the world, raising prices as it flows from place to place, the process consisting in all cases of the effort to get rid of an inconvenient surplus and one which cannot be permanently got rid of by transferring it from hand to hand, but only by a rise of prices.

This picture of the manner in which an increase of money causes a rise of prices is here given to show clearly that an increase in the amount of money (M) does not result in a mere decrease in its velocity (V). Its velocity depends, not on its quantity, but on the factors given in Chapter XI, 3, 4, 5- In the same way it might be shown that an increase in the quantity of money will not affect the velocity (V) of circulation of bank deposits nor the volume of trade (the Qs). It will merely affect the volume of deposits (A/) and the level of prices (P).

A change of M does not, of course, prevent other causes from at the same time affecting M, V, V, and the Qs, and thus aggravating or neutralizing the effect of M on the ps.

But these are not the effects of M. So far as M by itself is concerned, its effect is only on M and the ps and is proportional to its quantity. The importance and reality of this proposition is not diminished in the least by the fact that these other causes do not, as a matter of fact, remain quiescent and allow the effect on the ps of an increase in M to be seen separately from effects of other causes. The effects of changes in M are blended with the effects of changes in the other factors in the equation of exchange, just as the effects of gravity upon a falling body are blended with the effects of the resistance of the atmosphere.

Our main conclusion, then, is that we find nothing to interfere with the truth of the quantity theory: that variations in money (M) produce, normally, proportional changes in prices.

We have now finished with the principles determining the purchasing power of money. By the aid of these principles the student should be able to avoid hereafter most of the fallacies and pitfalls which beset the subject. He will find it a useful exercise to turn back to Chapter I and test himself by analyzing as many as he can of the money fallacies there stated. The others we hope to clear up in later chapters.

3. An Index Number of Prices

We have been studying the causes determining the purchasing power of money, or its reciprocal, the level of prices. Hitherto we have not defined exactly what a " general level" of prices may mean. There was no need of such a definition so long as we assumed, as we have usually done hitherto, that all prices move in perfect unison. But practically, prices never do move in perfect unison. If some /s do not rise enough to preserve our equation, others must rise more. If some rise too much, others must rise less. The case is further complicated by the fact that some prices cannot adjust themselves at all and some can adjust themselves but tardily. A price fixed by contract cannot be affected by any change coming into operation between the date of the contract and that of its fulfillment. The existence of such contracts constitutes one of the chief arguments for a system of currency such that the uncertainties of its purchasing power are the least possible. Contracts are a useful device; and an uncertain monetary standard disarranges them and discourages their formation. Even in the absence of explicit contracts, prices may be kept from adjustment by implied understandings and by the mere inertia of habit. And besides these restrictions on free movement of prices there are often legal restrictions; as, for example, when railroads are prohibited from charging over two cents per passenger per mile, or when street railways are limited to five-cent or three-cent fares. Whatever the causes of non-adjustment, the result is that the prices which do change will have to change in a greater ratio than they would were there no prices which do not change. Just as an obstruction put across one half of a stream causes an increase of current in the other half, so any deficiency in the movement of some prices must cause an excess in the movement of others.

Another class of goods, the price of which cannot fluctuate greatly with other prices, are those special commodities which consist largely of the money metal. Thus, in a country employing a gold standard, the prices of gold for dentistry, of gold rings and ornaments, gold watches, gold-rimmed spectacles, gilded picture frames, etc., instead of varying in proportion to other prices, always vary in a smaller proportion. The range of variation is the narrower, the more predominantly the price of the article depends upon the gold as one of its raw materials.

From the fact that gold-made articles are thus more or less securely tied in value to the gold standard, it follows also that the prices of substitutes for such articles will tend to vary less than prices in general. These substitute articles will include silver watches, ornaments of silver, and various other forms of jewelry, whether containing gold or not.

A further dispersion of prices is produced by the fact that the special forces of supply and demand are playing on each individual price, and causing relative variations among them, and although these variations cannot affect the general price level they can affect the number and extent of individual divergencies above and below that general level.

It is evident, therefore, that prices must constantly change relatively to each other, whatever happens to their general level. It would be as idle to expect a uniform movement in prices as a uniform movement for all bees in a swarm. On the other hand, it would be as idle to deny the existence of a general movement of prices because they do not all move alike as to deny a general movement of a swarm of bees because the individual bees have different movements. The general movement of prices is expressed by an "index number " which gives the average level of prices at any time as compared with some other time used for comparison.

Besides the changes in individual prices, there will be corresponding changes in the quantities of the commodities which are exchanged at these prices respectively. In other words, as each p changes, the Q connected with it will change also, because usually any influence affecting the price of a commodity will also affect the consumption of it.

We see, therefore, that it is well-nigh useless to speak of uniform changes in prices (/s) or of uniform changes in quantities exchanged (Qs). Therefore, instead of supposing such uniform changes, we must now proceed to the problem of developing some convenient method of indicating by an average the general trend of the changes in prices or in quantities. We must formulate two composite or average magnitudes: the price level (index number) and the volume of trade.

It is desired, then, in the equation of exchange, to convert the right side, Spq, into the form PT, where T measures the volume of trade, and P is the " index number " expressing the price level at which this trade is carried on.

T is conceived as the sum of all the Qs, and P as the average of all the ps.

To carry out these definitions in practice, suitable units of measure for the various articles must be selected. The ordinary units in which the various Qs are measured will not be the most suitable. Coal is sold by the ton, sugar by the pound, wheat by the bushel, etc. If we should merely add together these tons, pounds, bushels, etc., and call their grand total so many " units " of commodities, we should have a very arbitrary summation. It will make a difference to the result whether we measure coal by tons or hundredweights. The system becomes less arbitrary and more useful for the purpose of comparing price levels in different years if we use, as the unit for measuring any commodity, not the unit in which it is commonly sold, but the amount which constitutes a "dollars worth" at some particular year called the base year. Then every price in the base year becomes exactly one dollar, and the average of all prices in that year also becomes exactly one dollar. In any other year, the average price (i. e., the average of the prices of the arbitrarily chosen units which in the base year were worth a dollar) will be the index number representing the price level, while the number of such units will be the volume of trade. Thus, let us suppose, for simplicity, that there are only three commodities (bread, coal, and cloth), and let us use the table on the next page for facts to start with.

We wish to compare the average price or price level in the year 1912 with that in 1909 as the base year, and also to reckon the total volume of trade in 1912 in comparison with that in 1909. If we were not desirous of taking great pains to secure the best results, we could use the above figures just as they stand–averaging the prices and adding together the quantities. By this rough-and-ready method the average price per unit for 1909 would be (.10 + 5.00

Veax Prices (in Dollars) Quantities Exchanged
Bread (per Coal (per Ton) Cloth (per Yard) Bread (Ma-lions of Loaves) Coal (Mil-lions of Tons) Cloth (Mil-lions of Yards)
Lof)
1909. 1912. .10 5-00 6.00 1. 00 1. 10 too IO II 30 3S
IS 2IO
+ 1.00)-5-3, or 2.03; and for 1912 (.15 + 6.00 + 1.10)-3, or 2.42; the total trade for 1009 would be 200 + 10 + 30, or 240 million units; and for 1912, 210 + 1 1 + 35, or 256. That is, the price level would show a rise between 1909 and 1912 from 2.03 to 2.42, or a rise of nineteen and two tenths per cent, while the volume of trade would show a rise from 240 to 256, or six and six tenths per cent. But the simple method just used gives too much weight in the price comparison to coal, the price of which happens to be expressed by a large number simply because it is measured by a large unit. One way to remedy this disproportionate weighting is to measure all articles by one unit, as the pound; but a better way is that already described above, viz., to use as our unit" the dollars worth in 1909." The dollars worth of bread in 1909 was evidently ten loaves, the dollars worth of coal, the fifth of a ton, and that of cloth, the yard. Taking these units, we now have:–

Prices (in Dollars) Quantities
Year Bread (per Ten Loaves) Coal (per I Ton) Cloth (per Yard) Bread (Mil-lions of Ten Loaves) Coal (Mil-lions of i Tons) Cloth (Mfl-liona of Yards)
1909. 1. 00 1. 00 1. 00 2O 5 30
1912 1-5 1. 2O I. IO 21 55 35
The average price in 1909, on the basis of these new units, is simply 1, since this is the price of each individual article; while the average price in 1912 is–if we take the simple arithmetical average–(1.5o + 1.2o + 1.1o)-5-3, or 1.27. The total volume of trade in 1909 is (in millions of units) 20 + 50 + 30, or 100; and in 1912, 21 + 55 + 35, or 1n. Thus, according to this reckoning, the price level has risen from 1.00 to 1.27, or, as it is usually expressed, from a base of one hundred per cent to a height of one hundred and twenty-seven per cent–a rise of twenty-seven per cent; while trade has increased from 100 million units to 1n million units, an increase of eleven per cent.

We may slightly improve the above method by taking for 1912 a " weighted " average of prices instead of a simple average. It is found by dividing the total value of all the goods by their total quantity. This is a better method because, in. the result, it gives less weight to the commodities less dealt in, such as bread. The average for 1909 will still be 1.00, for that is the price for each individual commodity; but the average for 1912 will be slightly different. The total value is (in millions of dollars) 1.50 X 21 + 1.20 X 55 + 1.10 X 35, or 136 million dollars, and the total quantity is, as we have already seen, 21 + 55 + 35, or 11 1 million units; consequently the average price is 136-5. 111, or 1.23. According to this last and best method, then, the price level has risen from 1 (or one hundred per cent) to 1.23 (or one hundred and twenty-three per cent); this indicates a rise of twenty-three per cent. The index numbers are one hundred per cent for 1909 and one hundred and twenty-three per cent for 1912.

The results of the three methods of reckoning the average rise of prices differ slightly, showing respectively a rise of nineteen, twenty-seven, and twenty-three per cent. Other methods, of which many are possible, would also differ slightly. No method gives an absolutely perfect index of changes in price levels, but the last one worked out above is

as good as any. The main point in any system of averages is to give great weight to the great staples of trade, and little weight to the insignificant articles. Radium has fallen in price enormously in the last few years, but radium is so unimportant as an article of commerce that its great fall ought not to be allowed in our reckoning to have much effect on the index number for the general price level.

Introducing, then, our newly found magnitudes, P and T, into the equation of exchange, it assumes the form

$MV + MV = PT$, its right member being the product of the index number, P (or the average of prices), multiplied by the volume of trade, T (or the sum total of " units " sold).

4. The History of Price Levels It is impossible to have absolutely accurate index numbers, but those constructed for recent years by the United States Bureau of Labor are accurate enough for all practical purposes. For the remote past we have only very rough index numbers, because the records of prices in past times are so defective. These rough index numbers are sufficient, however, to show that the general trend of

prices during the last ten centuries has usually been upward. We may say that prices are now five to ten times as high as a thousand years ago. Since the discovery of America, prices have almost steadily risen. The successive opening of mines has been largely responsible for this rise.

For recent years (1896-1910) we are able to construct fairly accurate estimates of all the factors in the equation of exchange, M, M, V, V, P, T. The statistics of these magnitudes for the fifteen years mentioned are all presented in Figure 17. In this diagram the equation of exchange for each year is represented by the mechanical balance described in a previous chapter.

We note that in the years considered every factor has greatly increased. The quantity of money in circulation (M, represented by the purse) has about doubled; bank deposits subject to check (M, represented by the bank book) have about trebled; the volume of trade (T, represented by the weight at the right) has about doubled; the velocity of circulation of money (V, represented by the leverage of the purse, or its distance from the fulcrum) has increased slightly, and the velocity of circulation of bank deposits (V, represented by the leverage of the bank book) has increased considerably. As the net result of these changes, the index number of prices (P, or the leverage of the weight at the right) has increased about two thirds. As in the above illustration, the price level of 1909 is taken as 100. On this scale the price level of 1896 is 60, and that of the other years, as indicated. The volume of trade for any year is represented as the number of " dollars worth " on the basis of the prices in 1909. Thus the actual value of trade in 1909 was 387,000,000,000, or over a billion a day, i. e., 387 billion units of goods of various kinds, the units being such as to be each worth one dollar in 1909. The trade in 1910 was 399,000,000,000 of these same units (., such as were worth 1 in 1909). Similarly, the trade in 1896 was 191,000,000,000 of these units. As the index number of prices shows that the price level of 1896 was only about sixty per cent of the price level of 1909, the actual value of the trade in 1896 was only 114,600,000,000. This is PT for 1896, i. e., 191 billion units (each worth 1 in 1909) at 60 cents each, the price in 1896.

Let us express the matter in terms of cause and effect. The diagram affords a picture of the fact that the increases in money and deposits and in their velocities (represented, respectively, by the increased weights of purse and bank book, and their increased distances from the fulcrum) have necessitated an increase in average prices (represented by the increased distance of the tray from the fulcrum) in spite of the increased volume of business which has been transacted (represented by the increased weight of the tray).

It is interesting to observe the changes in all the factors before and after the crisis of 1907. These changes, it will be noted, fulfill the principles explained in the chapter on crises.

From 1896 to the present time, the extraordinary increase in the worlds gold production, chiefly in South Africa, Cripple Creek, and other parts of the Rocky Mountain Plateau, together with the Klondike region, has caused, and is still causing, a rapid rise of prices.

The history of prices has in substance been a race between the increase in media of exchange (M and M) and the increase in trade (T), while the velocities of circulation have changed in a much less degree. Sometimes the circulating media shoot ahead of trade, and then prices rise. Sometimes, on the other hand, circulating media lag behind trade, and then prices fall.

The outlook for the future apparently promises a continued rise of prices due to a continued increase in the gold supply and in the use of deposit banking.

The most careful review of present gold-mining conditions shows that we may expect a continuance of gold inflation for a generation or more. De Launay, an excellent authority, says, "For at least thirty years we may count on an output of gold higher than, or at least comparable to, that of the last few years." This gold will come from the United States, Alaska, Mexico, the Transvaal, and other parts of Africa and Australia, and later from Colombia, Bolivia, Chili, the Ural Province, Siberia, and Korea.

It is difficult to predict the future growth of trade, and therefore impossible to say for how long gold and deposit expansion will keep ahead of trade. That for many years, however, they will outrun trade seems probable, for the reason that there is no immediate prospect of a reduction in the percentage growth of money and deposits, nor an increase in the percentage growth of trade. Not only do mining engineers report immense workable deposits in outlying regions, but any long look ahead must reckon with possible and probable cheapening of gold extraction. The cyanide process, for instance, has made low-grade ores pay which did not pay before. If we let imagination run a little ahead of our times, we may expect similar improvements in the future whereby still lower grades may be worked, or the gold bearing clays of the South made to pay, or possibly even the sea compelled to give up its gold. Like the surface of the continents, the waters of the sea contain many thousand times as much gold as all the gold thus far extracted in the whole history of the world. We have seen that inflation is, in general, an evil, likely to culminate in a crisis. It is therefore to be hoped that the knowledge of how to get this hidden treasure may be secured but gradually,–unless its sudden acquisition may give the needed stimulus to governments to devise a more scientific standard of value than the yellow metal.

It is unfortunate that the purchasing power of money should be always at the mercy of every chance in gold mining. There are few enterprises more subject to chance than gold mining. There are always chances of finding new gold deposits, chances of their " panning out " well or ill, and chances of new methods of metallurgy. On these fitful conditions the purchasing power of money is dependent. Consequently every one interested in long-time contracts, whether debtor or creditor, stockholder or bondholder, wage earner or savings bank depositor, is made to some extent a partaker in these chances. In a sense every one of us who uses gold as a standard for deferred payments becomes a gold speculator. We all take our chances as to what the future dollar will buy. The problem of making the purchasing power of money stable so that a dollar may be a dollar–the same in value at one time as another–is one of the most serious problems in applied economics. As yet it has received very little attention. The advocates of bimetallism have claimed that " the bimetallic standard " possesses greater stability than either the gold or silver standard. Many other and very ingenious schemes for a more stable currency have been proposed, but have received very little attention. As the consideration of these schemes belongs to applied economics, we shall not discuss them here.

CHAPTER XV

SUPPLY AND DEMAND 1. Individual Prices Presuppose a Price Level

We have completed our study of the purchasing power of money, which, as has been noted, is really a study of price levels. Our next topic will be individual prices. Prices, as we find them in the market, are facts of everyday experience. As students of economics, we are seeking the explanation of these facts. Why, for instance, is the price of sugar six cents a pound at one time and seven or five at another?

It has already been shown (Chapter VIII, 1) that individual prices, such, for instance, as the price of sugar, presuppose a price level. This fact is one reason why we have considered price levels before considering individual prices. Before proceeding to the causes determining individual prices, it will be advisable to explain more fully this proposition that an individual price presupposes a price level.

The price of sugar is a ratio between sugar and money. Any one who buys sugar balances in his mind the importance of the sugar to him against the importance of the money which he has to pay for it. In making this comparison, the money stands in his mind for the other things which it might buy if not spent for sugar. If this general purchasing power of money is great, money will seem 258.

precious in his mind, and he will be more loath to part with a given amount of it than if its purchasing power is small; that is, the greater the power of money to purchase things in general, the less of it will be offered for sugar in particular, and the lower the price of sugar will therefore become. In other words, the lower the general price level, the lower will be the price of sugar. In still other words, the price of sugar must sympathize with prices in general. If they are high, it will tend to be high, and if they are low, it will tend to be low. Before the purchaser of sugar can decide how much money he is willing to exchange for it, he must have some idea of what else he could buy for his money. This explains why a traveler feels at first so helpless in a foreign country when he is told the prices of goods in terms of unfamiliar units. If the traveler has never heard before of kroner, gulden, rubles, or milreis, any prices expressed in these units will mean nothing to him. He cannot say how many of any one of these units he is willing to pay for any given article until he knows how the purchasing power of that unit compares with the unit to which he is accustomed. There must thus always be in the minds of those who use money some idea of its purchasing power. The sellers and buyers of sugar express the prices at which they are willing to supply or to demand in terms of money, and money means to them merely purchasing power over other things. It is often said that supply and demand of sugar or of any other commodity determine its price, and this is true, at a given price level; for those who supply or demand sugar, in deciding how much money they will take or give for it, are influenced by their idea of the general purchasing power of money. This needs emphasis because it is so often overlooked. Although the purchasing power of money is assumed, we are usually as unconscious of it as we are of the background of a picture against which we see and unconsciously measure the flgures in the foreground.

2. A Market and Competition

The terms " supply" and " demand," say, of sugar, thus imply a concealed reference to the purchasing power of money, i. e., to prices in general, as well as to the price of sugar in particular. As we have, through several previous chapters, already studied the subject of prices in general, we shall hereafter assume that the general level of prices has been determined in accordance with the principles set forth in those chapters relating to the equation of exchange. We are now ready to leave these general relations and to study the determination of a particular price (such as that of sugar) so far as this depends upon its own particular supply and demand in its own particular market.

A market for any good is any assemblage of buyers and sellers of that good. The buyers and sellers may be, and usually are, physically near each other, as on the New York Stock Exchange, or they may be merely connected by telegraph, telephone, or other means of communication, as in the stock market as a whole; for the stock market as a whole includes not only the members of the stock exchange, but also all other buyers and sellers of stock both in and out of the city. It is in the market that questions of supply and demand which we are about to discuss work themselves out.

Our study of price determination will fall under two heads, according as there is competition or monopoly. For the present we shall assume a condition of perfect competition; that is, we shall assume that there are a number of buyers and sellers each of whom offers to buy or sell independently of the others. Thus, if self-interest leads him to do so, a buyer will bid a higher price than others, irrespective of their wishes in the matter, and likewise a seller will ask a lower price if his independent self-interest so leads him.

When there is perfect competition, there is (in a given market) only one resultant price for all buyers and all sellers. This is evident; for if there were more than one price, no buyers would buy at any of the higher prices which had first been asked (and so these must fall), and no seller would sell at the lower prices which had been bidden (and so these must rise). The watchfulness of one competitor toward the others will eliminate differences in price. Even though not all buyers and sellers are careful to note slight differences in price, the more watchful bring about the same result by the operation of what is called "arbitrage." They buy at the lowest prices and sell at the highest. Their buying raises the lowest prices, and their selling lowers the highest.

In these ways differences in prices are reduced or entirely eliminated. It is true that in practice there often remain slight differences in price, even in the same or closely associated markets. This fact merely means that competition is often imperfect. In our discussion we shall not take account of those cases, but consider only the simple case where competition is perfect.

3. Demand and Supply Schedules

The terms " supply " and " demand " have a definite and technical meaning in economics, and the reader should note the following definitions carefully.

In any market there is a different demand for sugar at different prices. We may define the demand at a given price as the amount of sugar which people are willing to buy at that price. In the same way the supply at a given price is the amount which people are willing to sell at that price. If the price of sugar is 8 cents a pound, the demand for sugar in a given community at a given time may be, let us say, ooo pounds a week. If the price falls to 7 cents, the demand would increase, say, to 940 pounds. If the price falls to 6 cents, the demand would rise, say, to 1000 pounds; and so on.

The supply of sugar, we shall suppose, changes in the opposite way. At 8 cents it may be 1100 pounds; at 7 cents, 1050; at 6 cents, 1000; etc. The following table shows these figures and others, and constitutes what are called " schedules " of demand and supply in relation to various prices.

The schedule of demand is the second column considered relatively to the first. It shows the largest quantity which will be taken at each given price, or, what amounts to the same thing, the highest price at which a given quantity will be taken. When the relationship between the two columns is expressed in the latter of these two ways, it is more convenient to place the second column first, and the first, second; but their order is immaterial. It is their relation to each other which constitutes the demand schedule.

Puce Schedule or Dexand Schedule or Supply

.08 900 IIOO

.07.06 940 IOOO 1050 IOOO

.05 IIOO 900

.04 1250 73

In the same way the relation between the first and third columns constitutes the supply schedule. This tells us the largest quantities which will be supplied at stated prices, or, what amounts to the same thing, the lowest prices at which stated quantities will be supplied.

Running the eye down the table, we see that, although the supply at first exceeds the demand, as the price falls the demand increases and the supply decreases, until, when the price reaches 6 cents, supply and demand are

equal. For prices lower than 6 cents we find the reverse condition, demand exceeding supply.

If the foregoing figures represent the demand and supply schedules showing the amounts that buyers are willing to take and sellers to give at different prices, it is clear that there is only one price that will make supply and demand equal. That price is 6 cents, and that is the price that supply and demand will finally fix. The price cannot long be above 6 cents, for then supply would exceed demand, and the price would immediately fall. Nor can it be below, for then demand would exceed supply, and the price would rise. For instance, if the price were 8 cents, the supply (1100 pounds) would exceed the demand (900 pounds) by 200 pounds. Those wishing to sell this extra amount would then be unable to do so except by offering it at a lower price, and their competition would drive the price downukon the other hand, if the price were 4 cents, the demand (1250 pounds) would exceed the supply (750 pounds) by 500 pounds, (and those demanding this extra amount would be unable to get it except by bidding a higher price, and their competition would then drive the price up.

Since, then, the price cannot really be either above or below 6 cents, it must be finally fixed at 6 cents. A price which thus makes supply and demand equal is said to " clear the market," and is called the market price. The amounts supplied and demanded at the market price are called the amount marketed, i. e., the amount actually bought by buyers and sold by sellers. This amount marketed is, therefore, at once the market demand and the market supply.

4. Demand and Supply Curves

The relations discussed in 3 above can be seen more clearly by means of a diagram. In Figure 18 is represented the demand for sugar at different prices.

The two axes OX and OY are drawn simply for y

18 II IO
8 7 6 8 D
y
A
a
2
1 –
o BOO 4OO 600 BOO I000 1200 X
Fig. 18 (Demand).

reference, like the equator and the Greenwich meridian in a map. The intersection 0 of the two axes is called the " origin." The diagram is a "map" of demand on which the " latitude," or the distance above the line OX, represents any price; and the "longitude," or the distance to the right of the line OY, represents the amount demanded at that price. Let us, for instance, represent an assumed price, say 8 cents, by measuring off the " latitude" Oy from the origin 0. At this price of 8 cents, the demand, which we have seen to be 900 pounds, is represented by the " longitude " yd. We have thus located a point D, the " latitude " of which represents a particular price (8 cents), and the "longitude" of which represents the demand (900 pounds) at that price. It will be seen that the " latitude" is simply the elevation above the base axis OX, whether we measure this " latitude " by the line Oy or by xd. Likewise the " longitude " is simply the distance of D to the right of the axis OY, whether this distance be measured by yd or by Ox. Having found one point, D, the " latitude " and " longitude " of which represent, respectively, a price and the demand at that price, we may find in like manner other points, the " latitudes " and " longitudes " of which will represent other particular prices and the demands corresponding to those prices. Several such points are indicated in Figure 18. It will be seen that the lower in the diagram the points, the farther they are to the right. This represents the fact that the lower the price, the greater the demand. We may suppose the spaces between those various points to be filled by other points, all together forming what is called the demand curve.

A demand curve, then, is a curve such that the " latitude" of any one of its points represents a particular price, and the " longitude " of that point the particular demand corresponding to that price. Thus a demand curve is a graphic picture of a demand schedule.

In precisely the same way we may treat supply. In Figure 19 let us represent any particular price, say 8 cents, by the "latitude" Oy, and the supply corresponding to this price (1100 pounds) by the "longitude " ys. Thus we locate a point S such that its " latitude " (Oy or xs) represents a particular price, and the "longitude" (ys or Ox) represents the supply at that particular price. In like manner we may locate other points, the " latitudes" of which represent other prices and the " longitudes " of which represent the amounts which would be supplied at these respective prices. These points are so arranged that the higher their " latitude," the greater their " longitude."

This represents our assumption that the higher the price, the greater the supply. The curve which these points form is called a supply curve and is a graphic picture of a supply schedule.

```
  T
 12
  n
 10
  e S
  7
  e a
  4
  z i
  0 00 400 600 BOO IOOOXI20Q It
```
Flg. 19 (Supply).

In Figure 20 are drawn both the supply and the demand curves, the demand curve being DD, and the supply curve SS. We have seen that the demand curve shows many different demands at many different prices, and that, similarly, the supply curve shows many different supplies at many different prices; but that there is only one price at which supply and demand are equal. We can see this clearly in Figure 20; for there is only one point (P) in which the two curves intersect. The "latitude" (OP) of the intersection (P) of the curves DDf and SS represents the market price. The " longitude " of P represents the amount marketed, which is at once the supply at that price and the demand at that price. The point P may be called the market point.

The market price, OP, clears the market, and no other price will. If, for instance, we take a higher price, such as OP", the supply will be represented by the long line P"S", and the demand by the short line P"D", leaving the difference between them, or D"S", as the excess of supply over demand. The effort of sellers to get rid of this excess will drive the price down. Thus the market price cannot exceed OP. In like manner, the market price cannot be lower than OP. If, for instance, it were onlv OP", the demand would be P"D", and the supply only P"S", leaving an excess of demand over supply of D"S", which

Fig. 20.

at that price the buyers are unable to obtain. They will therefore bid up the price. We see, then, that the only real price is OP. The point P, at which the two curves intersect, is the only real point, the latitude of which represents the market price and the longitude the actual amount demanded and sold. All the other points in the two curves are hypothetical, representing, not what demand and supply actually are, but what they would be at other prices than the real market price.

All demand curves descend to the right. But they descend at different rates. Those demand curves which are steep–descend very rapidly–represent the demand schedules of those goods which are called necessities, for the rapid descent means that it requires a great fall of price to affect demand materially. They have an "inelastic" demand, which will "stretch" but little whatever the change in price. We know that the demand for a necessity such as salt does not change greatly, even if the price changes much. Otherwise expressed, a necessity has an " inelastic" demand which will "stretch" or expand but little for a given fall in price. At the other extreme are luxuries, the demand curves of which descend very slowly, thus interpreting the fact that a slight fall in price produces a great expansion in demand. Otherwise expressed, a luxury has an "elastic" demand which will "stretch" or expand much for a given fall in price. If the price of champagne, for instance, is slightly changed, the amount of it consumed will be materially affected.

In the same way supply curves may ascend at different rates, the steep ones representing commodities the supply of which is "inelastic," that is, cannot expand very much for a given increase in price. At the opposite extreme are the supply curves which ascend very slowly, being those of commodities, the supply of which is very "elastic"–can be greatly increased by a given increase in price.

Most of the articles produced in extractive industries such as agriculture or mining are of the rapidly ascending type, while manufactured articles often illustrate the slightly ascending type. It requires a great increase in the price of coal to affect materially the output of coal mines, but it requires only a slight rise in price of manufactured products to lead to an enormous increase in the output.

5. Shifting of Demand or Supply

Having represented supply and demand by curves, we are now in a position to understand more clearly what is meant by " increase of demand " or " increase of supply." These phrases are often used loosely, without realization that they are ambiguous. Sometimes we hear it said that " demand has increased " when the speaker merely means that demand has increased as a consequence of a fall in the market price; that is, the demand at a new and lower market price is greater than the demand at the old and higher market price, although the demand at this old price remains unchanged. Thus if the price of sugar falls from 8 cents to 5 cents per pound, the demand at the new market price, 5 cents, will exceed the old demand at the old market price, 8 cents, although the amounts demanded at 8 cents may remain unaltered and the amount demanded at 5 cents may remain unaltered. In this case the demand schedule remains unchanged. Only the particular demand in that schedule which corresponds to the market price is shifted downward in the second column (see 3).

Again, and more properly, we hear it said that " demand has increased " when the speaker means that the demand at a specified price has increased; as, for instance, that more sugar is demanded at 8 cents than formerly, and more, likewise, at 5 cents, or any other price; that in short the demand schedule has changed through the increase of the figures in the second column.

The two meanings which have been distinguished may be designated respectively as "increase of the market demand " and as " increase of the demand schedule." We have spoken only of changes in demand. But the same distinctions apply, of course, to two meanings F1G . " (Demand).

of the phrase "increase of supply," one, an increase in the market supply, and the other, an increase in the supply schedule.

We may see clearly the distinction between these two meanings of the phrase " increase of demand " and avoid their confusion if we express them by means of-y diagrams. Increase of demand may mean a mere shifting of the market point from one position A to another position B, farther to the right on the same demand Y curve (Fig. 21), or it may mean a shifting of the entire demand curve from the position A to the position B, farther to the right (Fig. 2 2). Both of these meanings are admissible, but they are entirely distinct. In the same way, "increase of " supply " may mean one of Fmj. 23 (Supply).

Fig. 22 (Demand).

two things, either a shifting of the market point A to another position B, farther to the right, on the same supply curve (Fig. 23), or a shifting of the entire supply curve from the position A to the position B farther to the right, as in Figure 24. We see, therefore, that an " increase of supply" or of demand may mean either a change of the market point on the same curve

B—

Fig. 24 (Supply).

or a change of the curve itself.

It will be seen that an

increase of demand in the market sense is nothing else than an increase of supply in the schedule sense; for we have already made it clear that there is only one point which is the intersection of the two curves, and that this point cannot be shifted to the right from A to B on the demand curve unless the whole supply curve has shifted so as to change the intersection. Such a shifting is seen in Figure 25. Here the demand has increased in the market sense, having changed from the longitude of A to the Flg 2j longitude of B on the same demand curve; but this increased demand comes about only because the supply has increased in the schedule sense, having shifted from the position of the unbroken supply curve to the position of the dotted curve.

To express these changes in terms of the schedules of 3, let us suppose that the supply schedule is changed by the addition of 200 pounds of sugar to each quantity given in the third column. It is evident that the market price will fall from six cents (at which supply and demand were each 1000) to five cents (at which supply and demand are each 1100). Thus the demand at the market price has increased from-. 1000 to 1100 as a con-sequence of the increases in the supply schedule.

Again, to say that supply has increased in the market sense is the same thing as to say that the demand has increased in the schedule sense. This is shown in Figure 26,- where the market point

Fig. 26. A on the supply curve has shifted to B on the same curve, because the demand curve had shifted from the unbroken to the dotted position. The same result can, of course, be expressed in terms of a change in the demand schedule of 3.

We should, therefore, be careful to know, when we speak of a change in demand or supply, whether we mean that the change is in the market sense or in the schedule sense. It seems odd at first to think that an increase of demand in one sense is really an increase of supply in another sense, and vice versa. Because of this ambiguity, when one person speaks of an increase of supply, it means the same thing as when another speaks of an increase of demand.

To illustrate the two meanings, let us suppose that the demand considered is the demand for automobiles, and that, given the same price, people would demand automobiles now no more and no less than they did a few years ago, but that the conditions of the supply have changed, so that now more automobiles can be supplied for the same price. That would mean that the supply curve had shifted to the right, so that its point of intersection with the same demand curve has also shifted to the right (Fig. 25). Therefore two things have happened on the demand side. The market price has fallen, and as a consequence of that fall of price the number of automobiles demanded has increased. The demand at the market price has increased, but the demand schedule has not changed at all. People are just as willing as before to take an automobile at any given price, but they are willing to take more automobiles at present low prices than at former high prices. There have been no changes in the conditions of demand, i. e., the demand schedule. What have changed are the conditions of supply, i. e., the supply schedule.

On the other hand, let us take as our illustration works of art. In the past few years there has been a great change in the attitude of Americans toward works of art. Of these we are much more appreciative than we used to be, and are willing to pay more, for instance, for a fine painting than previously. Thus, for works of art the demand schedule has shifted; the demand for works of art has increased in the schedule sense (Fig. 26). Consequently, the supply has increased in the market sense; namely, on account of the greater demand the price has risen, and therefore owners and makers of works of art have offered more for sale.

Thus increase of demand in the schedule sense brings about increase of supply in the market sense, and vice versa. An increase in the supply of automobiles in the schedule sense brought about an increase in the demand for automobiles in the market sense, while an increase in the demand for works of art in the schedule sense brought about an increase in the supply of works of art in the market sense. In either case the original change is in a schedule or curve. There can evidently be no change of points of intersection except by a change in at least one of the two curves. Hereafter we shall use the phrases " increase of supply " or " increase of demand " only in the sense of shifting to the right the supply or demand curve; in other words, of increasing the figures of demand or supply in the demand or supply schedules.

When we shift demand or supply curves, the effect on the intersection, i. e., on the market price, and the amount marketed, will, as is evident from the figures, depend greatly on the character of the curves; whether, for instance, one or both of them ascend rapidly or slowly. It will be instructive for the student to draw on paper various pairs of intersecting curves, making one or both nearly horizontal, and again one or both nearly vertical, and to observe the various effects then obtained, first, by shifting the demand curve a given distance to the right or left, and second, by shifting the supply curve a given distance to the right or left.1 In actual fact, demand and supply curves are constantly shifting, with the result that their point of intersection is constantly shifting, sometimes to the right, sometimes to the left, sometimes up and sometimes down. Consequently the market price and the amount marketed are changing from time to time.

The causes which shift the curves are innumerable. Changes in taste or fashion will affect demand curves, while changes in methods of production will affect the supply curves. For instance, fashion and outdoor sports, including motoring, have increased the demand for fur coats, and have, therefore, raised their price; while improved machinery has increased the supply of shoes and has consequently lowered their price.

1 Observe that when the demand curve is shifted, the change in price involved depends upon the steepness of the supply curve; and, vice versa, that when the supply curve is shifted, the change in price involved depends upon the steepness of the demand curve.

As to the variable point of intersection, we are more interested in its latitude than in its longitude, for the latitude represents the market price. This market price will evidently rise with a rise in either curve, and fall with a fall in either curve. It will also rise with a shifting of the demand curve to the right, or with a shifting of the supply curve to the left; and will fall with a shifting of the demand curve to the left, or of the supply curve to the right. In fact, by a leftward change in the demand curve or a rightward change in the supply curve, the price may fall to zero. A standard example of such a case is furnished by the air we breathe, the supply of which is so much greater than the demand that it bears no price. The same is often true of water and of. land of inferior qualities. There are millions of acres of land which may be had for practically nothing . (a fact of much importance to be emphasized in a future chapter).

One cause of. shifting demand and supply curves mentioned in a general way at the beginning of this chapter we wish especially to emphasize. This cause is a change in the general purchasing power of money. Let us suppose that we change our monetary unit so that what is now fifty cents should be called a dollar. This would mean that the purchasing power of a dollar had been cut in two, or that the level of prices had been doubled. We ought,

Fig. 27.

therefore, to find that the demand and supply of sugar will have been affected so as to double its price–the latitude of the point of intersection–and this will be, in fact, the result, unless prevented by some interfering cause. As soon as the half-dollar becomes a dollar, the price in " dollars " at which any given amount of sugar, such as Ox (in Fig. 27), is demanded, will evidently be doubled, becoming xb, which is twice xa. If previously people were willing to take Ox at one price, they are now willing to take it at double that price, because this double price means in purchasing power exactly the same thing as the original price. And, in fact, all points in the demand curve will be shifted to be twice as high as before.

In the same way and for the same reasons, those who have sugar to sell will require twice as high a price as before for a given amount; because, otherwise, they would not get the same purchasing power as before, in return. Thus, as indicated in Figure 28, each point, such as A, in the supply curve, will be shifted to twice as high an elevation above the base, OX.

When the two curves thus shifted are drawn on the same axes (see Fig. 29), it is evident that the new point of intersection, B, will be vertically over the old point of intersection, A.

The market price of sugar is therefore doubled, though the amount marketed is unchanged. Simply the doubling of the general price level carries with it a doubling in thf

Fig. 28.

price of sugar. While the supply and demand curves for sugar may change for many other reasons than the doubling in general price level, so far as this cause, taken by itself, is concerned, its effect on prices is to double them. Our analysis of demand and supply curves then brings us back to the fact already stated, that the price of any particular good, like sugar, depends partly on the general level of prices, or the purchasing power of money.

We can now see more clearly than before the shallowness of the idea that the supply and demand of each individual commodity fix its price independently of other commodities. According to this view, the general price level is regarded as the effect of innumerable individual pairs of supply and demand curves, each pair being supposed to completely determine some one price. The opposite is the truth. The general price level is not the result of the supply and demand of sugar in relation to money, but is itself one of the causes affecting the supply and demand of sugar in relation to money; for we have seen (Figs. 27, 28 and 29, and discussion) that, as the price level rises or falls, the price of sugar rises and falls correspondingly.

We end this chapter, therefore, with the statement with which we began; namely, that it is im-

Flg 2 portant to distin guish between the influences determining the general price level and the influences determining an individual price. The price level is determined by a comparatively simple mechanism, that of the equation of exchange. It is the result of the quantity of money and deposits, the velocities of their circulation, and the volume of trade. The general price level then helps to fix individual prices, although not interfering with relative variations among them, just as the general level of the ocean helps fix the level of individual waves and troughs without interfering with variations among them. The tides determine whether a wave shall be as a whole high or low, and so the general level of prices, while it does not fully fix the price of sugar, determines whether it shall be in general high or low. A rise in the general price level is one of the many causes raising the demand and supply curves of sugar; and, reversely, a fall in that level is a cause lowering those curves.

CHAPTER XVI

THE INFLUENCES BEHIND DEMAND 1. Individual Demand Schedules and Curves

We have seen that the market price of any particular good is that price in the demand and supply schedules which will just "clear the market." By this phrase is meant, of course, that the price will make supply and demand equal. Both the market price and the quantity marketed are determined by the intersection of the supply and demand curves. We have therefore explained how the market price (as well as quantity marketed) of any particular good is fixed by supply and demand.

But supply and demand are not the ultimate influences determining prices. They are only the proximate influences. Beneath and behind them lie influences more remote and more fundamental. In this chapter we shall trace back these influences so far as they have to do with the demand side of the market. We shall find (1) that the demand schedule explained in the last chapter is formed out of a large number of individual demand schedules, and (2) that each individual demand schedule is in turn formed out of two " desirability " schedules.

In the first place, then, what we have called the demand schedule is only an aggregate demand schedule. It is for the whole market, and resolvable into constituent demand schedules, one for each particular person in the market. The total demand at any price is merely the sum of the individual demands at that price. For instance, let the following table represent the demand schedules for coal of two in dividuals distinguished as Individual No. I and Individual No. II, at prices of from 12 to 2 per ton:–

Demand Schedules

Peice No. I No. II () Total (o + 4)

o)

12 I O I
10 2 0 2
8 3 O 3
6 4 I 5
S 5 2 7
4 6 3 9
3 7 4 11
2 8 6 14

The table tells us that at a price of 12 a ton Individual No. I will take only one ton, and Individual No. II will not take any; that at a price of 6 a ton Individual No. I will take four tons, and Individual No. II will take one ton; and so on. The last column gives the sum of the demands of these two individuals. If we should extend such a table to include the demands of all the individuals in the community, we would obtain in the last column the total demand in the community. The total demand schedule is thus merely the sum of the individual demand schedules found by adding together all the individual amounts demanded at any given price. Behind the total demand schedule, therefore, are a number of constituent demand schedules.

y l

7 6 J

K S

i s

S

4 3 d r) s n

y V v s

S

s, ri

2 1 rt H

O i a 3 4 s 6 7 a 9 10 j Mz 13 M-X -

F1G. 30.

The same relation, of course, holds between total and individual demand curves. In Figure 30 let the curve d d represent the demand curve for Individual No. I, and d the demand curve for Individual No. II. At a given price, represented by the vertical distance or " latitude," Oy, the demands of these two individuals are represented respectively by the horizontal distances or "longitudes," y and ydz. The sum of these two demands is represented by the longer horizontal distance, yd. Thus we add the longitudes of the two individual demand curves together to get the longitude of the combined curve DD. If, instead of two individual demand curves, we should have all the demand curves in the market, and should add together the longitudes corresponding to given latitudes, i. e., the demands corresponding to given prices, we should thereby obtain the total demand curve of the market.

We may pause here to note the fact that, ordinarily, any one individual plays so small a part in the demand for any commodity that he regards the price as beyond the influence of any act of his. He finds this price ready made in the market and adjusts his demand to it. To him the price is a fixed fact and entirely beyond his control, while his demand, the quantity he chooses to take at that price, is the only thing which he can adjust. It is of course true that each individual, however insignificant his demand,

Fig. 31.

has theoretically an influence upon the general price, but the influence is so small as to be practically negligible. While, for the market as a whole, price is effect and not cause, yet for the individual it is cause rather than effect.

To show more clearly these relations to the individual and to the total, we have drawn in Figure 31 an individual demand curve dd, the total demand curve DD, and the total supply curve SS. The intersection of the last two determines the market price P X (or OP, or px); and this price determines for the individual the amount, Pp (or Ox), which he will take at that price.

2. Desirability

We have now found that back of the demand curve or schedule in any market lie the individual demand curves or schedules of all the people who compose that market. The next step is to find what causes lie back of the individual demand curves or schedules. Taking, for instance, the demand curve of Individual No. I, we may ask: What are the conditions which determine its shape and size? The answer is that it depends upon the desires or " wants " of Individual No. I. It is true that a man may have a strong desire for something without having any demand for it in the economic sense. But this is simply because he desires still more the money he would have to spend for it. Every purchaser of goods balances two desires, the desire for the goods and the desire for the money they would cost. On the relative strength of these desires depends the price he is willing to pay. We have, therefore, to investigate these two desires, the one for goods, the other for money. We shall begin with the desire for the goods.

Desire for goods implies desirability in those goods. The term " desirability " is synonymous with what is usually called " utility " in textbooks. " Desirability " is preferred here as a better term to express the idea intended. If there exists a keen desire to purchase a certain piece of land, we say that the land is especially desirable or has great desirability. Likewise precious stones have great desirability to many people. Tobacco has great desirability to a smoker; silks and satins to ladies of fashion; books to scholars; and so on. The concept "desirability" is so important that it ought to be defined with great care. The desirability of any particular good, at any particular time, to any particular individual, under any particular conditions, is the strength or intensity of his desire for that good at that time and under those conditions. The desirability of any good is one of the most important factors in determining its price. The connection, however, between desirability and price was for a long time overlooked because of the puzzling fact that many of the most desirable articles are the cheapest, and many of the least desirable are the dearest. Thus water is so desirable as to be indispensable; yet there are few things which are cheaper. On the other hand, jewelry, which could easily be dispensed with, bears high prices. This paradox, however, is easily explained. While it is true that water as a whole is very desirable, the desirability of any one quart of water, to be added to or taken away from the whole amount, is negligible. This one quart could make little difference to anybody because there are so many other quarts which could take its place. Were any one quart of water indispensable, water would bear a high price. On the other hand, while all the jewels of the world could be more easily dispensed with than all the water, yet any one jewel is more desired than any one quart of water. The desirability of any one diamond, to be added to or taken away from the few which the owner possesses, is very great. Jewels are rare, and one jewel more or less may make a great deal of difference. It is the desirability of any one unit of water or of jewelry which influences its price and not the desirability of all the water in our possession or of all the jewelry.

We see, then, that the desirability of water or of any other sort of good may mean either (1) the desirability of the whole or (2) the desirability of one unit more or less. The desirability of the whole is called the total desirability; the desirability of one unit more or less is called the marginal desirability. The marginal desirability of any good is the desirability of one unit more or less of it. In economic science we have more to do with marginal than with total desirability, and it is therefore important that the concept of marginal desirability should be thoroughly understood.

3. Illustration

To illustrate in detail the distinction between total and marginal desirability, let us suppose a person wishing to furnish his house with chairs. As presumably he does not wish to sit or compel his friends to sit on the floor, it is extremely desirable that he should have some chairs; but each successive chair that he introduces will lessen the need for more. One chair is so highly desirable as to be almost indispensable. It provides a seat for at least one person. A second chair, though not quite so indispensable as the first, is also extremely desirable, as it is likely that he will often wish seating capacity for at least two. A third chair, though less urgently needed than the second, will be highly desirable; and so on–each successive chair having a lower desirability than the preceding. The number of chairs which he will buy will depend, among other things, upon their price. To fix our ideas, let us suppose that he decides to buy ten. Then the tenth chair is called the marginal chair of the ten, and its desirability is called the marginal desirability of the ten. It is this tenth or marginal chair which gives him the most concern when he attempts to decide how many to buy. He has no difficulty, for instance, in deciding that he does not want thirty or forty chairs; the question which requires careful consideration in his mind is whether he shall stop buying at the tenth chair or at a slightly earlier or later point. He will consider carefully what difference it will make whether he has nine chairs or ten, or what difference it will make whether he has ten or eleven. If he decides on ten rather than nine, it is because he thinks the tenth chair will make enough difference to him to be worth the price he pays, and if he decides against the eleventh chair, it will be because he thinks this will not make enough difference to compensate him for the price. For instance, let us suppose that the price of the chairs is 10 each; then the fact that he decides to take the tenth chair shows that this tenth chair has at least 10 worth of desirability, while the fact that he decides against the eleventh chair shows that this eleventh chair does not have as much as 10 worth of desirability. Practically money is used in just this way to measure the comparative desirabilities of various goods.

As has been stated, the last or tenth chair bought is called the marginal chair of the ten, and the desirability of this last or tenth chair is called the marginal desirability of the ten chairs. The total desirability, on the other hand, of the ten chairs is evidently quite another matter. This is not 10 X 10. It is the sum of the desirabilities of the first chair, second, third, etc., considered, as above, in succession up to the tenth. The householder will not ordinarily be as definitely aware of total desirability as he is of marginal desirability. As we have seen, he will, in order to decide how many chairs to buy, have to give careful attention to the desirability of the tenth chair; it is so easy to decide upon the first few chairs that he will not ordinarily stop to reckon exactly how desirable the ten chairs as a whole may be. Should he wish to reckon this desirability, he would do so by thinking how much difference it makes to him whether he has ten chairs or none at all. For instance, he might think that to have ten chairs rather than none at all is worth about 150 to him. Then 150 would measure the total desirability of the ten chairs, while the marginal desirability, that is, the desirability of the last or tenth chair, is only about 10. From what has been said it will be evident that the total desirability is of only theoretical importance, while marginal desirability is of great practical importance. It is of little practical importance to any purchaser to know how much is the total desirability of the chairs he owns; namely, how great is the difference in comfort and convenience between having the number of chairs which he actually does have and having none at all. He finds it difficult to imagine how it would seem to have none at all. Such a condition can be considered only hypo-thetically. It never enters into his calculations as a practical possibility.

On the other hand, marginal desirability enters daily into practical life. The question which every purchaser of goods asks himself is where to stop–where to draw the line or margin beyond which he will not buy. He has to fix a margin in every purchase, and in fixing it he has to settle the question whether one unit more or less is or is not as desirable as the money which he will have to pay for it. In other words, with the desirability of this unit he has to compare the desirability of the money which it will cost. He can only solve the question of how much to buy by weighing carefully in his mind the desirability of the last few units, balancing each against the desirability of the money which it costs. At last he decides to limit his purchase at a certain point beyond which the next unit would not be worth to him what it would cost. The preceding unit–the last which he decides to buy–is adjudged as barely worth its cost, affording, perhaps, a slight advantage or surplus desirability. On the unit next preceding, the advantage or surplus desirability is greater and so on backward; but the further back we go the less carefully are the desirabilities weighed.

4. Some Remarks on Desirability

The total quantity of goods whose marginal desirability is under consideration may be any specified quantity of goods whatever. It may be a specified quantity of goods now existing, or a specified quantity of goods in the future, or a specified flow of goods through a period of time. For instance, by the marginal desirability of coal to an individual may be meant the marginal desirability of the particular stock of coal in his bin at the present moment. If this stock consists of fifteen tons, its marginal desirability is the desirability of the flfteenth ton, or the difference to him between the desirability of having fifteen and of having fourteen tons. Again, if a person is consuming in his household fifteen tons of coal a year, its marginal desirability at any time is the desirability of the fifteenth ton, or the sacrifice which, in his estimation at that time, would be occasioned were he to reduce his yearly consumption from fifteen tons to fourteen. A stock of fifteen tons and a consumption of fifteen tons a year are evidently quite distinct. It is, therefore, necessary in each case to specify the particular quantity of goods referred to, whether it be a stock in the present or a stock in the future or a flow through a period of time.

Undesirability is the opposite of desirability. Often we may express the very same fact by either word. For instance, it does not matter whether we speak of the desirability of keeping money, or the undesirability of losing it.

One of the most important general facts in regard to marginal desirability is that an increase in the quantity of goods whose marginal desirability is under consideration results in a decrease in the marginal desirability. This we have noted in the case of the chairs. Each unit in addition is less desirable than the preceding unit.

Marginal desirability is, as we have seen, often expressed as the desirability of the " last" unit. But this word last " is used metaphorically and not in any literal sense of sequence in time. All of the supposed ten chairs may be bought at the very same instant. The desirability of the tenth chair simply means the difference in desirability between having ten chairs and having only nine. Any one of the ten chairs may be considered as the tenth.

A special and important instance of marginal desirability is the marginal desirability of money. The marginal desirability of money at any particular time, to any particular individual, under any particular conditions, has the same sort of meaning as the marginal desirability of any other good. It means, therefore, the strength or intensity of a mans desire for an additional dollar, or, what amounts to the same thing, his reluctance to part with it. Briefly, the marginal desirability of money to him is the desirability of a dollar to him. Whenever he thinks of making a purchase, this desire comes into play, and the question of whether or not to buy is, as implied in the preceding discussion, determined by his judgment as to whether or not the marginal desirability of the goods exceeds the marginal desirability of money multiplied by the price in money required to secure those goods.

5. Individual Demands derived from Marginal Desirabilities It is on such comparison of the marginal desirabilities of goods and money that the demand curve of each individual depends. We shall now illustrate in detail how demand depends on desirability by taking the desires and demand of a given individual (whom we shall call No. I) for a given good (such as coal). As in the case of the chairs, the price Individual No. I is willing to pay is simply the ratio between two marginal desirabilities, that of coal and that of money.

We are to find how each individual demand schedule, as given in 1, depends upon two antecedent schedules of " desirability." If Individual No. I thinks that one ton of coal is a dozen times as desirable to him as a dollar, he will evidently be willing to pay any price up to 12 for that ton. If the price is over 12, he will not buy even a ton of coal. If it is just 12, he is willing to buy /ms/ one ton. A second ton will be worth less, in his estimation, being, let us say, only ten times as desirable as a dollar. He will then be willing to pay up to 10 for this second ton. If, then, the price is 10, he will buy up to two tons; for at that price it will evidently be more than worth his while to buy the first ton and just worth his while to buy the second. If the desirability of a third ton is eight times the desirability of a dollar, he will be willing to pay up to 8 per ton for three tons; for at that price the first and second tons are more desirable than the money, and the third, just as desirable. If the desirability of the fourth ton is six times that of a dollar, he is willing to pay a price up to 6 per ton for four tons.1 1 He will stop buying at that point at which the last unit bought has slightly more desirability than the money it costs, and the next unit (left unbought) has slightly less desirability than the money it costs. Thus, if the price of coal is 5.50 per ton, he will buy four tons because the fourth ton is slightly more desirable than 5.50 (being, according to the figures supposed above, as desirable as 6.00) while the fifth ton is slightly less desirable than 5.50 (being only as desirable as 5.00). In the case of most purchases, the desirability of the last of the units bought and that of the first of those unbought differ so slightly that we may call either of them the marginal desirability. That is why we have spoken of marginal desirability as the desirability of one unit more or less. Strictly speaking, however, the margin lies between the last of the units bought and the first of those unbought, and the marginal desirability may be called a mean of the desirabilities of these two units rather than the desirability of either. In some cases the desirability of the last unit bought and the next unit (first unbought) are widely different. This is true when the units are large and are not subdivisible into smaller units. For instance, pianos are large units and not subdivisible. One cannot buy one and a half pianos, but must choose between buying one and buying two. Only one piano is usually bought by a family. A second piano would have little or no desira bility. In this case the difference between the desirability of the piano which is bought and that of the next which is not bought, is very great. The family might be willing to give 1000, if need be, to get one piano but only 10 to get a second, u In each case the highest price he is willing to pay for a given quantity is measured by the ratio of the desirability of the last ton to the desirability of a dollar. The consequent derivation of prices from desirabilities is summarized in the following table:–

Desirability Of Last Ton Purchased Desirability Op A Dollar Price Per Ton The Customer Would Be Willing To Pay

Tons Purchased (o) ())

I 12 I 12

2 IO IO

3 8 8

4 6 6

5 5 5

6 4 4

As indicated, the last column is found by taking the ratio of the figures in the second to those in the third; that is, dividing (a) by (b). As there are no standard units of desirability, it will not matter what unit we select. In the table, for simplicity of division, we have taken as our unit for measuring desirability the marginal desirability of money to Individual No. I himself. We thus derive the individuals demand schedule from his schedule of desirabilities. The resulting demand schedule is the fourth column considered with respect to the first column. It tells us the highest prices (column 4) Individual No. I is willing to pay for stated quantities of coal (column 1), or, what amounts to the same thing, the largest quantities of coal he is willing to take at stated prices. As shown in the preceding chapter, it does not matter which way the relation is expressed.

In the preceding table the numbers expressing desirabilities of coal and those expressing price are the same, because we arbitrarily represented the desirability of a dollar by " 1 "; i. e., we took the marginal desirability of money as our unit of desirability. In this case we may say that the marginal desirability of any point in the table is measured numerically by the money the individual is willing to pay for the marginal unit at that point. But imagine another individual (No. II)–an individual who has precisely the same intensities of desire as No. I for coal, but who, on account of relative poverty, prizes each dollar twice as much as does Individual No. I. In comparing the two men, we shall have to use the same unit of desirability, viz., the marginal desirability of money to Individual No. I. For Individual No. II the desirability of money is, therefore, two such units. The result is the following table for Individual No. II:–

Desirability 01 Each Successive Ton Desirability Of A Dollar Price Per Ton The Customer Would Be Willing To Pat

Tons Purchased () (4) (o-4)

I 12 2 6

2 IO 2 S

3 8 2 4

4 6 2 3

5 5 2 2.50

6 4 2 2

The first ton has a desirability of 12 units just as did the first ton for Individual No. I, but the desirability of a dollar to Individual No. II is twice as great as the desirability of a dollar to Individual No. I. Hence the first ton, instead of being twelve times as desirable as a dollar, is only six times as desirable. Therefore he is willing to pay only up to 6 for it. Just as in the case of Individual No. I, the prices in the last column are found by dividing the figures in the second column by those in the third. In this case, however, the figures in the last column are not identical with those in the second column, but are only half as great. And in general the higher the marginal desirability of money, the lower the schedule of prices which buyers are willing to give.

We see, then, that the two individuals, though they have precisely the same intensities of desire for coal, have very different demands for coal. If the price of coal is 5 a ton, Individual No. I will buy up to the fifth ton; for when he reaches the fifth ton, and not before, the marginal desirability of coal (5) to him will be just five times that of a dollar (1). But at this same price of 5, Individual No. II will buy only up to two tons; for in his case the second ton is the point at which the marginal desirability of coal (10) is five times the marginal desirability of a dollar (2). This contrast interprets the fact that the poor " cannot afford " to buy as much as the rich. The poor, like Individual No. II, have a relatively high marginal desirability of money.

It is easy to express these same relations by curves. A demand curve is, as we know, merely a graphic picture of a demand schedule. We may likewise draw desirability curves as graphic pictures of desirability schedules. And just as the demand schedule is derived by simple division from desirability schedules, so is the demand curve derived by simple division from desirability curves.

In Figure 32 the curve dd is the desirability curve of coal for Individual No. I; that is, it represents the desirability to him of each successive ton of coal as given in the preceding table. Thus the latitude or height (12) of d represents the desirability of the first ton. The height (10) of the next point to the right represents the desirability of the second ton; and so on to d, the height of which (5)

represents the desirability of the fifth ton. The desirability of the fifth ton is, as we know, the " marginal desira-H bility" of five tons, the desirability of the fourth, the marginal desirability of four tons, etc. That is, the latitude or height of each of the points from d to d represents the marginal desirability of the amount of coal corresponding to the longitude of that point. The heights of the points which form a horizontal s B x row one unit above the Pjq 32 base represent the marginal desirability of money.

From the heights of these two sets of points.–the upper ones representing the marginal desirability of coal and the lower ones representing the marginal desirability of money– by simple division of the numbers indicated, we derive the heights of the set of points constituting the demand curve for Individual No. I. As the divisor is in this case unity, the demand curve so derived will coincide with the curve dd. Hence dd will serve not only as the desirability curve for coal for Individual No. I, but also as the demand curve for Individual No. I.

Figure 33 represents the corresponding curves for Individual No. II, for whom, by hypothesis, there are precisely the same marginal desirabilities of coal, but for whom the marginal desirability of money is twice as great. The upper points, r to r, represent the marginal desirability of coal, and are at the same heights as the upper points d to d in Figure 32. The lower points in Figure 33, however, are now two units high instead of one. Hence, when we divide the numbers 12, etc., for rr by the number 2, we shall get as our demand curve a curve dd, which, unlike the demand curve for Individual No. I, will not coincide with rr, but will be everywhere only half as high.

We see, then, how to derive an individual demand schedule (or curve) by dividing, so to speak, one desirability schedule (or curve) by another. The resulting demand schedule (or curve) of coal will coincide with the schedule (or curve) of marginal desirability of coal if the marginal desirability of money be taken as unity. Otherwise the demand schedule (or curve) will have its figures all standing in a given ratio to those of the schedule (or curve) of marginal desirability of coal. In either case the demand curve is, or is equal to, a desirability curve translated into terms of money.

This is all true on the assumption that the marginal desirability of money for each individual remains constant, as represented in our tables or curves, being always unity for Individual No. I and always 2 for Individual No. II. In other words, we have assumed that the marginal desirability of money is not appreciably affected by a large or small purchase of coal. Of course, a purchase might be made so large and at so high a price that the marginal desirability of money would be appreciably affected. Theoretically, the marginal desirability of money increases with every expenditure; the less money there is left, the more precious it becomes. But there are so many ways to spend money, and the expenditure on any one thing, such as coal, requires ordinarily so small a drain on the total power to spend, that the

Y r
12 10 8
d.
. e.
6 X 6 " . J
3–. .
2 2 Z. 2 2
o 1 I 5 t .! X.
Flo. 33.

marginal desirability of money is not very different whether a man buys no coal at all or all the coal he can afford. Consequently in considering the purchase of any particular good, the desirability of a dollar may be regarded as practically a constant quantity, represented, as in Figures 32 and 33, by the heights of a horizontal row of points.

In the last chapter we considered the price of coal as the effect of supply and demand and expressed by two curves. In this chapter we have seen that one of these two curves, the demand curve, is in turn the result of innumerable individual demand curves; and, finally, that each of these individual demand curves is in turn the result of two desirability curves–one for coal and another for money–which characterize the given individual. These desirability curves are the ultimate curves lying back of demand, and the demand curve is, as it were, a desirability curve translated into terms of money.

6. Relation of Market Price to Desirability

We are now ready to see clearly that the market price of coal is equal to the ratio between two intensities of desire in the mind of each purchaser–the ratio of the marginal desirability of coal to that of money. No individual demander of coal can, of course, determine the market price of coal. On the contrary, to him the market price seems to be fixed, and all that he can do is to adjust his purchase to it. But this adjustment, when practiced by all the numerous persons who demand coal, constitutes the whole demand side of the market, and exerts, therefore, a very powerful influence on said existing market price. Market price, we have seen, must " clear the market," and, applied to the demand side of the market, this means that the market price must be such that when each individual on the demand side adjusts his purchase to it in such a manner that the ratio of his marginal desirability of coal to his marginal desirability of money is equal to the price, the sum total of all such purchases (i. e., the total demand) shall equal the total supply.

This principle that the market price of any good is equal to the ratio between its marginal desirability and the marginal desirability of money for each and every buyer is so important that it will be advisable to restate it in as many forms as possible.

Any one of the following statements will show where the stopping point of each purchaser is:– 1. Each purchaser buys until the ratio of the marginal desirability of the good to the marginal desirability of money is brought into equality with the price.

2. Each purchaser buys until the desirability of the marginal unit becomes equal to the desirability of the money spent for this marginal unit.

3. Each purchaser buys until his marginal gain (of desirability) is reduced to nothing.

4. Each purchaser buys until he makes his total gain (or surplus desirability) a maximum.

The last two may require further explanation.

Evidently it is the same thing to say that a purchaser stops buying when the desirability of the last ton purchased is equal to the desirability of the money paid for this last ton, as to say that he stops buying when the last ton has no excess of desirability over the desirability of the money paid for it.

Let us examine the nature of the gain which the purchaser makes, and which is thus reduced to zero on the last ton. Evidently he gains no money; on the contrary, he loses it. What he does gain is desirability. His gain in desirability and his " surplus desirability " is the difference between the total desirability of the coal he buys and the total desirability of the money he has to sacrifice.

If the price is 5 per ton, in which case Individual No. I, as his schedule (or curve) shows, buys 5 tons, the total de sirability of these 5 tons to him is 41 units of desirability, being the sum of the desirabilities as given in the schedule (or curve) for these 5 consecutive tons, viz., 12 + 10 + 8 + 6 + 5, or 41; the sacrificed desirability is the desirability of the 25 spent, which, as we assume that each dollar has 1 unit of desirability, is 25 units; the surplus desirability is the excess of the total over the sacrificed desirability, or 41−25 = 16 units.

Now this gain of 16 consists of diminishing gains on successive tons. On the first ton the gain is the difference between the 12 units which the ton is worth and the 5 units he must sacrifice to get it; this is 12–5, or 7 units. Likewise the gain on the second ton is 10–5, or 5 units; on the third, 8–5, or 3 units; on the fourth, 6–5, or 1 unit; and on the fifth, 5–5, or zero. He stops his purchase at this point, for, if he should extend it further, he would lose desirability. The sixth ton, for instance, would yield only 4 units and cost him 5, and the seventh and later tons would cause greater losses.

Likewise for Individual No. II, who can only afford to buy 2 tons, the total desirability of these two tons is 12 +10, or 22 units; the sacrificed desirability is the desirability of the 10 paid, which, as each dollar is supposed to have 2 units of desirability, is 20 units; and the surplus desirability is 22–20, or 2 units. This gain is all on the first ton, as the second is worth only its cost.

Individual No. I thus gains more than Individual No. II, though both gain something.

The last method of stating the principle was that each buys so as to make the greatest possible gain in desirability. Evidently, Individual No. I gets his greatest gain by buying 5 tons. His gains on these 5 tons were, respectively, 7,5,3, 1, and o units, making, as we have seen, an aggregate gain of 16 units. Had he stopped buying at the third ton, his gain would have been one unit less, i. e., 7 + 5 + 3, or 15 units. On the other hand, if he had bought 6 tons, he would have lost one unit on the sixth ton, which would have reduced his gain from 16 to 15. Thus by stopping at the fifth ton he gains the most he can.

The idea of something, not money, gained in a trade is important to grasp. By its aid we have no difficulty in understanding that both parties usually gain by a trade. Trade does not imply that one of the two parties gains at the expense of the other. This is true when one of the two parties cheats the other, but ordinary trade is not cheating. Nevertheless, the idea that only one party can gain by a trade is an old and persistent one. It was largely responsible for attempts to regulate prices in the Middle Ages, to make the price " just " and prevent one party gaining at the expense of the other; it was also largely responsible for the sentiment in favor of encouraging the export trade and discouraging the import trade,–a practice which implied that a nation was winning when it sold more than it bought, but losing when it bought more than it sold. In fact, the phrases " favorable balance of trade " and " unfavorable balance of trade," based on this idea, are still in use, although their original implication of gain or loss is gone. We now recognize that the country parting with money by buying goods from abroad may gain desirability just as the man who parts with money by buying coal gains desirability.

Those who were misled as to a balance of foreign trade being " favorable " or " unfavorable " were also misled as to the nature of domestic trade. They convinced themselves that trade within a nation was of no consequence to that nation. They said it merely changed money and goods from one mans hands to anothers in the same country, and therefore could not increase the wealth of the nation as a whole. They failed to see that every exchange affords " surplus desirability " to both parties engaging in it. Each man gets the goods he wants in preference to those he already has. The values of the goods exchanged

are equal and, as we saw in Chapter V, 6, these values may be canceled against each other when we are making up accounts involving values; but, as then stated, this does not imply that there is no gain of any kind. We now see dearly that there is actual gain and that this gain consists in "surplus desirability."

7. Importance of the Marginal Desirability of Money

The student will have noticed that the money element was present in all the stages of our study, and is still present even when we carry our analysis down to each individual mind. A halving of the purchasing power of money halves its marginal desirability to each person. But as we have seen in the desirability schedules (and curves) of Individuals I and II, the marginal desirability of money to the individual is a divisor to be divided into the marginal desirability of coal to him in order to give the price the individual is willing to pay for coal. Therefore, to halve this divisor for each individual will result in doubling the quotient–the price he is willing to pay. In other words, the prices in each individuals demand schedule (or curve) will all be doubled by halving the purchasing power of money. Consequently the same is true of the total demand schedule (or curve). This is merely restating what has been said before, except that before we considered the demand as a whole, whereas now we trace back the effects of a change in the purchasing power of money to each individual on the demand side of the market.

We can now see more clearly than in Chapter I how careful we should be when measuring values in terms of money. If our object is to compare desirabilities, we must correct our money comparisons for differences in the desirability of money. We must make allowance for differences in the importance of a dollar (1) among different people according to differences in wealth and needs, and (2) between different times or countries according to differences in purchasing power of money.

(1) If a millionaires wife pays 10,000 for a brooch, while her poor neighbor pays 10 for a gown, we should not infer that the rich woman prizes her brooch a thousand times as much as the poor woman prizes her gown. This would be true if the desirability of a dollar were the same in the two cases, but as it is likely that the poorer woman prizes a dollar more than a thousand times as highly as does the richer woman, it is altogether probable that the gown is of more importance to the poor woman than the brooch is to the rich one.

From the fact that the richer an individual is, the less the marginal desirability of money to him or her, it further follows that the difference in desirability of two fortunes is much less than their money values would suggest. A man whose income has increased from 1000 to 10,000 a year is better off than when it was 1000 a year, but he is not ten times better off. The extra 9000 may not be worth as much as the original 1000, in which case he is not even twice as well off. It is still truer that a man with a fortune of 500,000,000 is only slightly better off (if at all) than one with only 1,000,000. Were these facts better appreciated, " great riches," though desirable, would be less dazzling to those who have never possessed them.

In Figure 34, longitude represents the income of a man,

Fig. 34-

and latitude represents its marginal desirability to him. The curve is purely illustrative, as we do not know in figures what exact difference in the marginal desirability of money is caused by a given increase in a mans income. It is intended merely to express the fact that the marginal desirability of money (assuming a given purchasing power) decreases very rapidly with an increase in income; that is, the richer a person, the less–and very much less–he prizes an individual dollar. The curve probably continues to the right indefinitely, though approaching closer and closer to the base; no matter how rich a man becomes, an additional dollar will still have some desirability in his eyes. Man is literally insatiable.

(2) So much for the allowance to be made between different individuals. To illustrate the allowance to be made for differences in different price levels, we note that money wages in the United States are higher, for instance, than money wages in England; but that it is misleading to make any comparisons unless we first correct for differences in the price levels or purchasing power. In some occupations it would seem that the difference in wages only just corresponds to the difference in the purchasing power of money, so that in those cases the American workman is really no better off than the English. In such cases he has more money in wages, but its marginal desirability is so much less that he has no more desirable food, lodging, or comforts. In most cases, however, it is a fact that, after all allowances are made for difference in price levels, the lot of the American workman is better than that of the English.

8. Desires or Wants, the Foundation of Demand

Evidently desirability is a far more fundamental concept than the concept of mere money value. Human desires are very real economic influences, and the variations in their intensity are definitely registered by variations in the de mand for goods. Although, therefore, "desirabilities" of goods and money are somewhat elusive to grasp, they are by no means unreal, unimportant, or imaginary. Like the heights of the clouds they are difficult to measure, yet definite magnitudes. They are, however, magnitudes pertaining to separate individuals personally, not to society in the mass. It is not surprising, therefore, that as yet we have no means of measuring desirabilities by actual statistics except in terms of money, and such measurement is misleading because it takes no account of differences in the desirability of money to different people or to the same person at different times.

Moreover, to measure desirability in terms of money is merely to measure a cause by its effect; for all money valuations depend on desirabilities. Although desirability is extremely difficult of measurement, even for the individual concerned, it is sufficiently measurable to make its study of great and fundamental importance in economics. Each individual who buys is compelled, in fact, to decide upon the relative importance to him of the goods he buys and the money he pays for them. It is these decisions, based entirely on desirability, which among millions of human beings make up the forces on the demand side of the market, on which forces the market prices depend. While desirabilities seem fleeting and indefinite as compared with the "hard cash" in terms of which we daily express our valuations, yet these very cash transactions are simply the resultant of innumerable "desirabilities." While the individual desire is fitful, the resultant of the desires of all the purchasers is relatively steady,–just as, in physics, the force of the individual molecules of the atmosphere which bombard our bodies are variable and fitful, but the aggregate resultant atmospheric pressure is a steady fifteen pounds per square inch.

In this chapter we have endeavored to discover the influences at work behind demand. We have found, back of the demand schedule (or curve), the demand schedules (or curves) of individuals; and we have further found, back of each individual schedule (or curve), a pair of desirability schedules (or curves), one member of each pair representing the desirability of the good, and the other the desirability of the dollar. By comparing these two desirabilities, the individual finds how many dollars the good is worth to him. In other words, he translates the desirability of the good into terms of money, which is, as it were, the universal language of commerce.

In some cases the individual is saved the trouble of translating into money by the fact that he finds the translation has already been made. Thus a commission merchant, buying on an order from a customer who has already told him at what price to buy, has little difficulty in making up his mind as to how much money he is willing to give. He is willing to give the price at which he is to resell to his customer,–less, of course, a slight margin for his own commission. So, also, a wholesale dealer, in buying of a jobber, is guided largely in his decision as to what prices to pay by the prices which he expects to get from the retailer, and the retailer is similarly guided by what he expects to get from his customer. But even in such cases, so far as the dealer finds money valuations ready made for him, these must, of course, have been made by some one, such as the ultimate customer, through the painful process of comparing the marginal desirability of the good with the desirability of the dollar.

CHAPTER XVII

THE INFLUENCES BEHIND SUPPLY 1. Analogies between Supply and Demand In the last chapter we have seen that a total demand schedule (or curve) for any particular good is derived from innumerable individual demand schedules (or curves), and that each individual demand schedule (or curve) is derived from a pair of desirability schedules (or curves), one relating to the marginal desirability of the particular good under consideration and the other relating to the marginal desirability of money.

With certain exceptions to be explained later, precisely these same propositions are true of the supply side of the market.

First of all, then, the total supply at any price is merely the sum of the individual supplies at that price, as illustrated in the following " supply schedules " for coal for two individuals. As before, we distinguish them as Individual No. I and Individual No. II (without meaning to imply, of course, that they are the same individuals as those called No. I and No. II in Chapter XVI).

Supply Schedules. Tons Which
WOULD BE SUPPLIED BY INDIVIDUALS
Price Total
I n (o + 4)
(a) ( )
4 ISOO 2000 35
5 1600 2400 4000
6 1800 3000 4800
7 2100 3900 6000

The table tells us that at a price of 4 a ton, Individual No. I will supply only 1500 tons and Individual No. II, 2000 tons; that at 5 a ton Individual No. I will supply 1600 tons and Individual No. II, 2400 tons; and so on. The last column gives the sum of the figures in the two preceding columns. If we should include in our table not simply two but all suppliers in the market, we should obtain in this way the total supply schedule.

The same relations are indicated graphically in Figure 35, where 5 / is the supply curve for coal of Individual No. I, i. e., a curve such that if the latitude of any point on it represents a given price, the longitude of that point will represent the amount of coal the individual is willing to supply at that price. Similarly, szst shows the supply curve for coal of Individual No. II. If, as in the case of demand curves, we add longitudes (e. g., Sy = sly + s2yj, we obtain 55 as the curve representing the total supply of both individuals.

If, in like manner, we add together all the
Y
8 , . f .3
7 6 3 4. 3 2 1 / /
/ s / 3
r / J /
/ /

0 1000 2000 3000 4000 6000 6000 4

Fig. 35.

individual curves of all the individuals in the market, we shall obtain the total supply curve of the market.

Having thus derived the total supply schedule (or curve) from its constituent individual supply schedules (or curves), we next seek, as in the case of demand schedules (or curves), to derive each individual supply schedule (or curve) from a pair of desirability schedules (or curves). In the case of the seller, however, it is not desirability, but wwdesirability which needs to be considered,—the undesirability of the trouble and expense of supplying coal. Marginal undesirability is also called marginal cost.

The following table illustrates the derivation of the sellers undesirability curve or marginal cost curve. The figures in the last column, found from the second and third by simple division, give the prices a coal dealer would be willing to take in view of the undesirability of the trouble and expense involved in providing coal and the desirability to him of the money he seeks to get by selling coal. If the 1500th ton costs him 8 units of undesirability, and a dollar represents to him 2 units of desirability, he will evidently be willing to take 4 a ton up to the 1 500th ton; and so on for the other figures in the table.

Undesirability or Supplying Last Ton Desirability Of Price The Dealek Would Be Willing To Take

Tons Sold A DOLLAR

(o)	()	(a -ft)
1300	8	2 4
1600	10	2 5
1800	12	3 6
2100	H	2 7

The same relations may, of course, be represented graphically. In Figure 36, the latitudes of the points on the line rr represent the undesirability per ton of providing the coal, and those of the lower line mm represent the desirability per dollar of obtaining the money. The result of dividing the latitudes of the points of rr by those of mm (i. e., by 2) gives us the supply curve 5/, the height of which at different points will be proportional to the height of corresponding points of the curve rr. The lati-and . frf tude of the curve r/ represents the undesirability of the efforts and sacrifices of furnishing each successive unit, or

"marginal undesirability," and the latitude of the curve ssf represents, in terms of money, this same marginal undesirability or marginal cost of production; that is, the supply curve is the undesirability curve translated into money. This translation of undesirability into money may, X to a large extent, have 36 been already made for the dealer by others. In fact, it will usually happen that the larger part of any individuals costs are in the form of money expenditures,—expenditures for labor and for materials. But these money valuations have themselves come about by the process, in the minds of laborers and others, of comparing the undesirability of efforts with the desirability of the dollar. The prices or " latitudes " of the supply curve are found, therefore, by translating into the universal language of money miscellaneous undesira-bilities of all kinds. That is, marginal cost of production comprises everything undesirable involved in supplying the article under consideration, including all discounted future costs, the money equivalent of all labor and trouble, as well as all actual money expenses. The seller is more apt to think and talk in terms of money than the buyer, since the seller has to do with costs, and his costs, as above stated, are usually in the form of money costs. Ultimately, however, as we have seen in previous chapters, back of all money costs lie labor costs. Money costs in the last analysis are merely the accumulated translations into money of labor costs. Labor or human efforts thus

stand at the end of our analysis of supply just as satisfactions stand at the end of our analysis of demand. Supply and demand are thus, in a sense, the money equivalents of efforts and satisfactions.

2. Principle of Marginal Cost

Hitherto we have considered the marginal desirability of money as the same whatever the amount of coal bought or sold. Expressed in the terms of the diagram we have considered the marginal desirability curve for money as a horizontal straight line. As explained in the last chapter, this was essentially true for the purchaser; but for the seller it is often untrue. The purchaser of. let us say, sugar will prize a dollar substantially as much whether he buys ten or twenty or thirty pounds of sugar a week or none at all; the reason is that this one commodity cuts little figure in his total budget; it can make so little inroad on his income that it can scarcely affect the desirability of money to him. Even in the case of coal, where the expenditure may perhaps be large enough to pinch the purchaser appreciably, the desirability of a dollar would probably not be noticeably greater if ten tons a year are bought rather than five. Each consumer expends his money in so many different directions that the part he can, under ordinary circumstances, expend on any one commodity is too small to make him feel appreciably poorer as a consequence.

With the seller of sugar or coal, on the other hand, the situation is altogether different. Whereas the consumer expends his money in the purchase of a great many different goods, the producer receives his money by the sale of a very few. In fact, he may concentrate on one only. The coal dealer, for instance, usually makes his living by selling coal and nothing else. To him, therefore, changes in the amount of coal sold and in the price of coal will make a great difference in the total amount of money he gets, and therefore in its marginal desirability. If, for instance, the price of coal changes a dollar a ton, though to the purchaser this fact will not appreciably affect the marginal desirability of money, to the seller it may make all the difference between poverty and affluence.

Therefore, in treating supply, we cannot always assume that the marginal desirability of money remains constant and may be represented by a horizontal straight line. Instead, the greater the sales, and the more money consequently obtained, the less will be the marginal desirability of money. Therefore, the line mm, representing the marginal desirability of money, should, strictly speaking, descend to the right as the sales increase, and the rate of descent will depend on the price concerned. This descending character of the curve representing the marginal desirability of money will make the diagram less simple, but it will still be possible to derive the supply curve from the desirability curves of coal and of money.

The supply curves thus far considered ascend to the right. In such supply curves the price is a minimum relatively to the supply; that is, the curve shows the lowest prices at which given amounts will be supplied. Expressing this same truth the other way around, we may say that the supply is a maximum relatively to the price, i. e., the curve shows the greatest amounts which will be supplied at given prices.

We see, then, that the total supply curve, analogously to the total demand curve, may be derived from a number of individual supply curves (Fig. 35); that each such individual supply curve may be derived from (1) curves of marginal undesirability of furnishing the article, and (2) curves of marginal desirability of money; and that, therefore, the supply curve is, or is equal to, an undesirability curve translated into terms of money.

The important result is that the market price, as finally determined by supply and demand, is not only equal to the marginal desirability of getting coal for each buyer, but also to the marginal undesirability of furnishing it for each seller, both the desirability and the undesirability being measured in terms of money. Thus, if the price of coal is 5 a ton, the last ton bought by each buyer is worth barely 5 to him, while the last ton sold by each seller costs him about 5 worth of expense and trouble.

These equalities on the margin of all sales and purchases, and the fact that the price must be such as will equalize supply and demand, i. e., "clear the market," are among the fundamental principles which determine the market price of any particular good.

It may be worth while here to emphasize the fact that there is a separate market at each stage in the operations by which coal passes from producer to consumer. At each stage supply and demand fix a price for the market at that stage. The first market for coal is at the mine, the sellers being the producers and the buyers, middlemen, who later will resell. The market price at the mine is, of course, quite different from the market price later in the wholesale market, and the latter market price is different in turn from that in the retail market. But the same principles apply to all these market prices.

We may summarize these principles as follows:– (1) The equalization of all marginal desirabilities and undesirabilities (both being measured in money).

(2) The equalization of supply and demand.

We cannot neglect either of these two principles. Nor can we omit either half of the first principle; it is a mistake to think that price can be determined by marginal desirability alone or by marginal undesirability alone. It takes two sides to make a bargain and a market price.

The present chapter, however, is especially devoted to the supply side. On the supply side of the market, therefore, the great determinant of market price (in terms of money) is marginal cost (in terms of money).

These two determinants of price–marginal desirability and marginal cost–are, as has been explained, human desires translated into money. Marginal desirability represents the desire to secure something agreeable, while marginal cost represents the desire to avoid something disagreeable.

In this connection it is important to remember that both the " something agreeable " which we desire to secure, and the " something disagreeable " which we desire to avoid, lie in the future. When an intending purchaser of an orchard speaks of it as a desirable object, he means that he has a desire in the present for certain expected satisfactions in the future, –satisfactions from eating the apples or other future benefits which the ownership of the orchard is expected to bring. Likewise when the owner of a coal mine decides which leads or galleries he shall exploit, he bases his decision on what he expects the extraction of coal to cost. The marginal desirability to the purchaser of the orchard represents future satisfactions translated into present cash by the usual process of discount, and the marginal cost of coal extraction represents future expected costs translated into cash by the same process. Later, when the expected satisfactions or the expected costs have become past history, they no longer control marginal desirability or marginal cost. It is the costs of the future, and not of the past, which always control. After the coal miner has exploited the lead or gallery, and it turns out to have cost more than he expected, he will not on that account obtain a higher price for the coal than he originally calculated. Again, if a railway has been built and located unwisely, its value may fall far short of its original cost. It is important that the student should carefully avoid the error of believing that the prices and values are controlled by what things have cost to produce in the past. In the case of staple articles, however, which are constantly being reproduced, and of which the cost does not greatly vary from time to time, the price will come to be approximately equal to this cost; for the cost of reproducing in the future will be practically the same as the cost which has been experienced in the past. Even in these cases, however, it is the cost which is expected to continue in the future rather than the cost which has been experienced in the past, that furnishes the controlling motive to the producer in determining at what price he will supply his product.

We may here call attention to the fact that the principle of marginal cost applies to the particular case of gold as a commodity, priced in terms of wheat, or priced in terms of all other commodities in general–which is the same thing as saying, priced in terms of its general " purchasing power." During part of our discussion of money, we did thus treat gold as a commodity. If the student will turn to Figures 13-16, he will see that the distance below the line 00 of the highest outlet in operation from any bullion reservoir is simply what we would now call the marginal desirability of gold for use in the arts (measured in terms of general purchasing power over goods), and that the distance from OO to the lowest inlet in operation is the marginal cost of production or undesirability of gold (measured likewise in terms of general purchasing power over goods). That is, the mechanical representation there employed is merely another way of representing what we would now express in terms of supply and demand of gold.

We may now add that the differences in costs of producing gold, represented by the differences in heights of the inlets, are not altogether due to differences between mines, but also to differences in working the same mine. There is a marginal cost of production for each mine. The higher the speed of extracting, the higher the cost per ounce. This is called the law of increasing cost.1 It applies, of course, 1 It is also called the " law of diminishing returns." The two expres-1 are e-nt. Each statement expresses the effect of asing relation between product and cost. If with

more generally than to gold and silver alone. In this chapter we have taken coal as our typical example. We might have taken numerous other examples. If the price of wheat rises, its marginal cost will rise. Such a rise in price acts as an encouragement to the production of wheat. Just as we have seen that an encouragement in the production of gold leads to an opening of the poorer mines, so an encouragement to the production of wheat will lead to the cultivation of the poorer wheat lands. At a given price, there are always some lands on which it will not pay to produce wheat because of the prohibitive cost of production upon these lands. In gold mines, as in wheat fields, there is a marginal point of production beyond which production will not pay.

3. Upward Supply Curves which Turn Back In spite of the analogies we have noted between the supply and the demand side of the market, the differences between them are so great and important that the rest of this chapter will be devoted to them.

Practically all demand curves descend to the right, and we have hitherto assumed that all supply curves ascend to the right. But not all supply curves do ascend to the right. One peculiar type of supply curve grows out of the fact recently noted, that there is a descending curve of marginal desirability of money dependent on the price assumed. This fact, when combined with the ascending curve of un-desirability of efforts and sacrifices (as in Fig. 36), tends to bend the supply curve upward–sometimes so much as to cause it to curl back to the left, as in Figure 37. Such a curve, although it ascends, does not, throughout all its increasing production the ratio of cost to product increases it is the same thing to say that the ratio of product to cost decreases. The one form of statement is that there is greater and greater cost per unit of product returned; the other, that there is less and less product per unit of cost incurred.

70

.60

.58 .35

.30 .20 .15.10.05 course, ascend to the right. It applies especially to the supply of labor. The meaning of such a supply curve is that a rise of price does not always cause an increase of supply. At first it does, but beyond the point where the curve begins to curl back, a rise of price evidently results in reducing the supply.

If wages are low, a rise in wages will at first stimulate him to work longer hours, but after a certain point, he will prefer to rest on his oars. He earns so much in a few hours that he feels it is no longer necessary to work so hard. In South America, for instance, traders from Europe were once buying native-made baskets of a peculiar kind. In order to increase the supply of baskets, which was far less than they could market in Europe, the traders decided to raise the price that they would offer to the makers, thinking to stimulate the production of baskets by inducing the men to work more hours. Exactly the opposite result followed. As soon as these workmen were offered high prices for the baskets, they worked fewer hours and made fewer baskets than before; they could now get more money even for doing less work, and they did not need or want more money. Their wants were so few and simple that the marginal desirability of money to them decreased very rapidly with an increased amount of it; and their disinclination to work was so 2-i. 9 6 7 B 9 IO 1I 12 hours Fig. 37.

great that, combined with the feeble desirability of its rewards to them, they would supply less of it when the rewards were great than when they were small. Similar instances have been cited among the Filipinos and among the negroes in the South. Recent experiments in coal mines show that a slight increase in wages stimulates the men to work longer, but that a large increase (sixty per cent beyond the ordinary wage) results in irregularity of work and the desire to reduce the number of hours. That is (as shown in Fig. 37), as the price rose from the height of s to that of s", the supply of labor or number of hours spent in making baskets decreased from the longitude of s to the longitude of s".

Now this same principle applies to all labor. Experience indicates that as wages go up workmen demand shorter hours. The eight-hour movement of to-day is at bottom due to the fact that wages are high. When wages were low, men worked twelve hours a day; now that they are high, they work only ten, nine, or even eight hours a day. The same principle explains why men with the highest salaries, instead of working longer hours than others, usually work shorter hours. The most highly paid grades of workmen work the fewest hours and take the longest vacations.

The exact point in wages at which the curve begins to bend back, so that if wages are raised any higher the supply of work will diminish, depends on the particular conditions in each case, the size of the workmans family, the range and character of their wants or their " standard of living," and other similar conditions. The more wants a man has, the higher the point at which the curve begins to bend back, i. e., the less easily is he satisfied with more money.

4. Downward Supply Curves

The typical supply curve, with which we began, ascends continually to the right. A different type was just consid ered, one in which the rightward movement was arrested and turned into a leftward movement. A still different type is that in which the curve does not even ascend, but descends. Such descending supply curves are common under modern conditions of factory production. It is often found that a large product costs less trouble, per unit, than a small product. In such cases, the marginal undesira-bility of furnishing the good decreases with an increase of supply, and not only decreases, but decreases in a faster ratio than does the marginal desirability of money; so that the ratio of the one to the other, i. e., the marginal cost expressed in money, decreases with an increase of supply.

When the marginal cost decreases with an increase of supply, the supply curve also descends, but its relation to the curve of marginal cost is now quite different from what it was in the case previously considered in which the curves ascend. The supply curve is no longer the curve of marginal costs, but must be constructed on an entirely new principle. The principle that market price is equal to marginal cost will no longer hold true. Only when the supply curve ascends is it true that the price at which the seller is willing to supply a given amount is equal to its marginal cost, and is therefore derived from the curves of undesirability. Descending supply curves, which we are about to consider, depend not on marginal cost at all, but on average cost. The reason is that no seller is willing regularly to sell at a loss, and this is what he would be doing if he should offer to sell at prices corresponding to marginal cost when the marginal cost decreases with the amount sold. It is clear that, if the cost of supplying the 3000th ton of coal is 5, and the cost of all preceding tons is greater than 5, not even one ton of coal could be sold at 5 a ton without a loss, and if 3000 tons were sold at that price, there would be a loss on every ton except the last. Rather than sell 3000 tons or any less number at 5 a ton, the dealer would choose to sell none at all. Contrast this result with that which obtains in the case of an ascending curve. In this case, if the cost of supplying the 300oth ton were 5, the cost of all preceding tons would be less than 5, so that instead of a loss there would be a gain on each of these preceding tons. Not only could he afford at 5 to sell 3000, but this amount gives him the maximum profit–more, for instance, than if he should sell 2000 or 4000 tons.

Now whether the cost curve ascends or descends, it is clear that any dealer to sell at all, must expect to get back at least the total cost. This means that he must, therefore, charge a price at least as high as the average cost per ton. When the cost of each successive ton is greater than that of the preceding ton, the cost of the last, or marginal cost, is the greatest cost of all, and therefore exceeds the average cost. Consequently, the dealer is assured a profit when selling at a price equal to the marginal cost. But when the cost of each successive ton is less than that of the preceding ton, the cost of the last ton (marginal cost) is the least of all, and therefore is less than the average cost. To sell at a price equal to marginal cost would, in this case, mean to sell at a loss.

In either case, whether the curve ascends or descends, the seller will seek to determine his price on the basis of the higher of the two costs (marginal and average). Whichever of the two is higher will show itself in the supply curve. When the marginal cost increases with supply, marginal cost is the higher, and will rule supply. When the opposite is true, average cost is the higher, and will rule supply.

In the latter case the supply schedule (or curve) is a schedule (or curve) of average costs. We need not describe in detail how to construct such a schedule (or curve). This presents no difficulty, since we already know how to construct a schedule (or curve) of marginal costs which gives the cost individually of each separate ton. The simple average of any specified number of these is the average

cost of that number. This average-cost-curve will descend, though it will be higher than the marginal-cost-curve from which it is calculated.1 5. Resulting Cutthroat Competition

But, besides the fact that ascending supply curves are based on marginal costs, and descending supply curves are based on average costs, the two types of supply curves offer another and even more important point of contrast. The supply at a price is in the first case the maximum which the seller is willing to offer at that price, whereas in the second case it is the minimum. In the first case, the more the seller can sell, the more he charges. In the second, the more he can sell, the less he charges. When we consider simply ascending types of supply, we may express the relation between the price and supply in two ways, either– (1) Given the quantity, the price is the minimum price at which that quantity will be supplied; or (2) Given the price, the quantity is the maximum which will be supplied at that price.

The first of these two propositions still holds true when the supply curve is descending instead of ascending; but the second will not hold true until we have changed the word " maximum " to " minimum." In other words, when, as originally supposed, the supply curve ascends, the seller is willing at any given price to supply a certain amount or less; but, when the supply curve descends, he is willing at any given price to supply a certain amount or more.

1 The relation between cost and product represented by a descending supply curve is sometimes called the " law of decreasing cost" and sometimes the law of " increasing returns "; for, it is evidently the same thing to say that the ratio of cost to product

decreases as to say that. ratio of product to cost increases. The one form of statement is that there is less and less cost per unit of product returned; the other that there is greater and greater product per unit of cost incurred. These expressions are in antithesis to the " law of increasing cost" (or, the " law of diminishing returns") of 2. There is, theoretically, an intermediate condition called the " law of constant cost" (or "law of constant returns").

In the case of demand we found no such two classes as ascending and descending curves. In all cases demand decreases as price increases. Consequently we found only one sort of relation between price and demand. The amount demanded at a price is always the maximum amount which will be taken at that price; and the price is always the maximum price which will be given for that amount.

Let us then summarize our results, expressing each on the basis of a given price:–
I. At a given price, each buyer is willing to take a certain maximum amount or less at that price.

II. At a given price, each seller is willing (1) (in case marginal cost increases with an increase of supply) to offer a certain amount or less at that price.

(2) (in case marginal–and therefore also average– cost decreases with an increase of supply) to offer a certain amount or more at that price. The contrast between the two types of supply, II (1) and II (2), is illustrated graphically in Figures 38 and 39. Figure 38 illustrates case 1 and Figure 39, case 2. The curve in the first case is seen to be the maximum limit of longitude, and in the second case the minimum limit. The longitude of any point in the shaded area represents an amount which the seller is willing to supply at the price corresponding to the latitude of that point. Thus, if we take any given horizontal line, such as ab, in the shaded area of Figure 38, its latitude represents an assumed price at which the seller is willing to supply any amount, from nothing at the left end, a, of the horizontal line, to the maximum amount at the right end, b, where the line is limited by the curve. Taking any given horizontal line, such as ab, in the shaded area of Figure 39, the seller is willing to supply any amount from the minimum longitude (that of the point a at the left) up to an indefinite amount at j the right; or, dropping the symbolism of the curve, the seller is willing at a given price to sell any amount from a

Fig. 38 (Supply).

certain minimum upward.

In tie latter case, i. e., when the cost of each additional unit of product is less than that of the preceding unit, the more the seller can sell at a given price, the better he likes it. If he sells only the minimum which he is willing to sell at that price, he gets back only his average cost of production, and makes no profit. Any sales beyond this bring him a profit, and the larger the sales, the larger the profit. He stands ready to sell an indefinitely great amount at the given price.

Y

+ —. —-

s.

. . –

A V b

. .

```
V –
———
v –
–.—
1–
v –
. s—
ks
0 X
```

Flo. 39 (Supply).

This fact introduces us to an unexpected conclusion, viz., that if the total supply curve descends, the price represented at the intersection of the supply and demand curves, although it clears the market, is not a stable price, but tends always to fall. Whether the price is above, at, or below, the latitude of the intersection, it will tend to fall so long as the supply curve descends. Let us consider each of these three cases separately, i. e., the price above, at, or below the intersection, allowing the demand curve to s descend faster than the D supply curve. If the price X (Fig-40) is OP, higher Fig. 40. than the intersection, the demand exceeds the minimum supply and stimulates each supplier to furnish more than his minimum, which, of course, he is only too glad to do. Consequently, supply will soon overtake demand. Those competing to supply will strive to underbid each other, and the price will fall.

But it will not stop falling at the intersection. For, suppose it is below, as at OP. It is evident that it will continue to fall; because then even the minimum supply exceeds the demand, and ae who compete to supply will be very eager not to be left with unsold goods or unused productive capacity. A rise of price would, it is true, remedy the difficulty. But no individual can apply this remedy. The individual competitor cannot raise prices without securing the agreement of others; but to do this would be to create a combination which is contrary to our present hypothesis of independent action. If he should individually raise his price, he would be committing commercial suicide, for people would not buy

of him when they could buy more cheaply of his competitors. His only hope of achieving his purpose of increased sales lies in adopting the opposite course, and underselling his competitors, regardless of the consequences to them and to the market price. His hope is that before they can meet his cut in price, he may win the patronage he needs to make it worth his while to stay in the market, and that he may thus drive some of his competitors out of business. If he fails to get the needed patronage, he must go out of business himself. He therefore offers his wares at a price below OP. If at this point many of his competitors should go out of business, he could succeed; for though the total demand does not quite reach the supply curve, it will reach and pass his supply curve, which lies much to the left of the total supply curve shown in the figure. But his competitors remain, and under these conditions, as we have seen, there cannot be two prices in the same market at the same time. Hence all his competitors must reduce their prices to his.

Whatever the effect of this action may be on the individual who first cuts the price, the result on the whole is evidently to make matters worse; for, according to conditions shown in the diagram, the lower the price, the more will the supply exceed the demand.

We have here what is known as " cutthroat competition " or a " rate war," i. e., competition the effect of which is not simply to reduce profits, but to create losses.

6. Resulting Tendency toward Monopoly

But we have not yet reached the ultimate result of such competition. Some competitors must sooner or later see that there is no hope to secure the large sales necessary to make business worth while. They withdraw. This reduces the losses for the rest; for, by removing their supply curves, the total supply curve is reduced in longitude, i. e., is shifted leftward, and the discrepancy between supply and demand is lessened, if not done away with entirely. But even so, the tendency of the price to fall is not hindered; for we have seen that, as long as the supply curve decreases, competition forces the prices down on whichever side of the intersection the price may be. In the case of a descending supply curve, the intersection has nothing to do with the case. Competition with descending supply curves will always lower the price so long as there are any competitors with descending supply curves. No check to this fall is possible until either competition ceases or the supply curve ceases to descend. If the supply curve at some point at the right reaches a minimum point, this marks the lowest point to which the price can fall; or if the crowding out of competitors finally leaves only one supplier in the field, he at that moment becomes a monopolist, and the prices will cease falling on that account.

Not only may monopoly come about by this process of " the survival of the fittest," but it may also come about in another way, as already suggested, i. e., by combination. When there is cutthroat competition, the motive to combine is strong. No one of the competitors relishes the prospect of being crowded out any more than he relishes the prospect of continued cutthroat competition. Whether combination will actually result or not depends on a variety of circumstances. One or more of the competitors may flatter himself that the rate war will end in crowding out all suppliers except himself, and prefer to keep up the fight to the bitter end. Others may keep on from other motives, being prevented by pride or resentment either from withdrawing from the contest or from begging their rivals to form a combination. But for our present purpose it does not matter much whether the monopoly which finally results comes from the final survival of one supplier or from deliberate combination of many suppliers. In either case the result is monopoly.

We find, then, from our study of the supply side of the market that supply curves sometimes descend, and that in

such cases competition is " cutthroat " competition, and results in losses and tends toward monopoly.

In all our reasoning we have assumed perfect competition to start with. It should be noted that in actual fact competition is always somewhat imperfect. The slight undercutting of prices by one grocer will not ruin the trade of another in another part of the same town for the reason that the two are not absolutely in the same market. Each has a sphere which the other can only partially reach, not only because of distance, but also because each has his own " custom," i. e., the patronage of people who, from habit or from other reasons, would not change grocers merely because of a slight difference in price. Thus each is protected by his partial isolation. We see, then, that even when supply curves descend, competition may be so limited as to prevent any very fierce rate war, the rate war being prevented by partial or local monopolies among the suppliers in the first place. A rate war, therefore, is never a permanent or normal condition. If not avoided at first by imperfect competition or by partial monopoly, it is brought to an end eventually by the monopoly to which it leads.

7. Fixed and Running Costs

We have now to notice another peculiarity on the supply side of the market. The peculiarity referred to is the fact that there are often costs which do not vary with supply, but remain unchanged whether the supply is large or small or nothing. These are called the fixed costs as contrasted with the costs which vary with supply, which are called the running costs. If all costs are in the form of actual money expenses, the two classes are also called respectively fixed expenses and running expenses. The fixed expenses of a railway company, for instance, consist of the interest on its bonds. The running expenses consist of the salaries, wages, and payments for fuel, materials, etc. The only costs hitherto included in our discussions were running costs. The fixed costs were not included, because they have no effect on variations in supply curves. We shall now study fixed costs merely to show that they do not have any effect on supply after once they have been incurred, a fact at first surprising.

In general, fixed costs of production of any given goods consist simply of interest on past costs which have been " sunk " in the business, i. e., which cannot now be reimbursed to the owner except as the sale of his goods may reimburse him in part or in whole. As we have seen in a previous chapter, interest is not a cost to society, for it is merely a payment from one person to another, an interaction. (See p. 76.) To society as a whole the only cost is the " sunk " cost, which, in the last analysis, consists, as has been explained, of the labor expended at various times in the past. But to the individual supplier–and his is the only cost in which we are at present interested–interest is a cost. If he pays no interest, he must have incurred the " sunk " cost himself, in which case this past sunk cost constitutes his only fixed cost; there is then no fixed annual cost. In one of the two ways he must bear the burden of sunk cost. That is, either he must have borne it in the past directly, or he must now be paying interest to some one else who so bore it. The two ways are equivalent in the same sense that two goods are equivalent which exchange for one another. That is, a sunk cost of 100,000 is equivalent, if interest is five per cent, to a fixed cost of 5000 a year. Whether the individual person or company has sunk the 100,000 in the past or is paying 5000 a year to some one else who did–in neither case does this cost enter into the cost (or undesirability) curve, or the resultant supply curve, or the resultant price.

We shall cite some examples which have been almost literally realized in actual life. A man once sunk about 100,000 in a hotel on the top of a mountain. He found that so few guests wanted to go there that the most he could earn was 2000 beyond his running expenses. He never succeeded in recovering the sunk cost, and the fact that he had sunk 100,000 gave him no power to command prices high enough to enable him to succeed. Nor could he withdraw from the business and recover his 100,000. His building was worth nothing except for hotel purposes. He could only make the best of his mis-investment and run his hotel for 2000 a year. This was better than nothing at all, which would have been the result of going out of business. The 100,000 sunk in the past was sunk just the same, whether the hotel was run or not.

Another hotel keeper borrowed 100,000 on bonds and paid interest at five per cent, i. e., 5000 a year, to the bondholders. His business paid running costs, but only 2000 beyond those costs, so that he failed by 3000 to earn enough to pay his interest to the bondholders. The hotel was losing, in actual money expended, 3000 a year. But even in this case the hotel could not be abandoned. The only result was to change owners. The bondholders foreclosed their mortgage and ran the hotel themselves. As it still earned 2000 beyond running expenses, they found it more profitable to continue the business and get two fifths of their interest than to close and get nothing.

In either of these two cases, whether the hotel was built by the owner out of his own purse or whether it was built out of borrowed money, there was a loss equivalent to three fifths of the original cost, or, what amounts to the same thing, three fifths of the interest thereon. Yet this cost could not be avoided, whether the hotel business were large or small or abandoned altogether, and it " paid " to run at a loss rather than to close down at a greater loss. This paradox, that " it sometimes pays to run at a loss," is important to analyze and to understand.

A third hotel keeper made a lucky hit with his 100,000.

He got not only his running expenses and interest on the 100,000, but a handsome profit besides. But this fact did not affect the prices at which he was willing to supply accommodations. He still charged as much as he could.

The point to be emphasized is that in all three cases the past fixed costs had no influence on prices. Whether these costs are easy to carry, as in the last case, or burdensome, as in the other two, they have no influence on prices. In each case the owner tries to make the most he can. The fixed costs take out the same amount, whatever he does, and may therefore be disregarded in deciding what is best to do.

It follows that fixed costs will not even prevent prices, under the stress of competition, from going below what will pay those costs. A railway may be making money enough to pay both its running and fixed expenses and a handsome surplus besides, until a parallel road is built. Then each tries to take business away from the other; a rate war ensues, and prices of freight and passenger services are driven down. Each road is now running behind on its interest payments, yet neither can afford to stop running, for then it would run behind still further. We have here the same cutthroat competition as when the supply curve descends, except that in this case it is " cutthroat" because of the fixed costs. If also the supply curve descends, then there are two conditions tending toward cutthroat competition; namely, the existence of the descending supply curve and the existence of fixed costs. As a matter of fact, these two conditions are often united.

8. General and Particular Running Costs

The two costs–fixed costs and running costs–are not only often associated, but are at bottom very similar to each other. This may best be seen if we divide one of the two classes of costs, running costs, into two subclasses, " general " costs and " particular " costs. By general costs, also called " overhead costs," are meant costs which, though they could be got rid of if the business ceased, will not greatly vary whether the business is large or small. They include the labor of superintendence, salaries of the chief officers, rent of rented quarters, interest on short-time loans for stock carried, etc., power, lighting and heating, insurance and repairs. By particular costs are meant those which apply to each particular unit so that their total amount will vary almost or quite in proportion to the amount of product sold. They include cost of raw materials and ordinary wages.

Now when the supply curve descends, i. e., when running costs decrease with increase of supply, the reason is usually found in the " general costs." As the total " general costs " remain little changed by an extension of the supply, the general costs per unit supplied grow smaller, the larger the supply. These costs, added to the particular costs, which remain practically the same, evidently cause the total running cost per unit to decline with an increase in production. For instance, let us suppose a shoe factory in which the general costs (for office salaries, heating, lighting, rent, insurance, etc.) amount to 100,000 a year, while the particular costs for materials (leather, etc.) and labor applied to the materials (cutting, sewing, etc.) amount to 1 per pair of shoes. It is evident that the greater the product, the less the cost of shoes per pair. If 10,000 pairs are produced per annum, the share of the general costs (100,000) which each pair must bear will be 10. This, added to the particular cost for each pair (1), will make a total cost per pair of 11; but if the output of the factory is 100,000 pairs, the share of the general cost (100,000) which each pair must bear will be only 1, which, added to the particular cost (1 per pair), will make a total cost per pair of 2. Thus we see that the total cost per pair will in each case be the particular cost, 1, plus the share in the general cost, which will be large for a small output and small for a large output.

Now the reason that fixed costs were not treated like general costs and included in the computation of the average cost per unit, was that, as we have seen, fixed costs could make no difference in the price at which the supplier is willing to supply a given amount. The supplier is not willing to sell at prices below what is necessary to cover general costs, for he has the option to escape these general expenses by going out of business entirely. But he is willing, if need be, to sell at prices below what is necessary to cover fixed costs in addition to general costs; for from these there is no way of escape, not, at any rate, as long as the capital representing fixed costs lasts. He might have escaped them once had he not made the original investment, but now it is too late. The difference between fixed and general expenses, then, is chiefly one of dates. When a man is contemplating building a hotel, and forecasting his possible profits or losses, he will try to make his prospective prices cover fixed costs, for they are then in the future; but after the hotel is built, he will no longer do this. The fixed costs are then past and beyond recall, and he must let bygones be bygones.

Since, then, his running cost and supply curves are independent of fixed costs, the price which results from this supply curve and the demand curve will also be independent of the fixed costs. This conclusion is consistent with what has been said in previous chapters as to price and value being dependent on the future and not on the past. We have seen that, on the demand side, people who buy any good buy it on the basis of what benefit it will do them in the future; now we see that, on the supply side, those who sell it, sell it on the basis of what it will cost them in the future to continue in the business, and not on the basis of costs which were sunk in the past. The principle has been stated (somewhat imperfectly) as follows:–

"The price of any article (when once it has been produced) is not determined by its cost of production, but only by its

benefits." The imperfection in this statement is its failure to discriminate past from future. The costs of production, if they be future, do enter into value, precisely as future benefits enter. Future costs are estimated in advance just as future benefits are. For instance, the value of the great irrigation plants in the West now in process of construction is dependent upon their future expected benefits, taken in connection with the future expected cost of completion. Past elements are without significance. The future elements being given, the value of the irrigation will be the same whether the past cost was large or small, or nothing whatever. Of course it is true that the future expected cost of completing the plants is less than if some of the work had not been already accomplished, so that the greater the past cost has been, the less the future cost ought to be, and hence the greater the present value of the plants. But whatever causes may increase or decrease future benefits and costs, it remains true that the present value of anything depends exclusively on the future benefits and costs which it yields.

9. Monopoly Price

The supreme principle which guides economic action is the principle of maximum gain. This principle applies both to competition and monopoly, but its application is different in the two cases. In the case of competition the price set by a mans competitors is an important element which must be reckoned with by that man, while in the case of monopoly he has no such element to reckon with. In fact, monopoly is best defined as absence of competition.

In explaining the principle on which monopoly price is fixed, we shall first assume that competition is entirely absent, there being no fear even that high prices will lead to competition in the future.

Under these circumstances the monopolist will fix his price with an eye to the expected effect on demand. He will charge " what the traffic will bear," i. e., will put up his price to the point which will give him a maximum profit. The higher the price, the larger the profit per unit sold. But, if he makes his price too high, he kills the sales. If, on the other hand, he makes it too low, he kills his profit per unit. By trial and error or by exercise of his best judgment, he steers a middle course, and selects that price which he thinks will render his profit a maximum.

In general, the price under monopoly will be higher than under competition, but this will not always be the case if, as may happen, the costs under monopoly are less than the costs under competition. In some cases monopoly may result in lowering costs so much that the greatest profit is secured by setting the price lower than under competition. Such economies in cost come from getting rid of duplications in plant, management, and advertising, and by having the advantages in general of large-scale production.

When monopoly price exceeds price under competition, there is usually danger that competition will thereby be invited. Practically such danger is seldom absent. Competition which is feared, but not in actual existence, is called potential competition.

This potential competition has an effect similar to real competition, so that under monopoly the price is usually not quite " a// the traffic will bear," but something between that and the price that would result from actual competition. In general, prices are seldom determined under conditions either of perfect monopoly or of perfect competition. There is usually a partial monopoly, or, what is the same thing, imperfect competition.

There are many and obvious evils in monopoly. Some monopolies originate in a deliberate plan to do evil, in a "conspiracy" to raise prices and without any excuse from cutthroat competition. But the evils of high prices are among the least of the evils of monopoly. There are also the evils involved in the ruthless process of crushing competitors by first lowering prices and then raising them; there are the evils of discrimination, or charging different prices to different persons or localities. There are also the dangers of political corruption and control. The reader will have an opportunity in other books to study these evils and the proposed remedies; we cannot properly discuss them here. We may, however, take space to warn him to avoid the common but false conclusion that all monopolies are evil. In fact, a chief lesson from this chapter is that, on the contrary, competition itself is sometimes an evil, i. e., when it is of the cutthroat kind, for which some form of monopoly is the only remedy. When any business involves a large sunk cost or has a descending cost curve, and therefore a descending supply curve, competition becomes of the cutthroat kind. Even if we deny our sympathy to those producers who lose by such competition, we must not fail to note that in the end consumers will lose also. The reason is that when cutthroat competition is feared, producers will avoid sinking capital in the enterprise. It is largely in recognition of this fact and in order to encourage such investment that patents and copyrights are given. These are monopolies expressly fostered by the government. Herbert Spencer once invented an excellent invalid chair, and, thinking to give it to the world without recompense to himself, did not patent it. The result was that no manufacturer dared risk undertaking its manufacture. Each knew that, if it succeeded, competitors would spring up and rob him of most or all of his profits, while, on the other hand, it might fail. Enforced railway competition has sometimes resulted in killing railway enterprise. The rise of trusts, pools, and rate agreements is largely due to the necessity of protection from competition, precisely analogous to the protection given by patents and copyrights.

Combinations are largely the result of the two conditions we have been considering– the fact that the supply curve descends, and the fact that there is large invested capital. The antitrust movement, in so far as it aims to compel competition, does not take these facts into account; nor does it understand the necessities which have led to monopoly. So considerable are the lines of business in which either there is a large sunk capital or a descending supply curve, that if we do not allow some form of trade agreements many kinds of trade are to-day practically impossible. Restrictive measures should be directed toward the control of monopolies and combinations, not to the restoration of competition. At the present time the general tendency is towards those forms of production in which cutthroat competition figures and in which monopoly will ultimately rule. It must not be supposed, however, that all or even most of productive enterprise is of this character. There is an immense field in which the older form of competition still holds sway; that is, in which marginal cost increases with increased production so that the supply curve is of the ascending, not the descending, type. In such cases competition is still the " life of trade " and affords a safeguard for the consumer against exorbitant prices. Such competition needs no regulation, and in general is better off without it.

CHAPTER XVIII

MUTUALLY RELATED PRICES 1. Arbitrage

We have seen how the price of any particular good is determined under varying conditions of competition and under monopoly. In each case the particular price has been considered, quite apart from other prices. We found that each price was determined by its own supply and demand. But " supply and demand " were expressed by schedules (or curves) which in turn depend upon schedules (or curves) of desirability which themselves depend on innumerable outside conditions–among them being other prices than the particular price in question. In fact, we have seen that these separate curves are affected by the general level of prices. We now have to observe that they are also affected by other particular prices.

In the first place it is evident that the prices of the same article in different markets act and react on each other. Thus, the price of wheat in Chicago affects the price of wheat in New York, Liverpool, and elsewhere. The fact that wheat can be transported quickly and cheaply from one market to another prevents the possibility of great differences in prices. Any considerable difference in prices between two markets such as Chicago and New York will soon correct itself through the transportation of wheat from the cheaper to the dearer market. If all communication between the markets could be cut off so as to prevent absolutely such transportation of wheat, the supply and demand schedules or curves in each market would be independent of those in the other, and the resultant prices in the two would fluctuate independently of each other. But, given cheap and rapid transportation, the supply and demand in one market will closely affect and be affected by the supply and demand in the other, and there will be a tendency toward equalization of prices. In the two this tendency to equalization works itself out chiefly through a special class of men who make it their business to watch prices in different markets, endeavoring always to buy in the cheaper and sell in the dearer. Such transactions are called arbitrage transactions. These men engage in the business of arbitrage in order to take advantage of price differences; and while it is not their object or wish to equalize prices (for it is on the inequalities of prices that they live), nevertheless, to equalize prices is the effect of their action.

Suppose, for instance, that the price of wheat in Chicago is 75 cents per bushel and in New York 1 a bushel. Such a situation offers an opportunity for an arbitrage merchant to make money rapidly by buying wheat in Chicago at 75 cents and selling it in New York at 1. He therefore appears in Chicago on the demand side of the market, being willing to take a large amount of wheat at 75 cents per bushel. He appears in New York, on the other hand, on the supply side of the market, being willing to sell a large amount of wheat at 1 per bushel. Thus he increases the demand for wheat in Chicago and increases the supply in New York. The effect, as we have seen, must be to increase the price in Chicago and decrease the price in New York.

The former may rise from 75 cents to 80 cents per bushel, and the latter may fall from 1 to 95 cents per bushel. But, even at these prices, the arbitrage merchant will be able to reap a rich harvest and will continue to do so until the difference in price is sufficiently reduced. Instead of the prices remaining 80 cents and 95 cents, they become, let us say, 82 cents and 93 cents and then 84 cents and 90 cents. This leaves the merchant a margin or difference of only 6 cents. But as the cost of transporting wheat from Chicago to New York is, we shall suppose, about 6 cents per bushel, there is no longer profit to the arbitrage merchant, and thus the equalization of prices will be limited by the cost of transportation. The price in New York can never be above that in Chicago by more than 6 cents per bushel. For similar reasons, the prices in Chicago cannot exceed those in New York by more than the cost of transportation; otherwise the arbitrage merchant would buy wheat in New York and sell it in Chicago.

It is by such arbitrage transactions that the prices of the same commodity in different markets seek a common level, just as water flowing from one reservoir to another tends to equalize the levels of the two. The more the costs of transportation are reduced, the more nearly equal will be the prices of any commodity in different markets become. With the progress of civilization, and especially with the improved means of transportation by railway and steamships, the equalization of prices of transportable goods has proceeded with great rapidity. The commercial world still consists of a number of separate markets, but the communication between these markets is becoming constantly more cheap and rapid, so that, in a sense, the whole world almost forms one great market for certain staples like wheat, other grains, and the precious metals. For articles which are difficult of transportation, bulky, and otherwise subject to expenses of transportation large relatively to their value, the tendency to the equalization of prices is less striking. This is particularly true of human services by " labor," which can only be transported through migration. Nevertheless, there is a constant tendency for migration to take place in order to take advantage of differences in the price of labor. Both the European and Oriental workmen often leave their low wages for the higher wages in America or other new countries.

Before the days of rapid transportation it was not uncommon for wheat to command famine prices in one country, while, at the same time, it was a glut on the market in another.

It is evident that the equalization of prices is an advantage to the world as a whole, for it is better that there should be a moderate supply of wheat, and therefore of bread, throughout the world than that there should be in some places feast and in others famine. Therefore the intercommunication of markets and the resulting equalization of prices must be regarded as an advantage to society. It does not follow, however, that it is an advantage to every individual in society.

For instance, when the fertile lands of the Mississippi Valley were tapped by building railways from the East, the cheap wheat from these lands began to enter the markets of the East, where the price of wheat had been relatively high. The result was to lower the price of wheat in the East. This reduction in price injured the New England farmer. Such injury of individuals almost inevitably happens with every economic readjustment of conditions. Rapid and cheap transportation by connecting all lands and countries has, in spite of the general good accomplished for the world as a whole, injured great groups of producers by subjecting them to competition from which the barriers of nature had previously protected them. These producers have therefore asked the government to protect them by raising artificial barriers in place of the natural barriers which have been destroyed, and the protective tariff has as its chief source of popularity the fact that it protects the local producer of particular articles against the importation of such articles from abroad. The policy of protection is thus an attempt to interfere with the equalization of prices which the improvement in transportation is constantly producing.

But just as this progress of equalization of prices creates a special injury to some particular producers, it creates special benefits to others. The transcontinental railways have not only injured the owners of the rocky farms in New England, but have vastly benefited the owners of the alluvial lands in the Mississippi Valley; for they have given them an opportunity to sell their products to advantage in the more rocky parts of the world. In general we may say that the equalization of prices constantly going on through improvement in transportation facilities injures the producer in those regions where prices were previously high, but benefits the producer in regions where those prices were previously low. The former group have, therefore, an interest in protection; the latter, an interest in freedom of trade: the one, an interest which tends to prevent, and the other, an interest which tends to promote, the intercommunication of markets. Among consumers, on the other hand, opposite results ensue. Those particular consumers who were enjoying the lowest prices are injured by the rise which equalization brings to them, while those who had to pay high prices are benefited by the fall which equalization brings to them. In general, the inevitable effect on society as a whole is a gain, for the reason that a larger quantity of goods is obtained with a smaller expenditure of effort. It is evidently more economical for the world to grow its wheat in the Mississippi Valley than on the refractory soil of New England, and the transportation facilities which have brought about this condition have been of the same nature as labor-saving machinery.

It is not within the scope of this book to discuss the argument for or against the protective tariff, but the student can at this point realize that the movement for protection is of the same nature as the movement against labor-saving machinery, which is a protest against the cheapening processes which come from inventions, the protest being made by the special interests which are injured by the introduction of these processes.

2. Speculation

We have spoken of the equalization of prices as between different places. We have next to consider equalization of prices as between different times. Corresponding to the tendency to the equalization of the prices of a given commodity between different places, that is, between the places where it is abundant and cheap and the places where it is scarce and dear, there exists a tendency to the equalization of the prices of a given commodity at different times. Moreover, the method of equalization of prices between times corresponds somewhat to the method of equalization of prices between different places. Just as the equalization between places is accomplished by the transportation of commodities, so the equalization between times is accomplished by keeping the commodity from the time when it is abundant, and therefore cheap, to the time when it is scarce, and therefore dear. For instance, ice is abundant and cheap in winter, but scarce and dear in summer. Consequently much of it is stored in ice houses in winter and kept for use in the summer; that is, the part which is thus stored is subtracted from the winter supply and added to the summer supply. The effect tends to equalize the prices of ice at different seasons. In the same way many vegetables and fruits, such as potatoes and apples, which are abundant and cheap in the summer and fall, are to a large extent stored for use in winter when they will be scarce and dear. The effect is to subtract a certain quantity from use in the summer and fall and to add to the amount used in the winter.

Just as the equalization of prices between places is largely due to the work of a special class of business men who engage in arbitrage transactions, so the equalization of prices between different times is largely accomplished by a special class called speculators. A wheat speculator, for instance, svithdraws wheat from the market when it is abundant and cheap, and supplies it when it is scarce and dear. At the former times he appears on the demand side of the market as a wheat buyer; at the latter he appears on the supply side as a seller. By adding to the demand when the price is low, he tends to raise prices, and by adding to the supply when the price is high, he tends to lower prices, thus acting as an equalizing agent.

We need to distinguish two chief kinds of speculation according as the price of the given commodity is expected to rise or fall. Speculators who try to profit by any expected rise of price are called " bulls." Their operations consist simply in buying wheat in the present, keeping it until the future, and then selling it again at higher prices. Speculators, on the other hand, who try to benefit by an expected fall in prices are called " bears." Their operations are somewhat more complicated. It is easy to decrease the present consumption of any commodity and increase correspondingly future consumption, i. e., to withdraw certain stocks and hold them until the future. But when the reverse operation is needed, namely, to increase present consumption at the expense of future, the operation is more difficult. We cannot lay hold of a future stock of wheat before it exists. The best we can do is to use up our present wheat as completely as possible. This is what is needed when prices are falling. Speculators will then add to the present supply by selling out any stocks from previous holdings. They and all who deal in wheat will refrain as far as possible from intentionally carrying over any of the present stock of wheat into the period when they expect it to be abundant, and therefore cheap. But this is not all; the speculators will also speculate for a fall by " selling future wheat short." This operation of "selling short" consists in agreeing to sell wheat in advance of the time of delivery, depending on its expected fall in price to enable them to secure the wheat in time to fulfill their contracts. It is called " selling short," because the speculators are selling some thing which they do not yet possess, i. e., of which they are " short." The speculator who sells short hopes to make a profit by buying at a lower price than the price at which he sells short. If, for instance, in January the price of wheat is high, say 1 a bushel, he sells July wheat, that is, wheat deliverable in July, at 90 cents a bushel. This is because he expects that when July comes, wheat will be worth less than 90 cents a bushel, say 85 cents, so that he can buy it for 85 cents and sell it immediately to his customer for the 90 cents previously agreed upon.

The effect of selling wheat short is to encourage still further the using up of present supplies, the speculator thus guaranteeing the delivery of wheat to those who buy of him so that these persons will not need to accumulate the wheat in advance for themselves. Of course, the speculator must take good care that the wheat is available at the time agreed, but, being presumably an expert as to the conditions of wheat supply, he can manage to get the wheat in the nick of time or, at any rate, with less preliminary accumulation than those who are not experts. The effect is therefore to obviate the necessity of any ones keeping wastefully on hand any large stock. Where such a speculative market exists, a miller can, when wheat is scarce, use up his existing stock without replenishing it until the last minute, at which time he has the assurance of those who have sold him wheat short that the wheat will be on hand. Without such assurance from experts in wheat speculation, the miller would have feared to have run his stock so low and would have laid in wheat in advance even at high prices. He defers his stocking up by means of the short selling of wheat to him by the speculator.

In the same way a woolen manufacturer is enabled in a speculative market to lay in his supply of wool in the most advantageous manner. If the price of wool is falling, he will wait before stocking up, merely contracting in advance with a speculator for the immediate delivery of new wool, when his present stock is exhausted. In the same way builders use the speculative market to assure themselves of building materials when needed. The builder arranges in advance with dealers in building materials for the delivery to him of the lumber, bricks, and stones needed. By thus selling short or making contracts for delivery in advance of possession, and sometimes even in advance of the actual existence of the commodity sold, there is a great saving accomplished in the stocks which need to be carried. Without such selling of futures the miller, the woolen manufacturer, the builder, and great classes of merchants would be under the necessity of carrying far larger stocks than they now carry. In other words, the speculative operation known as selling short enables the community to economize its capital existing in the form of accumulated stocks of goods, especially at times when these goods are scarce and dear and most need to be economized. This selling short has the effect of deferring the demand for a commodity. The miller, the woolen manufacturer, the builder, and all others who buy futures–the wheat, the wool, the building materials, etc.–do so instead of buying present wheat, wool, building materials, etc. The fact that they find a speculative market in which they can buy futures has therefore, as its effect, less buying in the present. In other words, it reduces the present demand, and therefore reduces the present price, while it increases the future demand and the future price. Thus it tends to reduce the gap between the present high prices and the future low prices.

But while speculation normally tends to mitigate either an impending rise or fall of prices, its power to do so is limited, just as is the power of equalizing prices among different places by arbitrage. The latter operation does not pay when the difference in price is reduced to the cost of transporting from place to place. Likewise speculation does not pay when the expected difference in price becomes too small. One of the costs to the speculator for a rise is interest on the capital he locks up when he withdraws a commodity from the market and holds it for a certain period. Suppose, for instance, that he borrows money in order to speculate for a rise. The anticipated rise must be sufficient to cover the interest he pays and all the other costs involved in the operation. Otherwise the speculation promises a loss instead of a gain. Likewise, if he is to speculate for a fall, he must anticipate a fall sufficiently below the price at which he sells short to enable him to make a profit. Speculation, therefore, is a function in equalizing prices between times, very analogous to the function of arbitrage transactions in equalizing prices between different places. But there is one important distinction between speculation and arbitrage. Speculation, by the nature of the case, involves uncertainty in a far greater degree than arbitrage. The prices among different places can easily be known, but the prices between different times are far more difficult to know, for the future is always uncertain. All we can do is to predict according to the best information we can get. It therefore often happens that the speculator makes a mistake in his forecast of the future. He may believe that prices are going to rise when they are going to fall, or to fall when they are going to rise If, acting on a mistaken belief that prices are rising, he holds wheat for a rise, the result of his action will be to aggravate the fall; for buying in the present will raise prices now when they are already high, and selling in the future will lower them then when they will be low. In like manner, if he makes the mistake of selling short when prices are rising, he will aggravate the rise, for he will lower the prices in the present when prices are already low and raise them in the future when they are already high.

Therefore speculation may do either good or harm. It does good when it reduces the inequality of prices at different times. It does harm when it aggravates this inequality. Fortunately, the interests of the speculator and the public are to a large extent identical. It is evident that when the speculator is correct in his prognostications, he will make a profit. His object is to make a profit when prices are rising, but he can do so only by mitigating the rise. Likewise his object is to make a profit when prices are falling, but he can do so only by mitigating the fall. His profits are, as it were, a reward paid him by the community for mitigating price changes. If he makes a mistake in either form of speculation, he suffers losses, and these losses may be regarded as a sort of penalty he suffers for aggravating the inequalities in prices. Since the interests of the speculator and of the public are thus parallel, there is a premium put on wise and beneficial speculation and a penalty on unwise and injurious speculation.

It is unfortunately true, however, that in spite of the penalties for unwise and injurious speculation, much speculation is of this character. This is largely due to the fact that many engage in speculation who have no adequate equipment for so doing and no independent judgment as to the causes making for a rise or a fall in prices. The ultimate justification for speculation must rest in the wisdom and independence of those who speculate. Speculation which merely follows a " tip" has no independent value. If every person who speculates for a rise or a fall should do so on a basis of his own best independent judgment, the chances are that mistakes of those who are overconfident in either direction would largely offset each other.

During recent years the general public have been beguiled into the folly of entering the speculative market, but the public have no special knowledge of market conditions, and their participation in speculation is almost as apt to aggravate as to alleviate the inequalities in prices. In such cases speculation becomes mere gambling. In fact, it is worse than gambling, for the evils are more extensive, being shared by the consumers and producers and all who are affected by the price fluctuations thus caused. Such evils of

speculation are especially grave when, as usually happens, the general public speculate in a mass, i. e., all in the same direction. Like sheep, they tend to follow the same leader, and the great bulk of their mistakes are apt to be in the same direction, first in one direction and then in the other. The effect of their movements is like that of a sudden rush of the passengers of a ferryboat first to one side and then to the other,–it may cause a capsize.

We see, then, that the chief evils of speculation are largely the work of the unprofessional speculators, just as the chief evils of reckless automobile driving are due to untrained chauffeurs. It must not be supposed, however, that the professional speculator is always a public benefactor. Not only may he also make mistakes which cost him and society dear, but he may sometimes "rig the market" and manipulate prices. When a professional speculator merely attempts to take advantage of an impending rise or fall of prices, he is usually a public benefactor; but when he attempts to create the rise or fall, of which he is to take advantage, by false reports, by "cornering," or by other means, he is apt to be a mischief-maker.

This is not the place, however, to discuss the benefits and evils of speculation further than to warn the student against the wholesale condemnation of speculation so common in the public press. Like most other industrial operations, speculation may be either good or bad. So far as it is good or bad, the discussion of the two belongs to applied economics. Our object here is to show that speculation, so far as it is good, tends to equalize prices in time.

3. Prices of Goods which Compete on the Demand Side

As a result of our study of arbitrage and of speculation, we see that the price of any particular commodity at any time and place, though directly fixed by its supply and demand at that time and place, is indirectly affected by the supply and demand at other times and places; for these react upon supply and demand at the particular time and place under consideration. The price of wheat in Chicago on January 1, 1912, is determined by the intersection of the supply and demand curves in Chicago on that date; but those supply and demand curves depend, as we now see, upon the price of wheat in St. Louis, New York, Liverpool, and other places, and depend likewise on the prices of wheat on dates before and after January first. The price of wheat in Chicago on January first tends to be close to the price of wheat in neighboring places and at neighboring times.

Not only does the supply and demand of wheat at any time or place depend upon the price of wheat at other times and places, but it depends likewise on the prices of other things than wheat. In particular the price of wheat depends on the prices of substitutes for wheat. Substitutes for wheat will resemble wheat in affecting the price of wheat, but the effect will not be so direct if the substitutes are only substitutes on one side of the market; for instance, if they are like wheat so far as the use to the consumer is concerned, but unlike wheat so far as the cost to the producer is concerned. Thus sugar and honey are substitutes for each other to the consumer, for they serve similar needs so far as the consumer is concerned, though on the supply side they are produced in totally different ways.

Two sorts of wealth are said to be substitutes on the demand side when they fill similar needs. It follows that the satisfaction of needs by one of the two substitutes not only reduces its marginal desirability, but affects the marginal desirability of the other in a similar fashion. Consequently, the marginal desirabilities of the two tend to fall or rise in unison. Therefore also the prices of the two tend to fall or rise in unison. It is evident, for instance, that the price of coal will affect the demand for coke, since coal and coke are often substitutes, or competing articles. The more nearly either of the two articles comes to filling the office of the other, the more closely do their prices keep pace with each other. If two articles are absolutely perfect substitutes, they are, to all intents and purposes, the same article, and have the same price.

There is scarcely an article which does not have its substitutes. The two fuel substitutes, coal and coke, include numerous subclasses and varieties, such as anthracite and bituminous coal. Other fuel substitutes are wood, petroleum, gasoline, alcohol, and gas. A change in the price of any one of these tends to produce a similar change in the prices of the rest. Likewise the prices of food substitutes are sympathetic among themselves–the prices of such substitutes as wheat, corn, oats, rice, and barley; of fish, meat, and fowl; of the various fruits and the various vegetables. Similar sympathetic relations exist among clothing substitutes, such as woolen, cotton, linen, and silk; or among ornamental substitutes, such as diamonds, pearls, rubies, and amethysts.

The closest substitutes, though still sufficiently distinguishable to prevent their being quite classed as the same article, are the various " qualities," " grades," or " brands " of any particular class of articles. The various breakfast foods prepared from wheat are close substitutes. There are many grades of wheat, of sugar, of coffee, of meat, of silk, and, in fact, of almost any class of articles which can be named. Among different grades the prices are usually so closely parallel that trade journals often give the price of one staple grade only–as of a standard grade of coffee–leaving it to the reader to infer what the prices of the other grades must be. But the prices of different qualities of any good, though they rise and fall together, may be wide apart among themselves. Various qualities of land, for instance, bring very different prices, ranging from almost nothing to thousands of dollars per square foot. When the various "qualities" yield precisely the same sort of benefit, the only differences among them are differences in the quantities of benefits which flow from them. In this case the prices of the goods will evidently be proportioned to the net benefits they yield. Wheat lands, for instance, of different fertility, will be worth prices proportioned to the net value of wheat which they yield.

4. Prices of Goods which are Complementary on the Demand Side

Substitutes may be said to compete with each other. We now consider articles which complete each other or, in other words, are complementary. Complementary articles jointly serve the same want. We have seen that of two substitutes one is used instead of the other for a given purpose. But of two complementary articles one is used in conjunction with the other for a given purpose. Horses and mules are substitutes, so far as either may be used for the purpose of drawing loads. A horse and a cart are complementary, for this same purpose.

We have seen that the essential attribute of substitutes is the tendency of their marginal desirabilities to keep pace with each other, and the consequent tendency of their prices to correspond. In the case of complementary articles it is the quantities of the articles which tend to maintain a constant ratio. In the case of perfect substitutes the ratio of their prices is absolutely constant. In the case of perfect complementary articles it is the ratio of the units used that is absolutely constant. Table knives and forks are practically perfect complementary articles, as are cups and saucers or " hooks " and " eyes." A " hook " without an " eye " is of little or no use and the number of " hooks" and the number of " eyes " will always be substantially equal. The prices of two substitutes tend to move sympathetically, but the prices of two complementary articles tend to move inversely. If horses are abundant, and therefore cheap, the tendency is to make mules, which are a substitute, cheap also, but to make the complementary carts dear; for the more horses used, the more carts will be needed, and the increased demand for them will tend to raise the price.

Articles which are related to each other in this complementary fashion are almost as common as those which are related to each other in competitive fashion. Various articles of food are used in combination, as, for instance, bread and butter, or the elements of which a sandwich is composed. A daily diet is usually constructed with regard to the f1tting together of the different courses served, and of the meals as a whole. Similarly, the various parts of ones wardrobe are arranged with reference to one another; and again, a dwelling and its various furnishings are mutually adapted. The tables and chairs, crockery, knives and forks, beds and bedding, rugs and wall paper, are severally arranged in relation to one another in their respective groups, and to the house to which they all constitute a complement.

5. Similar Relations on the Supply Side

Thus far we have considered only goods which compete with each other, or complete each other, in respect to demand. Turning now to the supply side of the market, we find similar relations.

Two goods compete in supply when they occasion similar efforts or costs to those who sell them. Thus, hay and wheat–though far from being substitutes on the demand side, satisfying dissimilar wants–are to some extent substitutes on the supply side, for they require similar costs. Both require the use of farm land and the labor of mowing or reaping. The prices of such articles competing in supply, like those of articles competing in demand, tend to rise or fall together because their costs tend to rise or fall together. The best example of competition of costs is found in the services of laborers. The wages, or the prices paid for various kinds of work, tend to keep pace with each other. Man is so versatile a machine that one kind of workman can readily substitute for another. On a pinch, the same man may be a factory employee, a farm hand, a coachman, carpenter, mason, plumber, or clerk. Consequently, these various sorts of work, though filling very unlike wants on the demand side, compete on the supply side, and tend to bear similar prices. If the wages of clerks rise, the wages of carpenters will rise also, because otherwise many carpenters would want to become clerks. The consequence is that wages of all sorts usually rise or fall together. If labor of all kinds could be perfectly substituted, wages of all kinds would remain in absolutely fixed ratios to each other, i. e., would rise or fall together in exactly the same ratios. Such " perfect mobility of labor," however, never exists. On the contrary, labor may be classified into several more or less " noncompeting groups," such as brain work, skilled work, and unskilled work.

Two goods complete each other in supply, or are complementary on the supply side, when jointly they involve the same cost, i. e., when the supply of one tends to carry with it the supply of the other. The less important of the two is then called the by-product of the other. Tallow is a by-product of beef and hides. Other examples of articles completing each other in supply are mutton and wool; coal, coke, and gas.

The prices of two completing goods on the supply side tend to move in opposite directions, just as we saw was the case on the other side of the market. Consider, for instance, beef and hides. If the price of beef rises, the amount supplied at the higher price will increase. Hence the supply of hides will be increased at the same time. Consequently their price will fall.

We see, therefore, that two articles may be substitutes on the demand side by replacing each other in satisfying the same sort of desires, or on the supply side by requiring

the same sort of costs; and also that they may be complementary on the demand side by jointly satisfying the same desire, or on the supply side by jointly requiring the same costs.

6. Prices of Goods in Series In all the cases thus far considered, the relationship between articles is on the same side of the market. We next proceed to consider goods, the relation between which involves both sides of the market.

The supply of one article may have relationship to the demand of another. This is true of two articles, one of which is used in producing the other. Such goods may be called goods " in series," because one follows after the other in the process of manufacture. In this respect their relationship differs from the others discussed. Substitutes or complementary articles are, as it were, " abreast" of each other on the same side of the market, whereas wool and woolen cloth, for instance, " go tandem" on opposite sides of the market. Wool is used (as raw material) in producing woolen cloth. Hence the prices of wool and woolen cloth are intimately related to each other. The relation, however, is different from those relations hitherto considered. Wool and woolen cloth are neither substitutes nor complementary goods on the same side of the market. Their relation consists in the fact that the producers or sellers of woolen cloth are the consumers or buyers of wool. Both the demand and the supply side are involved. Certain people demand wool in order to supply woolen cloth.

The prices of goods in series move in sympathy. It is evident, for instance, that given a high price for wool, the prices in the supply schedule (or curve) for woolen cloth will be higher than otherwise, and as a consequence the market price of woolen cloth will rise. Conversely, given a high price for woolen cloth, the prices in the demand schedule (or curve) for wool will be higher than otherwise, and as a consequence the market price of wool will rise. Thus, any change in price of either of these two articles will tend, sooner or later, to make the price of the other move in the same direction.

In the same way cotton and cotton cloth are goods in series, and their prices are likely to move in sympathy with each other; likewise the prices of wood and houses, of wheat, flour, and bread; or of iron mines, iron ore, pig iron, rolled iron, steel, steel rails, and railways. This chainlike or serial relationship comprises many other elements than raw materials and finished products. Thus, steel is related to the labor and coal consumed in its manufacture in much the same way as it is to the iron ore out of which it is wrought. The price of steel therefore moves in sympathy not only with the price of iron, but with that of coal and labor as well and of all the other goods employed in its production. The series or chain of goods is the chain of productive processes already discussed under the head of successive interactions.

7. Efforts and Satisfactions the Ultimate Factors

This serial relationship enables us to see clearly the fact that, at bottom, supply rests on efforts, and demand on satisfactions. We have seen in economic accounting that all items of income and outgo cancel among themselves, except efforts and satisfactions. We now see this same truth in its application to supply and demand. As simple as this truth is, it is commonly overlooked, because people are blinded by the all-pervading presence of money receipts and expenses. The business man, reckoning in money, comes to think of money expenses and money receipts as though they were real costs and benefits in the productive process, whereas they are only the representatives of real costs (efforts) and real benefits (satisfactions). We disentangle ourselves from the meshes of this money snare when we see that the controlling factors in determining prices are satisfactions on the demand side and efforts on the supply side. Between efforts and satisfactions there may be innumerable intermediate stages, at each one of which supply and demand result in a market price; but each such price represents simply anticipated satisfactions or efforts translated into money valuations. Any dealer at intermediate stages, between efforts preceding him and satisfactions following after, has but little independent influence on price. He is like a link in a chain or a cogwheel in a machine, merely receiving and transmitting. If some real cost of production earlier in the chain, i. e., some effort (labor), is saved, he receives the cheapening effect from those of whom he buys, and passes it on to those to whom he sells. If some real benefit is reduced, i. e., some satisfaction diminished, as by a change of fashion, he receives the cheapening effect from those to whom he sells, and passes it back to those from whom he buys. The supply and demand of wheat in the Chicago wheat pit, for instance, is chiefly dependent on the labor of growing wheat and the satisfaction of eating bread. If a new labor-saving reaping machine is devised which reduces the actual effort of producing wheat, the effect is soon felt by the Chicago wheat dealer and transmitted to his customer. Or if people turn to a rice diet and no longer care much for bread, this effect is also soon felt by the Chicago dealer and passed back to the wheat producer.

An intermediate dealer may not know the ultimate causes of the changes in supply and demand which affect his business on either side, and sometimes he does not try to think beyond what he immediately observes. Wholesale merchants generally offer to their customers, the retailers, as an explanation of the rise in their charges, the fact that they have to pay higher prices to the jobber; or, again, they may offer to the jobber as an explanation of the fact that they cannot pay as much as before, the fact that they cannot get as much from the retailers. Any such explanation of prices is shallow, for it goes no farther than explaining one price by another in the next link in the chain of prices.

We see, then, that everything intermediate which happens in the economic machinery represents merely steps in the connection between effort and satisfaction. When Robinson Crusoe supplied his wants, there was a direct connection between his efforts in picking berries, for instance, and the satisfaction of eating them. To-day there are a number of links between these, but the same principle still applies. Supply and demand at intermediate points merely reflect final efforts and satisfactions.

CHAPTER XIX INTEREST AND MONEY 1. The Importance of Interest

We have seen that, in the last analysis, prices depend on comparisons between satisfactions, or efforts, or both. But, since these satisfactions and efforts are not all simultaneous, but are distributed in time, their comparison requires us to take account of interest. Consequently our study of prices will not be complete without a study of the rate of interest. It is only by means of the rate of interest, explicitly or implicitly employed, that the prices of most goods are reckoned. The rate of interest, as previously explained (Chapter VI, 1), is itself a sort of price. So far as it has been used in Chapter VI and elsewhere for capitalizing income, it was taken ready made just as all prices were taken ready made. We are now about to inquire how this peculiarly important price, called the rate of interest, is actually determined, just as we have already inquired how other prices are determined. And it is by far the most important sort of price with which economics has to deal.

Most people have an idea that the rate of interest is a technical Wall Street phenomenon, concerning nobody except money lenders or borrowers. This is partially true of explicit or contract interest. But there is implicit interest to be considered. An explicit rate of interest is the rate of interest explicitly stated in a contract. An implicit rate of interest is the rate of interest which an investor expects to realize who makes sacrifices at one time for the sake of compensating benefits at a later time. Implicit interest is also called profits. As was shown in Chapter VI, if we invest in a bond, the price that we pay carries with it the implication of a rate of interest we expect to realize on the investment. The implicit rate of interest, or the rate which we realize, is that rate of interest which, when used for discounting the income of the bond, will give the price at which we bought the bond. For instance, if a bond yielding 5 a year for 10 years, and then redeemable for 100, sells now for 102, we know that the rate of interest realized is not five per cent, as it would be if it sold at par. It is less than five per cent–about 4.8 per cent (see Chapter VI, 4). The implicit rate of interest we realize on such a bond may be found, as we have already seen, from a mathematical table. The man who buys the bond mentioned receives 4.8 per cent interest on his investment just as truly as though he had lent out his 102 at that rate. In fact, to buy a bond of a corporation or a government is often spoken of as " lending money" to that corporation or government. Again the buyer of land who pays " twenty years purchase " (for instance, 20,000 for land from which he expects an annual rental of 1000) is making five per cent just as though he were lending out his 20,000 at that rate. In the same way a man who buys stock realizes a certain rate per cent on his investment just as if he were lending money at interest. Similarly the purchaser of a house gets a return on the money he spent for it quite analogous to the return he would have received had he lent that money.

In short, every investment is analogous to a loan and involves a rate of interest on the purchase price just as truly as does the loan. As every purchase is really an investment of present money for future benefits in money or measurable in money, every purchase price implies a rate of interest. A man cannot even buy a piano or an overcoat or a hat without virtually discounting the value of the uses which he expects to make of that particular article.

The rate of interest, then, is not confined to Wall Street, but is something that touches the daily life of us all.

How, then, is this important magnitude, the rate of interest, determined? The problem of interest is one of the most perplexing problems with which economic science has had to deal, and for two thousand years people have been trying to solve the riddle.

2. A Common Money Fallacy

Among the earliest explanations of the rate of interest was that it is a payment simply for money, and that consequently it depends upon the quantity of money on the market. We commonly speak of interest as the "price of money," and the trade journals tell us that " money is easy" in Wall Street, meaning that interest is low, or that it is easy to borrow money. Or we are told that " the money market is tight," meaning that it is hard to borrow money. We often hear the argument that the present high cost of living cannot be due to any plentifulness of money, because, if money were really plentiful, it would be cheap, meaning that the rate of interest would be low. Probably the great majority of unthinking business men believe that interest is low when money is plentiful, and high when money is scarce.

This view, however, is fallacious, and the fallacy consists in forgetting that plentiful money ultimately raises the demand for loans just as much as it raises the supply, and therefore has just as much tendency to raise interest as to lower it. Suppose, for instance, a piano dealer wishes to stock up his store with pianos (the price of pianos being 200 apiece), and that he wishes to have a stock of 50 pianos in his salesroom. To accomplish this he evidently will have to borrow 10,000. He goes to the bank and borrows it. Now, let us suppose that money becomes twice as abundant. This man, wanting to borrow again, will have an idea that in some way he will this time get a lower rate of interest at the bank, because, he reasons, the bank will have more money in its vaults and will be more anxious to lend it out. What he forgets is that the result of the very abundance of money will be that prices in general will rise, and presumably the price of pianos in particular will rise; therefore, in order to get 50 pianos, he will have to borrow twice as much money to enable him to pay for his pianos at the doubled prices. In order to buy 50 pianos, he will need 20,000 instead of 10,000. Likewise every other borrowing tradesman will need to borrow twice as much to conduct the same business. The fact that the banker has twice as much to lend is therefore completely offset by the fact that the borrowers will want to borrow twice as much. The consequence is that, in the end, doubling the amount of money will not affect the rate of interest. It will simply affect the amount of money lent and borrowed.

We must remember that interest is not only the price of money, but it is the price in money. Interest is unlike any other price in that it is the price of money, but it is like all other prices in that it is the price in money. Thus the rate of interest is found by dividing, say, the 5 paid per year by the 100 cash for which it is paid. Both the numerator and the denominator of this fraction are expressed in terms of money. If we pay attention only to the denominator, we are apt to think that an increased supply of money should decrease the rate of interest. But if we are to have a one-sided view, we might just as well fix our attention only on the numerator, and maintain that an increased quantity of money, instead of decreasing the rate of interest, ought to increase it. The truth is, inflation of money ultimately works equally on both sides. In mechanics one of the first things we learn is that a man cannot raise himself by pulling up on his boot straps. The reason is that he is pulling himself down as much as up. The in flation of the currency pulls interest up on the demand side as hard as it pulls it down on the supply side.

We should beware of the phrase " the price of money," for it has two meanings. It may mean the rate of interest, which is a ratio of exchange between two moneys– the price of money-capital in terms of money-income; or it may mean the purchasing power of money over other goods–the amount of other goods for which a given amount of money can be exchanged. The abundance of money will, as we have seen, reduce its price in the sense of purchasing power over goods, but it need not on that account reduce its price in the sense of the rate of interest. Yet the idea that the plentifulness of money tends to make interest low is a persistent one among business men.

One reason for this idea is that bankers usually look upon money in relation to their reserves, and if bank reserves are low, they have to raise the rate of interest to " protect " those reserves. If the reserves are abundant, bankers reduce the rate of interest in order to get rid of the reserves. The banker is constantly watching his reserve, and has to adjust the rate of interest with respect thereto. One way to get rid of a plethora of money in the reserve is to lower the rate of interest, and one way to protect a depleted reserve is to raise the rate of interest. But the banker should not measure the amount of money circulating outside by the amount of money inside the bank vaults. What he forgets is that a larger reserve in his vaults does not necessarily mean more plentiful money in the country; nor when we have, as at present, for instance, a great quantity of money throughout the world, does this fact necessarily imply that Banker Smith will have more gold in his vaults. The money may get into the pockets of people flrst; it may in that way raise prices so high that the borrowers at banks may demand, for the reasons explained, larger loans. And yet, if for some reason a due share of the money has not at the start flowed into the banks, the result will be that Banker Smith will, for a time, have too little reserve in relation to the greater loans that are now demanded of him. The consequence, then, will be actually to raise the rate of interest. When, therefore, the banker says that more money lowers the bank rate of interest, he ought to say, "When bank reserves get an undue fraction of money, the bank rate of interest will be low; but when an undue fraction goes into circulation outside of banks, the rate will be high." In other words, an increase of money will operate in two different ways, according to where it happens to go first. Normally and eventually, as we have seen in a previous chapter, an increase of money distributes itself between pockets, tills, and bank reserves, so as not to disturb the normal ratios between them. When this happens, the rate of interest will not be affected at all.

This conclusion is not based merely on theory. As a matter of statistical fact, the rate of interest does not go up when money is scarce and down when money is abundant. For instance, an examination of the figures for per capita circulation of money in the United States for thirty-five years shows that in about half of the cases, when money grows more abundant, interest is higher, and in half of the cases it is lower. In other words, interest changes with absolutely no relation to the quantity of money in circulation.

3. Effect during Appreciation or Depreciation

We conclude, then, that an inflation of the currency does not affect the rate of interest, provided, however, the inflation affects the loan at the time the loan is made just as much as it affects the repayment at the time the repayment is made. But the loan and the repayment do not occur at the same time; there is an interval of time between them, and it may be that the degree of inflation is greater or less at the end than at the beginning of this period, in which case the change in the inflation may, through its effect on the values borrowed and repaid, affect the rate of interest during the process of change. While inflation is taking place there is an effect on the rate of interest, because the effect of inflation on the sum loaned is different from the effect on the sum repaid.

This brings us back to the consideration of the transition periods of rising and falling prices and discloses a phenomenon which we were not ready to discuss in Chapter X. This phenomenon is that the rate of interest tends to be high during a transition period when prices are rising from one level to a higher level and, reversely, that it tends to be low while prices are falling from one level to another. Suppose, for instance, that prices are rising at the rate of one per cent per annum. Then 100 lent to-day is equivalent in purchasing power, not to 100 repayable next year, but to 101 repayable next year. If prices had not risen, the borrower, when he paid back his principal of 100, would be paying back the same amount of goods as were represented by the 100 when he borrowed it. In terms of goods he would have been in the same position at the end as at the beginning, and so would the lender. But we are supposing that prices are rising. Then the lender, when he gets back his principal of 100, does not get back as much purchasing power as he lent, and the borrower does not pay back as much purchasing power as he borrowed. In other words, the fact that prices have risen during the year has made things easier for the borrower and harder for the lender. During the Civil War the United States government issued a great many " greenbacks." The result was an inflation of the currency and a consequent rise of prices, and the result of that was that men who had mortgaged their farms in the West found it very easy to pay back their loans. As they said, the mortgages on their farms "disappeared like smoke." Five thousand dollars paid back in 1864 for 5000 loaned in 1860 really represented only half as much purchasing power over goods, for prices had doubled; the inflation of the currency freed the borrowers from half their debts.

We see, then, that when prices are rising, the principal of a debt becomes less and less valuable. If prices are rising one per cent per annum, that is, if the principal of the debt, in terms of goods, is falling about one per cent, then the interest on the debt ought to be increased about one per cent in order that there should be the same burden on the borrower as there would have been if prices had not risen. If prices are rising two per cent per annum, two per cent would have to be added to the rate of interest in order to compensate for the rise; and so on for other rates of rise in prices. On the other hand, if prices are falling, we must reduce the rate of interest to offset the appreciation of the principal.

This ideal compensation in the rate of interest would occur if mans foresight were perfect. If we knew absolutely, for instance, that next years prices were going to be two per cent higher than this years, the rate of interest might be two per cent greater than otherwise. So also, if we knew absolutely that all prices would be one per cent less a year from to-day, than to-day, the rate of interest during the year might be, on that account, one per cent less than otherwise. As a matter of fact, an approximation at such adjustment does actually occur. A study of the periods of rising and falling prices in the United States, England, Germany, France, China, Japan, and India shows that, in general, when prices are rising, the rate of interest is high, and when prices are falling, it is low. But the adjustment is never perfect. Men never know the future exactly; they can only guess. People are apparently reluctant to believe that prices are going to change very much in either direction. The result of this inadequacy of foresight is that, when prices are rising, the rate of interest is usually high, but not so high as it should be to make a perfect

compensation for the rise; and that, on the other hand, when prices are falling, the rate of interest is usually low, but not so low as it should be to make a perfect compensation for the fall. Thus the rate of interest, though partially adjusted during transition periods, is not sufficiently adjusted to alter the essential fact emphasized in Chapter X; namely, that during rising prices the burden of debts grows lighter on borrowers, and that, consequently, "enterpriser borrowers" tend to be prosperous; while, reversely, when prices are falling, the same people lose, and " business is dull."

4. Effect of Unequal Foresight

Besides being inadequate, foresight is unequally distributed. Different persons differ greatly in their power to foresee; and, in general, borrowers foresee better than lenders. The great borrowers of to-day are not, as is often supposed, the ignorant poor, but the alert and well-informed rich. It is the function of these people to look ahead, and the consequence is that they foresee a rise or fall of prices more quickly than the lenders or bondholders, who are only silent partners in business. Now, a consequence of the superiority in foresight of borrowers over lenders is that the borrowers are willing, during rising prices, to pay a higher rate than they have to pay, whereas the lenders do not see any reason for raising the rate of interest. Suppose that the rate of interest, on a basis of stationary prices, is five per cent, and that prices are rising two per cent per annum. We know that the rate of interest ought to be seven per cent in order to make things even; but let us suppose that the borrowers foresee that prices are going to rise two per cent per annum, and that they are perfectly willing to pay seven per cent, where otherwise they would pay five per cent. Let us suppose, also, that the lenders are not alert enough to see why interest should be any more than five per cent. The consequence will be that the rate of interest will not rise as high as seven per cent, but will be something like six per cent. The consequence of this, in turn, is that the borrowers, who are willing to pay seven per cent to get the same loans that they used to get at five per cent, when they find that they do not have to pay seven per cent, but can get loans at six per cent, will increase the size of their loans. Thus borrowers are encouraged to borrow more. Likewise lenders are encouraged to lend more, for they find that they can get six per cent when they are willing to take five per cent. This six per cent is low in the eyes of the borrowers, but high in the eyes of the deluded lenders. The consequence, therefore, is an inflation of loans stimulated from both sides of the market.

In a previous chapter we saw that an increase of loans of banks produces an increase of deposits, inflates the currency, and makes prices rise further, and so on around the circle of inflation, loans, deposits, and inflation again. The circular process has to come to a stop sometime, but it never does come to a stop until the rate of interest is adjusted. As long as the rate of interest still stays too low, borrowing will continue too high. When presently people wake up to the danger of this condition of inflated loans and deposits, the rate of interest does go up, discouraging loans and precipitating a crisis. Then we have the back-flow: prices decreasing, interest falling, and discouragement of business. This has all been explained in a previous chapter. What needs emphasis here is that an essential factor in all these changes is the rate of interest. The rate of interest is the key to the situation. Were the rate of interest properly adjusted, there would be less trouble, if, indeed, there were any at all. Crises would be fewer, and they would be less severe.

How, then, can we get a better adjustment of the rate of interest? One way is to prevent these changes in price levels as much as possible. This we have already discussed. Another is to have men more alive to the future and more quick to predict what is going to happen to prices. Education on this line will go on and is going on through the trade journals. Still another way is through the removal of the existing prejudice against raising the rate of interest. We still inherit the old idea that interest is " usury " or robbery. If we could once get rid of the prejudice against allowing the rate of interest to rise high as well as to fall low, that is, could regard the rate of interest as properly subject to fluctuation and as being a market price changing day by day, like any other price, a long step would be taken toward preventing crises.

CHAPTER XX IMPATIENCE FOR INCOME THE BASIS OF INTEREST 1. The Productivity Theory In the preceding chapter we have considered the relation of money to the rate of interest. We saw that the money supply has no effect on the rate of interest, except during transition periods. The real riddle of interest, therefore, still remains unsolved. Why is there such a thing as a rate of interest, even when the purchasing power of money is constant, and what, then, determines that rate? What other factors besides changes in the purchasing power of money affect the rate of interest? We must now go back of money and study the supply and demand of loans.

In our study of prices we began by considering first the part played by money, and then undertook an analysis of supply and demand of goods. We are following the same order in our study of that peculiar price called the rate of interest. We have thus far considered only the part played by money, and now are ready to undertake an analysis of the supply and demand of loans. We shall find that, contrasted with the supply and demand of goods, which resolves itself in the last analysis into a comparison between different marginal desirabilities and undesirabilities, which are simultaneous, the supply and demand of loans resolves itself in the last analysis into a comparison between different marginal desirabilities and undesirabilities, which are not simultaneous, but are distributed at different points in time.

Before, however, we can fully justify these propositions, we shall need to clear the way by removing some of the many fallacies and pitfalls which surround the subject.

There is, perhaps, no other "nut" so hard to "crack "in all economics as this one of the rate of interest; and before most persons have grown old enough to consider the subject philosophically, they have absorbed, more or less unconsciously, a number of untenable and even conflicting theories.

Next to the money fallacies which were considered in the last chapter, one of the most persistent fallacies is that the rate of interest represents the " rate of productivity of capital." If a man who has never thought on the subject is asked why the rate of interest is five per cent, he will almost invariably answer, " because capital produces five per cent." A 100,000 mill will produce a net income of 5000 a year; a 100,000 piece of land will produce a net crop worth 5000 a year; and so on. When the rate of interest is five per cent, nothing at first sight seems more obvious than that it is five per cent because capital yields five per cent. Since capital is productive, it seems self-evident that an investment of 100,000 in productive land, machinery, or any other form of capital will yield a rate of interest proportionate to its productivity. This proposition looks attractive, but it is superficial. Why is the land worth 100,000? Simply because 100,000 is the discounted /value of the expected 5000 a year. We have seen in previous chapters that the value of capital is derived from the value of its income, not the value of the income from that of the capital. Capital value is merely the present or discounted value of income. But whenever we discount income, we have to assume a rate of interest. If we have wealth yielding a given perpetual income of 5000 a year and capitalize this income at five per cent, we get 100,000 as the value of the wealth. It would be reasoning in a circle to derive the rate of interest (five per cent) by dividing the 5000 by the 100,000; for this 100,000 was itself derived by assuming the rate to be five per cent in the first place. Again, if we have wealth yielding 1000 for 50 years, and capitalize it at five per cent, we find its present value to be 18,300. One year later, by the same process, its value will be 18,215, showing a depreciation of 85. If we subtract this depreciation from the 1000 of income, we obtain 915 as the interest accrued, which is exactly five per cent of the 18,300, but this result, five per cent, is a necessary consequence of the assumption of five per cent when we calculated the present value as 18,300 and 18,215. Had we assumed four per cent for this calculation, we would have gotten four per cent of accrued interest as a result. We always find at the end exactly what we assumed at the beginning; but if we are not careful, we delude ourselves into thinking that we are finding something new.

It is evident that if an orchard of ten acres yields 100 barrels of apples a year, the physical-productivity, 10 barrels per acre, does not of itself give any clew to what rate of return on its value the orchard yields. Even assuming a given value for the 100 barrels of apples as, say, 200, we are still unable to state what the rate of interest is. We can only say that the orchard yields 2 per acre. We cannot say it yields so much per cent. What then is the rate of interest yielded by the orchard? This question cannot be answered without a knowledge of the value of the orchard; and the value of the orchard cannot be obtained without assuming a rate of interest and using it in discounting the income which the orchard yields. The orchard produces the apples, but the value of the orchard does not produce the value of the apples; on the contrary, the value of the apples produces the value of the orchard.

The following diagram shows the typical relation between capital and the productivity of capital in the physical sense and also in the value sense–which latter sense is the important factor in studying the rate of interest.

Present Capital Fotuhe Income Instruments Benefits

Value of instruments-Value of benefits

This scheme signifies (1) Any physical instrument, such, for instance, as land, railways, factories, dwellings, or food, is the means for obtaining benefits in the future; this first step in the sequence pertains to the study of the " technique " of production, and involves no rate of interest. (2) The benefits are valued in money; this step pertains to the study of prices. (3) From the value of the benefits thus obtained is computed the value of the original instrument by the process of discounting; it is clearly with this last process that we are concerned in the study of interest.

The paradox that, when we come to the value of capital, it is value of income which produces the value of capital, and not the reverse, is, then, the stumbling-block of the productivity theorists. It is clear, of course, in any particular investment, that the selling value of the stock or bond is dependent on its expected income. And yet business men, although constantly employing this discount process in specific cases, usually cherish the illusion that they do so because their capital-value, if invested in some vague "other use," would actually produce interest. They fail to observe that the principle of discounting the future is universal, and applies to any investment whatsoever, and that in such a discount-process there is necessarily assumed the very rate of interest we are seeking to explain. It is futile to derive the rate of interest from the productivity of capital.

The futility of this productivity theory may be further illustrated by observing the effect of a change of productivity. If productivity makes interest, then a change in productivity ought to make a corresponding change in the rate of interest. Yet, if an orchard could in some way be made to yield double its original crop, though its yield in

the physical sense would be doubled, in the sense of the rate of interest its yield would not be necessarily affected at all–certainly not doubled. For the orchard whose yield of apples should increase from 1000 worth to 2000 worth would itself correspondingly increase in value. For some reason or other, people would find themselves calling it a 40,000 orchard instead of a 20,000 orchard; and the ratio of the income to the capital-value would then remain just what it was before, namely, five per cent. Of course it is true that if an orchard which had already been bought for 20,000 on the assumption that it would yield only 1000 worth of crops per year should in some way be doubled in productivity, the owner would be making ten per cent on his original investment, for his original investment was made before either he or the man who sold it to him knew that the orchard would increase in productivity. Had the purchaser known this fact in advance, he would have been quite willing to pay more than the 20,000 which we have supposed him to pay; and as soon as this new knowledge is acquired, he will revalue the orchard according to his new expectations. Realizations do not always or even usually correspond to expectations. Properly speaking, the rate of interest applies only to expectations. To raise the productivity of the orchard or of any other article of wealth will raise its value also. The idea of raising the rate of interest by increasing the productivity of capital is, therefore, like the idea of raising ones self by ones boot straps.

2. The Socialist Theory

So much for the productivity theory. We have next the socialist theory. The socialist has the idea that interest is robbery. He says " it is all wrong that the capitalist who does not lift a finger should get any pay; he is getting something for nothing, and that is interest; interest is robbery; interest is sucking the blood out of somebody else, viz., the workman." According to the socialist theory, especially as represented by Karl Marx, interest is exploitation. The socialists say that labor produces capital, and therefore produces the interest from capital, and therefore labor should get all the income from capital; and since the laborer does not get it all, it must be true that it is held back by somebody who is in a position of vantage to steal it. This is the key of so-called " scientific socialism." There are many motives for socialism, but so far as it has an economic theory behind it, this is that theory. According to it, the capitalist holds a club over the workman and virtually says: " If you will come to-day and work for me, I will give you half of what you produce; I have got the capital, and you cant get on without me, and therefore I am in a position to rob you. Take what you can get, or get nothing."

The socialist theory involves two propositions: first, that all income and all capital are practically produced by labor; and, secondly, that all the resulting income should be paid to the laborer. Now the first proposition is much more nearly correct than the second. We need not contest it in order to see the fundamental error in the theory of socialism. Let it be granted that practically every instrument of production is produced by labor; let it be granted that the capitalist is always living on the product of past labor; that a millionaire who gets his income from railroads, ships, and houses, all products of labor, is reaping what labor sowed; that the capitalists of to-day are receiving compound interest on the labor of bygone times.

It does not follow, however, that injustice has been done to the laborer. Let us consider the case of a tree which is planted with one dollars worth of labor, and twenty-flve years later is worth three dollars. The socialist virtually asks, "Why should not the laborer who planted the tree receive three dollars instead of one dollar for his work?"

The answer is that he may receive it, provided he will wait twenty-five years for it! As Bohm-Bawerk, an authority on interest, says: " The perfectly just proposition that the laborer should receive the entire value of his product may be understood to mean either that the laborer should now receive the entire present value of his product, or should receive the entire future value of his product in the future. But Rodbertus and the socialists expound it as if it meant that the laborer should now receive the entire future value of his product."

It would be a mistake to say that there is no exploitation of laboring men by capitalists, because we know the contrary to be a fact, but it would likewise be a mistake to condemn all interest on the ground of exploitation. The basis of interest is much deeper. It lies in the preference for present over future goods. Neither the employer nor the employee likes to wait a long time for the fruits of any enterprise in which he engages. But somebody must wait, and whoever does so is clearly entitled to some reward.

3. Impatience the Source of Interest

The essence of interest is impatience, the desire to obtain gratifications earlier than we can get them, the preference for present over future goods. It is a fundamental attribute of human nature; and as long as it exists, so long will there be a rate of interest.

Interest is, as it were, human impatience crystallized into a market rate. The market rate of interest is formed out of the various degrees or rates of impatience in the minds of different people. The rate of impatience in any individuals mind is his preference for an additional dollar, or one dollars worth of goods, available to-day, over an additional dollar, or dollars worth of goods, available a year from to-day. In other words, it is the excess of the marginal desirability of to-days goods over the marginal desirability of next years goods viewed from to-days standpoint. It can be expressed in numbers as the premium that a man is willing to pay for this years over next years goods. If, for instance, in order to get 1 to-day he is willing to promise to pay 1.05 next year, then his rate or degree of impatience is said to be five per cent. The present 1 is worth to him so much that in order to get it he is willing to pay for it five per cent more than 1 in the future; it is the willingness to do this to gratify ones impatience which causes the phenomenon of a rate of interest. A man will prefer to have a machine to-day rather than a machine in the future; a house to-day rather than a house a year from now; a piece of land to-day rather than a piece of land when he is ten years older; he would rather have some food to-day than wait until next year for it, or for a suit of clothes, or stocks or bonds, or anything else.

But what are these present and future "goods" which are thus contrasted? At first sight it might seem that the "goods" compared may be indiscriminately wealth, property, or benefits. But when present capital (whether capital-wealth or capital-property) is preferred to future capital, this preference is really a preference for the income of the first capital as compared with the income of the second. The reason why we would choose a present fruit tree rather than a similar fruit tree available in ten years is that the fruit of the first will be available earlier than that of the second. The reason we prefer immediate tenancy of a house to the right to occupy it in six months is that the uses of the house will begin six months earlier in the one case than in the other. In short, capital-wealth available early is preferred to capital-wealth of like kind available at a more remote time, simply because the income of the former is available earlier than the income of the latter. For the same reason early capital-property is preferred to late capital-property of a similar kind; for property is merely a claim to future income; and the earlier the property is acquired, the earlier will the income accrue, the right to which constitutes the property in question.

Thus, impatience for goods of any kind resolves itself into impatience for income,–i. e., preference for immediate in-I come over remote income. Moreover, the preference for immediate income over remote income resolves itself into the preference for present enjoyable income over future enjoyable income. The income from an article of capital which consists merely of an "interaction" is desired for the sake of the final income to which that interaction paves the way. We prefer present bread-baking to future bread-baking because the enjoyment of the resulting bread is available earlier in the one case than in the other. Present weaving is preferred to future weaving, because the earlier the weaving takes place, the sooner will the cloth be manufactured, and the sooner will the clothing made from it be worn by the consumer.

When, as is usually the case, exchange intervenes between the weaving and the use of the clothes, the goal in the process is somewhat obscured by the fact that the manufacturer regards his preference for present weaving over future weaving as due not to the fact that the clothes will be more early available to those who will wear them, but to the fact that he will be enabled to obtain a quicker income by selling the cloth earlier. To him early sales are more advantageous than deferred sales, because the earlier the money is received, the earlier can he spend it for his own personal uses,–the shelter and the comforts of various kinds constituting his real income. It is not he, but his customers, whose preference for present cloth over future cloth is based on the earlier availability of the clothes which can be made from it. But in both cases the minds eye is fixed on some ultimate enjoyable income, i. e., benefits, to which the interaction in question is a mere preparatory step.

The same principles apply where corporations or firms borrow and lend. Here the relation of enjoyable income is more indirect, and yet it is still the guiding force. For borrowing and lending, when directed by the directors of a company on behalf of the stockholders or bondholders, have reference to the enjoyable income, not of the directors, but of the stockholders and bondholders.

We thus see that all preference for present over future goods resolves itself, in the last analysis, into a preference for early enjoyable income over late enjoyable income. Every preference for present over future goods reduces itself, therefore, to this preference for present over future satisfactions.

The preference for present over future goods, when thus reduced to its lowest terms, rids the values of the contrasted present and future goods of the interest element, which, in all other attempts at explanation, is so unconsciously presupposed. When any other goods than enjoyable income are considered, their values already imply a rate of interest. When, for instance, we say that interest is the premium on the value of a present house over that of a future house, we still leave the problem of interest unsolved; for we forget that the value of each house–the future one not less than the present one–is itself based on a rate of interest. As we have seen, the price of a house is the discounted value of its future income, and in the process of discounting there always lurks a rate of interest. When we compare the values of present and future houses, therefore, both terms of the comparison involve the rate of interest. But when present enjoyable income is compared with future enjoyable income, the case is different, for the value of enjoyable income involves no interest whatever.

We have thus reduced the problem of determining the rate of interest to the problem of determining the premium which people are willing to pay for present enjoyable income in terms of future enjoyable income.

CHAPTER XXI INFLUENCES ON IMPATIENCE FOR INCOME 1. Differences in Impatience Due to Differences in Human Nature

Bur we have not yet wholly solved the problem of interest. It is not enough to know that the more impatient a people are, the higher will be their rate of interest, and the more patient they are, the lower will be their rate of interest. We must also know on what causes the degree or rale of impatience depends. It depends principally upon the character of the individual and the character of the income which he possesses. It is clear that the degree of impatience which corresponds to a specific income-stream will not be the same for everybody. One man may have a degree or rate of impatience of five per cent and another a rate of impatience of ten per cent, although both have the same income. The difference will be due to a difference in the personal characteristics of the individuals. These characteristics are chiefly five in number: (1) foresight, (2) self-control, (3) habit, (4) expectation of life, (5) love for posterity. We shall take these up in order.

(1) First, as to foresight. Generally speaking, the greater the foresight, the less the impatience, and vice versa. In the case of primitive races and uninstructed classes of society, the future is seldom considered in its true proportions. The story is told of a shiftless householder who would not mend his leaky roof when it was raining, for fear of getting more wet, nor when it was not raining, because he did not then need shelter. Among such persons impatience r present gratification is powerful because their comprehension of the future is weak. If we compare the Scotch and the Irish, we shall find a contrast in this respect. The Irish, in general, lack foresight and are improvident, and the Scotch have foresight and are provident. Consequently the rate of interest is high in Ireland and low in Scotland.

These differences in degrees of foresight produce corresponding differences in the dependence of impatience on the character of income. Thus, for a given income, say 1000 a year, the reckless might have a rate of impatience of ten per cent, when the forehanded would experience a rate of only five per cent. Therefore, impatience, in general, will be greater in a community consisting of reckless individuals than in one consisting of the opposite type.

(2) We come next to self-control. This trait, though distinct from foresight, is usually associated with it and has very similar effects. Foresight has to do with thinking, self-control with willing. A weak will usually goes with a weak intellect, though not necessarily, and not always. The effect of a weak will is similar to the effect of inferior fore-sight. Like those workingmen who cannot carry their pay home Saturday night, but spend it in a grogshop on the way, many persons cannot deny themselves any present indulgence, even when they know definitely what the consequences will be in the future. Others, on the contrary, have no difficulty in controlling themselves in the face of all temptations.

(3) The third characteristic of human nature which needs to be considered is habit. That to which one is accustomed exerts necessarily a powerful influence upon his valuations and therefore upon his impatience. This influence may be in either direction. A rich mans son who has been brought up with expensive habits, when he finds himself with a smaller income than his father provided him during his formative years, will be more impatient for income than a man who has this same income but who has climbed up instead of climbed down.

(4) The expectation of life will affect a mans degree of impatience. A man who looks forward to a long life will have a relatively high appreciation of the future, which means a relatively low appreciation of the present, i. e., a low degree of impatience; whereas a man who has a short life to look forward to will want it at least to be a merry one. " Eat, drink, and be merry, for to-morrow we die " is the motto applying to this type.

(5) The fifth circumstance is love for posterity. Probably the most powerful cause tending to reduce the rate of interest is love for ones children and the desire to provide for their good. When these sentiments decay, as they did decay at the time of the decline and fall of the Roman Empire, and it becomes the fashion to exhaust wealth in self-indulgence and leave little or nothing to offspring, the rate of impatience and the rate of interest will be high. At such times the motto, "After us the deluge," indicates the feverish desire to squander in the present, at whatever cost to the future. A noted gambler, who had led a wild and selfish life, once said, when life insurance was first explained to him, "I have seen many schemes for making money, but this is the first time I have seen a scheme where you had to die before you could rake in the pile." That man did not care for a payment which would come in after his death. But there are many men who do, and in fact care much more for it than for anything else in the world. This care leads them to insure their lives in order that they may leave the money to their families. Their desire to provide for those who survive them tends to make them more patient, i. e., tends to reduce their impatience to enjoy income immediately. Life insurance, by training people to provide for posterity, is acting as one of the most powerful means of lowering the rate of impatience and therefore the rate of interest. At present in the United States the insurance on lives amounts to 20,000,000,000. This represents, for the most part, future income to be received by the next generation by reason of sacrifices of income made by the present generation. These sacrifices spring from a low rate of impatience, and tend to produce a low rate of interest.

Thus we see that men may differ in many ways which affect the rate of interest and the rate of impatience. We may contrast two extreme types of men. Men who are shortsighted, or weak willed, or have the habits of a spendthrift, or look forward to a short or uncertain life, or are selfish and have no regard for posterity, will (other things equal) have a high degree of impatience. Men who possess foresight, self-control, habits of thrift, confidence in length of life, and altruism with respect to posterity, will (other things equal) have a low degree of impatience.

2. Differences in Impatience Due to Differences in Income

But not only does impatience vary as between different individuals; it varies also for the same individual according to circumstances. The most important circumstance affecting a persons degree of impatience is the character of his expected income in the immediate and in the remote future. Ones impatience for satisfactions will vary inversely as the abundance of his immediate as compared with his remote satisfactions. If the future satisfactions which he expects and looks forward to are very great, and his present satisfactions are very small, he will be impatient to hurry from his present scarcity and arrive at the expected future abun dance; that is, he will have a high rate of preference for present over future satisfactions. This is on the same principle that prices are high when goods are scarce. The preference for present satisfactions is high if present satisfactions are scarce. Now ones impatience to bring future satisfactions nearer the present will depend on ones whole future stream of satisfactions, i. e., what we call his final enjoyable income. It will depend on three chief characteristics of that income: first, as just said, it will depend on its distribution in time, i. e., the relative abundance of his immediate as compared with his remote satisfactions; secondly, on the amount of the income, i. e., whether his satisfactions are, as a whole, scant or abundant; thirdly, on the uncertainties of the income, i. e., to what extent his satisfactions throughout future years are subject to chance, that is, may turn out to be greater or less than he first expected.

3. Influence of the Distribution in Time of the Income-stream

We have first to 2 0 consider the in-2400 fluence which the 220 distribution in 200 1800

tIme of Income I600 has upon the im-1400 patience for in-I20 come. Three dif-1C ferent types of distribution in 400 time may be 200 distinguished: uniform income, IO II "12 re 14 "IS 16 17 Fig. 41.

consisting of equal yearly items, as represented by the dark lines in Figure 41 (in which, as in previous diagrams, the heights of the successive vertical lines represent the amounts of the successive installments of income, say 1900 a year); increasing income, as represented in Figure 42 (in which the income is supposed to increase from 1200 a year in 1911 to nearly 3000 in 1917); and decreasing income, as represented in Figure 43 (in which the income is supposed to decrease from almost 3000 in 1911 to about 1200 in 1917).

The effect of possessing an increasing income (Fig. 42) is, as we have already indicated, tomake the possessor impatient to get the larger income which the future holds or keeps back. A man who is now enjoying an income of only 1000 a year, but expects in ten years to be enjoying one of 10,000 a year, will be impatient 3000 2000 26OO 24OO 2200 2000 I800 1600 I4OO

1200 1000

aoo

600

4-00 200 1

IS MO II 12 I3 14 15 16 I7

Fig. 42.

V 3OOO 2800 26OO 2400 2200 2000 I8OO I6OQ 1400 IZOO IOOO 8OO 600

4OO

aoo IS

HO II I2 13 "14 IS i6 I7

Fig. 43.

to have those ten years elapse. He has " great expectations." He may, to satisfy his impatience, borrow money to eke out this years income, and make repayment by sacrificing from his more abundant income ten years later.

Reversely, a gradually decreasing income (Fig. 43), making, as it does, the earlier income relatively abundant, and the remoter income relatively scarce, tends to reduce impatience, or the preference for present as compared with future income. The man with a descending income already has a high income without being compelled to wait for it. With him there is little reason for impatience–there is nothing to be impatient for; on the contrary, the future does not look at all inviting. The outlook, so far from tending to make him borrow, tends to make him wish to save from his present abundance to provide for his coming need.

The extent of these effects will, as we have already seen, vary greatly with different individuals. Corresponding to a given ascending income, one individual may have a rate of impatience of ten per cent and another of only four per cent. What we need here to emphasize is merely that, in the case of both of these individuals, a descending income causes a lower degree of impatience than an ascending income.

4. Influence of the Size of the Income-stream

We have considered the dependence of impatience for expected income on the distribution of that income in time. Our next topic is the dependence of impa-f tience on the size of income. In general, it may be said that the smaller the income a man has, the higher is his preference for present over future income. It is true that a small income implies a keen appreciation of future wants as well as of immediate wants. Poverty bears down heavily on all parts of a mans life, both that which is immediate and that which is remote. But it enhances the desirability of immediate income even more than of future income.

This result is partly rational, because of the importance of supplying present needs in order to keep up the continuity of life and the ability to cope with the future; and partly irrational, because the pressure of present needs blinds one to the needs of the future.

As to the rational side, it is clear that present income is absolutely indispensable, not only for the present, but even as a precondition to the attainment of future income. One break in the thread of life is sufficient to destroy all future enjoyment. It is of the utmost importance, therefore, to keep up life. As the phrase is, " a man must live," and in the present a man must keep his hold on life in order to have any life in the future. If, then, a man were on a desert island and had only such rations as would last a few months, he would naturally prefer to use them immediately–sparingly, but immediately–rather than to put off their consumption ten years; because if he put off consuming them he could not consume them at all; he would die in the meantime. And in general, a man who is poor, and upon whom poverty presses so as to make it hard to make both ends meet, will always have a higher realization and appreciation of the present than a man who is rich.

As to the irrational side, the poorer a man, the more his eyes are blinded to future needs. He is too much occupied with the need of the present, and shuts his eyes to the future. To him " sufficient unto the day is the evil thereof." We all suffer from lack of perspective, and tend to exaggerate the needs of the present. Poverty especially tends to distort the perspective. Its effect is to relax foresight and self-control, and tempt one to " trust to luck " for the future, if only the all-absorbing clamor of present necessities may thus be satisfied.

We see, then, that a small income tends to produce a high degree of impatience, partly from lack of foresight and self-control, and partly from the thought that provision for the present is necessary both for itself and for the future as well.

5. Influence of Uncertainties of Income

The next influence on impatience and therefore on the rate of interest consists in the risks or uncertainties attaching to prospective incomes. Now uncertainties affect impatience in several different ways. In general, risks tend! to raise the degree of impatience. There are four ways in which risk tends to increase impatience, and one in which j it tends to decrease impatience.

First, we know that if a loan is risky, the rate of interest 1 has to be high. If the repayment of a loan is regarded as uncertain, this uncertainty to the lender will have to be offset by an increase in the rate of interest, and produces a correspondingly high rate of impatience in the case of risky loans. The rate of interest on risky loans thus includes, as it were, an element of insurance against loss. Strictly speaking, such a rate is not pure interest; for we have denned a rate of interest as the premium paid for present money in future money, on the assumption that both sums are certain.

But even the pure rate of interest–the rate in riskless loans–will be raised by risk in certain ways. One way in which risk tends to raise the rate of impatience has already been mentioned in 1, namely, when the risk is of life,–that is, of its terminating before the lender finds himself able to enjoy the fruits of his loan. This acts like the risk in the loan itself. You may tell a man he is perfectly sure of being repaid his loan fifty years from now. But will he live so long? It is cold comfort to tell him he is sure to get his money after he is dead! A sailor is a type of man who is constantly taking this fact into account. He knows that almost any day he may be shipwrecked, and the consequence is that he prefers money ready to spend to-day to money available only next year. Sailors are proverbial spendthrifts and have a proverbially high degree of impatience.

The third case is where the receipt of the income itself , is uncertain, its uncertainty applying alike to all times. Such a condition largely explains why salaries and wages are lower than the average earnings of those who work for themselves. Those who choose salaries rather than profits are willing to accept a small but sure income in order to get rid of a precarious though possibly larger one. Since a risky income, if the risk applies evenly to all parts of the income-stream, is nearly equivalent to a low income, and since a low income, as we have seen, tends to intensify impatience, risk, if uniformly distributed in time, must tend to increase impatience.

The fourth way in which risk tends to increase impatience is seen where immediate income is risky as compared with remote income. A man in time of war, when there is prospect of peace in the future, looking forward to a relatively safe income in the future, will have a high degree of impatience for that future to arrive, because the present risky income is in his eyes not equivalent to the future safe income. These, then, are four ways in which risk tends to increase impatience. There is, however, one way in which ; risk tends to decrease impatience. The instance just given is one in which income in the immediate future is risky, but income thereafter safe. That sometimes happens, as just indicated, where in time of war man expects peace in the future, or in time of sickness he expects to get well and resume his regular earning power. Nevertheless, there are numerous examples of the opposite type, where the risk applies to the future and not to the present. If a ship owner, for instance, has his ship in port to-day, but is going to sail within a few months, his risks are high in the future as compared with the present. His future looks dubious, and that will cause him to be less impatient, because a risky future income is like a small future income, and we have seen that a small future income tends to lessen impatience. An income which gets more and more risky in the future is therefore like an income which gets smaller and smaller in the future. In actual fact, such a type is not uncommon. The remote future is usually less known than the immediate future. This means that the risk connected with distant income is greater than that connected with income near at hand. The chance of disease, accident, disability, or death is always to be reckoned with, but under ordinary circumstances is greater in the remote future than in the immediate future. Consequently there is usually a tendency, so far as this influence goes, toward a low degree of impatience. This tendency is expressed in the phrase to " lay up for a rainy day."

Risk, then, operates in diverse ways according to diverse circumstances. We see that risk tends in some cases to increase and in others to decrease the degree of impatience. There is a common principle, however, in all these cases. Whether the result is a high or a low degree of impatience, the primary fact is that the risk of losing the income in a particular period of time operates as a virtual impoverishment of the income in that period, and hence increases the estimation in which it is held. If that period is a remote one, the risk to which it is subject makes for a high appreciation of remote income and a low degree of impatience; if the period is the immediate future, the risk makes for a high appreciation of immediate income and a high degree of impatience; if the risk is in all periods of time, it acts as a virtual decrease of income all along the line and promotes a high degree of impatience. From a practical point of! view, there is no factor affecting the rate of interest more important than the factor called risk. This is because interest always has to do with the future and the future is always uncertain.

6. Summary

The impatience of any individual depends, then, partly on the character of that individuals income, i. e., on three characteristics of income:– (1) its distribution in time, (2) its amount, (3) its uncertainties.

This proposition–that the preference of any individual for immediate over remote income depends upon the nature of his prospective enjoyable income–corresponds to the proposition in the theory of prices, that the marginal desirability of any article depends upon the quantity of that article; both propositions are fundamental in their respective spheres.

We see, then, that a mans impatience depends (1) upon his nature, and (2) upon his income. In the following illustrative table we see contrasted the supposed extreme types of income and of human nature, and see how impatience will differ among the four extreme cases here represented.

Description Of Incohx Corresponding Rate or Impatience To An Individual Wbo 1s

Short-sighted, weak-willed, accustomed to spend, without heirs Far-sighted, self-controlled, accustomed to save, desirous to pro-vide for heirs

Small Large Increasing Decreasing Precarious Assured 20 5 1

5

If we compare the figures in the same vertical column, we see that the lower figure is the smaller, expressing the influence of the character of income. If we compare the figures in the same horizontal line, we see that the right-hand figure is the smaller, expressing the influence of human nature. But a man may have an income-stream of a kind which tends to inflame his impatience, and at the same time a nature of a kind which tends to allay his impatience. The result will then be a compromise rate of impatience, say five per cent. Or a man may have an income-stream which tends to keep his impatience low, and a nature which tends to keep it high. Thus five per cent is found twice in the table forming a diagonal. The other diagonal shows the contrast between the extreme where both the character of the income and the nature of the individual conspire to make a very high degree of impatience, and the opposite extreme where they conspire to make a very low degree of impatience. The same individual may, in the course of his life, change from one extreme of impatience for income to the other. Such a change may be due to a change in the persons nature (as when a spendthrift is reformed or a man, originally prudent, becomes, through intemperance, reckless and thriftless), or to a change in his income, whether in respect to size, distribution in time, or uncertainty. Every one at some times in his life doubtless changes his degree of impatience for income. In the course of an ordinary lifetime the changes in a mans degree of impatience are probably of the following general character: As a child he will have a high degree of impatience because of his lack of foresight and self-control. When he reaches the age of young manhood he may still have a high degree of impatience, but for a different reason, viz. because he then expects a large future income. He expects to get on in the world, and he will have a high degree of impatience because of the relative abundance of the imagined future as compared with the realized present. When he gets a little farther along, and has a family, the result will be a low degree of impatience, because then the needs of the future rather than the endowment of the future will appeal to him. He will not think that he is going to be so very rich in the future; on the contrary, he will wonder how he is going to get along in the future because he will have so many mouths to feed. He looks forward to the future expenses of his wife and children with the idea of providing for them–an idea which makes for a high relative regard for the future and a low relative regard for the present. Then when he gets a little older, and his children are married and gone out into the world and are taking care of themselves, he again has a high degree of impatience for income, because he expects to die, and he thinks, "Why shouldnt I enjoy myself during the few years that remain instead of piling up for the remote future?"

CHAPTER XXII

THE DETERMINATION OF THE RATE OF INTEREST z. Equalizing Marginal Rates of Impatience by

Borrowing and Lending In the preceding chapter we saw that the rate of preference for present over future goods is, in the last analysis, a preference for immediate over remote income; that this preference depends, for any given individual, upon the character of his income-stream,–its size, its distribution in time, and its uncertainties; and that the nature of this dependence varies with different individuals.

The question now arises: What relation do these different " rates of preference " of different individuals have to the rate of interest?

For the moment let us assume a perfect market, in which the element of risk is entirely lacking, both with respect to the certainty of the expected income-streams belonging to the different individuals, and with respect to the certainty of repayment for loans. In other words, we assume that all individuals are initially possessed of foreknown income-streams, and are free to exchange any parts of them, that is any present or immediate income for any future or remote income. Prior to such exchange, the income-stream is supposed to be fixed in size and distribution in time; that is, the capital instruments which the individual possesses are each supposed to be capable of only a single definite series of benefits contributing to his income-stream.

Under these hypothetical conditions, the rates of impatience for different individuals would become perfectly equalized.

For if any particular individual has a rate of impatience above the market rate, he will sell some of his surplus future income to obtain (i. e., " borrow") an addition to his present meager income. This will have the effect of decreasing the desirability of his present income and increasing the desirability of the remaining future income. The process will continue until the rate of impatience of this individual is equal to the rate of interest. In other words, a person whose impatience rate exceeds the current rate of interest will borrow up to the point at which the two rates will be equal. Reversely, a man who, with a given income-stream, has a rate of impatience below the market rate, will sell (i. e., " lend ") some of his abundant present income to eke out the future, the effect being to increase his rate of impatience until it also harmonizes with the rate of interest.

To put the matter in figures, let us suppose the rate of interest is five per cent, whereas the rate of impatience of a particular individual is at first ten per cent. Then, by hypothesis, the individual is willing to sacrifice 1.10 of next years income in exchange for 1 of this years. But in the market he is able to obtain 1 for this year by sacrificing only 1.05 of next years income. This ratio is, to him, a cheap price. He therefore borrows, say, 100 for a year, agreeing to return 105; that is, he contracts a loan at five per cent when he would be willing to pay ten per cent. This loan, by increasing his present income and decreasing his future, tends to reduce his rate of impatience from ten per cent to, say, eight per cent. Under these circumstances he will borrow another 100, being now willing to pay eight per cent, but actually paying only five per cent. This loan will still further reduce his rate of impatience. He will continue to borrow until his rate of impatience has been finally brought down to five per cent. Then for the last or " marginal " 100, his rate of impatience will agree with the market rate of interest. As in the general theory of prices, this marginal rate, five per cent, being once established, applies indifferently to all his valuations of present and future income. Every comparative estimate of present and future which he actually makes must be "marginal," i. e., relative to small additions to or subtractions from his present and future income.

In like manner, if another individual, entering the loan market from the other side, has at first a rate of impatience of two per cent, he will become a lender instead of a borrower. He will bewilling to accept 1o2 of next years income for 100 of this years income, but in the market he is able, instead of the 102, to get 105. As he can lend at five per cent when he would gladly do so at two percent, he jumps at the chance to get five per cent and invests, not one 100 only, but another and another. His present income, being reduced by the process, is now more highly esteemed than before, and his future income, being increased, is less highly esteemed. The result will be a higher relative valuation of the present, i. e., a higher rate of impatience, which, under the influence of successive additions to the sums lent, will rise gradually to the level of the market rate of interest.

In such an ideal loan market, therefore, where every individual could freely borrow or lend, the rates of impatience for all the different individuals will become equal to each other and to the rate of interest.

To illustrate these principles by diagrams, let us suppose a man has a given income-stream, as indicated in Figure 44. It is assumed that his income-stream is an ascending one, as between one year and the next; that is, that the income for the year 1910 is relatively small and that for 1911 is relatively large. It may be that in 1910 he is ill, and therefore does not earn his usual amount of money, but that the year after he expects to get an unusual income from some particular source. This man will then probably be impatient to get the large income he anticipates. He does not wish to wait till next year if he can avoid waiting.

I00 . o 5 F ct urr 1C(i

ov ec

0 1910 191I

Fig. 44- 19I2 10I3

His impatience is due to a scarcity of income this year and an abundance of income next year. He will wish to adjust his income or rectify the disparity by increasing this years income at the expense of next years income. He will borrow, but borrowing changes the distribution in time of his income-stream. His original income in the. first year is 300, indicated by the dark line for the year 1910. Next year his income is 600, indicated by the dark line for that year. The effect of borrowing will be to elevate the first line by 100 and to depress the second by 105. These two adjustments will lessen both the scarcity of this years income and the abundance of next years income. This will therefore modify the distribution in time of his income and lessen the valuation he puts on a dollar this year as compared with next year. This reduces the premium he puts on this years dollar, i. e., his rate of impatience. By increasing his loan he can evidently reduce this premium to conform to the rate of interest. He can also make other loan contracts, or plan to make them later, by which he can increase or decrease any years income at the expense of an opposite change in that of some other year or years. In this way he can alter the distribution in time of his income-stream at will, and he will always so alter it as to make his rate of impatience equal to the rate of interest. He began with a rate of impatience greater than the market rate of interest, but ended in harmony with that rate.

Figure 45 represents the income-stream of a man supposed to have a rate of impatience at first less than the rate of interest. If we choose, we may suppose that he has just received a small legacy which makes this years available income unusually large, say 600, while he expects next year to have an unusually small income. Looking forward to next year, he sees that it will be hard to get along comfortably, while this year he has more than he needs. He therefore invests some of his present abundance to the extent of 100 in order to eke out his future scarcity by 105. He will do so, however, only provided his rate of impatience is less than the market rate of interest, five per cent, and he will do so only up to the point which will reduce his rate of impatience to the level of this rate of interest.

The two men started out with rates of impatience different from the market rate of interest. The market rate was five per cent, while the first man had a rate of impatience above this, and the second a rate of impatience below this. But when they finished their loan operations or readjustments of the distribution in time of their income-streams, they brought their rates of impatience each into harmony with the rate of interest and therefore with each other. Therefore, as long as there is a market in which everybody can borrow or lend at will at five per cent, everybody will have at the margin a rate of impatience of five per cent. Nobody will have a rate of impatience above five per cent, because, if it is at first above it, he will borrow enough to bring it down to the market rate; and nobody will have a rate below it, because, if it is at first below it, he will lend enough to bring it up to the rate of interest.

TOO 6OO "and

snt–.

400 300 1

3 kic 5 e ru . n d

o 1910 49U T9I2 1913

Fig. 45.

Even men of widely different natures as to foresight, self-control, etc., will have the same marginal rates of impatience. If such different men start with precisely the same sorts of income, they will have different rates of impatience. But in that case they will not continue to have the same sorts of income. They will severally modify their income-streams until equal degrees of impatience are effected. They will then have, instead of different degrees of impatience, different sorts of income-streams.

2. Equalizing Marginal Rates of Impatience by

Spending and Investing It must not be imagined that the classes of borrowers and lenders correspond respectively with the classes of poor and rich. Personal and natural idiosyncrasies, early training, and acquired habits, accustomed style of living, the usages of the country, and other circumstances will, by influencing foresight, self-control, regard for posterity, etc., determine whether a mans degree of impatience is high or low, and whether he becomes a borrower or a lender.

It should be noted that borrowing and lending are not the only ways in which ones income-stream may be modified. The same result may be accomplished simply by buying and selling property; for, since property rights are merely rights to particular income-streams, their exchange substitutes one such stream for another of equal value but differing in distribution in time, or certainty. This method of modifying ones income-stream, which we shall call the method of sale, really includes the method of loan; for a loan contract is at bottom a sale; that is, it is the exchange of the right to present or immediately ensuing in come for the right to more remote or future income.

A borrower is a seller of a note of which the lender is the buyer. A bondholder is regarded indifferently as a lender and as a buyer of the bond.

The concept of a loan may therefore now be dispensed with by being merged in that of sale. At bottom every " loan" is a sale. Thus when a bank " lends" to a customer, it really buys that customers note, i. e., buys (for present cash) the right to receive a sum of money in the future. In the same example the customer or " borrower " is really a seller of future income for present cash; he sells his note which is a promise of a future payment. In short, every so-called " loan " is merely an exchange of present money for future money. These two moneys are, of course, not the same; so that only by a fiction is the original money " lent" and afterward " returned." The original money is not actually lent but absolutely transferred, never to be actually returned, but simply to be replaced by other money.

By selling some property rights and buying others it is always possible to transform ones income-stream at will, whether the transformation be in respect to distribution in time or in respect to certainty. Thus, if a man buys an orchard, he is providing himself with future income in the use of apples. If, instead, he buys apples, he is providing himself with similar but more immediate income. If he buys " securities," he is providing himself with future money, convertible when received into final or enjoyable income. If his security is a share in a mine, his income-stream is less lasting, though it may be larger, than if the security is stock in a railway.

Purchasing the right to remote enjoyable income is called investing; purchasing the right to immediate enjoyable income is called spending. The antithesis between " spending " and " investing " rests upon the antithesis between immediate and remote income. The adjustment between

the two determines the distribution in time of ones income-stream. Spending increases immediate income, but robs the future, whereas investing provides for the future to the detriment of the present.

From what has been said it is clear that by buying and selling property an individual may change the conformation of his income-stream precisely as though he were specifically lending or borrowing. Thus, if a mans original income-stream consists of 1000 this year and 1500 next year, and if, selling this income-stream, he buys with the proceeds another income-stream yielding 1100 this year and 1395 next year, he has not, nominally, borrowed 100 and repaid 105, but he has done what amounts to the same thing–increased his income-stream of this year by 100 and decreased that of next year by 105, the 100 being the modification produced in his income for the first year by selling his original income-stream and substituting the second one, and 105 being the reverse modification in next years income.

3. Futility of Prohibiting Interest

We may now note that interest taking cannot be prevented by prohibiting loan contracts. To forbid the particular form of sale, called a loan contract, would leave possible other forms of sale, and, as has been shown, the valuation of every property right involves interest. If the prohibition should leave individuals free to deal in bonds, it is clear that virtually they would be still borrowing and lending, but under the name of "sale"; and if "bonds" were tabooed, they could merely make the slight change to "preferred stock." It can scarcely be supposed that any prohibition of interest-taking would extend to the prohibition of all buying and selling; but as long as buying and selling of any kind were permitted, the virtual effect of lending and borrowing would be retained. The possessor of a forest of young trees, not being able to mortgage their future return, and being in need of an income-stream of a less deferred type than that receivable from the forest itself, would simply sell his forest, and with the proceeds buy, say, a farm with a uniform flow of income, or a mine with a decreasing one. On the other hand, the possessor of a capital which is depreciating, that is, which represents an income-stream great now but steadily declining, and who is anxious to " save " instead of " spend," would sell his depreciating wealth and invest the proceeds in some such instrument as the forest already mentioned.

It was in such ways, as, for instance, by " rent-purchase," that the medieval pro-hibitions of usury were rendered nugatory. Practically, at the worst, the effect of restrictive laws is simply to hamper and make difficult the finer adjustments of the income-stream, compelling would-be borrowers to sell wealth yielding distant returns instead of mortgaging it, and would-be lenders to buy the same, instead of lending to the present owners. It is conceivable that " explicit " interest might disappear under such restrictions, but" implicit" interest would remain. The young forest sold for 10,000 would bear this price, as now, because it would be the discounted value of the estimated future income; and the price of the farm bought for 10,000 would be determined in like manner. The rate of discount in the two cases must tend to be the same, because, by buying and selling, the various parties in the community would adjust their rates of impatience to a common level–an implicit rate of interest thus lurking in every contract, though never specifically appearing therein. Interest is too omnipresent a phenomenon to be eradicated by attacking any particular form; nor would any one undertake it who perceived the substance as well as the form. In substance, the rate of interest represents the terms on which the earlier and later elements of income-streams are exchangeable against each other. Interest can never disappear until present and future dollars will exchange

at par. This would imply that human beings were no longer impatient, but consid-ered it no hardship to wait indefinitely. We have hitherto supposed, for simplicity, that the income from each instrument is fixed in size and distribution in time. But often the same article may be used in any one of several ways producing any one of several different income-streams. In such a case the owner merely chooses the particular way which gives the capital the highest value. Since any mans income may be transformed as to its distribution in time by the process of borrowing and lending or buying and selling, he need not be deterred from selecting an income by an inconvenient distribu-tion in time. He can choose it exclusively on the basis of maximum present value and later correct any inconvenience of its distribution in time by borrowing and lending or buying and selling.

4. Clearing the Loan Market

We have seen that from the standpoint of the individual, when a rate of interest is given, he will adjust his rate of impatience to correspond with that rate of interest.

For him the rate of interest is a relatively fixed fact, since his own rate of impatience and resulting action can affect it only infinitesimally. All he can do is to adjust his rate of impatience to the rate of interest as he finds it. For society as a whole, however, these rates of impatience determine the rate of interest. This corresponds to what was said as to the determination of prices. We have seen that each individual regards the market price, say, of coal, as fixed, and adjusts his marginal desirability or undesirability to it; whereas, for the entire market, we know that these marginal desirabilities and undesirabilities fix the price of coal. In the same way, while for the individual the rate of interest determines the rate of impatience, for society the rates of impatience of the individuals determine the rate of interest. The rate of interest is simply the rate of impatience upon which the whole community may concur in order that the market of loans may be exactly cleared. Supply and demand will work this out.

To put the matter in figures: if the rate of interest is set very high, say twenty per cent, there will be relatively few borrowers and many would-be lenders, so that the total extent to which would-be lenders are willing to reduce their income-streams for the present year for the sake of a much larger future income will be, say, 100,000,000; whereas, those who are willing to add to their present income at the high price of twenty per cent interest will borrow only, say, 1,000,000. Under such conditions the demand for loans is far short of the supply, and the rate of interest will therefore go down. At an interest rate of ten per cent, the present years income offered as loans might be 50,000,000, and the amount which would be taken at that rate only 20,000,000. There is still an excess of supply over demand, and interest must needs fall further. At five per cent we may suppose the market cleared, borrowers and lenders being willing to take or give, respectively, 30,000,000. In like manner it can be shown that the rate would not fall below this, as in that case it would result in an excess of demand over supply, and cause the rate to rise again.

Thus the rate of interest is the common market rate of impatience for income, as determined by the supply and demand of present and future income. Those who are very impatient strive to acquire more present income at the cost of future income, and tend to raise the rate of interest. These are the borrowers, the spenders, the buyers of goods which afford immediate gratification, the sellers of property yielding remote income, such as bonds and stocks. On the other hand, those who–being relatively patient–strive to acquire more future income at the cost of present income, tend to lower the rate of interest. These are the lenders, the savers, the investors.

The mechanism just described will not only result in a rate which will clear the market for loans connecting the present with next year, but, applied to exchanges between the present and the remoter future, it will make similar adjustments. While some individuals may wish to exchange this years income for next years, others wish to exchange this years income for that of the year after next, or for income several years in the future. The rates of interest for these various periods are so adjusted as to clear the market for all the periods of time for which contracts are made. That is, supply and demand must be equal, so as to clear the market for every period of time.

5. The Conditions Determining the Rate of Interest

We have sketched the main principles determining the rate of interest. Some have not been mentioned save by implication. In summary we may say that the rate of interest, considered independently of fluctuations in the monetary standard, is determined by six conditions. Those which we have above considered and explained are the following three: (1) the dependence of impatience upon prospective income–its size, distribution in time, and uncertainties; (2) the tendency of the rates of impatience for different individuals to seek a common level in the resulting rate of interest; (3) the fact that supply and demand must be equal so that the modifications in the income-streams of individuals, through buying and selling, or borrowing and lending, must " clear the market."

Of the remaining three determining conditions the most important may be stated in the following form: (4) of all the optional uses to which a man may put his capital he will choose that one which at the market rate of interest makes the present value of his capital the largest possible. Thus a farmer may have the option of using a certain piece of land as wheatland or as woodland. If he uses it as wheatland, he can get an income from it every year; but if he plants a young forest on it, he must wait perhaps a generation before receiving any return. To compare the relative merits of these two uses of the land, he will need to calculate, as well as he can, the total present values of the incomes he would get in the two ways. If he reckons that the present value of the future income he can get by growing wheat is about 10,000, but that the present value of the future income he can get by growing timber is 12,000, he will prefer to grow timber. Evidently these calculations of present value can be made only by employing a rate of interest, and, if the rate of interest falls, the comparison may be reversed; timber-growing might then become more profitable than wheat-growing. Thus the farmers decision as to which of the optional uses of his capital is the best will depend, in part, on the rate of interest. Reciprocally the rate of interest in the community will depend in part on the choice of uses of capital. Thus, if a fall in the rate of interest leads many people to abandon wheat-growing in order to take up the timber business, this shifting of part of the income of the community from the immediate to the remote future will tend to check the fall in the rate of interest on the principle already explained–that an increase of a remotely future income increases human impatience. To be more specific, if a fall in the rate of interest makes timber-growing pay, where before it was unprofitable as compared to wheat production, then many of the farmers who turn to timber will need to borrow money while they are waiting for their slow-growing crop. They will therefore add to the demand for loans, and tend to raise the rate of interest. Thus we see that the choice between different uses of capital is one of the influences determining the rate of interest.

The remaining two conditions are very obvious ones; one condition being that (5) what is borrowed at any time by some persons equals what is loaned at that time by other persons, and the other condition being that (6) what any person borrows at one time must be repaid by that person at another time with interest at the market rate.

These six conditions would fully determine the rate of interest under the assumption we have made of a perfect loan market. But in practice these conditions are somewhat modified. For instance, the last or sixth condition (that the loan is to be repaid) is not always actually met, and the fear that it may not be met affects the rate of interest and often decides whether at the outset a loan shall be made or not. Some sort of security is required for almost every loan. Here, as in other instances, the element of risk is intertwined with the rate of interest. 11 Again, the second condition (that the degrees of impatience of all persons become equal to the rate of interest) may not be fully met;

for a would-be borrower may not be able (owing to lack of security satisfactory to the lender) to secure a large enough loan to reduce his impatience to equality with the market rate of interest. Or he may be affected by laws restricting loans. Those thus shut out of the loan market will continue to have an impatience for income higher than the market rate of interest. 1 Again, the fourth condition (that the use of ones capital chosen will be that use of which the present value is greater than the present value of any rival use) is not always met, either because the owner is mistaken in his forecasts or because he is unable to obtain a loan by which to finance his choice. For instance, certain land may be worth most as timberland and yet actually used as grazing land, because the owner cannot provide by loans or otherwise for the lean years which must pass while the timber is growing. One result of these and other imperfections in the loan market is that there are really many rates of interest instead of one rate only. One rate, or rather group of rates of interest, is that realized on bonds; another is that used in short-time bank loans; a third, that in "call" loans. Perhaps the most representative rate of interest is the rate on two or three months loans at banks on indorsed notes of merchants called " commercial paper."

Another result of the imperfections of the loan market is that the minor fluctuations in any particular rate of interest are more often due to varying imperfections of the market adjustment than to variations of income, human impatience, and the other factors enumerated as the fundamental conditions determining the rate of interest. For instance, the rate of interest on bank loans varies from time to time with the changes in the ratio of reserves to deposits, especially if there be a legal requirement as to this ratio. A bank may refuse a loan to avoid increasing its deposits (in relation to reserves) above the legal ratio or, before this becomes necessary, it may raise its rate in anticipation. Thus the Bank of England raises its rate when necessary to "protect" its reserve. The daily variations in bank rates are usually due more to the need of readjusting the ratio of reserves to deposits than to changes in its customers impatience or in their incomes.

But in the long run the rate of interest is a fairly faithful register of human impatience as modified by mutual loans and borrowings in conformity with the six conditions mentioned. While the surface causes mentioned in the preceding paragraph are necessary to explain slight local variations of interest as between New York and Boston, or to explain slight daily or monthly changes of interest rates by a fraction of one per cent, the differences in human impatience in incomes and in price movements are the underlying influences which explain why the rates in America or China are several per cent higher than in England or Holland, and why the rates in one epoch of history are two or three times as high as in some other epoch. In short, interest rates are like the ocean, the level of which is slightly and temporarily influenced by winds, but more fundamentally by great tidal forces.

6. Historical Illustrations

We have now completed our study of the causes determining the rate of interest. If they are correct, we should find that the rate of interest is low (1) if in general the people are by nature thrifty, farsighted, self-controlled, or thoughtful for the future welfare of their children, or (2) if they have large or descending income-streams; and that it is high (1) if the people are shiftless, shortsighted, impulsive, selfish, or (2) if they have small or ascending income-streams.

History shows that facts accord with these conclusions. The communities and nationalities which are most noted for the qualities mentioned–foresight, self-control, and regard for posterity–are probably Holland, Scotland, England, and France. Among these people interest has been low. Moreover, they have been money lenders; they have the habit of thrift or accumulation, and their instruments of wealth are in general of a durable kind.

On the other hand, among communities and peoples noted for lack of foresight and for negligence with respect to the future are China, India, Java, the negro communities in the Southern states, the peasant communities of Russia, and the North and South American Indians, both before and after they had been pushed to the wall by the white men. In all of these communities we find that interest is high, that there is a tendency to run into debt and to dissipate rather than accumulate capital, and that their dwellings and other instruments are of a very flimsy and perishable character, built for immediate, not remote, gratifications. This is true even where, as in China, the people are industrious. Industry without patience will result in hard work, but this work will be for immediate and not remote gratifications.

These examples illustrate the effect on the rate of interest of differences in human nature. We now turn to illustrations of differences in the distribution in time of incomes. The most striking examples of increasing income-streams are found in new countries. It may be said that the United States has almost always belonged to this category.

In America we see exemplified on a very large scale the truth of the theory that a rising income-stream raises, and a falling income-stream depresses, the rate of interest, or that these conformations of the income-stream work out their effects in other equivalent forms. A similar causation may be seen in particular localities in the United States, especially where changes have been rapid, as in mining communities. In California, in the two decades between 1850 and 1870, following the discovery of gold, the income-stream of that state was increasing at a prodigious rate. During this period the rates of interest were abnormally high. The current rates in the " early days " were quoted at one and one half to two per cent a month. " The thrifty Michael Reese is said to have half repented of a generous gift to the University of California, with the exclamation, Ah, but I lose the interest, a very natural regret when interest was twenty-four per cent per annum." After railway connection in 1869, Eastern loans began to flow in. The decade 1870-1880 was one of transition during whlch the phenomenon of high interest was gradually replaced by the phenomenon of borrowing from outside. The residents of California were thus able to change the distribution in time of their income-streams. The rate of interest consequently dropped from eleven per cent to six per cent.

The same phenomena of enormous interest rates were also exemplified in Colorado and the Klondike. There were many instances in both these places during the transition period from poverty to affluence, when loans were contracted at over fifty per cent per annum, and the borrowers regarded themselves as lucky to get rates so " low." In general the pioneer is willing to pay a high rate of interest so long as he cherishes the " great expectations " characteristic of new countries.

7. Interest and Prices

We have seen that the rate of interest is not a mere technical phenomenon, restricted to Wall Street and other " money markets," but that it permeates all economic relations. It is the link which binds man to the future and by which he makes all his far-reaching decisions.

The rate of interest is itself a sort of price and plays a central rôle in the theory of other prices. It operates in the determination of the price of wealth, property, and benefits. It enters into the price of securities, real estate, and commodities, as well as into rent, wages, and the value of all " interactions." As was shown in previous chapters, the price of any article of wealth or property is equal to the discounted value of its expected future benefits. If the value of these benefits remains the same, a rise or fall in the rate of interest will cause a fall or rise respectively in the value of all instruments of wealth. The extent of this fall or rise will be the greater, the farther into the future the benefits of wealth extend.

As to the influence of the rate of interest on the price of benefits, we first observe that benefits may be interactions or satisfactions. The value of interactions is derived from the succeeding future benefits to which they lead. For instance, the value to a farmer of the benefits of his land in affording pasture for sheep will depend upon the discounted value of the benefits from the flock in producing wool. The value of the wool output to the woolen manufacturer is in turn influenced by the discounted value of the output of woolen cloth to which it contributes. In the next stage, the value of the production of woolen cloth will depend upon the discounted value of the income from the production of woolen clothing. Finally, the value of the last named will depend upon the expected income which the clothing will bring to its wearers–in other words, upon the use of the clothes.

Thus the fInal benefits, consisting of the use of the clothes, will have an influence on the value of all the anterior benefits of tailoring, manufacturing cloth, producing wool, and pasturing sheep, while each of these anterior benefits, when discounted, will give the value of the respective capital which yields it; namely, the clothes, cloth, wool, sheep, and pasture. We find, therefore, that not only all articles of wealth, but also all the " interactions " which they render, are dependent, for their value, upon final enjoyable uses, and are linked to these final uses by the rate of interest. If the rate of interest rises or falls, this chain will shrink or expand. The chain hangs, so to speak, by its final link of enjoyable benefits, and its shrinkage or expansion will therefore be most felt by the links most distant from these final benefits. At the close of Chapter VI it was shown that a change in the rate of interest only slightly affects the value of a suit of clothes, the benefits from which are soon realized, but greatly affects the value of land, the benefits of which stretch out into the distant future. So a change in the rate of interest will affect but slightly the price of making clothing since the final benefits from making clothing will occur in a short time, but it will affect materially the price of pasture for sheep since the final benefits from the pasturing will require a long time.

A study, therefore, of the theory of prices involves (1) a study of the laws which determine the prices of final benefits on which the prices of anterior interactions depend; (2) a study of the prices of these anterior interactions, as dependent, through the rate of interest, on the final benefits; (3) a study of the price of capital-instruments and capital-property as dependent, through the rate of interest, upon the prices of their benefits. The first study, which seeks merely to determine the laws regulating the price of final benefits, is relatively independent of the rate of interest. The second and third, which seek to show the dependence on final benefits of the anterior

benefits and of the capitals which bear them, involve and depend upon the rate of interest.

In the theory of prices we found that the ultimate elements supplied and demanded were satisfactions and efforts. But we now see that there is involved in each price another special price, viz., the rate of interest. Without the rate of interest we may only compare simultaneous satisfactions or efforts. With it we may compare all that exist. By means of the rate of interest any future satisfaction or effort is discounted, and thus translated into terms of present value. It enables us to pause at every step and appraise the interactions and capital which anticipate future satisfactions. In other words, by it we capitalize income and form our capital accounts.

Interest, then, is the universal time-price, linking impending and remote satisfactions, or efforts, or both. It is literally the previously missing link necessary for a complete comparison of efforts and satisfactions at all points of time.

The study of the rate of interest, therefore, rounds out and completes our study of prices.

8. Classification of Price Influences

We may now fitly review the theory of prices by enumerating the various possible causes which might decrease the price of, let us say, pig iron in New York. Its price might fall for any one or more of the following reasons:– I. A rise in the marginal desirability of money due either to

A. A rise in the purchasing power of money through 1. A decrease in money or deposit currency, or 2. A decrease in their velocities, or 3. An increase in the volume of trade; or to

B. An impoverishment or reduction of incomes.

IL A fall in the marginal desirability of pig iron due either to

A. An increase in the amount of pig iron used, through 1. Importation of pig iron from other places where its

price is lower than in New York, or 2. Short sales of pig iron for future delivery in expectation of a fall of price, thus releasing to present use such stocks as would otherwise be held over for the future, or 3. A decrease in its cost by a. A saving of waste, b. A saving of labor, c. A decrease in the price of iron ore or other prices entering into its cost, d. An increase in the price of by-products, or 4. A trade war; or to

B. A fall in the marginal desirability of a given quantity of pig iron, through 1. A decrease in the price of iron products through a decrease in the marginal desirability of the satisfactions they yield, because of a. An increase in their amount, b. A change in fashion, etc., or 2. An increase in substitutes for pig iron, or 3. A decrease in complementary articles, or 4. An increase in the rate of interest whereby the value of pig iron is obtained (by discounting the value of iron products) through an increase in the marginal rates of impatience, a. From a change in human nature (1) By decreasing foresight, (2) By decreasing self-control, (3) By increasing shiftless habits, (4) By decreasing regard for posterity, or b. From a change in incomes (1) By shifting their distribution in time toward the future.

(2) By reducing their size, (3) By increasing their uncertainties.

Back of these causes lie other causes, multiplying endlessly as we proceed backward. But if we trace back all of these causes to their utmost limits, they will all resolve themselves into changes in the marginal desirability or undesirability of satisfactions and of efforts, respectively, at different points of time, and in the marginal rate of impatience as between any one year and the next.

CHAPTER XXm INCOME FROM CAPITAL 1. Distribution according to Agents of Production and according to Owners

We began this book with a study of economic accounting. In this way we obtained a birds-eye view of the whole field of economic science. At that time we had to take ready-made the material for constructing our capital and income accounts. This material consisted of the values of various items, whether of capital or of income. These values are, in each case, the product of two factors, the quantity of the good valued and the price of that good. We have now finished the study of one of these two factors, price, and there remains for us only the study of the other, quantity. We have explained how the price of instruments, property rights, and benefits, which enter into capital and income accounts, is determined. We have still to explain how the quantities of instruments, property rights, and benefits are determined. What determines, for instance, the quantity of wheat which a given wheat field will produce; what determines the quantity of the wheat fields; what determines the quantities of human beings on a given area; what determines the quantities of the necessities, comforts, luxuries, and amusements of life which a nation or an individual possesses? Once we can explain these quantities, we have completed our task of explaining economic quantities, prices, and values. We shall then be able to explain–at least in general terms–why, for instance, the quantities and values of the capital or income, in capital-accounts or in income-accounts, of some communities or individuals are so great, and those of others so little; why the benefits flowing from one piece of land are so great, and from another so small; and so forth.

Our purpose is not so much to reach absolute, as relative, results. We care less about the absolute population of the globe than about population relatively to land. We care less about the worlds total yield of wood than about the yield per capita, or per acre; less about the total yield of cloth than about the yield per capita or per loom. In general, we care less about the total amount of the yield from the aggregate of any kind of capital than about the yield per capita and per unit of that particular kind of capital.

Our present search, then, is for relative quantities, or for relative values. There are two sets of such quantities, or of such values, which are of special importance in our study. One is the quantity and value of income per unit of capital which yields the income, and the other is the quantity and value of income and of capital per human being who owns the capital and the income from it. The first represents the distribution of income relatively to the agents which produce it. The second represents the distribution of income and of capital among their owners. The study of the first will occupy our attention in this and the following chapter. In the present chapter we shall consider income produced by capital (in its narrow sense, i. e., exclusive of human beings); in the following chapter we shall consider income produced by labor, or human beings.

It is well to bear in mind that income is usually a joint product of labor and capital; for labor and capital are usually " complementary" to each other, each helping the other to produce the joint product of both. It is convenient, however, in thought to separate the two.

Our immediate task, therefore, is to study the ratios of income to capital. We take up first the ratio of the value of the income to the quantity of capital which yields it.

This ratio is called rent. Rent as here used means the value of income yielded per physical unit of capital. Thus, land may yield a "rent" of 10 a year per acre; or houses, of 1000 a month per house. The concept of rent here employed is somewhat broader than the popular concept; for it includes, besides the rent explicitly named in a lease between landlord and tenant, the rent which is implicit when there are not two persons involved, but landlord and tenant are one and the same person. Explicit rent is rent in the usual and strict sense of the term. Implicit rent is often called capitalists profits. That is, rent is explicit when the income is stipulated; it consists of a definite payment for the use of the instrument. This occurs when the owner of the instrument sells its use, i. e., "lets" or "rents" it to another person and gets from it a definite money-income. Implicit rent occurs when the income is not stipulated, and therefore can only be appraised. When a landlord rents his land to a tenant for 1000 a year, the rent is explicitly 1000 a year; when, instead, he works the land himself and makes from it an income which consists in the production of crops, the rent is only implicit. Before he can state its amount he must appraise the crops, including both those portions which he sells and those consumed by himself and his family. If he appraises the crops and other benefits which he receives from the land at 3000 and the costs at 2000, his net income is 1000, and therefore his implicit rent is 1000. A " rented " house bears explicit rent, but a house lived in by the owner has an implicit rent, i. e., whatever benefits it yields to the owner reckoned over and above its costs.

The most common kind of instruments explicitly rented is real estate, although many other more or less durable commodities, such as furniture, horses and carriages, telephones, pianos, typewriters, and even clothing, may sometimes be explicitly rented.

Explicit rent, being stipulated, is usually fixed and certain
—at least for all practical purposes; implicit rent, on the other hand, is variable and uncertain.

2. The Rent of Land

Although a piece of real estate is usually rented as a whole, including both land and improvements thereon, sometimes the land and the improvements are rented separately. Thus a man may lease an empty building lot and then make a supplementary contract to lease a building to be erected thereon by the landlord. The rent of land separately is called ground rent. Even when ground rent is not separated in contract, it may, for purposes of discussion, be separated in thought; so that all land bears ground rent, either explicit or implicit. Ground rent has been the subject of a vast amount of discussion. It underlies, for instance, " the single tax " propaganda, which advocates that taxes shall be laid on ground rent alone.

There are two important peculiarities of land which are shared by very few other instruments. One of these peculiarities is that, practically speaking, the land in the world is fixed in quantity. Except-by filling in tidal lands, as in Holland, and in a few other instances, we cannot add to the worlds acreage; nor can we subtract from it. It is true that in some cases we may materially increase its productivity by irrigation, fertilizing, etc., on the one hand, or decrease it by erosion and exhaustion of the soil and other abuses on the other. These alterations in land are more important than has sometimes been recognized, and their importance is increasing. For the present, however, we shall assume a community in which the land remains unchanged, both in quality and quantity, possessing, as Ricardo expressed it, " natural and indestructible powers of the soil." For our purpose it is enough to assume that the land is indestructible. Whether it be natural or not is a matter of indifference; precisely the same principles of valuation apply to the land which was wrested by our ancestors from the wilderness as apply to land which was solely a gift of nature.

The second peculiarity of land is that its different qualities cannot, in most cases, be as fully separated and classified as the different qualities of most other kinds of wealth. We can sort wool, for instance, into different kinds or categories and label and sell each kind separately. The same is true of wheat or coffee or automobiles. Each separate kind is then regarded as a separate commodity. But it is not practicable to sort different kinds of land, because the different kinds are inextricably intermingled and cannot be moved apart, and because one element in the character of land–its situation–differs materially with every individual piece of land. Any classification which would really " standardize " lands,–that is, make the lands in any one class sufficiently homogeneous as to bear substantially the same price per acre,–would have to be too minute a classification to be of any practical value. In the case of ordinary commodities which are "standardized " there exists but one price for each category. But the price of land differs with each individual piece, varying almost continuously from nothing up to 870 a square foot, the record recently set in New York City.

The prices of land, for. the most part, follow the principles of substitutes or competing articles. It is true that the various lands are not all substitutes. A city building site is not a substitute for wheat land, nor is it a substitute for forest or mineral lands. But here, again, for the sake of simplicity, we first consider only wheat lands, and shall assume that all these wheat lands are incapable of any other product and differ only as to productivity of wheat. We therefore assume:– (1) That these wheat lands are fixed in quantity.

(2) That they differ in quality (i. e., productivity) by continuous gradation from very fertile to very infertile lands, each fixed and invariable as to wheat productivity and having no other product.

(3) That the cost of tilling each acre is likewise fixed and invariable, say 10.

(4) That the lands are substantially equal in accessibility (thus being in a common land-market and contributing wheat to a common wheat-market).

Let us suppose, as represented in Figure 46, an island fulfilling the three conditions above mentioned. In order

Fig. 46.

further to simplify the picture, let us suppose the most fertile land situated in the center capable of producing 25 bushels of wheat per acre per year, and the other lands arranged around it spiral fashion in the order of descending productivity. If there is a superabundance of the 25-bushel-per-acre land so that it can be had merely for the trouble of occupying it, and there is no prospect that any inferior grades will ever need to be used, the land will be, like air, without value, and will yield no rent. The reason is that the supply of land of the first quality, which may be had free, exceeds the amount demanded. We have seen that under such extreme conditions of supply and demand the price is low. No one will pay for the use of land when, without traveling farther than across a field, there is plenty of equally good land to be had for nothing. The wheat, however, will have a price equal, as previously explained, to its marginal desirability measured in money and also to its marginal cost measured in money. But we have already assumed that this cost is fixed for each grade of land and is the same for every bushel. Consequently tf1e price of wheat is in this case simply equal to the marginal cost of producing the wheat. For, if sellers should try to sell above this cost, buyers would prefer to grow the wheat at that cost themselves. Hence the value of a bushel produced on an acre of the first-grade land is only just equal to the cost of producing wheat there, which, at 10 per acre for 25 bushels, is 10-5-25, or 40 cents per bushel. But if the population so changes as to create a demand for wheat which cannot be supplied from the most fertile land, some of the next grade of land will be used, yielding 24 bushels per acre. What was before true of only the first-grade land will then be true of this second-grade land. It will be valueless, and will yield no rent. But no longer will this be true of the first-grade land. It will have a value and yield a rent. For there will be a rise in the price of wheat. The price will still be equal to the marginal cost, but now the marginal cost is the cost of producing a bushel on the second-grade land. The value of the 24 bushels produced on this land will now be equal to the cost of producing 24 bushels on that land, i. e., 10. The marginal cost is, therefore, 10-5-24, or 41.6 cents a bushel.

But since there cannot be two prices for the same article in the same market, the price of the wheat produced on the first-grade land must be the same as that produced on the second grade. Consequently, the owners of the first-grade land now have a crop worth more than the cost of producing it, and can now, if they choose, obtain a rent for it equal to the excess, i. e., one bushel per acre; for a tenant paying the equivalent of one bushel per acre would have 24 bushels for himself, which is exactly the same as he would get if he took up a claim for himself on the second-grade land; and if the landlord should attempt to charge more, he would lose his tenant, as the latter would then be better off on the second-grade land. If he charged less, he would be besieged by applications, and would put up his price. The market would be cleared by a rent of one bushel per acre. In money this is 41.6 cents per acre. If the owner does not rent his land to another, but enjoys the product himself, he is still said to obtain 41.6 cents an acre of implicit rent.

If the population changes again so as to require a resort to the third-grade land, the price will be still higher, viz., 10 -t-23, or 433 cents per bushel; and the rent of the first-grade land will rise to equal the difference between its productivity and that of the third-grade land, viz., 2 bushels per acre or 2 x 43! cents, i. e., 87 cents per acre. Likewise the second-grade land will now bear a rent equal to its superiority over the third grade, viz., one bushel per acre, or 435 cents. In the same way we may reckon the rent under other states of land-occupation. In each case the rent of any grade of land is the difference between its productivity and the productivity of the worst or marginal land occupied. If, for instance, the lowest grade of land occupied is that indicated in the table as having a productivity of 9 bushels per acre, the rent of the first grade is now 25–9, or 16 bushels per acre; that of the second grade, 24–9, or 15 bushels per acre; that of the next, 23–9, or 14 bushels per acre; and so on down to the worst land, which bears no rent. Since the price of wheat is, in all cases, its cost of production on the worst, or no-rent land, it will now be 10 for 9 bushels, or 1.11 per bushel. Therefore in money the rents of the various lands from the best to the worst will be:– 16 X 1.11 or 17.76 per acre,

15 X 1.11 or 16.65 Per acre,

14 X 1.11 or 15.54 per acre,

etc.

The last, worst, or no-rent land, is sometimes also called the " Ricardian acre " in honor of Ricardo, who first stated this doctrine of land rent. Its scientific designation is " marginal acre "; that is, it is the last acre whose cultivation can be made to pay. This marginal land in a sense forms a standard by reference to which the rent of all other land may be measured, and the cost of producing wheat on this marginal land sets the price of wheat for all lands,–for there can be but one price of wheat in the same market.

We have reached, then, two important results true under the conditions supposed,–

(1) The price of wheat is equal to its cost of production on the margin of cultivation.

(2) Ground rent of any land is the difference between the productivity of that land and the productivity of land on the margin of cultivation (i. e., the poorest land cultivated).

With an increase of population, then, the price of wheat and the rent of wheat land will rise, and the owner of good land will become gradually wealthier merely through the increase in population. He receives an increase in rent; and therefore the value of land–i. e., the capitalized or discounted rent–will increase also. This increase in the value of the land is sometimes called the " unearned increment " because it is due to no labor on the part of the landowner. (It should be noted, however, that during the transition of rents from low to high, those who foresee a rise in rent will discount in advance the larger future rents; not all so-called " unearned increments " are unexpected.) These conclusions hold absolutely under the conditions assumed. But in the actual world these conditions are never exactly realized. Instead, we find:–

(1) Land is not absolutely fixed in quantity.

(2) The productivity of any piece of land is not fixed, but varies from time to time both in kind and in degree, and this productivity will vary with the price of its product, e. g., wheat.

(3) The cost of tilling land is not fixed, but varies with different land, and, indeed, as we shall presently show, is influenced by the price of the product.

(4) Some lands are much more distant to reach and occupy than others and their product much more difficult to bring to market.

(5) The land may be capable of more than the one use of wheat-growing, and a change in the price of wheat may shift the use to which certain lands are put. No theory of land rent is complete which assumes that the difference in quality among lands is merely a matter of different amounts of one product, like wheat.

We have already discussed the first of these points and find it to be of little practical importance. The second is that the productivity of land is not solely a matter of natural fertility. This might be the case with some mineral springs or oil wells; but in most cases each piece of land may be more or less intensively cultivated, and a rise in the price of wheat will stimulate wheat production on all lands, the better grades included. Thus, if the first grade produced 25 bushels when no other land was in use, it would, with more outlay, produce more than 25 bushels as soon as the next grade was in use; and the poorer the worst grade was, and the higher the price of wheat, the greater would be the amount grown by those cultivating the superior grades of land. In other words, a change in the price of wheat would not only affect the amount of land under cultivation, but would affect also the intensity of cultivation of each piece of land. The productivity of each acre is not a constant quantity, but is indirectly dependent on the price. Each acre will be cultivated up to that degree of intensity at which the last dollars worth of cost will barely repay itself. That is, not only is there a margin of cultivation as to acres–in other words, a last acre which it pays to cultivate–but there is also a margin of cultivation for every acre, good or bad, i. e., the last degree of effort or cost which it pays to put forth on that acre. Each acre will be tilled until this marginal cost of tilling agrees with the market price as determined by the cost of production on the most inferior land.

Again, as to the cost of tilling land per acre, this is by no means a constant quantity for all lands, both good and poor; nor is it constant even for the same land. The cost of tilling per acre may be either higher or lower on good land than on poor land; and, as implied above, the cost on any land will vary with the price of the product, just as the product itself varies with the price. The farther cultivation is extended to poorer and poorer lands or the more intensively the same land is cultivated, the greater will be the marginal cost. This is the law of increasing cost applied to agriculture. It is also often called " the law of diminishing returns "; for to say that, as cultivation is either extended or intensified, the cost of producing a given amount of wheat continually increases is, turned about, evidently the same thing as to say that the amount produced at a given cost continually diminishes. In an absolutely correct theory the numbers expressing productivity in Figure 46 must be conceived as increasing slightly as the margin of cultivation is extended, and the numbers expressing cost will not be simply a con slant 10 per each acre, but will differ among different kinds of land according as the soil is rocky or not resistant to the plow and harrow, level or uneven in surface, containing obstructions such as trees, or free of obstructions. Moreover the cost will not be invariable even for a given land but will increase slightly as the margin is extended.

Again, lands differ so widely as to accessibility that tenants are reluctant to leave English lands, for instance, to take up lands in the Mississippi valley. A slight advantage in the latter over the former will not suffice to produce emigration from the English to the American lands and to reduce the rents of the former. Only when the advantage is considerable will emigration ensue. The readjustments of population are therefore not as delicate as the readjustments of water between two connecting reservoirs seeking a common level. They resemble, rather, the readjustments of a viscous fluid like pitch which requires a considerable difference of level before the fluid will flow at all. The same viscosity applies in a less degree to the products of lands. These do not compete on even terms, for some lands are distant and others near the common market, and some have good and others poor transportation facilities. These differences are especially important in the case of bulky products such as hay which, for the reasons just given, differs very widely in price in different localities.

While, therefore, the theory of rent as above given is correct under the ideal conditions assumed, it is not absolutely correct under the actual conditions we find in the world. But the modifications necessary to make the theory of ground rent true to life are so slight as not materially to change the practical results. It still remains substantially true that the rent of any wheat land is equal to the difference between its productivity and the productivity of the worst wheat land under cultivation in the neighborhood.

3. Rent and Interest

The principles of ground rent apply also to house rent, piano rent, or rent of any other kind, except that much greater divergencies from such stereotyped figures as we gave for ground rent will be necessary in these cases. In particular, houses, pianos, etc., are not essentially fixed in quantity, but their quantity will be changed according to their rent and their price (which is the discounted value of their rent). The difference, then, between the rent of land and the rent of other instruments is a difference in the character of the supply. The supply of land is relatively fixed; other instruments are reproducible.1 It is important to understand this difference and also not to confuse it with a common fallacy that land rent alone is truly rent, and house rent and other rent are really interest. It is easy to see that land rent may be equal to interest on the capital-value of the land just as truly as house rent may be equal to the interest on the capital-value of the house. In that case both are rent and both are interest; they are simply two different ways of measuring the same income-value. Rent is measured per unit of physical capital, as for instance per acre; interest is measured per cent. That is, rent is income considered in relation to the quantity of the capital yielding it; it is expressed as so many dollars per acre or per piano or other rented unit of wealth. Interest is the same income considered relatively to the value of the capital yielding it; it is expressed as so many cents of income on the dol 1 This practical difference between ground rent and other rent, such as house rent, has an important application in taxation. It is not within the scope of this book to consider problems of taxation. In treatises on taxation it is shown that a tax on ground rent falls on the landlord and does not appreciably affect the tenant, because it cannot affect the supply of land, which is practically fixed by nature; whereas a tax on house rent is borne partly by the tenant, because it discourages house building and affects the supply of houses.

lar of capital, "., as a simple percentage, such as five per cent.

To illustrate, let us suppose a quantity of land–ten acres–to have a value of 1000, and that 50 a year is paid for its use. This 50 is both rent and interest. It is the rent on the ten acres and the interest on the 1000. The rent is 50 per year for 10 acres, or 5 per acre per annum. The interest is 50 per year for 1000, or five per cent per annum. In precisely the same way, let us suppose a quantity of houses–ten houses–to have a value of 100,000, and that 5000 a year is paid for their use. This 5000 is both rent and interest. It is the rent on ten houses and the interest on 100,000. The rent is 5000 per year for ten houses, or 500 per house per annum, and the interest is 5000 per year for 100,000, or five per cent per annum.

The erroneous belief that land bears only rent, and that other instruments bear only interest, is to a large extent responsible for the narrow definitions of capital which are so often given and which are so framed as specifically to exclude land. A true analysis justifies the usage of business men who apply the term " rent " as freely to income from houses as to income from land, and the term " interest " as freely to income from land as to income from houses.

4. Four Forms of Income: Interest, Rent, Dividends, and Profits If now we gather together what was said in regard to explicit and implicit rent and the relations between rent and interest, we shall see that there are four chief forms in which men receive income from capital. These are ordinarily known as interest, rent, dividends, and profits. In order to distinguish them clearly, let us suppose four brothers, each of whom inherits a fortune of 100,000. The first invests his 100,000 in a land company in one hun dred 1000 bonds at par bearing five per cent interest. He then receives 5000 a year, which is interest in the narrow or explicit sense of the term. The next brother invests his 100,000 in a ranch of a thousand acres, which he rents to a tenant for 5 an acre. He then receives an income of 5000 a year, which is rent in the narrow and explicit sense. The third brother invests his 100,000 in a hundred shares of stock in a land company, buying them at par, or 1000 per share. This stock we shall assume yields him five per cent, and he receives an income of 5000 in dividends (also called profits). The fourth brother invests his 100,000 in a ranch of a thousand acres, which he proceeds to operate himself. Supposing that he succeeds in securing a net income of 5 per acre, he will be receiving 5000 a year of profits. Each of these brothers is receiving an income of 5000 a year from capital in the form of real estate; but they are all receiving their income under different conditions. The four types of income may be arranged as follows:–.

(1) Interest per cent. (3) Dividends (or profits) per cent.

(2) Rent per acre. (4) Profits per acre.

In the upper line, namely for brothers (1) and (3), the income is expressed as a percentage of the value of the capital. In the lower line, namely, for brothers (2) and (4), the income is expressed per acre. As we have seen, either expression can be translated into the other.

Again the first column, namely for brothers (1) and (2), represents the explicit or assured income, while the second column, namely, for brothers (3) and (4), represents the implicit or uncertain income. The first two brothers have an assured or stipulated income of 5000. The last two have an uncertain or precarious income which, though we have supposed it to be 5000, may, and probably will, fluctuate from time to time. There is a fundamental difference between the first two and the last two brothers in regard to the risk involved. The first two are supposedly relieved of risk, some one else assuming the risks of managing the land of the company or of running the ranch, and guaranteeing to these brothers a certain stipend of 5000 a year each. Corresponding to this fundamental difference in risk is a fundamental difference in variability. The incomes of the first two brothers are regular; those of the last two are irregular. Where there are risks or chances to be taken there is irregularity of income as a consequence.

It is evident that some one must assume these risks. Uncertainty attaches to the future product because we can never know absolutely the conditions as to weather, blight, fire, labor conditions, etc. Nature never offers a perfectly safe investment. What is called a safe investment is always in the form of a contract between one man and another by which one man takes risks and guarantees another man against risks. Even then the guarantee is not perfect, so that the most " gilt-edged security " involves a slight element of risk, while in many cases little dependence can be placed upon a guarantee because of the unreliability of the person making it.

Nevertheless, it remains true in a general way that explicit income promised to the holder of a note or bond is comparatively certain, while the income to a stockholder is uncertain. Investors, therefore, are naturally divided into two groups: those who are unwilling to assume the risks of business, or bondholders, and those who are willing to assume these risks, or stockholders. Most modern enterprises are financed by both of these two classes of investors, part, often half, being owned by the bondholders and the remainder by the stockholders. As we have seen in the study of capital accounts, the stockholders share is the residuum after the value of all other obligations is deducted; and this residuum acts as a sort of a buffer or guarantee that the assets shall cover the liabilities. The smaller the fractional part assumed by the stockholders, the less adequate is this margin or guarantee and the greater the risk of large losses to the stockholders or even of complete bankruptcy. Therefore, in any proper financiering of an industrial project, care should be taken to provide that enough of the first cost should be paid by stockholders to fully guarantee the bonds. Exactly what constitutes a safe proportion will depend on the particular circumstances of the business. Experience, however, has determined certain fairly definite proportions for stocks and bonds of different enterprises. These should be ascertained by the intending investor before entering into any particular project.

The question now arises: What determines the rate at which the risk takers in a business, those who receive dividends and profits, shall be rewarded? Will all four brothers normally receive the same income? To this our answer is, first, that those who assume risk may receive either a larger or a smaller income than those who do not, and probably over a long period of time will receive a fluctuating instead of a steady income. Probably on the average the risk takers will receive a larger income than those guaranteed against risk; for risk is, or should be, regarded as a burden and will not be undertaken unless the chance of unusually large returns outweighs the risk of unusually small ones. The daring spirits who assume the risk of embarking their capital in ships, railways, and other enterprises and guarantee to their fellow-investors, the bondholders, a fixed return, not only deserve, but in general receive, a higher return. Those who voluntarily assume risks, as the stockholder, do so not because they like the chance of taking risks, but because they hope hi the long run to be sufficiently rewarded for so doing. They may, of course, be disappointed where bad luck has been unusually persistent or where the investors have been unusually sanguine and lacking in caution.

At the extreme of incaution are the gamblers and reckless speculators to whom a small chance of great gain out

weighs a great risk of moderate losses; and where men of this temperament predominate, as is often true in mining camps, the average profits or dividends are apt to be less than the interest and rent which the cautious, conservative investor receives.

5. Avoidance of Risk

Uncertainty being regarded as an evil by practically all normal persons, there is a constant effort to avoid or reduce uncertainties of income. Not only do bondholders avoid risks by shifting them to other persons, but those who thus assume risks also strive to reduce them to a minimum. This they accomplish in various ways, of which the following are important: (1) by increasing their knowledge of the future, (2) by employing safeguards against mischances, (3) by insurance, (4) by speculative contracts, especially " hedging." We shall take these up in order.

(1) Risk, being simply an expression for human ignorance, decreases with the progress of knowledge. The chief lines of progress in industry at the present time may be said to be those which tend to lift the veil which hides the future. Countless trade journals exist principally to enable their readers to forecast the future more accurately than they otherwise could. This the journals accomplish by supplying data as to past and present conditions, as well as by instructing their readers in the relations of cause and effect. Our government weather bureau supplies weather forecasts which somewhat reduce this form of uncertainty for the farmers. Government reports of crop conditions and information as to diseases of plants and animals are more important influences in the same direction. Again the prediction as to the amount of ore to be obtained from a mine and the cost of obtaining it is to-day far less uncertain than ever before. Whereas formerly the mining prospect consisted of wild statements of the ore " in sight," and the time and cost required to mine it, to-day the graduate of a mining school can, through his knowledge of economic geology and metallurgy, make forecasts with some degree of certainty.

(2) Safeguards of many kinds have been invented to reduce the risk of shipwreck, fire, explosion, burglary, etc. A modern ship is built in compartments as a safeguard against shipwreck; fire escapes are a safeguard against loss of life by fire; safety valves against explosions; and burglar alarms and safety deposit vaults against burglary.

(3) Insurance consists in consolidating risks, i. e., in offsetting one risk by another by consolidating in one insurance company a large number of chances. Relative certainty is, as it were, manufactured out of uncertainty. Insurance, unlike increase of knowledge and safeguards, does not directly decrease the risks for society as a whole, but by pooling these risks it has the effect of steadying the income of individuals and spreading the burden of risk more evenly over all. The owner of a house would receive, if it were not insured, a net annual income of, let us say, 500 until the house was burned, after which he would suddenly find himself without any house

to have an income from; whereas if he insures, he will be receiving annually an income slightly less than before because of the insurance premium he will have to pay; but when a fire occurs, he will receive an indemnity enabling him to restore the house and continue his income almost unabated. The same method of steadying ones income is obtained by marine insurance, steam-boiler insurance, burglar insurance, plate-glass insurance, live-stock insurance, hail and cyclone insurance, accident and fidelity insurance, employers liability insurance, and even life insurance. If a wife holds insurance on her husbands life, she avoids the evil, when widowed, of being left relatively destitute; for the insurance provides her with an income which is a partial substitute for that formerly received from her husband. He and she prefer to sacrifice a yearly premium during his lifetime to avoid the risk of the sudden complete loss of income to her at his death. In short, the effect of pooling risks through insurance frees the individual of the large fluctuations in income which would otherwise be suffered. The income of society fluctuates less, relatively speaking, than that of the individuals composing society. This is true because the evils which form the extraordinary catastrophes in individual lives constitute a regular stream of events in the life of society. Death in a family is an unusual catastrophe, but the number of deaths in a community forms a regular and predictable series of events. To the owner of only a few vessels the shipwreck of one of them is an extraordinary catastrophe, but the shipwrecks of the world constitute a regular and predictable series of events. The same is true of accidents and mischances of all kinds. They are irregular for the individual and regular for society. When, therefore, society through insurance companies and otherwise consolidates these risks, the individual gains an advantage by securing greater certainty and regularity in his individual income, even though the average income of the individual is not increased at all, in fact is decreased, by the cost of conducting the insurance companies.

In this last connection it should be noted that insurance indirectly leads to the reduction of risk; for insurance companies find it to their interest to reduce the risk against which they insure. Marine insurance companies expect the ships to secure the installation of safety devices. Fire insurance companies do likewise, and to-day even life insurance companies are beginning to advise their policy holders how to reduce the chances of death.

In view of all that has been said, it is evident that insurance is one of the grandest of human devices in the warfare against risk. As its importance has gradually been appreciated, its use has been steadily extended, and in some cases, as in Germany, its employment (in certain cases affecting workingmen) has been made compulsory.

(4) It seems at first to be a curious fact that speculation, although dealing in chances, may be used to reduce chance to some persons who use it for this purpose. We have already seen how short selling reduces the risk to the person sold to. A building contractor when taking a large contract was asked whether he was not taking a large risk, since he could not know in advance what the costs would be. He replied, "No, I am taking no risks at all except on labor; I have made contracts to be supplied with material when needed at fixed prices." In other words, dealers had sold him future building materials " short." They had each assumed the risk of fluctuation in those special materials in which they dealt, thus relieving the contractor of the necessity

of informing himself of the special market conditions on stone, brick, timber, etc. Similar results follow from short sales of wool to the woolen manufacturer previously cited in another connection.

An important method of shifting risks is " hedging," whereby a dealer, for instance in transporting wheat, may be relieved of the risk of a change in price. He buys wheat in the West intending to ship it to New York and sell it there at enough to cover cost of transportation and a small profit. He aims to make a gain in the form of " arbitrage," that is, a gain due to a difference in price between different places; but as the transportation requires time, he finds himself running the risk of a loss–or gain–due to a difference in price between different times. By hedging he eliminates the time gain or loss and retains the place gain. If he did not " hedge," he might, in consequence of a sudden fall in price, find all his profit wiped out; or he might, on the other hand, by a rise in price, make much more than normal profits. Being of a cautious disposition, he prefers an intermediate course–a small profit which is sure, rather than the chances of both gain and loss. Consequently he " hedges " against loss. " Hedging " against a loss from the risks of ones business is speculation so ar ranged that if the man loses in his regular business he will win in his speculation, or if he gains in his regular business he will lose in his speculation. It is like betting on both sides of a contest at the same time. The result eliminates largely the effect of risk so that he neither gains nor loses from mere chance. Thus let our supposed wheat dealer enter into some speculative market, such as Chicago, knowing that its prices will move in sympathy with the New York market, and there " speculate " for a fall, or sell " short." If the price of wheat happens to fall he will lose on the wheat which he has transported, but he will gain in his speculation. Evidently this man is running a double set of chances. A fall in price will bring him loss on the wheat he is transporting to New York; but, on the other hand, it will bring him gain in his speculation in Chicago. Contrariwise, if the price rises, he will gain on his wheat transported, but lose in the speculative market. He can draw his speculative contrast in such a way and for such an amount that for every cent per bushel of fall of price he will gain a cent per bushel in his speculation, and for every cent per bushel of rise of price he will lose a cent per bushel in his speculation. In this way he will practically eliminate all loss as well as all profit arising from a change of price in time and keep intact the profit arising from a difference in price between places, i. e., he retains the arbitrage gains of his regular business and foregoes the speculative gains or losses, which are not his business. He only obtains his normal profit, commission, or percentage on the actual wheat handled, throwing the burden of risk of speculation on the speculative dealers to whom he sells short.

Now it is evident that the effect of the short sales we have mentioned and of hedging is to shift the risk from those less able and willing to those more able and willing to bear it. Those grain merchants who hedge, for instance, are relieved of a big risk which they would suffer if they did not hedge. Thus, strange as it may seem, they run less risk by speculating through " hedging " than by not speculating at all; and as they thus reduce the risk of their business they are enabled to reduce their margin of profit. Consequently, the public in the end receives a benefit in cheaper grain. The case is thus very similar to that of the builder and the woolen manufacturer. Short selling and hedging, binding the future and the past, enable the student of special risks to guarantee the future to the general public. Risk is one of the direst economic evils, and all of the devices which aid in overcoming it–whether increased guarantees, safeguards, foresight, insurance, or legitimate speculation–represent a great boon to humanity.

If risk could be completely eliminated, the profit of the stockholder would be more certain and steady and would average the same rate as the returns of those who receive explicit interest and rent. But, although there is a continual effort and tendency to reduce and consolidate risks, we can never expect in this world absolute certainty, and, as long as risks exist, there will be an important practical distinction between the income received in explicit interest and rent by such persons as the first two brothers and the profits and dividends received by those represented by the last two brothers. The former will always receive a certain and steady but small income, while the latter will receive a fluctuating but, on the average, a relatively large income.

CHAPTER XXIV INCOME FROM LABOR 1. Similarity of Rent and Wages

We have seen that income always has a source, and that this source is either labor or capital, or, more usually, both jointly. We thus have two great agents in the production of income, labor and capital.1 The income from capital we have called " rent." The income from labor is called " wages."2

Corresponding to the distinction between explicit and implicit rent, we may distinguish between explicit and implicit wages, explicit wages being wages actually paid to a hired person, called the employee, by the person hiring him, called the employer; and implicit wages being the earnings of a person who does not sell his services, but enjoys them himself. Such a person we have already called an enterpriser.3 The earnings which the enterpriser secures (so far as he secures them by working as an enterpriser) are called enterprisers profits.

1 As has been previously stated, " capital" is used in this book to include land. Land is so important and peculiar a kind of capital that many writers prefer to make of it a special category and therefore to distinguish three agents of production–labor, land, and capital. It is also common to restrict the term " capital" still further by excluding goods in the hands of consumers or by other restrictions. The terminology here adopted is believed to be the most serviceable and also to conform more closely than most other textbook terminologies to the usage of business men.

! The term " wages " is here used to include those forms dignified as " salaries." The usual distinction between wages and salaries is merely one of degree, and has no scientific significance.

Sometimes the French term " entrepreneur" is used. The English equivalent " undertaker," in the sense of one who undertakes an enterprise, was formerly in vogue, but has fallen into disuse, perhaps because of its special application to funeral directors. 2 F 433

The income of a community may therefore be classified into rent and wages, and each of these subdivided into explicit and implicit classes. We thus have four great branches of income–explicit rent, explicit wages, implicit rent (or capitalists profits), and implicit wages (or enterprisers profits).

Moreover, since the income included under rent (explicit or implicit) may be measured with reference to the value of the capital producing this income, it may also, as we have seen, be regarded as interest (explicit or implicit).1

Practically, therefore, we may divide the income of a community into six main parts simply by separating out from rent, whether explicit or implicit, the part which is reckoned in terms of the value of capital, i. e., that part which is interest, whether explicit or implicit. While it is true that all rent may be translated into interest, only part of rent is, in the actual world of business, so expressed. We therefore find in the modern world six great branches of income considered in reference to the source from which it comes. These are commonly called wages and enterprisers profits, rent and capitalists profits, interest and dividends. The first pair are measured per man, the next pair per acre or other physical unit of capital, and the last pair as a percentage of capital-value. All six branches of income may be arranged as follows: 2– 1 In order to make a corresponding measurement of wages, i. e., wages relatively to the value of the men who earn them, we should need to appraise the value of free human beings. As this is both difficult and of little practical use, it will here be disregarded.

2 The classification of income here given corresponds closely to that of business men, but differs somewhat from that in most other textbooks. A very common textbook classification of income divides it into rent, wages, interest, and profits. Of these four terms " wages " is generally employed in the same sense as in this book. But the terms "rent" and " profit" are in many books employed in other senses. Thus the term " rent " is usually restricted by economists to income from land. It excludes, for instance, the rent of houses. The term " profits " is used in many different senses, but is often restricted to enterprisers profits.

The student of economics needs to accustom himself to study carefully the terminology of each economic writer. Otherwise the conflict among these writers and the discrepancy between most of their concepts and the usage of business men may be found confusing.

Explicit Implicit

From Capital IInterest P61"cent Profits Per cent (dividends) I Rent per acre I Profits per acre

From Labor Wages per man Profits per man

The principles governing the rate of wages are, in a general way, similar to those governing the rate of rent. The rate of a mans wages per unit of time is the product of the price per piece of the work he turns out multiplied by his rate of output in that time. His productivity depends on technical conditions, including especially his size, strength, skill, and cleverness, while the price per piece of his services depends upon the general principles of supply and demand as already set forth.

The productivity of any capital, whether human or external, will differ with the capital. Men differ in quality, i. e., in productive power, as truly as lands or other instruments differ. Some men have a high degree of earning power and some have not. Some men can work twice as fast as others. Some men can do higher grades of work than others. The result is that we find men classified as common manual laborers, skilled manual laborers, common mental workers, superintending workers, and enterprisers. Just as we can measure the rent of any land by the difference in productivity between that and the low-rent, or no-rent, land, in exactly the same way we can measure the difference in productivity between men. There is no grade of workmen called the " no-wages men," but there would be such a grade if it were customary for their employer to pay for their cost of support (as the employer of land pays for its cost), so that only the excess above this cost were to be called wages. There are, indeed, men so incompetent that their net earning power is nearly zero, and they can

barely earn enough to support themselves. These incompetents may be unfortunates, as in the case of invalids and imbeciles, or blameworthy, as in the case of indolents. But whatever the cause may be, they roughly correspond in economic analysis to no-rent land.

2. Peculiarities of Labor Supply

But owing to the fundamental fact that a laborer, unlike any other instrument, is owned by himself and not, except in slavery, by another, there are certain peculiarities of wages as compared with rent. These peculiarities lie in the supply curve. We shall note four of these peculiarities.

In the first place, the supply curve of human services ascends very rapidly and often even " curls back," as previously explained (Chapter XVII, 3). This peculiarity, as we saw, was due to the fact that a mans desire for more money (marginal desirability of money) decreases rapidly with an increase of his earnings. Beyond a certain point the more he is paid, the less he will work. We may state the same fact in the reverse direction, and say that under certain circumstances the less a man is paid, the harder he will work. The shape of his supply curve will depend in very large measure on whether or not he has other sources of income besides his work.

Figure 47 exhibits this fact. The curve SSS" represents the supply curve of work for a well-to-do or rich man who has income from other sources than his work, and the curve sss" that for a poor man, who has to depend on what he can earn. The " rich " man represented in the diagram will not work at all for any wages below a certain price, say 1 an hour, or 05. Any price above this will induce him to work a little. Thus for 1.20 an hour he will work about two hours; for 1.40 an hour, about three and one half hours; and for 2 an hour, about five hours. But if the price exceeds a certain height, and, represented in the diagram as 2 an hour, the result will be that he will work less rather than more. These relations correspond with observed facts. A millionaire will not work for a day laborers wages. He may work a few days in the year for 100 a day, and work more days for 500 a day, but 1000 a day may lead him to work fewer days, 2.eo and devote more time to vacations and to enjoying his large income.

The poor man will be guided by similar considerations. His curve will be lower vertically, but wider horizontally–. if the measure of work in each case is in hours of work. Owning little or nothing besides his person, he cannot afford to be idle. Unemployment for him is seldom voluntary. So long as he can get a price for his work sufficient to keep him out of the poorhouse, he will work for that price. Thus, the minimum price which is necessary to induce him to work rather than become a tramp or beggar is represented in the diagram by Os, the very small sum of ten cents an hour. We note that it takes only a relatively slight rise in that price to induce him to work a full day. The height of 5 represents the price at which he will work the greatest number of hours. Above this he will prefer slightly shorter hours. As already stated, it is probable that the eight-hour move ment to-day is partly due to the fact that wages are high enough to enable the laborer to afford some leisure instead of being so low as to " keep his nose close to the grindstone."

I 234.56788 10 II 12 hours

Fig. 47.

A reduction in wages works in the opposite way, making workmen willing to work longer hours. Only when the price falls much below the elbow at 5 will they refuse longer to endure the low wages and long hours. They will then prefer, if not to starve, to throw themselves upon the mercy and charity of the community. The general level of the curve between the elbow, s, and the beginning, s, represents their minimum standard of living which they require if they work at all.

Now, if wages keep high and the workmen have a sufficiently low degree of impatience for income to enable them to accumulate savings, they become more " independent," which, as applied to their supply curve sss, means that it shifts a little toward the rich mans supply curve SSS". The result is a higher minimum wage necessary to induce the laborer to work and a smaller maximum number of hours which he is willing to work. The intersection with the demand curve will therefore tend to be higher and may be farther to the left; that is, the market rate of wages may be higher and the hours worked fewer.

This result is not du2 to any reduction in the number of workmen, but simply to a reduction in their intensity of desire for money. Savings, therefore, making workmen more independent and less necessitous, will–by lessening their desire for money–both increase their wages and shorten their hours.

A second peculiarity in regard to wages is that, except under slavery, the earnings of a laborer are seldom discounted for the purpose of ascertaining his capital-value. The reason for making any appraisement usually has reference to some proposed sale; and, as working men and women are no longer for sale, their capital-value is seldom com puted. For this reason, wages, unlike rent, are not often regarded in the light of interest on the capital-value of the agents earning them.

A third peculiarity of wages is one already alluded to, viz., that in practice they are always reckoned as gross and never as net. This is because the wages are reckoned from the standpoint of the employer who pays them, and not of the laborer who receives them. Under slavery the case was different, and the net income earned by a slave was computed in the same way as the net income earned by a horse–by deducting from the value of the work done the cost of supporting the slave. But under the system of free labor which now prevails, the employer has no such cost. The laborer assumes his own support, and furnishes only his work to the employer. The wages of the laborer are therefore reckoned gross. His net wages, if they are to be computed at all, are to be found by allowing for the irksome-ness of his work, i. e., the real costs which he bears of labor and trouble. At the margin–i. e., for the last unit of work done–this cost is, as we have seen, equal to the wages received for it; but on all earlier units of work there is a gain of desirability which might conceivably be appraised in money. The net wages thus reckoned will be only a part of the wages as ordinarily quoted.

When, therefore, we compare the 500 a year which a workman gets by selling his work with the 500 a year which a bondholder gets as interest, we must not forget that the workmans 500 is really less valuable than the bondholders 50x3, and for two reasons. One is the reason just given, that the workmans 500 is obtained only by the sweat of his brow, while the bondholders is all clear gain; the other reason is that the workmans 500 will cease at his death or disablement, while the bondholders goes on forever.

A fourth peculiarity concerning wages is that the supply of wage earners differs from the supply of any other instru

mer1t. Except in slavery, workmen are not bred like cattle on commercial principles. A rise in the price of the services of a draft horse will increase the demand for draft horses, and the result will be that both the market price and the amount supplied at that price will be increased. Those who supply draft horses will breed them to take advantage of the higher prices of them and their services. A rise in the price of human services will not act so simply. It is true that a rise in wages usually increases the number of marriages and often increases the birth, rate, but such is not always or necessarily the result; and even when births do increase in number, they do not increase on the same commercial principles as the draft horses. It is an exceptional father who can think or say as did a cynical old farmer who had raised a large family and thriftily turned their child labor to early account for his own benefit: " My children have been the best crop I ever raised." Ordinarily parents view their children not as potential earning power, but as objects of affection, and either do not attempt to regulate their numbers, or do so with reference to consideration for their own or their childrens comfort. The principles which regulate the number of laborers are part of the principles regulating population in general, and will be considered in the next chapter.

3. The Demand for Labor

Turning now from the supply to the demand side of the market, we find that the demand of employers for the services of workmen is in general quite analogous to their demand for the services of land or of any other productive agent. Sentiment and humanity have a little influence, but not enough to require special attention on our part. Wages are paid by the ordinary employer as the equivalent of the discounted future benefits which the laborers work will bring to him–the employer–and the rate he is willing to pay is equal to the marginal desirability of the laborers services measured in present money. We wish to 1. emphasize the fact that the employers valuation is (1), marginal, and (2) discounted. The employer pays for all his workmens services on the basis of the services least desirable to him, just as the purchaser of coal buys it all on the basis of the ton least desirable to him; he watches the " marginal " benefits he gets exactly as does the purchaser of coal. At a given rate of wages he " buys labor" up to the point where the last or marginal mans work is barely worth paying for. This marginal unit of work is a sort of barometer of wages. The employers problem in buying labor is the same as the householders problem in buying coal discussed in a previous chapter. He is constantly balancing in his mind the desirability of the work of his employees against the undesirability of the wages he pays for that work. If, say, he decides on one hundred men as the number he will employ, this is because the hundredth or marginal man he employs is believed to be barely worth his wages, while the man just beyond this margin, the one hundred and first man, is not taken on because the additional work he would do is believed to be not quite worth his wages.

Secondly, wages which the employer pays are the discounted value of the future benefits he receives. Thus, the shepherd hired by the farmer to tend the sheep in the pasture renders benefits the value of which to the farmer is estimated in precisely the same way as the value of the benefits of the land which he hires, i. e., by discounting the value of the future yield of wool or other benefits toward the production of which the shepherds work contributes. To take another example, suppose a landowner is contemplating the planting of 10,000 trees which he believes will be worth as lumber in twenty years about S10, o00, or one dollar per tree planted. His problem is: How much is it worth his while to pay per tree for the planting? The answer depends on the rate of interest. If this is three and a half per cent, it is worth his while to pay 50 cents per tree planted, for the present value (1 discounted for twenty years at three and a half per cent) is $1-=-(1.0)20$, which is 50 cents (Chapter VI, 4). As some trees may require more and some less labor, the landowner will limit his tree planting at that point or margin where the cost of the labor amounts to about 50 cents per tree. It follows that wages, like rent, are dependent upon the rate of interest.

Every employer, in deciding whether his workmen are worthy of their hire, takes account of the probable future product and the time he must wait for it. If he undertakes to put up a sky scraper, he discounts the rent he expects to get for it when finished. On that basis he decides whether or not he can afford to build it at current wages, and his decision will tend to affect those wages. The same is true of the manufacturer making cloth or the organizers of a railway construction company. In every case the employer of labor must discount the expected value of the product of labor. In fact an employer of labor has justly been called a " labor-broker," paying present cash for work which leads to future benefits.

A rise in the rate of interest will tend to produce a fall in the rate of wages by lowering the discounted value of the final benefits from the work of laborers, and therefore lowering the prices which employers are willing to pay. Contrariwise, a fall in interest produces a rise in wages. Thus if the rate of interest in the case of the landowner planting trees rises from three and a half per cent to six per cent, he can no longer afford to pay 50 cents per tree for the sake of getting back a dollars worth of lumber in twenty years; for 1 discounted at six per cent for twenty years is worth only 31 cents. Consequently, the prospective landowner will diminish his demand for tree planters, and their wages will fall.

In Chapter VI, 5, we have seen that, the value of capital being the discounted value of future uses, a rise or fall in the rate of interest produces a fall or rise, respectively, in the value of capital, and that the more remote the future uses, the more pronounced is the effect of a change in the rate of interest.

By this same reasoning, the dependence of wages on the rate of interest is the more pronounced, the more remote are the ultimate benefits to which the work of the laborer leads. In a community where the workmen are largely employed in enterprises requiring a long time, such as digging tunnels and constructing other great engineering works, the rate of wages will tend to fall appreciably with a rise in the rate of interest, and to rise appreciably with a fall in the rate of interest; whereas in a country where the laborers are largely engaged in personal and domestic service or in other work which is not far distant from the final goal of enjoyable benefits, a change in the rate of interest will affect the rate of wages but slightly.

Moreover, a change in interest will divert laborers from one employment to another. If interest rises, it will divert labor from enterprises which require much time and in which, therefore, the high interest is a serious consideration, and turn it into enterprises which yield more immediate benefits. For example, the higher the rate of interest, the less relatively will laborers be employed in planting slow-growing trees, and the more relatively will they be employed as domestic servants, and vice versa.

We have now considered the supply and demand of labor, or, to be exact, of the services of laborers. The rate of wages in each occupation will be such as will make the supply and demand equal, i. e., will "clear the market."

One corollary of the principle of clearing the market as applied to labor is that unemployment tends to correct itself. In the particular trades in which unemployment may, for a time, exist, the rate of wages will tend to fall.

The fall in wages will call forth an increased demand for labor which will tend to absorb the unemployed. So long as any unemployment continues, wages will tend to fall until the demand for labor again equals the supply. It must, of course, be remembered, however, that in practice this equalization of supply and demand works itself out slowly and imperfectly. No market is a perfect market, least of all the labor market. For instance, the reluctance of a laborer to change his residence in order to get a new job, or his ignorance of the existence of jobs which he might have, impedes the free working of the machinery of supply and demand.

What has been said applies only to wages under conditions of competition. Under competition they are determined–like any other competitive price–by the familiar principles of supply and demand. If, instead of competition, we have conditions of more or less perfect monopoly, wages will be determined according to the principle of monopoly price previously explained (Chapter XVII, 9). If employers form combinations called trusts, or if laborers form combinations called trade-unions, there will be an effect on the rate of wages. These combinations tend to render bargaining collective instead of competitive, and the effects on the two sides of the market are worked out through struggles called strikes and lockouts. But the consideration of these subjects belongs to applied economics.

4. The Efficiency of Labor

We have seen how the price of the laborers services is determined. But the total income of a workingman will depend not only on the price he receives for each unit of work, but also on the number of units of work he turns out. His capacity to turn out work is called his efficiency. In general the greater the efficiency of workingmen, the greater will be the amount of real income they receive. This is perfectly obvious in the case of implicit wages, and every independent worker is so fully aware of it that he is constantly aiming to improve his own efficiency. The farmer, for instance, knows that the more work he can accomplish in a day, the greater the income which he will enjoy. The more wheat he can gather this year with a given expenditure of time and effort, the greater will be this years income. He will, therefore, endeavor to gather as much wheat as possible with a given amount of effort, or, in other words, to put forth as little effort as possible to gather a certain amount of wheat. The more he can reap with a given amount of effort, the greater will be this years income in relation to the cost or outgo; and the more he can sow with a given amount of effort, the greater will be next years income in relation to this years outgo. His problem is always to minimize labor and to maximize the product of labor, and his prosperity depends upon his so doing.

The same principle applies, in general, to wage earners, even when their wages are explicit, since the products of their labor will, to a great extent, be consumed by other laborers. While the interests of workmen lie chiefly in increased wages, these wages can only be obtained by rendering adequate services. Wages are not the gift of the employers, but the product of the workmens own exertions. To attempt to get great wages without rendering great services in return is to fight the best interests of those other workmen who use the product. The more efficient the hired men on the farms in the West, the greater will be the wheat crop and the more abundant and therefore cheaper will be the bread bought by the employees in the shoe factories in the East; just as the more efficient the employees in the shoe factories in the East, the more abundant and cheaper will be shoes for the farm laborers in the West. It is, therefore, to the best interests of each workman that all other workmen should produce as much, and as economically, as possible. Moreover, while a workman may temporarily injure his employer by a policy of wastefulness, in the long run the employer will largely recoup himself for such wastefulness by charging higher prices for his products and thereby raising the general cost of living. Thus in the end the wasteful workman injures himself and his fellow-workmen.

We have seen, then, that for the ultimate prosperity of all classes, including the laborers themselves, it is of the utmost importance that workingmen should do the largest possible amount of work in the most efficient manner in a given time. The efficiency of laborers can be increased in three chief ways: first, by improvement in physical and mental vitality; second, by improvement in trade education; and third, by improvement in organization and division of labor.

It is obvious that if a laborer performs his tasks under conditions which tend to impair his vitality, there will be a resulting injury to his prosperity and to that of the community of which he forms a part. The public is beginning to realize that there are many factors in a workingmans life which tend to lower his vitality and thus greatly to reduce his earning and producing powers. Some of these factors are due to his personal habits, some to the lack of proper public health regulations in the community in which he lives, and still others to certain conditions under which he works. Among the personal habits which are very harmful to the wage earner should be mentioned the use of alcoholic beverages. As employers are becoming more and more conscious of this fact, they are beginning to require temperance and sometimes total abstinence of their employees, particularly when those employees occupy positions which make them responsible for the safety of property and of lives. Sea captains, locomotive engineers, and those charged with conveying telegraphic signals are often required to be total abstainers, and this requirement is being constantly extended to other classes of labor. Wrong habits of diet among work ingmen are also often the cause of impaired vitality, and consequently of impaired efficiency. Some of these, such as the use of ill-balanced rations deficient in or containing an excessive amount of tissue-building elements, are the result of ignorance on the part of the workingman. Others, such as the use of injurious foods, like tuberculous meat, infected milk, or canned foods containing harmful preservatives, while due in part to the ignorance of the workingman, are more largely due to the failure on the part of the lawmakers of a community to enact and enforce laws which shall prevent the sale of such foods.

There are many other ways in which lack of proper laws and regulations in a community endangers the health of the workingmen of that community. Among these is exposure to infection from those having infectious diseases, whether among neighbors, fellow-employees, or children in school. Housing conditions, especially as to ventilation, are particularly objectionable and are at present the subject of much discussion and study on the part of social reformers. A recent investigation has shown that without increasing the expense to a community in the construction of houses for working people, it would be possible to secure for them sanitary conditions far superior to those which they now ordinarily enjoy.

Still other causes of the impairment of the laborers vitality are certain conditions under which he works. The fight against excessively long working days, which is being carried on both by workingmen themselves and by others interested in their welfare, is gradually being won. Experiments in reducing the hours of labor from the present average of about ten hours a day to nine hours, or in many cases eight, have often resulted in an increased productivity not only per hour, but per day. We are still suffering from the tradition handed down from the days of slavery when often the employers whole effort was to " drive " his employees to the utmost. In many trades to-day an example of this " driving " is seen in the " pace maker " or fast worker selected for his ability to work fast and employed to set a rapid pace for the other workmen. As laborers vary greatly in the rapidity with which they can turn out work this struggle to live up to an excessive speed standard, while it may result temporarily in an increased output per man per day, often results ultimately in producing chronic diseases and in injuring the health of the men in other ways to such an extent that their future earning capacity is greatly unpaired. Trade-unions protest, and rightly, against the abuse of pace making; but curiously enough, they strive to substitute another kind of inefficiency, the " go easy " plan of purposely reducing output. They do not yet realize that workmens prosperity depends on workmens efficiency.

We have seen how the efficiency of laborers can be increased by improvements in their physical vitality. We shall next consider how it may be increased by improvements in trade education. When the apprentice system was prevalent, a long technical training was required of workmen entering any trade. But modern division of labor has reduced the amount of education needed. When a laborers work is so specialized that he only needs to make one or two motions–to turn a crank, or push a lever, or feed raw material into the hopper of some great machine–it is clear that no long course of training is necessary. A weeks or a months experience suffices to fit him for his particular little job. Consequently the apprentice system of preparation for the complete mastery of a trade has fallen into disuse. Recently, however, a reaction has manifested itself and the need of trade education has been felt. With the advent of intricate machinery–of electrical apparatus in particular–there has grown a need of a great number of technically trained workmen. This need is being supplied by trade schools rather than by the old system of shop experience by apprenticeship. The discussion of trade schools does not belong in a textbook on the principles of economics, but they are mentioned as indicating one of the promising methods of improving workmens efficiency and, therefore, improving their condition.

It is true that a scarcity of trained workmen of any particular sort, such as electricians assistants, will tend to keep their particular wages high, and that a greater abundance of such workmen, as would result from trade schools, would reduce their wages. But it will improve the condition of the newcomers who otherwise would have been compelled to have remained unskilled and low-paid workmen, and, by withdrawing some of the number of unskilled workmen, it will tend to raise the wages even of the unskilled workman. It will improve the general average for all, because it will increase the total productivity of society.

We come now to improvement in workingmens efficiency through organization and division of labor. In the earlier and simpler stages of division of labor, an individual workman limited himself merely to a single trade. Thus one workman became a tailor, another a baker, a third a shoemaker, etc. The more constantly each practices at his particular trade, the greater becomes his dexterity in that trade. This obviously becomes much greater than that of a man who attempts to carry on several different occupations. "A jack at all trades is good at none." When labor becomes still more minutely subdivided so that the work of one individual becomes reduced to one movement or group of movements repeated over and over again, the workman not only becomes more skillful but the movement gradually becomes almost automatic. "Practice makes perfect." Shoemaking becomes a manufacturing affair consisting of dozens of separate processes with special men to attend to each. One group cut leather, another drive pegs or sew, etc. Even these operations are reduced to tending machinery which does most of the work.

Besides dexterity from practice, another advantage resulting from division of labor is the adaptation of work to the qualities and abilities of the laborers. This is especially true in the case of mental workers. If a man who has ability for leadership turns over the less difficult and the mechanical parts to subordinates, devoting himself to the work which he alone can do or can do better than any one else, he becomes much more productive.

Besides personal division of labor there is geographical division of labor. This, as indicated in Chapter II, 1, is partly because of special adaptation of certain climates and soils for the production of certain crops, partly because of the location of mineral deposits and water power, and partly because of the advantages of grouping estab-lishments carrying on operations of a related kind. Thus Pittsburg is an iron and steel producing center largely because of its situation, being near deposits of iron and coal.

The division of labor, both personal and geographical, means, of course, that the persons who perform the various operations of a certain branch of industry combine—whether consciously or unconsciously—to bring about the final result. The final product of modern industry is peculiarly a joint product of many hands and minds in many different parts of the world.

While noting the advantages which result from division of labor, it is important that the student should realize an attendant disadvantage which should be understood and overcome, if possible, by trade education. This disadvantage comes about through the fact that mere specialization, while it fits the laborer for his special task, does not qualify him to meet the requirements of a world where industrial conditions are rapidly changing. The fact that specialization prevents a workman from being able to change from one occupation to another lies at the basis of the complaints against labor-saving machinery. Probably the best results will be secured by com

bining special trade education and special trade experience on the one hand, and general education and general trade experience on the other. The more the laborer can have of a general grammar school or even high school education, the more adaptable he will be; and if at any time he is thrown out of his special employment by changes, he will have less difficulty in adapting himself to the new employment which this change almost inevitably brings about.

The importance of general education for the workman is widely recognized, but it is not yet realized that a certain amount of general experience is likewise valuable. If employers could see an advantage in changing the tasks among workmen from time to time, it is probable that the temporary loss from such changes would more and more be offset by the greater intelligence and efficiency of the workmen which would result.

The full discussion of the methods of increasing efficient production by workmen belongs to applied economics, and if the student wishes to follow these important and interesting subjects, he will find them in books on Labor Laws, the Housing Problem, Public Health, Hours of Labor, Child and Woman Labor, Technical Education, Factory Sanitation, Workmens Compensation, Workmens Insurance, etc.

5. The " Make-Work " Fallacy

The blindness of workmen and others to the fact that the greater the efficiency of workingmen, the greater their own ultimate prosperity, is sometimes responsible for the " make-work " fallacy. According to this erroneous belief, the welfare of workmen depends, not on their productivity, but on their having jobs. On this basis they advocate great public works by the state in order to "make work" for the unemployed. According to this philosophy, a snowstorm blockading a city is an advantage to workmen, as it " makes for the snow shovelers. If we carry this logic a little farther, we should have to conclude that it would be an advantage to workingmen to destroy the houses of a community in order to make work for carpenters; to break windows in order to make work for glaziers; to burn up the stock of the clothier and the shoe dealer to make work for those employed in tailoring and shoe manufacturing; and in general to destroy all products of industry in order to make more work for those who produce. We could go even farther and advocate that without waiting for a snowstorm to blockade the streets, a city could benefit its workmen by engaging them to deliberately obstruct the street with dirt and then to shovel it away again,–thus "making work" not only in the removal, but also in the placing of the obstruction in the street.

The make-work fallacy grows out of neglecting the goal at which work is aimed. Work is not pursued for its own sake, and has no justification except as it fulfills actual human wants. Mere aimless work cannot in the end benefit workmen. To produce things merely to be destroyed, or to shovel dirt back and forth with no useful object, will in the end reduce and not add to the real wages of workingmen; for it reduces the volume of the products of labor which constitute the real wages. If shoes and clothes are destroyed, the main effect will be not to increase wages of shoemakers and clothiers, but to make workmen in general go ill-shod and ill-clothed. To break windows or to destroy houses will, as its main effect, not increase the wages of glaziers and carpenters, but decrease the quantity and the quality of shelter which workmen enjoy. No matter how complicated the organization of society, we cannot get rid of the simple fact that our welfare depends on our producing the largest possible output at the smallest possible cost, thus maximizing the final satisfactions of life and minimizing the effort by which they are obtained. The type of economic production may be pictured by Robinson Crusoe picking berries. He will not try to " make work" for himself by destroying the berries he has picked; he will not try to limit the amount of berries he picks; he will entertain none of the other fallacies which in modern complicated conditions workmen so often do entertain. He will simply try to pick as many berries as he can with the least amount of effort and waste. Modern conditions of exchange and industry do not modify this essential relation between satisfactions and efforts. They do, however, obscure the relation and as a result, lead to the make-work fallacy. This fallacy vitiates a great deal of the reasoning employed by trade-unions and by the uninstructed public. It is very analogous to the money fallacies which have been previously discussed, that confuse the mere medium of exchange with the goods exchanged thereby. It is almost as crude an error to suppose that workmen can be enriched by " making work " for them as that they can be enriched by issuing paper money. Work and money are merely means to an end. In order to rid ourselves of the money fallacy and the make-work fallacy, we must fix our attention on the end, and not on the means.

One of many manifestations of the make-work fallacy is the prejudice of workmen against labor-saving machinery. They see themselves thrown out of work by the introduction of a labor-saving device. For instance, linotype typesetting machines threw out of employment many professional typesetters and rendered almost worthless their skill laboriously acquired through years of practice. But it tended to increase the quantity and decrease the price of printed matter, including newspapers, and in this way to benefit workingmen in general. Another of the offsprings of the make-work fallacy is the policy of " protecting" a home industry against foreign competition. Thus the make-work fallacies, like the money fallacies, have been employed in aid of the protective fallacy. Whatever else of good may be said in favor of protection, the argument that it does good by making work for those employed in the

protected industries is fallacious. The argument is quite analogous to the argument against labor-saving machinery. In fact, free trade may be thought of as a sort of labor-saving machinery, and the objections to free trade, which many instinctively feel, are quite analogous to the objections which many workmen instinctively feel against labor-saving machinery. According to this argument we ought not to try to secure goods as cheaply as possible if by a greater expenditure of effort we can manufacture them at home; for this home manufacturing will give employment to workmen. According to this argument, instead of importing woolen cloth from abroad, it is better to protect woolen manufacturers at home in order to " make work " for spinners, weavers, etc., in American woolen mills. Here again we come in contact with applied economics, and it is not within the scope of this book to discuss at length the pros and cons of protective tariff further than as it illustrates the make-work fallacy.

The reasoning back of the make-work fallacy has been illustrated by supposing that a farmer driving his wagon to market should convince himself that to put sand in his axles would enable him to get to market faster. He might reason: " The harder the horse pulls, the faster the wagon will go; if I put sand in the axles the horse will have to pull harder, and therefore will get me to market faster! " To "make work" is to put sand in the axles of the industrial wagon. It makes labor pull harder without getting on any faster. What we need is to grease the axles to reduce the effort required for a given result. Then with the same effort as before, or even less, we shall get a greater result.

6. Wages and Enterprisers Profits

What has been said applies to income received through wages in general, including both explicit and implicit wages, but implicit wages or enterprisers profits need to be more particularly considered. Profits are in practice seldom called wages; for the term "wages" is usually employed in the narrow sense of explicit or stipulated wages.

The peculiarity of profits lies in the element of chance. Stipulated wages are supposedly certain, while profits are, by the nature of the case, uncertain. Many a worker has the option of hiring out to some one else or of being his own employer. In the former case he foregoes the chance of gain and the chance of loss. In the latter case he secures the chance of gain at the expense, however, of assuming a risk of loss. As a consequence, workmen classify themselves into two groups–wage earners or employees and enterprisers or employers–entirely analogous to the two groups into which we have seen that capitalists classify themselves; namely, bondholders and stockholders. And just as the bondholders consist of those who wish to avoid chance and the stockholders of those who are willing to assume risks, so also the employees are those who wish to avoid chance and the employers those who are willing to assume risks. And just as the stockholder stands sponsor to the bondholder for a stipulated income from capital, so the employer stands sponsor to the employee for a stipulated part of the income from labor–or usually from labor and capital jointly considered. This is a consequence of the fact that those become enterprisers who believe themselves to be especially adapted to the responsibilities which their position involves.

The employee or recipient of explicit wages does not usually require foresight in any great degree, while one of the chief functions of the profit taker or enterpriser is to make forecasts. Again, a man, in order to be an employee, does not require any accumulation of capital, while an enterpriser is far better equipped for his position if he is the fortunate possessor of a considerable fund of capital. It therefore happens that while theoretically an enterpriser may have little or no capital, practically he is usually a capitalist as well as an enterpriser.

Profits stand in a double relation to (explicit) wages; for the work of the enterprisers and the work of the wage earners are to some extent substitutes and to some extent mutually complementary. So far as the two kinds of work are substitutes for each other, they compete, and the price of the one tends to correspond to the price of the other. If, for instance, wages of plumbers go down, it will often happen that a few enterprising plumbers, rather than take these low wages, will set up for themselves as independent plumbers and employ other plumbers at these low wages. The transfer of these men from the ranks of the employees to the ranks of the employers tends, by diminishing the supply of plumber employees, to raise their explicit wages. On the other hand, by increasing the supply of plumber employers, it tends to diminish the implicit wages of the latter; in other words, to diminish the disparity brought about by the supposed fall in plumbers (explicit) wages.

If, on the contrary, the wages of plumbers rise, it will often happen that the same or other men will move back from the ranks of employers to the ranks of employees. Finding that they can make only a small and precarious living as employers, either because there is too much competition among the independent plumbers or because of their own personal shortcomings or misfortunes, they now prefer to accept the high wages which plumbers are getting rather than to continue the fight any longer.

There is a similar competition between the carpenter employer and the carpenter employee; in fact, between the " boss" and the "man" in every trade or walk of life. If there were no difference in abilities, there would be a tendency for wages and profits to be almost equal, although there would usually be a slight difference in favor of profits owing to the fact that men in general regard uncertainty as an evil and require higher compensation for assuming it. Just as in general and normally a stockholder gets a higher average return than the bondholder, so the profit taker will in general and on the average get a higher return than the wages guaranteed to the employee.

But in actual life the difference in superiority of profits is still further increased by the fact that the enterprisers form a select class. While almost every enterpriser is capable of being a wage earner, not every wage earner is capable of being an enterpriser. Therefore the supply of enterprisers is always somewhat restricted, and this fact tends to elevate their profits. Moreover, enterprisers are also a select class in tha, t they are capitalists. While the possession of capital is not always an absolutely necessary qualification for becoming an enterpriser, it is so great an advantage as very materially to limit the number of those best equipped to be employers. While the possession of capital does not prevent a man from being a wage earner, the lack of it tends to prevent his becoming an employer. This still further limits the supply of employers and tends to elevate still further their profits. In short, the employers or enterprisers profits tend to be high for three reasons: (1) because these persons assume risks and responsibilities which few are able or willing to take; (2) because for that very reason qualities of foresight, courage, and exceptional ability, which few possess, are required; and (3) because the work of the enterpriser usually requires, for its success on a large scale, the possession of capital.

Partly as a consequence of these peculiarities of enterprisers and partly because of the general conditions of modern industrial organization, the relation between employers and employees is not altogether or even generally competitive, but is to a large extent complementary. This complementary relationship is more obvious and important than the competitive relationship just described. We may say that, in general, the employer and the employee in the same establishment do not usually stand to each other in a competitive,

but rather in a complementary, relation. The work of each is necessary for the efficient work of the other. The enterpriser could not accomplish very much if he worked merely by himself; he requires for the best use of his abilities a large number of employees. Conversely, the employees cannot receive a guaranteed wage unless they find some employer who is willing to make the guarantee. The two stand in a relation similar to that existing between any two complementary commodities, as, for instance, the relation of the engine to the train it draws.

To the extent that enterprisers and wage earners are complementary, the earnings of the one tend to move not in unison with, but in opposition to, the earnings of the other. The lower the wages of the employee in any establishment, the more in general will be the profits of the employer, and vice versa. We see, therefore, that the relation between the employer and the employee is a complicated one, being partly competitive and partly complementary, and that therefore their interests, though partly allied, are largely opposed. The net result is usually that profits are far greater per capita than wages.

But, while this is true of the average rate of profits, we must remember that, as the very nature of profits requires an element of chance, they vary enormously, and that in many instances the individual enterpriser may make less than the wage earner, or even less than nothing at all, while in other extreme cases he may make his fortune.

7. Profits and Distribution Generally

Hitherto we have spoken separately of the capitalist who is a profit-taker and of the employer who is a profit-taker, but, as has been indicated, often one and the same person is both capitalist and enterpriser. In fact those who receive profits as employers of labor usually receive profits also from capital which they own, although the converse is not so universally true. Those who wish to receive income through their capital without any work become bondholders rather than stockholders; while those who wish to get income from their work without investing (or perhaps even possessing) capital prefer to work for wages or salaries. If a man wishes to become a stockholder, he usually is actively interested enough to do a certain amount of work, if it is no more than investigating the relative prospects of different companies offering chances for investors. And it is still truer that those who wish to take the responsibility of conducting an enterprise wish not only to put their effort into it, but their capital also.

It thus usually happens that the profits which a man receives cannot be easily classified into profits from his capital and profits from his own exertions. Generally his profits are the joint product of both his labor and his capital. The profit-takers– who are, of course, also loss-takers–are, then, the risk-takers of society. Some men risk only their capital (and receive dividends per cent or profits per unit of physical capital according to the form of their investment), others risk their own labor (and receive earnings of management), while most risk both their capital and their labor and receive the joint earnings of their capital and labor. These enterpriser-capitalists are well called the " captains of industry." They take the initiative in enterprises of all sorts, and on their judgment will depend whether not only their own capital and labor, but the capital and labor of others (to whom they undertake to pay stipulated interest or rent, on the one hand, and wages on the other), shall be economically or wastefully employed. When their leadership proves wise they make large profits for themselves, but these may be said to be a well-deserved reward for the general good their sagacity brings the public. When their leadership proves unwise, they suffer a loss, and this may be said to be a deserved penalty for wasting the capital and labor of society. The men, like Commodore Vanderbilt, who have built railways which were needed, have made fortunes. Those who have built railways which had to be abandoned have lost fortunes. There is, then, to some extent, a justification of our system by which we put a premium on enterprises which turn out well for society and a penalty on those which turn out ill.

It is, however, also true that just as there are types of successful speculators which should be condemned, so there are types of successful enterprisers which should be condemned. Those clever promoters who gain at the expense of the public through the frauds of " high finance " are among the worst forms of public enemies.

The enterpriser-capitalist then is the leading figure in modern industry. He gathers round him other capitalists and laborers and jointly they produce the income of society. After paying them the parts of this income agreed upon, he takes for himself whatever may be left, large or small as the case may be. Their parts are the earnings of capital (in the two forms of rent and interest) and the earnings of labor (in the form of wages). His own part is the earnings of his own capital and labor (in the form of profits jointly on his capital–whether measured per cent or per unit of physical capital–and on his own labor).

We cannot too much emphasize the fact that though each of the various laborers (both employers and employees) and instruments of capital (land and other instruments) which jointly produce income, is credited with a certain part, it could not produce this part alone, or by itself. The earnings of a railway company are due, for instance, to the joint services of the stockholders, bondholders, officers, employees, locomotives, cars, roadbed, and terminals. These are not independent, but mutually complementary, instruments and laborers, and their services are complementary services. We impute to each a certain part, determined according to the principles which regulate the prices of complementary goods.

The sum of all these items–that is, all the interest, rent, wages, and profits, in any community in any given period of time is, of course, the total income of that community. An inventory of these would show what quota was contributed to this total by or imputed to human beings, land, and other instruments. As a matter of fact by far the larger part is contributed by human beings. Professor Nicholson of Edinburgh has estimated that the income from what he calls " the living capital" of Great Britain is five times as great as that from the " dead capital." In less wealthy countries the preponderance of man-produced income is probably still larger. Of the part produced by " dead capital" the larger portion is from land.

In a new country the rent of land is apt to be low, but rent of other things and wages high. For in such a country land is abundant, but other forms of capital, including laborers, relatively scarce. As a country grows older and more populous, land becomes scarce relatively to population, or, in other words, the demand for land increases without any increase in supply. Therefore land rent tends to rise, and other rents and wages to fall.

Progress in scientific knowledge causing an increase in productivity of land is like the rejuvenation of a country. Any increase in general productivities, whether of land or of other agents of production, has a tendency to make the rate of wages increase. For (1) by increasing the wealth of employers and thereby diminishing the marginal desirability of money, there is a tendency to increase their demand for everything, including the services of workmen; and (2) so far as workmen themselves are owners of houses, implements, and other instruments of any kind, and thus share in the increased affluence, the supply of work they offer is decreased, as we have seen.

Such a result is probably the chief general effect of so called labor-saving machinery. It increases the income of other classes than laborers, and with it their power to buy work of laborers. The first effect, however, is for the labor-saving machine to displace laborers, with which, in fact, it is a competing article, and we have seen that the increase in one of two competing articles or substitutes tends to lower the price of the other. The individual laborers thus displaced are likely to be injured by the improvement, being unable to learn another trade without undue loss of time. It is even conceivable that labor-saving machinery might become so automatic and so fully a substitute for human work that there would be no need and no demand for such work. But such an effect seems very improbable. The human machine is so much more versatile than other machines that its relation as substitute for labor-saving machines is not so important as its complementary relation to them. As a matter of history, so-called labor-saving machinery, while it " saves " or displaces laborers from one sort of work, often, if not usually, produces new needs for them in another sort of work. If horses and carriages were introduced into China, they would largely dispense with the need of coolies, who now carry passengers in sedan chairs, but they would call for coachmen and grooms. When, in turn, stagecoaches give place to railways, the trade of drivers of stagecoaches becomes obsolete, but the new trades of locomotive engineers, firemen, conductors, and brakemen are created. In fact, the very names of these occupations, as of hundreds of others, show that the demand for these kinds of work arises from the existence of machinery. In other words, while labor-saving machinery is always, as its name implies, a competing article with the human machine with respect to some of the many-sided capacities of a human being, it is usually also a complementary article with respect to some other capacity; and we have seen that an increase in the quantity of one of two complementary articles tends to increase the price of the other.

In the present chapter as in the preceding, we have considered income as distributed among the agents which produce it,–. labor and capital, including land. We are now ready to turn to the other sort of distribution,–the distribution among the owners. A decrease in the amount of capital which laborers own will, as we have already seen, make them willing to take lower wages than otherwise. In fact, the chief reason that there exists a wage class is that those constituting it have little or no capital apart from their own persons. Wage earners are chiefly " prop-ertyless " persons–persons who have either never had any property, or have lost what they did have, as, for instance, through too high a degree of impatience. We see, therefore, that the question of wages depends, among other things, on the distribution of the ownership of wealth. This will be the subject of the next chapter.

CHAPTER XXV

WEALTH AND POVERTY 1. The Problems of Wealth and Poverty

The first half of our study of distribution has been presented in the two last chapters. It dealt with the distribution of income relatively to the agents or instruments which produce that income. In the present chapter we shall take up the second half of the study–i. e., the distribution of this same income relatively to those who own and enjoy it. The two sorts of distribution are quite different, although there has been a tendency to confuse them. This was natural, for in the early days of economics people were classified roughly according to the sort of instruments they owned. There was the landlord class, whose chief income was ground rent; the non-landed capitalist, whose chief income was from other capital than land; and the laborer, whose chief income was wages. It was then natural to imagine that the incomes produced by laborers, by land, and by other capital, were also the incomes enjoyed by laborers, by landlords, and by other capitalists. But even were such a classification possible and duly made, it would still fail to tell us anything whatever as to how large was the per capita share within each class, or whether the amounts enjoyed by different individuals were or were not very unequal. The best we could say would be that certain land yields a rent of 10 an acre, and other lands more or less than this; that certain houses rent for 1000 a year, and others for more or less; that money lenders make five per cent on their loans; and that ordinary wage earners get 2 a day. But these data, however detailed, would not tell us the relative income enjoyed by different persons, except in the case of the common laborer, and then only on the assumption that he derived no income from any other source than from his work. Furthermore, to-day there are only small traces left of the old social stratification, and correspondingly little excuse for confusing the distribution of income with reference to the capital which yields it and its distribution with reference to the persons who own it.

But, though the two sorts of distribution are distinct, each is needed to understand the other. The problems now before us–of distribution relatively to owners–may be described as the problems of the total income of a nation, of the average income of its inhabitants, and of the relative numbers of people owning incomes of various sizes.

The last-named problem is the problem of grading the population according to income–the problem of discriminating the relatively rich and the relatively poor. No other problem in economics has so great a human interest as this, and yet scarcely any other problem has received so little scientific study. Since income necessarily comes from capital or from labor, the problem of "distribution" of income is largely that of the "distribution" of capital. Our problem may therefore be stated in two ways: either as the problem of the personal distribution of income or as the problem of the personal distribution of capital and of labor-power. It is what is popularly known as the problem of " the distribution of wealth."

For the purpose of comparing the incomes or capitals of different persons or nations, values are more important than quantities. If we know that As income is worth 1000 a year and Bs, 10,000, we may say that Bs income is ten times As in the sense that the elements composing Bs income are worth in exchange ten times the elements com posing As income; or, if we know that X is " worth " (i. e., owns capital worth) 1,000,000 and that Y is " worth " 10,000,000, we may say in like sense that Ys capital is tenfold Xs.

In order to compare the incomes or capitals of widely distant times or places, a correction may need to be made for differences in the purchasing power of money, and if the rate of interest is also different in the two cases, the result of the comparison will not necessarily be the same for the capital as for the income. A millionaire worth 1,000,000 in California half a century ago, the rate of interest being twelve per cent, commanded an income equivalent to that of a multimillionaire to-day, worth 3,000,000; for the present rate of interest is only one third as high. If, therefore, we were to compare the possessor at that time of 1,000,000, having an income of 120,000, with the possessor now of 2,000,000 having an income of 80,000, we should have to say that though the first was only half as rich in capital as the second he was fifty per cent richer in income. Another point of difference between comparisons of capital-value and comparisons of income-value lies in the fact that while capital-values differ only in size, income-values differ also in distribution in time as well as in certainty. For this reason a man rich in lands from which there happens to be little immediate income–but only prospects of income in the distant future–is sometimes called " land poor," having much land, but little immediate income.

But when we are seeking to compare the absolute comforts which different persons or nations enjoy, it is more important to consider quantities than values. In fact, as noted at the outset of our study, money valuations are apt to be misleading. A country where water is scarce will put a higher money valuation on its water supply than a country where water is so abundant as to have no price. Thus, a large quantity of water shows more affluence in the sense of " desirability " than does a large value of water.

Practically, however, if we confine our attention to modern times and conditions in western Europe and America, it is true, in a general way, that of two nations or individuals the one which is richer in capital-goods is richer also in income-goods, in income-value, and in capital-value. For simplicity we shall hereafter assume that these four comparisons are thus similar. We may say that a man is " rich " if he has a large amount of capital-goods of various kinds–lands, houses, stocks, bonds, etc.; or a large money-value of such goods; or a large amount of benefits of various kinds–nourishment, clothing, shelter, amusements, etc.; or a large money-value of such benefits. A man is "poor" if he has small amounts of all these things.

Of course, the two terms " rich " and " poor" are purely relative, and represent no deeper scientific meaning. A man who is rich according to one standard may be poor according to another. But the two terms are very convenient to designate relative conditions. Corresponding to the adjectives " rich " and " poor " are the nouns " wealth " and " poverty "; for, as noted in the first chapter, the term " wealth " is especially used to indicate a large amount of wealth, just as the term " poverty " is used to indicate a small amount. Our subject, then, in this chapter is comparative wealth and poverty, both of nations and of individuals.

2. National Wealth or Poverty

We may divide this subject into two heads: the wealth or poverty of nations and the wealth or poverty of individuals. We shall first consider the wealth or poverty of nations.

"The wealth of nations " depends upon two things: their labor and their capital, including their lands and the other capital the people have produced. The income earned by the people of a nation always far exceeds the income earned by all its capital. Yet people do not earn income without at least land. Given laborers and land, we have the only two real requisites of producing income. Other capital springs from these two. It is sometimes said that labor is the father, land the mother, and the other kinds of capital the children. A nation, then, is the richer, the larger the number of its inhabitants, the greater the extent of its territory, and the greater the amount of its accumulated products.

These three factors depend each on somewhat different conditions. The amount of land and its power to produce is largely a question of natural resources. It may be taken as a given quantity presented to man by nature. It is now becoming recognized, however, that land is not so definitely constant in its power to produce as was once imagined. One of the most important results of the recent "conservation movement" in this country has been to show conclusively that land is not altogether a constant source of income, but that it is possible by the impoverishing and washing away of top soil greatly to impair or destroy absolutely the productivity of land; while, on the contrary, by proper fertilization, keeping land fallow, rotation of crops, etc., it is possible to increase the efficiency of land just as it is possible to increase the efficiency of other instruments.

The dominion over land by any given group of men may depend on wresting it by military force from another group. In fact, one of the chief objects of war has been to increase national wealth by adding to territory. This was a chief object of the Roman Empire and of the colonial system of Great Britain. These and other nations have had what is called " earth hunger." The wealth of the British Empire to-day lies for the most part outside of the British Isles; for it includes, besides England, a number of important colonies–Canada, India, Australia, and parts of Africa. Except for the war of the Revolution, the

British Empire would now include also the territory occupied by the United States.

Turning from the quantity of land or the " natural resources" of a nation to the number of inhabitants, we note that this itself depends in turn upon the extent of the territory as also on the past history of the nation and on other, conditions which will be considered later in this chapter. Many nations have sought to increase their wealth and power by increasing their population. In fact, a chief reason for extending a nations territory has been to fill it with colonists. A country is usually alarmed at the prospect of a stationary or decreasing population. France is now trying to conserve its population, recognizing that national strength for future war or for future political position among the nations of the earth depends largely on the number of fighters and of workers. The productiveness of these people, as well as the productiveness of the lands they keep, will depend largely upon their condition as to vitality and accumulated knowledge.

We come last to the amount of accumulated products. This depends on two chief" qualities: first, thrift, which, as we have seen, leads to savings; and, secondly, inventiveness, which has led to the creation of income-producing instruments.

3. Per Capita Wealth or Poverty

We have considered the conditions determining the aggregate wealth of nations. We may pass now to the more important subject of the wealth or poverty of individuals. This subject may be divided into two parts: the study of average or per capita wealth, and the study of its distribution or the relative wealth and poverty among different individuals. By the per capita wealth of any nation is meant the quotient found by dividing the total national wealth by the number of inhabitants. It is evident that two nations may compare very differently as to aggregate and as to per capita wealth. The small countries, Holland and Switzerland, when compared with the large countries, India and China, are far poorer in aggregate wealth, but far richer in per capita wealth. The per capita wealth in any nation will thus increase with an increase in the total wealth (the population remaining the same) and decrease with an increase in population (the total wealth remaining the same).

With the advent of democracy in politics has come a greater emphasis on per capita as compared with aggregate wealth. Under autocracies the aim was to increase the wealth of the nation as a whole, partly for the mere aggrandizement of the autocrat or potentate, who often regarded himself as a sort of owner of the nation (" Ietat, cest moi "), and partly because the popular sentiment of national greatness was satisfied in this way. Under these conditions an increase in population was almost invariably welcomed and encouraged. But since the individuals of the nation have become its rulers and, so to speak, shareholders, they have regarded increase of numbers with mixed feelings; for while on the one hand they welcome an increase in the total wealth which a greater population brings, on the other hand they do not relish a decrease in the per capita wealth which may ensue. In the democratic ideal, therefore, an increase of population is usually welcomed only in a new country where there is plenty of land, or in a country acquiring colonies to provide room for a surplus population.

The effect of an increase of national wealth on per capita wealth will evidently depend upon the ratio between land and population. In a sparsely settled country an increase of population will not only increase the aggregate, but also the per capita wealth; for each new worker adds, by his cooperation, to the efficiency of workers already on the ground. A very few men cannot work together to as great advantage as a moderate number. The cooperation and division of labor incident to a moderate increase in population more than outweigh the fact that the greater population will require more nourishment, clothing, and other items of income. In short, though there be more mouths to feed, each additional mouth means an additional pair of hands; and the added capacity of the new hands to produce exceeds the added capacity of the new mouths to consume. The history of new countries shows that an increase in population is a blessing individually and collectively.

When, however, the country is settled and filled up with population to a certain point, the opposite becomes true, and a fresh increase of population, while continuing to increase aggregate wealth, will decrease per capita wealth. It then happens that each new pair of hands adds less to production than each new mouth subtracts in consumption. This fact sets a sort of elastic limit to an increase of population. That there must be such a limit is evident, since an indefinite number of people cannot be supported on one acre of land. We know as a generalization from ordinary observation that the billion and a half people now living on this planet could not be supported if all were packed into the state of Rhode Island and dependent on Rhode Island for sustenance. Per capita poverty would then be so intense that people would die of actual starvation. Famine, with the plagues which usually follow it, would decimate the population. Overpopulation in India and China often results in famine and plague. But in western civilization much milder instances of insufficiency of food are found. Long before such a starvation point is reached, every increase of population beyond a certain point results in an increased death rate. In fact, statistics show that the death rate increases as per capita wealth decreases. This fact is due to the unsanitary conditions which poverty necessarily brings–conditions which pertain not so much

to the quantity of food as to its quality and to the quantity and quality of housing and other comforts and conveniences of life, and perhaps above all to conditions of employment, especially hours of labor. These unsanitary conditions incident to poverty result in fatigue, malnutrition, infection, diseases such as tuberculosis, and deaths. We have, then, ample evidence that when the ratio of population to land becomes excessive, the death rate is increased, and consequently the further increase of population is checked. This law of per capita wealth is chiefly based on the anterior fact that land is an essential agent in production, and that each successive increase in the productivity of land is acquired at increasingly great cost–or, expressed otherwise, that, with each successive increase in cost, the return diminishes. This is the familiar law of diminishing returns in agriculture. There is, then, based on facts, a general law of per capita wealth in relation to population. It may be stated as follows: Given a particular stage of knowledge and of the arts and of other conditions that determine productivity, an increase of population up to a certain point increases the per capita wealth, after which a further increase of population decreases the per capita wealth.

4. Population in Relation to Wealth

The population of any country may be increased either by births or immigration and decreased either by deaths or emigration. The population of the world, as a whole, can be increased only by births and decreased by deaths. As we are more interested in general than in local increases or decreases in population, we may overlook the questions of emigration and immigration, assuming for the area under consideration that they are either absent or balance each other.

With this proviso, we may say that population will decrease if the death rate exceeds the birth rate, and will increase if the birth rate exceeds the death rate. As we have already stated, the facts show that the death rate increases with a decrease in per capita wealth. The birth rate, on the other hand, tends to decrease with a decrease in per capita wealth. There are exceptions to this last statement, but these exceptions will be ignored for the present.

If we assume what history has almost invariably shown to be the fact, that in a sparsely settled country the birth rate exceeds the death rate, so that the population tends at first to increase, we are now in a position to state what will happen to the population of that country in future generations, quite apart from any increase in immigration. By hypothesis the population will increase at first and, as at first each increase in population brings an increase in per capita wealth, it will continue to increase as long as this condition continues. But, as we have seen, it will ultimately happen that per capita wealth will cease to increase and will begin to diminish. It will then happen that the death rate will increase and the birth rate decrease, so that the increase of population will be slackened and ultimately cease altogether. Under these conditions, then, population in a new country will increase up to a certain point at which it will cease to increase. The population is then in a sort of equilibrium, the birth rate equaling the death rate because the per capita wealth has been reduced to such a point as to bring this equilibrium about.

The laws of population, therefore, may be stated as follows: 1. An increase in population will tend to increase aggregate wealth but less rapidly than population. That is, the increase in population tends to decrease per capita wealth.

2. A decrease in per capita wealth will tend to increase the death rate and decrease the birth rate. That is, the decrease in per capita wealth checks the increase of population.

In accordance with these laws the sequence of events is usually as follows: In a new and sparsely settled country, population at first increases. As the country fills up this increase is slackened and finally comes to a standstill when the death rate equals the birth rate. This stationary state is reached when the people are either unable or unwilling to lower the standard of subsistence. Such a stationary state has been nearly reached in India, where people are unable to lower the standard of subsistence, and in France, where they are unwilling. In most countries, population is still increasing and will probably continue to do so until the vast areas opened up by exploration and colonization in the last four centuries shall have been filled up. These areas include North and South America, Australia, and parts of Africa. The rendering available of these continents to occupation by Europeans constitutes the greatest economic event of modern times and has relieved for a season the pressure of population on subsistence. Similar relief has been afforded by great labor-saving inventions which enable a given population to secure increased subsistence. Future inventions may be expected to increase this process. But ultimately there must be a limit to the capacity of the world to support population.

This limit on human population is the same sort of limit which nature sets on animal and plant population. Blades of grass multiply until they cover the ground on which they grow. When grass is sown on a grass plot, it multiplies with great rapidity, but after the whole plot is covered and there is no room for more, the number of blades remains nearly stationary. There is a struggle for life constantly going on, and the death rate thus produced is great enough to balance the birth rate which the capacity of the soil allows. Out of this struggle for existence among animals and plants comes what Darwin called natural "selection," and it is interesting to know that Darwins first idea of such a struggle came from reading the economist Malthus, who first wrote an important treatise on Population. Population may then be said to be limited by the means of subsistence.

Since Malthuss day there has come into more definite operation what he called the "preventive check" on population. While it is still true that among the poor it usually happens that an increase in per capita wealth tends to increase the birth rate by encouraging marriages or making them earlier or increasing the number of children per marriage, it has become unfortunately true that among the wealthier classes an increase in wealth tends sometimes in the opposite direction. Instead of wealth being then thought of as a means of supporting children, it comes to be thought of as a means for gaining or maintaining " social position," and the more wealth gained, the more ambitious are its possessors that its enjoyment may not be interfered with by childbearing, or that it shall not be decreased by subdivision in the next generation. The result is that the wealthier classes often have, on the average, smaller families than the poorer classes. We must, therefore, modify the law of population so as to read that an increase in per capita wealth, instead of tending always to increase the birth rate, tends first to increase it and then, after the increase of wealth passes a certain point, to decrease it. This wealth check to population is peculiar. It is quite different from the poverty check. The poverty check works automatically so as to check population when it is too large and not to check it when it is too small. But the wealth check acts in the opposite way–or rather it would do so if it were sufficiently strong and general, which is not yet the case. Then it would come about that the greater the per capita wealth, the more would population be checked, and as the check to population usually tends

to increase per capita wealth, this would still further decrease population. The logical result is depopulation or " race suicide."

At present, however, this wealth check is confined to certain parts of the population, and results, for those parts only, in " race suicide." These parts include particularly the so-called " better classes " of the population. Statistics show that the children of college graduates are less numerous than the graduates themselves. Thus, besides depopulation, there is another danger, degeneration. If the vitality or vital capital is impaired by a breeding of the worst and a cessation of the breeding of the best, no greater calamity could be imagined. But while the risk of such a result undoubtedly exists, this is not immediate, and an increasing realization of its possibility, we may hope, will lead to some way of counteracting it. A method of attaining the contrary result–namely, reproducing from the best and suppressing reproduction from the worst–has been suggested by the late Sir Francis Gallon of England, under the name of " eugenics." This movement, which promises to become a strong one, aims to prevent (by isolation in public institutions and in some cases by surgical operations) the possibility of the propagation of feeble-minded and certain other classes of defectives and degenerates, and also to develop a public sentiment which shall condemn marriages in which either husband or wife has a transmissible disease, or any inheritable taint of epilepsy, insanity, etc., or is otherwise unfit to become a parent.

5. Distribution of Wealth

Having considered aggregate and per capita wealth, we come finally to the distribution of wealth among different individuals. Although a whole nation may be rich or poor relatively to another nation, the widest differences between nations are small as compared with the differences within any one nation. Every nation has its extremely poor, its extremely rich, and its classes in intermediate conditions. In the United States there are many wage earners who cannot earn 1 a day, and who have no income except what they earn by labor, while at the opposite extreme are the multimillionaires who receive incomes of over 1,000,000 a month.

What are the reasons for such prodigious inequalities in the personal distribution of wealth? Are such inequalities injurious? If so, are they preventable? If so, by what means? These are some of the most burning questions of the day. Out of them spring many reform movements, and especially socialism. But these, like other practical problems, are applications of economic principles, and cannot be discussed in a book designed to treat only of economic principles themselves. Suffice it to say that no proper answer can be made to the last question–how to cure the unequal distribution of wealth–until we have answered the first question–what causes this unequal distribution. As often happens, more study has already been devoted to cure than to diagnosis, and with the usual ineffective result of quack remedies.

Our present object will be to set forth the causes which affect the relative personal distribution of wealth. Whatever these causes may be, they are evidently fundamental and universal; for we find that extremes of poverty and riches have existed at all times and places. They are mentioned in the Bible and other histories of peoples in all ages and stages of civilization. It is probable that the degree of inequality differs as between the Oriental civilizations, like China and India, on the one hand, and the Occidental, like England and France, on the other, and also as between the older settlements of western civilization, like Russia and Italy, and the newer, like the United States and Canada. But the fact of inequality and also its causes are nearly the same everywhere. Distribution differs in some degree, it is

true, according to political institutions, as, for instance, between Germany and England. There is a comparative absence of extreme poverty in Germany as contrasted with England and the United States; a comparative prevalence of poverty in Russia and Italy; and a comparative frequency of extreme opulence in Holland. Nevertheless, Professor Pareto, a Swiss economist, has found that, as between different countries for which statistics are available, and as between various periods of time, the statistics of inequality in the distribution of wealth show a remarkable correspondence, more close, in fact, than that shown by the statistics of mortality.

The causes which have produced the present inequalities of wealth are largely historical; that is, they lie in the past. It usually takes more than one generation to affect greatly the economic standing of a family. For this reason some people have foolishly imagined that if to-day we could once correct the inequalities in wealth handed down to us from the past, the problem would be solved, and with a new and even start we would be forever rid of great poverty by the side of great wealth. We shall soon see, however, that if wealth were once equally divided, it would not remain so. The analysis of what would happen will serve as the best introduction to our study of distribution.

6. Equality of Distribution an Unstable Condition

Let us suppose that, through some communistic or socialistic law, the wealth in the United States were divided with substantial equality. It is proposed to show that this equality could not long endure. Differences in thrift alone would reestablish inequality. We cannot suppose that human nature could be so changed and become so uniform that society would not still be divided into " spenders " and " savers"; much less can we suppose that different people would all spend or all save in exactly the same degree. So

long as there are any differences whatever between people in regard to their degrees of impatience under like conditions, they will be led by these differing degrees of impatience to exchange present and future incomes among themselves. As a consequence there will ensue differences in spending and saving, and therefore differences in capital.

The larger the amounts saved or spent, the more rapidly is capital gained or lost. As we have seen, the process by which individuals thus gain or lose fortunes by saving or spending consists, in the last analysis, of an exchange of present and future income. If two men have to start with the same income of 1000 a year, but one has a rate of impatience above the market rate of interest and the other has a rate below, the first will continue to get rid of future income for the sake of its equivalent in immediate income, and the other to do exactly the opposite. Such substitutions of immediate for remote, and of remote for immediate income may take place by means of loans, sales, or changed uses of capital. The man with spendthrift tendencies will borrow, i. e., pledge future income for the sake of present income; or he will sell any durable goods which offer remote income, such as farms or forests, and buy perishable goods which offer immediate income, such as champagne, clothing, horses, and carriages; or he will change the uses to which he puts his capital, avoiding those which require improvements, and choosing instead those on which he can realize quickly, thus letting his property run down.

The man with saving tendencies, on the other hand, will lend or invest present income for the sake of future, will sell perishable and buy durable goods, and will make far-sighted uses of his capital. He will invest in stocks and bonds and in real estate capable of large future income. Both men will pursue their respective policies up to the point where their marginal rates of impatience harmonize with the rate of interest.

These effects on capital are worked out by the principles of Chapter VII. If a modification of the income-stream is such as to make the present rate of realized income exceed the "standard" rate, capital is being depleted to the extent of the excess, and the person will grow poorer. Individuals of the type of Rip Van Winkle, if in possession of land and other durable instruments, will sell or mortgage them in order to secure the means for obtaining enjoyable services more rapidly. The effect will be, for society as a whole, that these individuals who have an abnormally low appreciation of the future and its needs will gradually part with the more durable instruments, and that these will tend to gravitate into the hands of those who have the opposite trait.

It requires only a very small degree of saving or spending to lead to comparative wealth or poverty, even in one generation. It is remarkable how much may be saved in a lifetime by thrift. Cases are sometimes found of day laborers who, by saving and putting at interest, accumulate within a lifetime a small fortune, and in the meantime rear a family. As Micawber said, a man with an income of one pound a week will reach ultimately poverty if he spends just one penny more, and reach opulence if he spends just one penny less.

A central rôle in the distribution of wealth is thus played by the degrees of preference for present over future income and the rate of interest. The existence of a general market rate of interest to which each man adjusts his rate of preference supplies an easy highway for the change in his capital in one direction or the other. If an individual has spendthrift tendencies, their indulgence is facilitated by access to a loan market; and reversely, if he desires to save, he may do so the more easily if there is a market for savings. The irregularities in the distribution of capital are thus due in part to the opportunity to effect exchanges in the present and future parts of the income-streams of different people. The rate of interest is simply the market price for such exchanges. By means of this market price, both those who wish to barter present for future income and those who wish to do the reverse may satisfy their desires. The former will gradually increase, and the latter gradually diminish, their capital. If all individuals were hermits, it would be much more difficult either to accumulate or to dissipate fortunes, and the distribution of wealth would therefore be much more even. Inequality arises largely from the exchange of income, carrying some individuals toward wealth and others toward poverty. In short, the inequality of wealth is facilitated by the existence of a loan market. In a sense, then, it is true, as the socialist maintains, that inequality is due to social arrangements; but the arrangements to which it is due are not, as he assumes, primarily such as take away the opportunity to rise in the economic scale. On the contrary, they are arrangements which facilitate both rising and falling, according to the choice of the individual. The improvident sink like lead to the bottom, while the provident rise to the top.

But thrift, important as it is, is not the only road to wealth, nor thriftlessness the only road to poverty. Besides differences in the rates of impatience, there are equally potent differences in ability, industry, luck, and fraud. By ability is meant ones capacity to earn; by industry, the use of this capacity. Examples of getting rich from ability and industry are very common. Almost all the rich men in this country who have made their fortunes have done so, in part at least, through ability and industry. Often luck has aided greatly. There are many examples of miners who got rich in Colorado by simply stumbling on a gold mine. Luck plays a larger role in the accumulation of fortunes than many are inclined to believe. The " unearned increment " is usually a case of luck. Unforeseen increase in ground rents has given rise to large fortunes from time immemorial. It is also unfortunately true that some men have really got their start, if not their larger accumulations, through fraud. This has sometimes occurred through " high finance," which consists very largely in making contracts with ones self at the expense of others whose interests the double dealer, as director, trustee, etc., happens to control. If a man is a director in a corporation, and votes to have it buy materials of himself at any price he sets, he naturally can become rapidly wealthy at the expense of the stockholders. Also through political "graft," and especially through getting city franchises for gas and waterworks and street car companies, and through special tariff legislation, many men have become wealthy. Poverty, on the other hand, has often resulted not only from thriftlessness, but from incompetence, i. e., lack of ability, slothfulness (lack of industry), and misfortune or bad luck, and from having been defrauded by others.

We conclude, therefore, that equality of wealth is an unstable condition and, even if once established, would not endure, because of unequal forces of thrift, ability, industry, luck, and fraud.

But inequality once established tends, by inheritance, to perpetuate itself in future generations. The workman who accumulates a few thousand dollars from nothing makes it easier for his children to accumulate more. He gives them a start or a " nest egg." Recently four sons of a Connecticut farmer met in a family reunion. Many years previously the father had sent them into the world to make their fortune, giving each 700 to start with. When they met at the recent family reunion, all were worth thousands. The well-known woman millionaire, Mrs. Hetty Green, is an example of a person who inherited a large fortune and then accumulated more, by virtue of her low " degree of impatience," i. e., her preference to accumulate for the future rather than to spend in the present. A fortune of 6,000,000 was bequeathed her, and now her fortune is reputed to be worth 100,000,000.

Likewise poverty may be passed down from generation to generation. A special cause for handing down inequality of fortunes lies in the reduction of the birth rate among the rich. As we have explained, the tendency to-day is for the poor to have a high birth rate, and for the rich to have a low birth rate. There results a tendency toward an increase in the numbers of the poor and a decrease in the numbers of the rich. This result tends to exaggerate the differences in the per capita wealth between the two classes; for in the upper classes there will be a relatively larger share for the few who inherit fortunes, and in the lower classes there will be an increasingly smaller share for the many.

We see, then, that there is at least a tendency for the rich to grow richer and the poor to grow poorer. We may even go so far as to say that the richer a man or family becomes, the easier it is to grow richer, and that the poorer a family becomes, the more difficult it is to keep from growing poorer. Large fortunes often grow without effort. All that is necessary is for their owners to refrain from squandering. On the other hand, a family once caught in poverty is apt to be drawn deeper into the mire. Overwork, anxiety, and unsanitary surroundings bring on disease or disability, which robs the family of what little it once had. The opportunity of the wealthy is their wealth, and the curse of the poor is their poverty. " To him that hath shall be given, and from him that hath not shall be taken away even that which he hath."

7. The Limits of Enrichment and Impoverishment

Yet there are limits to enrichment and impoverishment. The ordinary downward limit is reached when a man loses all his capital. He has then no source of income left except his own labor. When a man has succeeded in losing all his capital, the process usually comes to an end, because society, in self-protection, decrees that it shall go no farther. He is in most civilized lands not allowed to sell himself or to pledge much of his distant future services. But where there is no such safeguard, the unfortunate victims may sink into even lower stages, such as the debt servitude in the Malay Archipelago or Russia, and to some extent in Ireland; or they may even sell themselves or their families into slavery. In most countries the poor come to be a large and permanent as well as a helpless class.

Next, as to the upper limit. We have seen that the opportunity to increase ones wealth depends upon the market for present and future goods, i. e., the loan and investment market. A hermit cannot become immensely wealthy; nor can any of the inhabitants of a small island, if cut off from the rest of the world. The utmost that a man in an isolated community can own is the capital which that community has or can get–its land, dwellings, means of locomotion and of manufacture, etc. These are necessarily limited by the size of the community. As the market widens, the limits to the growth of large fortunes widen also. To-day there is no limit to what one man may accumulate except that he cannot more than " own the earth."

This relationship between the possible size of individual fortunes and the size of the market to which the owner of the fortunes has access is important. Practically it means that in these modern times, when almost the whole world is one great market, the possibilities of individual fortunes are greater than ever before. Few people realize this fact; for most people imagine that at any time in the worlds history any fortune could have increased at compound interest. But a fortune is capital-value, and, as we have seen, capital-value has no power to produce income, but, on the contrary, is merely the discounted value of anticipated income. The only way a mans fortune can increase at compound interest is by his constantly reinvesting income as it comes in; that is, exchanging it for other and later income at the discounted values of the latter. But evidently he must find sellers of some such other and later income before he can buy it. His income has no power whatever of itself to create other income. In short, an extreme upper limit to the growth of any individual fortune is set by the scarcity of income-producing instruments available.

The common idea that " money has power to breed money " leads to absurdity when applied to compound interest. Were it true, any person might leave fortunes to posterity far exceeding the possible wealth which this earth can hold. The prodigious figures which result from reckoning compound interest always surprise those who make the computation for the first time. One dollar put at compound interest at four per cent would amount in one century to 50, in a second century to 2500, in a third century to 125,000, in a fourth century to 6,000,000, in a fifth century to 300,000,000, in a sixth century to 15 billions, in a seventh century to 750 billions, in an eighth century to 40 trillions, in a ninth to 2 quadrillions, and in a thousand years to 100 quadrillion dollars. Now the total capital in the United States is only about 100 billions, and that in the world at large–even assuming that the per capita wealth elsewhere is as large as the United States, which is an absurdly large allowance–must be less than 2 trillions, which is only one fifty-thousandth part of what we have just calculated as the amount at compound interest of 1 in 1000 years. Yet 1000 years is only half the time since the Christian era began. In 2000 years the 1 would amount to 100 quadrillion times 100 quadrillions, which is many, many times as much as a world composed of solid gold. Needless to say, such a prodigious increase of wealth could never actually take place, for the simple reason that this is a finite world. The difficulty lies, not simply in the reluctance of people to provide for accumulation several centuries after their death, but also to the fact above mentioned, that large accumulations would reduce oppor tunities for reinvestment and therefore reduce the rate of interest. The attempt, for instance, to invest trillions every year would drive up the prices of all investable property, i. e., all capital. To invest such sums would practically require the purchase by the rich man of all existing railways, steamships, factories, lands, dwellings, etc. But many of the present owners of these, having already sold a large portion of their property and thus reduced their degrees of impatience to equality with the prevailing rate of interest, would not part with more except at prices so high that the purchaser would make little or no profit or interest on his investment. Thus, the approach toward the limit of investment would reduce the rate of interest and retard, and finally altogether prevent, further accumulation.

There are some interesting examples of long-continued reinvestments. Benjamin Franklin at his death, in 1700, left 1000 to the town of Boston and the same sum to Philadelphia, with the provisos that they should accumulate for a hundred years, at the end of which time he calculated that at five per cent each legacy would amount to 131,000. In the case of the Boston gift, it actually amounted, at the end of the century, to 400,000, and has since accumulated to about 600,000. The sum received by the city of Philadelphia has not increased so fast.

Another interesting case of accumulation is that of the Lowell Institute in Boston, which was founded in 1838 by a bequest of 200,000, with the condition that ten per cent of the income from it should be reinvested and added to the principal every year. A peculiarity of this provision is that it applies in perpetuity. There is, therefore, theoretically, no limit to the future accumulation thus made possible, and it would be interesting to know what will be its history in future centuries. The fund, after only 67 years, amounted to 1,100,000. Another example is the " Sailors Snug Harbor" of New York, which has outgrown the work orginally intended and is now applying to the courts for relief.

8. The Cycle of Wealth

With a world market for investment, we have every prospect of a great increase in private fortunes in the next few centuries. But practically the limit reached in the history of most large fortunes is only a very small part of the high limit we have set, that of " owning the earth." There is usually a reaction against the desire to accumulate. Each reduction in the rate of interest tends to check the desire to accumulate. Moreover, this desire soon palls. A multimillionaire recently left his fortune to accumulate until 21 years after the death of his youngest heir, with the intention of accumulating by that time the largest fortune on record. But his heirs much preferred to use it during their own lifetime, and succeeded in breaking the will. Even had they not succeeded, those who finally came into the fortune would probably have begun, at least in a few generations, to dissipate it; for the usual effect of great wealth is to produce habits of spending.

It has already been noted that ones rate of impatience for future income, given a certain prospective income-stream, will be high or low according to ones past habits. If a man has been accustomed to simple and inexpensive ways, he finds it fairly easy to save and ultimately to accumulate a considerable amount of property. These habits of thrift, being transmitted to the next generation, result in still further accumulation, until, in the case of some of the descendants, affluence or great wealth may result. But if a man has been brought up in the lap of luxury, he may have a keener desire for present enjoyment than if he had been accustomed to the simple living of the poor.

The effect of this factor is that the children of the rich, who have been accustomed to luxurious living, and who have inherited only a fraction of their parents means, and often lack their ability and business training, will, in attempting to keep up the former pace, be compelled to check the accumulation and even to start the opposite process of the dissipation of their family fortune. It requires a certain amount of ability merely to maintain a fortune. Bad investments carelessly entered into are often the means of impairing or even annihilating a fortune. And then the unfavorable effects of luxury begin. A few years ago there came to this country an Englishman who had inherited a large fortune, but who had also inherited the desire to indulge himself in the present to the full extent of his capacity. To defeat the effects of this desire, his parents had left him only the income of their wealth " in trust " (and it is not an unusual thing in England, where there are spendthrift sons, to leave property so that they may use only the income). Nevertheless, this man contrived, by chattel mortgages and in other ways, to spend a good deal more than the interest annually accruing, and he was always in debt and in trouble. The product of such a course is, sooner or later, what is called a " shabby genteel " class. Eventually people in this class will have to overcome their pride, go to work, and become laborers–and often common laborers. After a few generations of poverty and the illiteracy which goes with it, the wealth-holding ancestry is forgotten. It is said that examples of such ancestry are common among laboring men, and would be more generally recognized were it not for the loss of records which is the inevitable accompaniment of illiterate poverty.

Thus the limits set by scarcity of investments (i. e., scarcity of purchasable instruments or shares in them) to the possible growth of large fortunes are always far higher than the vast majority of fortunes ever approach. Most fortunes rise and then fall, the turning point being due to the abandonment of thrift and the substitution of thriftlessness which the fortune itself sooner or later engenders. An old adage has put this observation in the form, "From shirt sleeves to shirt sleeves in four generations." We have no inheritors to-day of the fortune of Croesus, who, in his day, was supposed to be a wealthier man than Rockefeller, not only in proportion to the wealth of his time, but absolutely. A man with a start of that kind ought to have been able to make the fortune increase rather than decrease with the future, and yet we know of no heirs to that fortune. To-day we have a large number of wealthy families in this country, but most of them are only one generation old! Thus the very rich families, so far from growing rich indefinitely, usually do not even continue rich more than a few generations, but grow poor, arriving, too, at that condition without the vitality or the character necessary to retrieve themselves.

Likewise, at the opposite extreme, it does not always happen that the poor grow poorer or even remain poor. Just as wealth often relaxes thrift, poverty sometimes stimulates thrift. The children of the poor then become fired with ambition to get on in the world simply because they are poor. These people rise from the ranks, and rise rapidly. It should be noted, however, that unlike the downward movement of large fortunes, this upward movement is the exception, not the rule. It may be that ninety per cent of large fortunes reach a maximum and decline, but it is doubtful if one or two per cent of the poor reach a minimum and rise. Many fall into pauperism or die. The vast majority simply remain poor.

We see, then, that while it is very easy for those who have once reached the top of the economic strata to stay at the top, this result seldom occurs, chiefly because of their conversion from savers to spenders; and while reversely it is very easy for those who once reach the bottom to stay at the bottom, they do not always do so, chiefly because of their conversion from spenders to savers.

9. The Actual State of Distribution

The churning up of society resulting from saving and spending and the other causes above mentioned neutralizes the tendency we have mentioned for the rich to grow richer and the poor to grow poorer, and, what is more important, it prevents–to some extent–the establishment of wealth-castes by continually changing the personnel of wealth and poverty. The individuals of society are like goldfish in an aquarium. Those once started upward continue to ascend for a time, whereupon they start down again. Those once started downward continue to descend until perhaps they reach the bottom, whereupon they (may) start up again. To complete the figure, we must suppose the shape of the aquarium to be like a bell, very small at the top and very large at the bottom. There is room for only a few at the top, and the struggle of many to get there makes it difficult for any, while it makes it easy for all to descend. There is most room at the bottom, and consequently there is less change there than anywhere else. Reversely, at the top there is most change. The constant changing of position in this bell jar, while of great moment to the individual, does not greatly affect the distribution of society as a whole. There will always be about the same proportion of fish at each successive stratum. Professor Pareto has, in fact, represented the distribution of wealth by a bell-shaped figure which he calls the social pyramid. This is shown in Figure 48. The number of people having an income between Oa and Ob is represented by the contents of the bell-shaped vessel between the plane of aa" and the plane of bb". The social pyramid represents the fact that the larger the size of a fortune, the smaller the number of people who have it. There are many more at the bottom than at the top. We have no exact statistics for this country, but a rough popular estimate states that over half of our population have incomes of less than 600 per year, and of the remaining half about half (i. e., one fourth of the whole population) enjoy incomes between 600 and 1200, and the other half (i. e., the remaining fourth of the whole population) have incomes over 1200.

10. The Inheritance of Property

The frequency of changes in fortunes, whether up or down, will differ greatly in different countries according to the ages of the countries, and their laws and customs. Among these factors the laws and customs as to the inheritance of property are of great importance. If there is an equal distribution among the children of the rich, the fortune is pretty sure to run itself out in a few generations or centuries; but in England this result is prevented by giving to the oldest son the bulk of the estate and cutting everybody else off with small stipends. The effect of this custom is to maintain the family dignity and the integrity of the large estate. In this country there are signs that we are gradually changing toward this English custom by which a rich man, instead of dividing his fortune evenly, leaves the bulk of it to one of his heirs. Such a change in testamentary custom will furnish a new and powerful tendency for existing inequalities to be accentuated and perpetuated.

One of the special problems connected with inheritance is that of the control over wealth a man should be allowed to exercise after he has died. This problem has frequently been under discussion. It is sometimes called the problem of " the dead hand." Out of this problem grew the "statutes of mortmain "; and also the common law rule that no testator can " tie up " his estate beyond " lives in being "at the time of his death plus 21 years. This common law rule applies, however, only to so-called " private " bequests. To escape its operation a rich man very often leaves his fortune to some " charitable " foundation. But as it is ill advised to leave a fortune in the hands of private persons for a number of generations, so it has been found ill advised to leave fortunes in perpetuity in any shape whatever; for the result is that after a few generations it is impossible to carry out the instructions of the donor without doing harm–however good his intentions. Conditions will have come about which the donor could not foresee or provide for. In Norwich, England, for instance, there was left many generations ago a small sum to support a preacher for the Walloons, who should utter a sermon in Low Dutch every year at a certain time. That provision is still carried out, although there are no longer any Low Dutch in this place. There is no one to understand the sermon, and yet it is preached every year. Recently the preacher has learned one sermon by heart and repeats it every year in order to receive his remuneration. In 1862 a lady died in England and left a fortune to be used for the teaching of the doctrines of Joanna Southgate. The latter had had a large religious following in England, but at this time, 1862, there was not a single soul in England who believed in her doctrines. Here was the curious spectacle, therefore, of a fortune being left in the hands of trustees, no one of whom could be found who believed in these doctrines. In 1587 a certain man died leaving to the almshouse of Suffolk certain real estate, the income of which was then 113. The income at present is 3600, far more than the institution can use, and the trustees do not know what to do with it. The result has been to make the almshouse a mecca for all poor people for miles around and to pauperize the neighborhood.

The custom of making wills is one that is handed down to us from the Roman days. Regarding wills, there were no laws in ancient Germany, no provisions in the Levitical laws of the Jews, none among the Hindus, and only slight traces among the ancient Greeks. When we talk of the sacredness of private property and the right to dispose of it by will, we are merely expressing our loyalty to the particular custom under which we now happen to live. F It may be that in the future a remedy for some of the present evils connected with the ownership of wealth may be found by limiting or regulating the inheritance of wealth as to time or amount, by inheritance taxes, by limiting private ownership in certain perpetuities, by substituting leaseholds for perpetual franchises or for unencumbered titles in mineral lands, or even in all lands. There is much to be said on both sides of these proposals, but it is no part of our present task to enter upon their discussion.

CHAPTER XXVI

WEALTH AND WELFARE 1. True and Market Worth

An often-quoted passage from the Bible states that " the love of money is the root of all evil." Another states that "it is easier for a camel to go through the needles eye than for a rich man to enter into the kingdom of heaven." On the other hand, poverty has always been regarded as an evil. Agur prayed that he should be given neither riches nor poverty. This is the theory of the golden mean. Still another view is that while, absolutely, wealth is good and the more of it per capita the better, yet its unequal distribution is an evil. This is the view of the socialists.

In all these views there is some truth. Extreme wealth and extreme poverty are alike evils, and the disparity between the extremes is also an evil. Moreover, besides these evils dependent on the quantities of wealth are other evils dependent on the qualities of wealth. But how can it be that wealth, which is merely the physical means for satisfying human wants, can ever do harm? We have escaped this question hitherto because we have accepted wealth, so to speak, at its market valuation. As was explained at the outset, prices are determined by the actual desires of men, and, when seeking to explain prices as they are, we were not obliged to inquire as to whether the desires which explain them are foolish or wise, good or bad. There was no need to distinguish between the desires which fix the prices of Bibles and those which fix the prices of obscene literature. Now, however, we propose to go a little deeper and to point out instances in which " desirability " is shortsighted and foolish, and in general to point out the various ways in which market valuations fail to give a true picture of actual worth. As we have seen, market valuations of fortunes do not even show their comparative desirabilities, because of the wide differences between the marginal desirabilities of money to different people. The marginal desirability of money decreases rapidly with an increase of wealth, so that–beyond a comfortable competence–the addition of millions means little that is really desirable. In fact, to some men like Mr. Carnegie, swollen fortunes become a burden and responsibility rather than an addition to personal gratification.

2. Evils Connected with the Quantity of Wealth

That extreme poverty is an evil needs no proof. We shall, therefore, not discuss the problem of poverty. The chief causes of poverty we have already shown, and its remedies lie beyond the scope of our discussion. Suffice it to say that the problem is the greatest of all practical economic problems and is justly claiming a large share of the attention of philanthropists and reformers. Among the remedies or partial remedies suggested are socialism, old-age pensions, compulsory workmens insurance, regulation of hours of labor, better housing, abolition of disease, education in thrift, profit-sharing, cooperation, monopolization and regulation of labor by trade unions.

At the opposite extreme lie the opposite dangers and evils of great wealth. If the poor are too hard working, the rich are too idle. If the poor are underfed, the rich are overfed. If the poor have the discomforts of squalor and shabbiness, the rich have the discomforts of excessive attention to personal appearance. If the poor suffer from overcrowding, the rich suffer from the burden of overgrown establishments. If the poor drink alcoholics to get rid of fatigue, the rich drink them to get rid of ennui.

Not only does each extreme have its evils and dangers, but the unequal distribution of wealth has evils and dangers of its own. One of these is the perverted use of great wealth in a manner to humiliate, degrade, or demoralize the poor. Unequal distribution of wealth produces a caste feeling, breeding contempt for the poor by the rich, and envy of the rich by the poor. Corresponding to differences in wealth grow up differences in the mode of living, education, language, and manners, differences which distinguish the " gentleman " and " lady " from the common herd, and which gradually become confused with innate differences, which are quite another matter. Aristocracies are almost always founded on wealth and are therefore almost always on a false basis. There are undoubtedly wide differences between men. If so-called aristocrats were really all the name would imply, the " best " in body, mind, and heart, much could be said in favor of their segregation from the " vulgar " crowd, and the development from them of a better race of men. But a plutocratic aristocracy is based, not on what men are in themselves, but on what they possess outside of themselves.

Because of the differences in wealth, the poor serve the rich. The relation of master and servant is not simply a commercial relation. It also represents a supposed difference in caste.

Probably the worst demoralization of the poor, growing out of inequalities of wealth, is the prostitution of the daughters of the poor for the sons of the rich. Competent students of prostitution believe that it rests on this economic basis. For the white-slave traffic most people are blaming those who engage in it, just as for drunkenness most people blame the saloon keeper. Doubtless these agents have their share of moral responsibility. Yet they are merely the brokers in the business. The demand and supply are the important factors, and the demand and supply arise chiefly because of the unequal distribution of wealth.

Next to the poor selling their souls comes selling their votes. Bribery and political corruption are largely due to differences in wealth. In a democracy we have the ideal conditions for such perverted uses of wealth. In a democracy there are two great powers, the power of the ballot and the power of the purse. The power of the ballot rests with the poor because of their numbers. The power of the purse rests with the rich. Nothing could be more natural than that the unscrupulous representatives of these two powers should contrive to get together for mutual advantage. They need not meet directly. The perverted politician intervenes as a broker. Many of the city governments of the United States exemplify this condition. These politicians make, on the one side, a business of controlling the votes of the poor, partly by bribery, partly by dispensing " charity," and partly by activity in party organizations; and, on the other side, they make a business of " holding up " the capitalists who want franchises for street railways, water, gas, electric light, or telegraph or special tariff legislation. The unscrupulous capitalist finds it advantageous to pay toll to the politician, either by actual bribery or by stock in corporations, or by what a politician recently called " honest graft " in the form of " tips " or inside information as to the stock market, real estate transactions, etc. Some of the politicians in our state legislatures and even in our national Congress are of this character. Some are avowed or secret representatives of capital or "the interests"; others, of voters or "the people." In this case the conflict between plutocracy and democracy becomes more direct and visible. But it always exists and will continue to exist, in some form, unless one of the two powers shall some day completely vanquish the other. Here is one of the great practical problems of the day. 3. Forms of Wealth Injurious to the Owner

We have seen several of the evils of wealth, and in particular some of the misuses to which wealth may be put. We can better understand the nature of these and other misuses if we reemphasize the fact that wealth, in its narrow sense, does not include the most precious of our possessions, ourselves. The evils of wealth consist largely in an increase of external wealth at the sacrifice of what may be called internal wealth. Emerson said: " Health is the first wealth." The founder of Christianity asked, "What shall it profit a man if he shall gain the whole world and lose his own soul?" Many a millionaire would willingly give all his millions for youth, health, or even freedom from pain. Many uses of external wealth practically injure our internal wealth. The injury may be physical or moral or both. It is in this regard especially that " satisfactions," in the economic sense, fail to measure real welfare. Indeed, as regards the body, we may classify satisfactions into self-benefiting and self-injurious. Many articles of wealth, though possessing commercial value, are really injurious to those who use them. In some cases the articles of wealth referred to are used almost exclusively by the rich, in others, almost exclusively by the poor. Among examples of self-injurious satisfactions or uses of wealth are the consumption of unwholesome food or the wearing of constricting clothing or the use of dwellings injurious to the health; the practice of unhygienic or immoral amusements, the use of narcotics, such as opium in China, hashish in India, absinthe in France, whisky in Ireland, and alcoholic beverages in western civilization generally. These may be called perverted uses of wealth, but they are very common, so common as to give commercial value in millions of dollars to disease-producing food factories, distilleries, saloons dives, gambling houses, low dance halls, and theaters, houses of prostitution, immoral and degrading literature. The perverted satisfactions here represented are capitalized like any other satisfactions. They are often paraded to show how wealthy a nation is, but as they weaken the stamina of the people and shorten their lives, they really lessen its satisfactions in the end. In any complete view of the subject they should be recognized as sources of national weakness, not strength. This is recognized in the great reform movements–housing reform, temperance reform, and the movement to abolish the " white-slave " traffic.

4. Forms of Wealth Injurious to Society

Other evils of wealth consist in its use by one person to injure another. Just as we classified some satisfactions into personally beneficial and injurious, so other satisfactions may be classified into socially beneficial and injurious. Examples of socially injurious satisfactions are of many kinds. Robbery, fraud, embezzlement, arson, and other criminal acts are too obvious to need more than mention. A burglars " jimmy " is an article of wealth, but it nevertheless is a means of injury to society.

Of less obvious examples one is the exploitation of gold mines when their product depreciates the currency. As we have seen, the production of gold at a sufficiently rapid rate tends to raise prices. Here we find great gold fields, stamp mills, assay and smelting works, etc., standing in our accounts as important items of national capital. Yet, when they produce fluctuations and uncertainty in our monetary standard, they are injurious, rather than beneficial, to the country. While they afford means and opportunities for their individual owners and exploiters to make great private fortunes, they do not enrich a nation or the world; for their effect is merely to change the numbers in which prices are expressed. Thus, much of the labor and capital invested in gold mines may be said to be socially wasted. A small amount of money is as good a medium of exchange as a large amount. If gold flows out of the gold mines fast enough to raise prices, the result is social harm rather than good, disturbing the distribution of wealth and continually tending to precipitate a crisis.

The gold miners fortune is thus often made, not by an addition to the worlds real wealth, but by an abstraction from the worlds wealth for his benefit. In addition there is a waste of labor in mining. When gold can be profitably mined far in excess of what is necessary to maintain a constant price level, the gold miner is, as it were, robbing society. Thus, even the most genuine gold brick, as to which there is no thought or intent to defraud, may prove in the end a swindle.

Other examples of socially injurious wealth are such nuisances as the " smoke nuisance," privy vaults in a city, and " pests " of various kinds. A factory which defiles the household linen and the lungs of the neighborhood is not an unmixed benefit. If all the injury it caused could accrue to the factory owner, he would put in a smoke consumer, or else most willingly suffer a great deduction in the value of his plant. Instead, he causes a great loss of value thinly distributed over blackened houses and an injury, never capitalized or measured, in the health of his fellow citizens. Such cases, where social interests and individual interests do not run parallel, justify legal interference. We cannot allow bonfires or bad sanitation in a crowded city merely because many individuals want the " freedom " to have them, nor can we allow freedom of movement on the part of those carrying infectious diseases.

5. Forms of Wealth Used for Social Rivalry

The other examples of socially injurious uses of wealth we shall mention are all cases of social rivalry or racing. Three special cases will be considered.

The first relates to warfare and the preparation for war. It is usually conceded that actual warfare is economically injurious. The best that the apologists for war can say is that it is inevitable. But it is not so well recognized that the economic preparation for war is an example of world waste, albeit an effort toward economy on the part of each individual nation. When Germany invested millions in armaments, she merely stimulated France to do the same. The two nations have been racing with each other ever since, as have other countries, including England and the United States. Each battleship which costs 12,000,000 in the end adds practically nothing to the worlds effective capital. Its object is to benefit one nation by increasing its military strength relatively to other nations. But it does not even accomplish this object. On the contrary, as soon as this movement is met by the other rival nations and a similar battleship is added to their navies all the advantage which it was sought to gain is lost again and the various nations are in precisely the same relative position as before any battleships were built at all. Preparation for war is a species of cutthroat competition. If six world powers, instead of investing each 12,000,000 in a battleship, should agree not to do so, the result would be to save 72,000,000 from being wasted. The case would be very different if the ships belonged to the merchant marine. In that case, the building of 72,000,000 worth of ships would add that much to the worlds productive capital. The utility of merchant ships is absolute, that of battleships is relative.

Thus, for the most part, the " capital " of nations, in the form of armaments, represents economic waste, although no one nation could afford to dispense with it as long as other nations do not.

Our second example of socially injurious rivalry is commercial cutthroat competition. We have seen that what is often to the interests of individual producers is against the common interests of producers as a group. We may now add that it may be injurious to the interests of society as a whole. In fact, we have already noted that a patent and copyright have their justification in the fact that the play of unprotected individual interests would practically result in discouraging or suppressing inventions and books. The same must often be true in other instances. Telephone competition is not only injurious to the telephone companies but to each subscriber, who either has to have two or more telephones in his house, with all the expense and annoyance which that arrangement implies, or has to remain in want of proper and easy connection with subscribers to systems other than the one he happens to employ. Our third example of socially injurious rivalry is perhaps the most important and pervasive, although the most subtle, of all. It concerns rivalry in wealth itself, and introduces us to the subjects of luxury, extravagance, social ambition, and vanity. Thackerays novel, "Vanity Fair," is a satire on the sort of economic rivalry referred to. Vanity may be defined as a desire to obtain the approval of others, and vanity leads to social rivalry. This may be considered as rather a broad definition of vanity, and it is one which does not always or necessarily imply any slur. The important part played by vanity in economic affairs is seldom realized. A case of pure vanity is seen when a man wants merely the badges of distinction. For instance, the badge of the Legion of Honor which Napoleon established in France is much desired, merely as a means of obtaining the approval of other people. It has no intrinsic desirability. It is not because it is beautiful that it is desired; it is not because the badge can keep one warm or appease ones hunger or fulfill any of the primitive and individual desires of men. It merely appeals to the instinct to attain distinction in the eyes of other people. Most cases of vanity, however, are not so pure, but are mixed with a substratum of actual utility.

For instance, a diamond is desired chiefly out of motives of vanity, but it is desired also because it appeals to the aesthetic sense. It is a curious fact that as soon as we mix vanity with some other motive, people begin to hide behind this other motive and conceal the vanity of which, for some reason, they seem to be ashamed. When a woman wears a diamond hatpin, and can never, by virtue of its position, see it herself, what real motive is there except vanity? Of course it may be said that she is an altruist in attempting to provide an article of beauty for other people to admire; but the real object, however she may condone or conceal it, is to display this diamond to other people and to show thereby that she is in the fashion or leading it and able financially to do so. Most articles of ornament pander chiefly to this form of vanity and come into existence largely and chiefly for this reason, although the admiration of actual beauty is a secondary element and a subterfuge.

The amusements of mankind are almost always, or to a large extent, mixed with the motive of vanity. For instance, automobiling to-day is not always indulged in for the sake of sport alone, but also for the sake of display. Equipages have always been one of the means of displaying wealth. Narcotics have always been objects desired not merely for their drug effect, but also for the effect of display. The habit of using "fine wines" an expensive drinks in entertaining has long been one of the methods of social display. Clothing even, and housing, are very often objects of vanity. In fact, historically, clothing originated as ornament, like jewelry, rather than as an actual protection from the weather. Even food is a matter of vanity to a certain extent. Feasts have been favorite occasions for the exercise of this instinct.

A few extreme examples of ostentation will help us to understand the nature of vanity. Some years ago there was an American in Florence who carried the idea of display in his equipage to the extreme of getting a chariot and having sixteen horses to pull him through the narrow streets of the city. Ordinarily an attempt to gratify vanity results in the approval which is sought by the individual, but in extreme cases like this it often results in disapproval, and this man was known in Florence for years as " that fool American." A well-known French count, who through marriage became possessed of means, gratified the instincts of vanity by proceeding to spend untold sums in building a large and useless colonnade of pillars, simply to show that he was able to do so. A person not long ago left a will providing 1,000,000 for the erection of his own tomb. Cleopatra once showed what she could afford by drinking a dissolved pearl. Pliny states that after Cleopatra did this she was imitated by the son of a famous actor, and the practice of drinking pearls became a sort of fashion in Rome, as to-day some men of a less subtle vanity light cigars with 5 bills. It was probably this practice which led to the phrase "money to burn." In Philadelphia not very long ago a lady had a carpet made with a special design, and when the carpet was completed she was careful to have the design destroyed lest any one else should have a carpet like hers. A well-known speculator is said to have bought for his wife for 30,000 a particular carnation, in order that it might be called by her name. In Holland, centuries ago, there was a furor over tulip bulbs which took such a hold on the people and led to such extravagantly high prices that in 1639 one bulb sold for what would be approximately 2000 in our money.

The powerful influence of vanity is illustrated by the admiration people have for foreign importations. Many people really delude themselves with the idea that they care for an imported cigar or wine because they believe it to be superior to the domestic article. Nor is this the only species of vanity appeased by the purchase of foreign goods. An art dealer in San Francisco found that certain people preferred to pay 4000 in Paris for the same picture which they could buy in San Francisco for 2000, in order that they might state that they bought it in Paris. Some artists of San Francisco found it advisable, therefore, to take their pictures to Paris, in order that they might get higher prices from Americans. California wines go to Europe to be returned as " imported " wines. Not long ago an American who lives in a well-known cheese-making district in New York paid a very high price for an imported cheese and took great delight in the fact that it was imported. As a matter of fact, it had first been exported from his own town. New York cigars are shipped to Key West to be reshipped from there as " Key West " cigars.

The effort to produce imitations is found in the case of almost all articles of vanity, though the superiority of the " genuine article " is strenuously maintained. This is well illustrated in jewelry. A paste imitation of a diamond can never fetch the same price as a real diamond except when its character as an imitation is fraudulently concealed. If a chemical method should be developed of making a real diamond cheaply, the desirability of diamonds would be destroyed; they would immediately go out of fashion; the invention would be self-destructive, and the price of diamonds and the use of diamonds destroyed. That is, diamonds are desired because they are scarce and a badge of economic power of the people who possess them. This is why imitation jewelry is regarded as a sham. Paste diamonds may be quite, or nearly, as beautiful as real diamonds, but they can never be so valuable. Those who use. them do so not because they regard them as beautiful, but usually in order to make people believe they are " real" and that the possessor can afford to buy them. Sometimes they are worn as symbols of real diamonds kept for safety in bank vaults. The owners then appear at the opera with the imitation jewels. When spoken to of their jewels, these people will say that they are not real jewels, but are an exact imitation of real jewels which are in

the safe deposit vaults. In such cases the imitation jewels serve purely and simply as badges of ownership. There is then supposed to be no pretense involved. The wearers would be thought " cheating " if they possessed only the paste. Their virtue consists in actually having the " real thing," which the paste replica proclaims. A wealthy woman seriously argued the question of whether a poor woman had a right to wear an imitation diamond. Her thought was that, since the poor person could not afford to have a real diamond to wear, the imitation diamond amounted to deceit.

6. The Cost of Vanity

Now the efforts to satisfy vanity are like the efforts of nations to secure armaments. The chief advantage that social racing gives to an individual is relative and this implies putting other people at a relative disadvantage. So far as society is concerned, the cost of keeping up the race is a total waste. This cost consists in the labor expended on the gratification of vanity, and shows itself in the high prices of articles for that purpose. The tax thus laid by society upon itself is enormous, and a part of it may be measured roughly by the annual purchases of articles of pure vanity. Yet people seldom complain, for the individual can see little or no difference between the good he gets from an article of vanity and the good he gets from any other article. He does not care much about the pace he may be setting for others, and he does not hold any other particular person or persons responsible for the pace which has been set for him. He looks at the worlds fashion as an inevitable fact, and adjusts his own actions to it. Our task, however, is to look at the social effects of his actions on others, and of others actions on him. His expenditures for vanity may give him the satisfaction of " climbing," but by as much as he gets ahead of others the others are left behind. They are all in a social race to get ahead. In the scramble all are at great effort or expense, and in the end there is a loss of economic power similar to the loss by nations racing for military supremacy. Undoubtedly the race stimulates the racers, and may do them some good as a mode of exercising their abilities, and even lead to useful inventions. The same maybe said of war. But our present purpose is to point out the cost, which is usually overlooked. If the true cost could be expressed in figures, it would doubtless amaze people who have never stopped to see the extent to which luxury and luxurious rivalry is carried. Almost all expenditure is more or less colored by it.

We have called the extravagance which is created by the desire of a man to compete with his neighbor in vanity social racing. Now when fashion enters into the matter, as it almost always does, this race becomes more like a chase. There are leaders and followers, and the followers try always to overtake the leaders. When they do so, the leaders turn in their course in order to elude their pursuers. The consequence is that fashions are constantly changing at the hands of the leaders of fashion. The leaders of fashion are usually from among the richest people in the community, and whatever they consume, those beneath them in the social or economic scale wish to consume also.

We may take, as an example, the case of russet shoes, which are constantly coming in and going out of fashion. A few years ago a gentleman was surprised to find that only the highest grades of russet shoes were carried on the market. When he asked the reason, he was told that russet shoes had gone out of fashion only a year or two before; that now they were coming in, and the only way by which they could be got in was by putting the highest grades on the market first, because if the lowest and cheapest grades were put on, then the leaders of fashion would not want them, and if the leaders did not want them, then followers would not want them either. Consequently the demand at the top is the one to be first supplied. After this initiatory demand has been satisfied, the shoes are imitated in cheaper grades, until finally russet shoes become so common that the leaders refuse to wear them longer and they go out of fashion–only to come back again in a few years, after which the same cycle is repeated.

Vanity is literally insatiable. Without vanity there would be little use for the fortunes of multimillionaires. Beyond a modest fortune more wealth would be to them entirely superfluous. Therefore the use to which they put their millions is of much more moment to society than to themselves. If they use it to set standards of luxury, they are using it in a socially injurious manner. They produce the same effect on society as though they levied a tax on all persons poorer than themselves.

The individual can emancipate himself from the expense of social racing by asserting his independence and " living the simple life " regardless of his neighbors or their opinions of him. An interesting book called " One Way Out" describes how one family " ran away from its neighbors " in order to start life afresh in a less expensive environment. By such a step the cost of living could probably be cut in two or reduced in an even greater ratio.

But to most men and women such Spartan measures would seem a hardship rather than a saving. For them, no remedy for their own extravagance would be adopted which did not carry with it a remedy for the extravagance of their neighbors also.

7. Remedies for the Evils of Vanity

We have seen that the natural remedy for cutthroat competition in business is combination. In the same way if there could be a general " disarmament," as it were, or agreement between the social competitors, it might solve the problem of social rivalry.

This declaration of truce has, indeed, been put in operation on a small scale in schools, colleges, and clubs. A good instance is to be found among womens sewing circles. When such a circle is first organized, the hostess gives a very simple entertainment. At the next meeting a rival hostess gives something a little more elaborate, and presently the members of the circle are madly racing in the effort to supply the best entertainment. A reaction becomes necessary and the ladies finally agree explicitly " not to serve more than two kinds of cake."

An example of how this general disarmament works was seen in San Francisco at the time of the earthquake. There the people who lived formerly on Nob Hill in fine houses had to live in tents or out of doors. So far as this loss was concerned, it was no loss at all–at any rate, no loss at first–because each man was perfectly willing and liked to live out of doors, provided his neighbor lived in the same way. Yet before the earthquake any one of these people would have been ashamed to live in a tent because he knew that his neighbor would wonder or criticise.

Very similar to social disarmament is compulsion by the government. The Dutch government, for the sake of the nations resources, finally took a hand in the tulip craze, and the traffic in bulbs was stopped. History contains many examples of sumptuary laws designed to check social racing.

One cure was suggested by John Rae (a Scotch economist writing in 1834) which is ingenious, although it has never been consciously put into use. He says, and wisely, that we cannot change this inherent ambition in human nature. All we can do is to turn it to some good account instead of letting it run to waste. He suggested that social racing could be made to yield a revenue to a government by taxing imported luxuries so as to make them expensive, and therefore desired by the wealthy and out of the reach of their imitators. A case in point is that of the cheap wines of France being dear in England because of the tariff and cost of importation across the channel, and reversely, the cheap wines in England being dear in France. Each was fashionable in the country of the other, but unfashionable at home. Now if a tax is able to create a fashion in this way, through making an article exclusive, the government can get a revenue by creating a fashion, and the tax imposed on society by fashion could thus be made to accrue to the government.

Another way is to change the fashion of fashion, so to speak, so that it may be made to run in more useful channels. One of the better forms of vanity is that which does not satisfy itself by display in the usual sense, but seeks to make a record of power in the financial world. In these days a man may advertise his wealth in other ways than by high living. To be known as the largest stockholder in a railway is one of the coveted distinctions. Again, by publishing names and amounts contributed, the newspapers give distinction to the large contributors to charity. It is now known that more money can usually be raised by a public subscription list than by a church collection, where the contributor obtains no public notice. The publicity of tax lists even stimulates a desire, though still weak it is true, to have ones name near the top of the tax list. Private display is also taking on healthier forms. One wealthy American is distinguishing himself by buying works of art and loaning them to the great art galleries of Europe and America. In fact, in spite of many evidences to the contrary, there are some indications that display, in the old sense, is decreasing, especially among men. There was a time when men bedecked themselves in diamonds and expensive silks. But to-day men seldom wear jewelry or gaudy clothing. Business distinction takes the place of these. Even women are becoming ambitious to lead in other ways than in " society." They seek distinction in their womens clubs or as executives in charitable effort. There is, as a matter of fact, no reason why rich men and women should not try to distinguish themselves by doing good, and the tendency in America to-day is exactly in this line. Rich men are gradually trying to distinguish themselves by their large benefactions instead of by their large expenditures. They create great philanthropic foundations and endow hospitals, sanatoria, libraries, and universities. A few years ago, in the city of Pittsburg, two wealthy men vied with each other in erecting fine buildings for the good of the city of Pittsburg, and one, in order to triumph over the other, who had put up imposing buildings in a certain square, purchased the square immediately adjacent at a very high price for the purpose of erecting a still finer public building. Social racing of this sort may be socially beneficial and is an encouraging sign of the times. At present, however, great wealth is as a rule either running to waste or taxing those who cannot keep up with it. Perhaps some day it may–like other great wastes–be caught and harnessed and made to do some of the worlds work.

8. Recapitulation

We have now completed our brief review of the elementary principles of economics, or the study of wealth. It has fallen under three heads: (1) the " foundation stones," (2) the determination of prices, and (3) the principles of distribution. Under the first head were set forth the great concepts of the science, namely, wealth itself, the central theme, and the closely connected concepts of property, benefits and costs, price and value, capital and income. We saw how these concepts are defined, and, what is more important, how they are related to each other. In particular, we saw that property rights always have a basis in tangible wealth or persons; that wealth is a means, and property a right, to future benefits and costs; and that those present valuations called " capital " are the net discounted values of future benefits less costs called net " income."

These relations were found to be illustrated by the principles of accounting. We found two methods of combining different accounts, whether of capital or of income. By the method of balances we saw what part of capital or income belonged to the particular person or wealth to which the separate accounts relate; whereas, by the method of couples, we saw wherein the final total capital or income consists. The method of couples, when all accounts of society are included, brings us back to the fundamental truth that capital consists of concrete, physical objects (including in its broader sense human beings) and that income consists of final satisfactions. The "couples" which finally cancel themselves out are, however, for the individual accounts, very important. They are, for capital accounts, the debts between man and man and, for income accounts, the interactions between instrument and instrument.

We found a fundamental relation between the variations in the income from any species of capital and the variations in the value of that income; namely, that if the income realized exceeds the interest accrued, the capital will depreciate by the difference; and, reversely, if the income realized falls short of the interest accrued, the capital will appreciate by the difference.

Our second task grew out of the first. The formal concepts and relations had furnished us tools of thought, but they had not explained the facts with which they dealt. They had shown us what prices and values are, but not how they are determined. The determination of prices thus became next the focal point of study. We found the problem of price-determination to be twofold,–the problem of determining price levels and the problem of determining individual prices. The former is the problem of the purchasing power of money, and depends, for its solution, on the study of the "equation of exchange." We found that the price level is normally proportional to the quantity of money, and in versely proportional to the volume of trade; it was also noted that the volume of deposits subject to check (relatively to the money in circulation) and the velocities of circulation of money and of deposits are important factors in the problem, and that the disturbance of the normal condition of the magnitudes in the equation of exchange has much to do with periodical crises and depressions of trade. The other problem (individual prices) was again subdivided into two, the one relating to the prices of individual goods, and the other to the rate of interest. The chief key to the first was found in "marginal desirability," and to the second, in "marginal impatience," or excess of the desirability of a present dollar over the desirability of a future dollar.

Having seen the principles which rule the markets of the world, we were ready for our third and last task,—to study the larger results of these forces on the distribution of income, relatively to its sources and owners. We found that the distribution of income according to sources fell into several parts, differing in mode of measurement and in degree of certainty. These parts may be summarized as: profits (whether the profits are from capital or work or both), capitalists stipulated income (whether interest or rent) and labors stipulated income (wages).

The distribution by owners we found depends on inheritance constantly modified by thrift, ability, industry, luck, and fraud. The topic of distribution by owners led to a consideration of the effects of the ownership of wealth on social welfare.

Throughout the book we have confined ourselves to the study of principles,—the principles by which capital and income are related, the principles by which prices are f1xed, the principles by which wealth or poverty is produced, the principles by which men and women waste wealth in useless rivalry. The whole study has been, as a study of scientific principles should be, cold and impartial. The practical application of the principles was not included, and the stu dent was warned at the outset against taking any partisan position on economic questions until he had some grounding in economic principles. Now, however, that he has studied these principles, he is strongly advised to continue the subject in other books devoted to practical applications. The chief use of a study of principles is as a preparation for the study of their application; and, unless educated men use their knowledge of principles as a means of influencing public opinion on economic problems, the solution of these problems will be left to those who neither understand nor recognize the existence of any economic principles. Every educated man owes it to the community to use his education for intelligent leadership. To-day is a time of reform movements, and never before was there greater need of intelligent leadership in those movements. This book will nothave fulfilled its function if it does not induce the readers to apply its principles to their own lives and to the life of the nation of which their lives are a part. Its chief object is to put them in a position to study and help solve the great problems of money, tariffs, trusts, labor unions, hours of labor, housing and hygiene, and, above all, the problems of wealth and poverty. These are great problems and it will be well worth the readers while to take up some one of them for thorough study. He will find that such a study will lead him into ever broadening fields of human interest. In fact, practical economic problems are seldom restricted to economics proper, but lead into the great realms of law, politics, and morals. This is because economics is only one branch of a greater subject,–Sociology.

Printed in the United States of America.

Lightning Source UK Ltd.
Milton Keynes UK

178743UK00001B/228/P